D1715430

OXFORD MEDICAL PUBLICATIONS

Oxford American Handbook of
Psychiatry

Published and forthcoming Oxford American Handbooks

Oxford American Handbook of Anesthesiology
Oxford American Handbook of Clinical Dentistry
Oxford American Handbook of Clinical Medicine
Oxford American Handbook of Critical Care
Oxford American Handbook of Emergency Medicine
Oxford American Handbook of Nephrology and Hypertension
Oxford American Handbook of Obstetrics and Gynecology
Oxford American Handbook of Otolaryngology
Oxford American Handbook of Pediatrics
Oxford American Handbook of Psychiatry
Oxford American Handbook of Pulmonary Medicine
Oxford American Handbook of Surgery

Oxford American Handbook of **Psychiatry**

Edited by

David J. Kupfer, MD

Michelle S. Horner, DO

David A. Brent, MD

David A. Lewis, MD

Charles F. Reynolds, III, MD

Michael E. Thase, MD

Michael J. Travis, MBBS, MRCPsych

All: Western Psychiatric Institute and Clinic
University of Pittsburg Medical Center
Pittsburg, Pennsylvania

With

David Semple
Roger Smyth
Jonathan Burns
Rajan Darjee
Andrew McIntosh

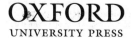

OXFORD
UNIVERSITY PRESS

OXFORD

UNIVERSITY PRESS

Great Clarendon Street, Oxford OX2 6DP

Oxford University Press is a department of the University of Oxford.
It furthers the University's objective of excellence in research, scholarship,
and education by publishing worldwide in

Oxford New York

Auckland Cape Town Dar es Salaam Hong Kong Karachi
Kuala Lumpur Madrid Melbourne Mexico City Nairobi
New Delhi Shanghai Taipei Toronto

With offices in

Argentina Austria Brazil Chile Czech Republic France Greece
Guatemala Hungary Italy Japan Poland Portugal Singapore
South Korea Switzerland Thailand Turkey Ukraine Vietnam

Oxford is a registered trade mark of Oxford University Press
in the UK and in certain other countries

Published in the United States
by Oxford University Press Inc., New York

© Oxford University Press, 2008

The moral rights of the author have been asserted
Database right Oxford University Press (maker)

First published 2008

British Library Cataloguing in Publication Data
Data available

Library of Congress Cataloging in Publication Data
Data available

Typeset by Newgen Imaging Systems (P) Ltd., Chennai, India
Printed in Italy
by L.E.G.O. S.p.A. Lavis (TN)

ISBN 978–0–19–530884–6

10 9 8 7 6 5 4 3 2 1

Preface

The dynamic field of psychiatry is constantly evolving. Pathophysiologically driven definitions for disease and developments in treatment are replacing the once symptom-based classifications and serendipitous discoveries of medication. Within medicine as a whole there is an increasing emphasis on integration across specialties and between treatment modalities. Psychiatry is at the forefront of these developments.

The Oxford American Handbook of Psychiatry serves to bring the reader up-to-date and prepare them for these advancements while providing the core essential knowledge required for today's complex clinical practice.

Covering the whole breadth of psychiatry, this American handbook has been thoroughly revised and updated from the Oxford Handbook of Psychiatry, to reflect US perspectives, procedures and practice. We have used a team of authors, led by a group of experts in the field. The handbook has been prepared with the assistance and input of faculty and residents at the Western Psychiatric Institute and Clinic, part of the University of Pittsburgh Medical Center.

The handbook incorporates the latest advances and hottest topics in psychiatry. Unique coverage on increasingly relevant subjects such as Integrated Medicine in Psychiatry, Eating Disorders, Reproductive Psychiatry and Sleep Disorders is also included. Additional features of this handbook include combined psychotherapy and psychopharmacology by disorder, an easily referenced glossary of psychiatric terms and an associated "Oxford American Pocket Notes" booklet.

With clear indexing and a simple layout, this book is an essential quick reference for students and residents, as well as experienced clinicians and allied health professionals. Designed for use at the bedside, while rounding or in clinic, the Oxford American Handbook of Psychiatry contains the key facts required for shelf and board examinations, integrated with sufficient detail to inform the comprehensive assessment and care of all patients presenting for psychiatric services.

David J. Kupfer, MD
Michelle S. Horner, DO
Michael E. Thase, MD
David A. Lewis, MD
David A. Brent, MD
Charles F. Reynolds, III, MD
Michael J. Travis, MBBS, MRCPsych

Acknowledgements

We would like to thank all of the Faculty and Residents of WPIC, UPMC and Medical Students of the University of Pittsburgh who acted as reviewers and advisors on the manuscript at various stages, as well as all the trainees and faculty who contributed to the success of this Handbook. In particular we would like to thank Julie Kmiec, D.O., Cyrus A Raji, Ph.D., and Mary Amanda Dew, Ph.D.; also Ryan Herringa, M.D., Ph.D, Olapeju Simoyan, M.D., Michelle Landy, B.S., Alexis Fertig, M.D., Kristen Dalope, M.D., Cynthia Miller, M.D., Petronilla Vaulx-Smith, M.D., Ph.D, Roger Haskett, M.D., Isabella Soreca, M.D., Soledad Romero, M.D., Allan Zuckoff, Ph.D., Melissa Kalarchian, Ph.D., Rameshwari Tumuluru, M.D., Umapathy Channamalappa, M.D., Tammy Chung, M.D., Sanjay Paidisetty, M.D., Tiberiu Bodea Crisan, M.D., Candace Good, M.D., April Fields, M.D., Lin Ewing, Ph.D., Meredith Chapman, M.D., Aalap Chandrakant Shah, M.D., Lee Haselkorn, Ph.D. and Alex Strauss, M.D.

We would also like to thank the authors of the UK edition of the Oxford Handbook of Psychiatry and the Faculty and Residents of the Department of Psychological Medicine, University of Edinburgh.

We are grateful to the following residents at the University of Chicago, Elias Dakwar, M.D., Deepak Kumar, M.D., Theodote K. Pontikes, M.D., and Sarah Riaz, M.D. for reading the initial finished drafts of the US Edition.

In addition, we would like to acknowledge the assistance, guidance and patience we received from the publishing team at Oxford University Press, both in New York and in Great Clarendon Street. The team included, Bill Lamsback, Kevin Kochanski, Nicola Williams, Anita Petrie, Katherine Davey and Andrea Seils.

This book is dedicated to Thomas P. Detre, M.D., Emeritus Distinguished Senior Vice Chancellor for Health Sciences, former Chairman of the Department and past President of UPMC. The departmental collaboration essential to this book was made possible by his tireless work and overarching vision. His knowledge, generosity, and panache inspire the generations of physicians and scientists who have been privileged to learn from Dr. Detre. We all continue to gain from his advice, insights and knowledge.

Contents

All contributing authors are from the Western Psychiatric Institute and Clinic,
University of Pittsburgh Medical Center, Pittsburgh, Pennsylvania.

Detailed contents

Symbols and abbreviations

5-HT	5-hydroxytryptamine or serotonin
5-HTR2A	5-hydroxytryptamine (serotonin) receptor 2A (gene)
5HTT	5-hydroxytryptamine (serotonin) transporter
5HTTLPR	Promoter region of the human serotonin transporter
a.c.	before meals
AA	Alcoholic's Anonymous
AACAP	American Academy of Child and Adolescent Psychiatry
AACWA	Adoption Assistance and Child Welfare Act
AAID	American Association of Intellectual and Developmental Disabilities
ABA	applied behavior analysis
ABC	Autism Behavior Checklist
ABFP	American Board of Forensic Psychiatry
ABPN	American Board of Psychiatry and Neurology
ACh	acetylcholine
ACP	American College of Physicians
ADHD	attention deficit hyperactivity disorder
ADI-R	Autism Diagnostic Interview-Revised
ADLs	activities of daily living
ADOS	Autism Diagnostic Observation Schedule
AFP	alpha-fetoprotein
AIDS	acquired immune deficiency syndrome
AIMS	Abnormal Involuntary Movement Scale
a.m.	before noon (from Latin, *ante meridiem*)
AMA	American Medical Association
AN	anorexia nervosa
ANA	anti-nuclear antibody
ANCOVA	analysis of covariance
ANOVA	analysis of variance
APA	American Psychiatry Association
APA	alpha-linolenic acid
ARR	absolute risk reduction
ASD	acute stress disorder
ASDI	Acute Stress Disorder Interview
ASDS	Acute Stress Disorder Scale

ASFA	Adoption and Safe Families Act
ATP	adenosine triphosphatase
AUA	American Urological Association
B_1	vitamin B_1 (thiamine)
B_2	vitamin B_2 (riboflavin)
B_6	vitamin B_6 (pyridoxine)
BAI	Beck Anxiety Inventory
BCL2	B-cell CLL/lymphoma 2 (gene)
BD	bipolar disorder
BDI	Beck Depression Inventory
BDNF	brain-derived neurotrophic factor
BDZ	benzodiazepine
BFI	behavioral family intervention
bid	twice a day (from Latin, *bis in die*)
BiPAP	bilevel positive airway pressure
BMI	body mass index
BMP	blood metabolic profile
BP	blood pressure
BPD	borderline personality disorder
BPD-Scale	Borderline Personality Disorder Scale
BPRS	Brief Psychiatric Rating Scale
BT	behavioural therapy
BUN	blood urea nitrogen
CADSS	Clinician Administered Dissociative States Scale
CAM	complementary and alternative medicine
cAMP	cyclic adenosine monophosphate
CAPS	Clinician Administered PTSD Scale
CAPTA	Child Abuse Prevention and Treatment Act
CARS	Childhood Autism Rating Scale
CAT	Cognitive Analytic Therapy
CATIE	Clinical Antipsychotic Trials of Intervention Effectiveness
CBC	complete blood count
CBCL	Child Behavior Checklist
CBT	cognitive behavioral therapy
CCK	cholecystokinin
CD	conduct disorder
CDC	Centers for Disease Control
CDD	childhood disintegrative disorder
CER	control event rate
CHAT	Checklist for Autism in Toddlers

CHF	congestive heart failure
Chol	cholesterol
CI	confidence interval
Cl	chlorine
CISD	critical incident stress debriefing
CNS	central nervous system
CO_2	carbon dioxide
COBRA	Consolidated Omnibus Budget Reconciliation Act
COPD	chronic obstructive pulmonary disease
CPAP	continuous positive airway pressure
CPK	creatine phosphokinase
CPS	Child Protective Services
Cr/creat	creatinine
CREB1	cAMP responsive element binding protein 1
CRF	corticotropin releasing factor
CRS	Conners' Rating Scale (for ADHD)
CSF	cerebrospinal fluid
CST	craniosacral therapy
CSTC	cortico-striatal-thalamo-cortical
CT	computed tomography
CVT	comprehensive validation therapy
CY-BOCS	Children's Yale-Brown Obsessive Compulsive Scale
CYP	cytochrome
D2	dopamine receptor, subtype 2
DA	dopamine
DBT	dialectical behavior therapy
DDIS	Dissociative Disorder Interview Schedule
DES	Dissociative Experiences Scale
DEX	dextro-amphetamine
DHA	docosahexaenoic acid
DIB	Diagnostic Interview for Borderline Patients
DID	dissociative identity syndrome
DIPD-IV	Diagnostic Interview for DSM-IV Personality Disorders
DIS	Diagnostic Interview Schedule
DKA	diabetic ketoacidosis
DMST	dexamethasone suppression test
DMV	Department of Motor Vehicles
DNRI	dopamine-norepinephrine reuptake inhibitors
DO	doctor of osteopathic medicine
DOD	Department of Defense

DRO	differential reinforcement procedures
DS	Down syndrome
DSH	deliberate self-harm
DSM	Diagnostic and Statistical Manual of Mental Disorders
DSS	Depersonalization Severity Scale
DUP	duration of untreated psychosis
DZ	dizygotic (fraternal twins)
DY-BOCS	Dimensional Yale–Brown Obsessive Compulsive Scale
e.g.	For the sake of example (from Latin, *exempli gratia*)
EBM	evidence-based medicine
EBMH	evidence-based mental health
ECG/ EKG	electrocardiogram
ECT	electroconvulsive therapy
ED	erectile dysfunction
ED	emergency department
EEG	electroencephalogram
EER	experimental event rate
EMDR	eye movement desensitization and reprocessing
EMG	electromyography
EMW	early morning waking
EMTALA	Emergency Medical Treatment and Active Labor Act
EOG	electrooculography
EPA	eicosapentaenoic acid
EPDS	Edinburgh Postnatal Depression Scale
EPS	extrapyramidal symptoms
ER	emergency room
ERP	exposure and response prevention
ES	effect size
et al.	and others (from Latin, *et alii, et aliae* or *et alia*)
ETOH	abbreviation for "drinking" alcohol
FAS	fetal alcohol syndrome
FDA	Food and Drug Administration
FFD	fitness for duty
FGA	first generation antipsychotic
FHWA	Federal Highway Administration
fMRI	functional magnetic resonance imaging
FSH	follicle-stimulating hormone
FTT	failure to thrive
FXTAS	fragile X-associated tremor/ataxia syndrome
GABA	gamma-aminobutyric acid

GABHS	group A beta-hemolytic streptococcal infection
GAD	generalized anxiety disorder
GH	growth hormone
GI	gastrointestinal
GnRH	gonadotrophin-releasing hormone
GRIK4	glutamate receptor, ionotropic, kainate 4 (gene)
GU	genito-urinary
GYN	gynecology
H&H	hemoglobin and hematocrit
H&P	history and physical
h.s.	at bedtime (from Latin, *hora somni*
H/A	headache
H1	histamine receptor, subtype 1
HAM-A	Hamilton Anxiety Scale
HAM-D	Hamilton Rating Scale for Depression
Hb	hemoglobin
HCG	human chorionic gonadotropin
HCT	hematocrit
HDL	high density lipoprotein
HFA	high-functioning autism
HGB	hemoglobin
HIPPA	Health Insurance Portability and Accountability Act
HIV	human immunodeficiency virus
HPA	hypothalamic-pituitary-adrenal
HPI	history of present illness
HPRT	hypoxanthine-guanine phosphoribosyltransferase
HPV	human papillomavirus
HR	heart rate
HRV	heart rate variability
HSV	herpes simplex virus
HT	Healing Touch
HTN	hypertension
IADL	instrumental activities of daily living
i.e.	that is (to say) (from Latin, *id est*)
ICD	International Classification of Disease
ICDs	impulse-control disorders
ICER	incremental cost-effectiveness ratio
IDDM	insulin-dependent diabetes mellitus
IDEIA	Individuals with Disabilities Education Improvement Act
IED	intermittent explosive disorder

IES	Impact of Events Scale
IM	intramuscular
IPDE	International Personality Disorder Examination
IPT	interpersonal therapy
IQ	intelligence quotient
IV	intravenous
K	potassium
kg/d	kilograms/day
K-SADS/ Kiddie-SADS	Schedule of Affective Disorders and Schizophrenia for School-age Children
LD	learning disorder
LDL	low density lipoprotein
LFTs	liver function tests
LGBT	lesbian—gay—bisexual—transgendered
LH	luteinizing hormone
LLD	language and learning disorders
LMP	last menstrual period
LP	lumbar puncture
LSD	lysergic acid diethylamide
Lytes	electrolytes
M1	muscarinic receptor, subtype 1
MADRS	Montgomery-Asberg Depression Rating Scale
MAO	monoamine oxidase
MAOI	monoamine oxidase inhibitor
MBP	Munchausen syndrome by proxy
MBSR	mindfulness-based stress reduction
mcg	microgram
MCMI	Millon Clinical Multiaxial Inventory
MDD	major depressive disorder
MDE	major depressive episode
MERRF	myoclonic epilepsy with ragged red fibers
mg	milligram
MI	motivational interviewing
MI	myocardial infarction
MMSE	mini mental status examination
MND	Motor neurone disease
MPH	methamphetamine
MPH	methylphenidate
MR	mental retardation
MRA	magnetic resonance angiogram or angiography
MRI	magnetic resonance imaging

MRS	magnetic resonance spectroscopy
MS	multiple sclerosis
MSE	mental status examination
MSLT	multiple sleep latency test
MTA	Multimodal Treatment Study of Children with ADHD
MZ	monozygotic (identical twins)
NA	Narcotics Anonymous
NA	noradrenaline/ norepinephrine
Na	sodium
NAMI	National Alliance on Mental Illness
NARIs	noradrenaline/norepinephrine reuptake inhibitors
NaSSA	noradrenergic/norepinephrinergic and specific serotonergic antidepressant
NCCAM	National Center for Complementary and Alternative Medicine
NDP	Norrie Disease Protein
NDRI	noradrenergic/norepinephrinergic and dopaminergic reuptake inhibitor
NE	norepinephrine/noradrenaline
NIDDM	non-Insulin-dependent diabetes mellitus
NIMH	National Institute for Mental Health
NMDA	N-methyl-D-aspartic acid
NMS	neuroleptic malignant syndrome
NMS	neuromusculoskeletal
NNH	number needed to harm
NNT	number needed to treat
NOS	not otherwise specified
NPV	negative predictive value
NREM	non-rapid eye movement
OB	obstetrics
OB/GYN	obstetrics/gynecology
OCD	obsessive-compulsive disorder
OCPD	obsessive-compulsive personality disorder
OCS	obsessive-compulsive spectrum
OD	overdose
ODD	oppositional defiant disorder
OMT	osteopathic manipulation therapy
OR	odds ratio
OSA	obstructive sleep apnea
p.c.	after food (from Latin, *post cibum*)
po	orally (from Latin, *per os*)

p.r.	rectally (from Latin, *per rectum*)
PANDAS	pediatric autoimmune neuropsychiatric disorders
PANSS	Positive And Negative Syndrome Scale
PAS	Personality Assessment Schedule
PCF	Pediatric Condition Falsification
PCL-R	Psychopathy Checklist—Revised
PCL-SV	Psychopathy Checklist—Screening Version
PCP	primary care physician
PCP	phenylcyclidine
PD	personality disorder
PDAC	Psychopharmacologic Drugs Advisory Committee
PDD	pervasive developmental disorder
PDQ-IV	Personality Disorder Questionnaire
PDW	passive death wish
PE	physical education
PE	pulmonary embolism
PET	positron emission tomography
PICO	problem, intervention, comparison, outcome
PLMD	periodic limb movement disorder
PLT	platelets
p.m.	*post meridiem* (Latin, after noon)
PMD	Pelizaeus–Merzbacher disease
PMDD	premenstrual dysphoric disorder
PMH	past medical history
PMS	premenstrual syndrome
PMT	parent management training
PPD	post-partum depression
PPV	positive predictive value
PSG	polysomnography
PTSD	post-traumatic stress disorder
PWACR	Prader-Willi/Angelman critical region
q	every (from Latin, *quaque*)
qam	every morning (from Latin, *quaque ante meridian*)
qod	every other day
qd	each day (from Latin, *quaque die*)
qhs	every bedtime (from Latin, *quaque hora somni*)
qid	four times a day (from Latin, *quater in die*)
QOLI	Quality of Life Interview
RAD	reactive attachment disorder
RBC	red blood cells

RCT	randomized controlled trial
RDC	research diagnostic criteria
REM	rapid eye movement
RF	rheumatoid factor
RIMA	reversible inhibitor of monoamine oxidase A
RLS	restless legs syndrome
ROS	review of symptoms
RR	relative risk
RRR	relative risk reduction
RTI	respiratory tract infection
SAD	seasonal affective disorder
SADS	Schedule for Affective Disorders and Schizophrenia
S-allele	generally refers to the short allele for the serotonin transporter
SANS	Scale for the Assessment of Negative Symptoms
SAP	Standardized Assessment of Personality
SAPS	Scale for the Assessment of Positive Symptoms
SARI	serotonin antagonist reuptake inhibitor
SBP	systolic blood pressure
SCI_PANSS	Structured Clinical Interview for the Positive And Negative Syndrome Scale
SCID-I	Structured Clinical Interview for DSM-IV Diagnosis, (Axis I)
SCID-II	Structured Clinical Interview for DSM-IV Personality Disorder
SCID-D-R	Structured Clinical Interview for DSM-IV Dissociative Disorders—Revised
SCN	suprachiasmatic nucleus
SGA	second-generation antipsychotic
SI	suicidal ideation
SIADH	syndrome of inappropriate antidiuretic hormone secretion
SIB	self-injurious behavior
SIB	Schedule for Interviewing Borderlines
sig	write on the label (from Latin, *signa*)
SIDES	Scheduled Interview of Disorders of Extreme Stress (SIDES)
SIDES-SR	Self-report Inventory for Disorders of Extreme Stress
SIPD-IV	Structured Interview for DSM-IV Personality Disorders
SLE	systemic lupus erythematosus
SM	selective mutism

SMR	standardized mortality ratio
SNRI	serotonin and norepinephrine reuptake inhibitor
SOB	shortness of breath
SP	social phobia
SPECT	single photon emission computed tomography
SPET	single photon emission tomography
SR	systematic review
SRS	sex reassignment surgery
SSD	social security disability
SSP	Schedule for Schizotypal Personalities
SSRI	selective serotonin reuptake inhibitor
STAR*D	Sequenced Treatment Alternatives to Relieve Depression
Stat	immediately, without delay (from Latin, *statim*)
STD	sexually transmitted disease
STM	short term memory
STEPPS	Systems Training for Emotional Predictability and Problem Solving
SUD	substance use disorder
SWS	Sturge-Weber syndrome
T3	liothyronine
T4	thyroxine
TAG	triacylglyceride
TB	tuberculosis
TCA	tricyclic antidepressant
TD	tardive dyskinesia
TEAS	treatment emergent affective switching
TFTs	thyroid function tests
TG	triglyceride
t.i.d.	three times a day (from Latin, *ter in die*)
TLE	temporal lobe epilepsy
TMS	transcranial magnetic stimulation
TPN	total parenteral nutrition
TSH	thyroid-stimulating hormone
TT	therapeutic touch
UA	urinalysis
UDS	urine drug screen
USSC	United States Supreme Court
UTI	urinary tract infection
vCJD	variant Creutzfeldt-Jakob disease
VNS	vagus nerve stimulation

VPA	valproic acid
WBC	white blood cells
WHO	World Health Organization
WISPI	Wisconsin Personality Disorders Inventory
Y-BOCS	Yale–Brown Obsessive Compulsive Scale
YGTSS	Yale Global Tic Severity Scale

Thinking about psychiatry

Psychiatry: Past and present

Now is the most exciting time to be working in the field of psychiatry. Since the beginning of recorded history, mental or psychiatric illnesses (or disease) have been regarded with fear, disbelief, and superstition. These attributions have often been accompanied by fantastic descriptions of both the causes and treatments of these illnesses.

Unfortunately, there exists a false separation of psychiatric illnesses from "physical illnesses," despite conclusive proof that all of the core psychiatric diseases are associated with changes in brain function or structure or both. This separateness means that psychiatry remains dogged by stigma, even from our colleagues in other medical specialties.

Psychiatric diseases are more common than almost any other type of disease and among the most serious chronic conditions from which a person can suffer in terms of morbidity and shortened life expectancy. The important World Health Organization (WHO) and World Bank studies and analyses continue to substantiate this point of view.

To truly understand psychiatry, one has to consider the centrality of the brain and its functioning to the organism as whole. Furthermore, the brain is an organ that develops and changes throughout life. Everything that an individual experiences in their life, every emotion, every memory, every interaction is processed by this changing organ. The human body comprises a system of pumps, filters, glands, conduits and mechanical systems whose primary aim is to support the brain, the organ that controls the system as a whole and the complexity of whose function makes us human.

To separate mind from body is akin to trying to divorce the function of the heart from that of the lungs, since disease in one can lead to malfunction and disease in the other. The brain is as intimately connected with all the organs of the body as the right ventricle is to the pulmonary arteries. It, therefore, follows, and is clear from the literature, that there are psychiatric sequelae from physical illness just as there are physical sequelae from psychiatric illness.

One of the perceived problems with psychiatry has been that the majority of diagnoses and treatments are based on the subjective description of symptoms by the sufferer and, therefore, somehow, the diseases are less valid than those where a rapidly available test can indicate the presence or absence of disease. Nevertheless, one needs to ask,

• What would be the consensus on the diagnosis in a malaised male patient describing nausea, acute right lower quadrant abdominal pain and a reluctance to move because of the pain'?
• How is that different from the consensus on, an ill-kempt patient describing low mood and hopelessness over the last month accompanied by a loss of appetite and concentration, and waking at four every morning?
• Further, would you tell the patient with acute appendicitis to pull himself together?

Much of our diagnosis in medicine as a whole is still conducted on the basis of the history from the patient. A physical examination is little different from a mental status examination in its attempt to elicit or observe further symptoms and signs of illness to confirm or refute the diagnosis based on the history. Laboratory procedures are important in medicine, but such procedures need to be integrated with the rest of the information often obtained from the patient and family members.

The complexity of the brain in comparison with the relative simplicity of the other organs in the body make a simple test for disease more intellectually challenging to discover but not impossible. The primary challenge is the fact that the brain is several orders of magnitude more complex than any other organ in the body. Furthermore, unlike the heart or the kidney, the brain cannot be easily studied in isolation, without reference to the organ systems that the brain controls and that in turn affect the brain's own functioning. Nevertheless great strides have been made over the last 20 years. The growth in our understanding of the complexity of the challenge and the possible answers has grown exponentially with the integration of different modalities of investigation.

Psychiatry: The future

The next 20 years will see key opportunities for further understanding of the causes and treatments of psychiatric illness and, as importantly, how this relates to the health of the rest of the human organism and the reciprocal nature of this interaction. In tandem with these discoveries, the study of brain development and physical development through the lifespan will lead to a reconceptualization of health and disease in all organ systems including the brain.

This reconceptualization is an ongoing process that probably formally started with ensuring that populations had access to clean water to prevent cholera and has progressed to the modern day. Today, people are placed on a medication because the level of cholesterol in their blood is raised above a certain threshold and/or are advised to reduce their stress levels in order to prevent a vascular event.

Similarly, the further understanding of the ordinary development of the brain and the changes in cortical processing that are associated with diseases of all kinds will lead to preventative interventions, many of them lifestyle based, and where these are not possible, to more effective treatments of disease.

Psychiatry and psychiatrists, because we are physicians, will be at the forefront of this endeavor.

The seven ages of man—"The Psychiatric Lifespan"

All the world's a stage,
And all the men and women merely players;
They have their exits and their entrances,
And one man in his time plays many parts,
His acts being seven ages. At first, the infant,
Mewling and puking in the nurse's arms.
Then the whining schoolboy, with his satchel
And shining morning face, creeping like snail
Unwillingly to school. And then the lover,
Sighing like furnace, with a woeful ballad
Made to his mistress' eyebrow. Then a soldier,
Full of strange oaths and bearded like the pard,
Jealous in honour, sudden and quick in quarrel,
Seeking the bubble reputation
Even in the canon's mouth. And then the justice,
In fair round belly with good capon lined,
With eyes severe and beard of formal cut,
Full of wise saws and modern instances;
And so he plays his part. The sixth age shifts
Into the lean and slippered pantaloon
With spectacles on nose and pouch on side;
His youthful hose, well saved, a world too wide
For his shrunk shank, and his big manly voice,
Turning again toward childish treble, pipes
And whistles in his sound. Last scene of all,
That ends this strange eventful history,
Is second childishness and mere oblivion,
Sans teeth, sans eyes, sans taste, sans everything.

From William Shakespeare, *As You Like It*, 2. 7. 139–167.

What is disease?

Most psychiatric diagnoses have had their validity questioned at several points in their history. Diagnosed by physicians on the basis of symptoms alone, some people found their presence difficult to accept in a field that had been almost universally successful in finding demonstrable physical pathology or infection. With recent findings from neuroimaging, neuropathology, and genetics, it has become increasingly clear that there is a definite but very complex and heterogeneous pathology underlying many mental diagnoses.

It must also be remembered that disease in medicine as a whole was not always based on pathology. The microscope was developed long after doctors began to make disease attributions. Thomas Sydenham developed the medico-pathological model based on symptoms, but it has grown to incorporate information obtained from postmortem and tissue examination. This model of disease has become synonymous in many peoples' mind with a model based solely on demonstrably abnormal structure. Thomas Szasz (📖 p. 25) criticized psychiatry in general by suggesting that its diseases fail when this model is applied.

This argument that psychiatric diagnoses are invalid still strikes a chord with many doctors and nonmedical academics. The British Medical Journal conducted a survey of nondiseases[1] (Fig. 1.1). Many people thought depression to be a nondisease, although schizophrenia and alcoholism fared somewhat better. It is clear from the graph that many conditions rated as "real" diseases have a characteristic pathology, although some do not (alcoholism, epilepsy). Similarly, many people regard head injury and duodenal ulcer as non-disease, although their pathology is well described. In a more recent update to this, a list of 20 non-diseases was created using a similar method. These are listed in Table 1.1. None of them are psychiatric diseases.

Table 1.1 Top 20 nondiseases (voted by bmj.com readers) in descending order of "nondiseaseness"

1. Ageing	12. Allergy to the twenty-first century
2. Work	
3. Boredom	13. Jet lag
4. Bags under eyes	14. Unhappiness
5. Ignorance	15. Cellulite
6. Baldness	16. Hangover
7. Freckles	17. Anxiety about penis size/penis envy
8. Big ears	
9. Grey or white hair	18. Pregnancy
10. Ugliness	19. Road rage
11. Childbirth	20. Loneliness

From Smith R.: BMJ, 324(7342). April 13, 2002. 883–885.

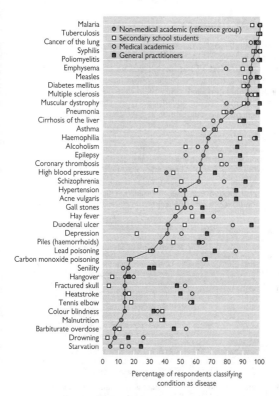

Fig. 1.1 Percentage of respondents classifying a condition as a disease Figure appears in Campbell, E.J., Scadding, J.G., Roberts, R.S. (1979). The concept of disease. *BMJ* **29**, 757–62; reproduced with permission of BMJ Publishing Group.

Models of disease

There are several models of disease in existence (see Table 1.2). No single model is adequate by itself, and diseases may move from one group to another. Most of the models can be said to be nominalist or descriptive. That is, they take a cluster of symptoms and signs, often with the course of the illness, and group them together into disease entities. To this may or may not be added laboratory analyses or postmortem findings, which may aid but cannot in themselves make or refute the diagnosis. More recently, there have been calls to move toward a more "essentialist" or etiological concept of disease.[1] In these models the cause of the disease is paramount in its definition. A combination of these two models is probably most useful especially as the evidence for specific causative pathways increases. The reality may be that "disease" is a concept that will tend to change over time as our knowledge base changes and has no real existence in itself. Within psychiatry these changes will have a profound effect on our concepts and classification of disease.

Table 1.2 Models of disease

Model	Summary of assumptions
Genomic (Temple *et al*, 2001)	Disease is a state that places individuals at adverse risk of consequences. Treatment is given to those with a disease to prevent or ameliorate adverse consequences.
Medical-pathological definition (Sydenham 1696; Szasz 1960)	Assumes diseases are associated with a necessary cause (e.g., bacterial infection) or have a replicable morbid anatomy.
Biological disadvantage (Scadding 1972)	Assumes that sufferers from a disease have a common characteristic to place them at a biological disadvantage.
Plan of action (Linder 1965)	Assumes disease labels are justifications for treatments and further investigations.
Syndrome with characteristic symptoms/outcome (Kendell 1975)	Assumes diseases represent circumscribed concepts distinguished from others by a bimodal distribution of scores on a discriminant function.
Disease as imperfection (Cohen 1943, 1953)	Assumes diseases are quantitative or qualitative deviations from a desirable norm.
Disease as concept (Aristotle)	Assumes diseases are man-made abstractions with no independent existence.

Recommended further reading

Campbell, E.J., Scadding, J.G., Roberts, R.S. (1979). The concept of disease. *BMJ* **29**, 757–762.

The role of the psychiatrist

Psychiatrists remain physicians, and to them falls the unique opportunity to deal with the effect of the brain on the rest of the body and the effect of illness in another part of the body on the brain. To do this, they must understand the concepts of illness and fully integrate the subjective experiences of the patient with the more physical aspects of their presenting symptoms.

What is illness?

Physicians, being generally practical people, busy themselves with the diagnosis and treatment of various types of illness. It is increasingly important, nevertheless, to ask "What is illness?" or "What is health?" For several reasons, psychiatrists have been at the forefront of this type of questioning:

• In all branches of medicine and surgery, the initial presentation and interview are based on the subjective experience of the patient. From this the doctor gains information that guides subsequent investigation and management.

• Within psychiatry, however, the patients' subjective experiences are currently more central to diagnosis than physical investigations.

• There is a nonabsolute, value judgment involved in the diagnosis of mental disorder—e.g., wheeze and dyspnea are abnormal and a sign of disease, but some degree of anxiety at times is a common experience, and the point at which it is pathological is based more on the effect that anxiety has on the patient.

• Mental illnesses have legal consequences.

• It is important that psychiatrists are clear in themselves about which behaviors and abnormalities are their responsibility. Psychiatrists are especially prone to involvement in human rights abuses in states around the world when the definitions of mental illness were expanded to take in political insubordination.

Disease, sickness, and illness behavior

The distinction between disease (or disorder) and sickness should be understood. Disease encompasses either the specific tissue lesion or characteristic constellation of symptoms. Sickness, on the other hand, encompasses the suffering and functional deficit consequent on symptoms. One may exist without the other—e.g., a patient with undiagnosed, asymptomatic breast cancer undoubtedly has disease but is not sick; a patient with a conversion (hysterical) disorder may see themselves (and be considered) as sick, but does not have an identifiable lesion.

Patients generally present complaining of symptoms, and this process is called illness or illness behavior. Patients need not be suffering from a disease or disorder in order to do this, and sometimes illness behavior may be abnormal (even when the patient does have a disease). Subject to certain social conventions (e.g., seeing a doctor), they are then afforded the "sick" role, which allows them to relinquish some of their normal obligations. This is a man-made concept, encompassing the special rights and expected behavior of both someone who is sick and the doctor who is treating them (see box). Difficulties arise when a person adopts the sick role to gain the rights afforded to them while neglecting their duties. Another concern relates to the process of diagnosis—causing someone who is not currently ill to adopt the "sick" role. Physicians should understand their special responsibility to act in the patient's best interests and not to stray outside the medical arena.

The rights and duties of patients and doctors

Patient

Rights

- Exemption from blame
- Exemption from normal duties while in the sick role
- To expect the doctor to act in their best interests

Duties

- To seek help
- To be open and honest
- To comply with treatment
- To give up the sick role once well

Doctor

- To be considered an expert
- To have privileged access to patient information and person
- To direct (and sometimes insist on) a course of action
- To validate the sick role

- To act in the patient's best interests
- To maintain confidentiality
- To keep up-to-date
- To act, where possible, in society's interests

Clarity of roles

It is all too easy for psychiatrists to slip into other roles for which they are untrained. Psychiatrists have special training and experience in mental disorder, and should avoid being drawn outside this specialty in their professional role. These other roles can include: substitute parent, friend, guardian of public morals, predictor of future criminality, or arbiter of normal behavior.

Mental health and mental illness

Psychiatrists are properly occupied in the business of diagnosing and treating significant psychiatric disorders. As providers of mental health resources there are often pressures to validate distress or create a diagnosis for normal experience. Saying that someone does not satisfy criteria for a specific mental disorder does not mean that they do not have significant problems; rather, it means the problems do not fall within the scope of psychiatry and would probably be best dealt with by help or advice elsewhere. In general, psychiatrists should not spend their time advising people on how to live their lives—this is the self-appointed specialty of popular psychology.

Diagnosis in psychiatry

Labels

People have a natural enthusiasm to be seen as individuals rather than as members of a class: "I'm a person, not a label." This desire for the recognition of individuality and uniqueness is a part of the public reaction against race-, class-, and gender-related value judgments.

At the same time people do like to belong to and identify with groups. They also like to classify and to have labels for things as this can bring order to life or comfort in a horrible situation. Physicians are no different. Labels in medicine are based on characteristic combinations of symptoms and signs, but these are viewed differently by patient and doctor. Symptoms are important to patients because of their individual nature; that this strange and atypical thing is happening to them. Symptoms are important to doctors because they indicate diagnosis and are features that make this patient similar to others we have seen or read about. Giving something a name has benefits for both.

Diagnosis

The naming of something is the first step toward understanding it. We seek to identify disorders (diagnosis) in order that we should be able to suggest treatments (management) and predict their course (prognosis). Ultimately, the aim is to identify the physical abnormality (pathology) and the cause of the disease (etiology) and so develop means of prevention and cure.

The ideal diagnostic system labels diseases according to a combination of clinical information and etiology. The etiology of most mental disorders was unclear and so current diagnostic systems are based on:
- common clinical features,
- shared natural history and disease course,
- common treatment response,
- or a combination of all three.

Diagnosis leads to the consideration of individual diseases as members of groups contained within a hierarchy, a form of classification system. Classification systems will change over the coming years as our knowledge base on the genetic and neural basis of psychiatric illness grows. (see The future of psychiatric research and classification, 📖 *pp. 32–35*).

Why make a diagnosis?

Just as in all branches of medicine there are compromises and a loss of information in allocating a patient, with their individual and unique history, experience, and range of signs to a single label.

Any diagnosis must be justified on a general and an individual basis. Generally, the process of establishing a diagnosis is essential:
- to allow succinct communication with colleagues,
- to help predict prognosis,
- and to carry out valid research on pathological mechanisms and on treatments.

Remember, however, that allocation of a patient to a diagnostic category can only be justified if it will bring them benefit, not harm.

Current classification in psychiatry

Over the past century within psychiatry there has been a debate about the value and method of psychiatric classification.

On one hand, the academic and biological psychiatrists worried that psychiatric diagnosis was insufficiently reliable and valid, with a wide variety of terms being used in imprecise or idiosyncratic ways; on the other hand, psychodynamic practitioners emphasized the importance of unique patient factors and the degree of detail lost by the reductionism of the diagnostic method.

The first concern was tackled by the development of operational criteria—clearly defined clinical descriptions of the disorders, together with explicit inclusion and exclusion criteria and details of the number and duration of symptoms required for diagnosis. The second concern was partially addressed by the development of multi-axial diagnosis, where, in addition to the primary mental disorder coded on axis-I, additional axes code information about the patient's psychosocial problems, personality factors, medical health, and degree of disability.

International classification

In psychiatric classification, there are two systems in use worldwide: the International Classification of Diseases (ICD-10), produced by WHO; and the Diagnostic and Statistic Manual of Mental Disorders (DSM-IV-TR), produced by the American Psychiatric Association. DSM-IV-TR is the classification system used clinically and for research in the United States. While DSM-IV-TR describes only mental disorders, ICD-10 is a wider general medical classification. The two classifications are broadly similar, having undergone a degree of convergence and "cross-fertilization" with subsequent revisions. DSM-IV-TR disorders and codes with corresponding ICD-10 codes are given on *p. 1151.*

The Diagnostic and Statistical Manual of Mental Disorders (DSM-IV-TR)
Coding—DSM-IV-TR uses a closed, numeric coding system of the form xxx.xx (mostly in the range 290–333.xx). A single version of DSM-IV-TR is used for both clinical and research purposes, although there are a series of "research" disorders and codes that are not in general diagnostic use.

Axial Diagnosis—DSM-IV-TR is a multi-axial diagnostic system using five axes.
- Axis 1 describes the clinical disorder or the current clinical problem.
- Axis 2 describes any personality disorder and any mental handicap.
- Axis 3 describes general medical conditions.
- Axis 4 describes current psychosocial problems.
- Axis 5 describes a global assessment of functioning.

The International Classification of Diseases (ICD-10)
The ICD-10 is a general medical classification system intended for worldwide, multispecialty use. It includes 21 chapters, each identified by a Roman numeral and an Arabic letter. Psychiatric classification is

Chapter V, and psychiatric disorders are identified by the letter F. An index of the disorders described in this book, together with their ICD-10 coding, is given on 📖 p. 1151.

Coding—The disorders are identified using an open alphanumeric system in the form Fxx.xx. The letter F identifies the disorder as a mental or behavioral disorder; the first digit refers to the broad diagnostic grouping (e.g., psychotic, organic, substance-induced); and the second digit refers to the individual diagnosis. The digits that follow the decimal point code for additional information specific to the disorder such as subtype, course, or type of symptoms. When used as second or third digits, the number 8 codes for "other" disorders whereas the number 9 codes for "unspecified."

There are separate Clinical, Research, and Primary Care versions of ICD-10.

Axial Diagnosis—The multi-axial version of ICD-10 uses three axes to broaden the assessment of the patients' condition.
- Axis 1 describes the mental disorder (including personality disorder and mental handicap).
- Axis 2 describes the degree of disability.
- Axis 3 describes current psychosocial problems.

Treating patients against their will

The power of the psychiatrist

Psychiatric patients may have treatment, hospitalization, and other measures imposed on them against their wishes. The power to impose such measures does not sit comfortably with the usual doctor–patient relationship, and psychiatrists may find the involuntary commitment of patients unpleasant.

The existence of these powers means that under some circumstances psychiatrists will be:

• damned if they do (criticized for being agents of social control, disregarding a person's autonomy, and being heavy handed) and
• damned if they don't (neglecting their duties, not giving patients the necessary care, and putting the public at risk).

Although it may not seem so, the involuntary commitment of a patient may, in fact, be a very caring thing to do. Such a paternalistic view may appall some people, but historically, paternalism has had a major influence in the field of health generally and in this area in particular.

When we consider why it is that we have such powers, we might argue that because psychiatric illness may affect insight and judgment (i.e., a person's capacity) sometimes patients might not be capable of making appropriate decisions about their care and treatment. Although to modern ears this may sound ethically sensible, there have been various forms of mental health legislation in the United States for as long as it has existed.

Although there is no single piece of overarching federal legislation governing the treatment of the mentally ill, there are state and federal provisions and regulations for different facets of mental health care. These have usually arisen out of case law over the years. This case law is always precipitated by a violation of civil liberties or individual rights as protected by the Constitution or, more specifically, the Bill of Rights.

For example, certain practices in regard to the mentally ill patient at one point were the norm and were justified by local legislation or a state's mental health code. Then, someone, often an advocacy group, sees the violation of a right (such as the lack of due process in older commitment procedures), and brings a case. The case works its way into the State Supreme Court or the U.S. Supreme Court. When the decision is for the plaintiff, the individual mental health codes are changed to comply with the decision. Case law is considered in more depth in Chapter 17, 📖 p. 807.

On a general theme and in most states, is it right that psychiatric patients can be treated against their wishes even when they have capacity to make such decisions? This does seem to raise interesting ethical questions about whether interventions can ever be justified by principles of paternalism or public protection, when a mentally disordered person has capacity.

The public health argument

There remains the "public health" argument of public protection. It is true that some psychiatric patients may also pose a risk to others just as many people without a psychiatric disorder pose such a risk. However, most people with mental disorder (even severe cases) are never violent; violence is difficult to predict, and many other people who pose a public risk (those who drink heavily or drive fast) are not subject to such special measures. Potentially dangerous behavior is not in itself a justification for the existence of mental health legislation, but instead provides one criterion for the use of such measures when a person meets other criteria (namely having a mental disorder) and needs care and treatment.

We need to be very wary of how our special powers to detain and treat patients against their wishes might be extended and misused. It is not the role of psychiatric services (including forensic psychiatric services) to detain dangerous violent offenders and sex offenders just to prevent them from re-offending. That is not to argue that psychiatrists should not have a role in the assessment and management of such individuals, but that we should not have primary responsibility for their "care." This is a current area of controversy, particularly with the expansion of forensic psychiatric services envisioned in the United States over the next few years, which should be aimed toward the treatment of inmates suffering from mental illnesses.

The way forward

In the 21st century we should be clear of our role: to care for individuals with psychiatric illnesses, without necessarily being paternalistic. We should treat our patients in such a way as to prevent harm to them and to others, but this should not be our sole reason for being. The primary justification for the existence of mental health legislation should be to ensure the provision of care and treatment for people who, because of mental disorder, have impaired ability to make appropriate decisions for themselves. We should not be able to forcibly intervene unless this is the case and, when we do, our interventions should be for our patients' benefit as well as for society.

By the same token, any mental health legislation should protect people with mental illness from being incarcerated in jails or prisons without adequate access to psychiatric care. Similarly mental health legislation should prevent the judicial murder by execution of offenders who committed their offense while mentally ill and/or had diminished capacity.

Perceptions of psychiatry

The public perception

What does the public think about psychiatry? When the public gives the discipline any thought at all, they usually conjure up images from television or movies: psychiatrists who treat patients with hypnosis or years of talk therapy, occasionally effecting miracle cures on people with mental illness who are unpredictable, violent, traumatized, and hopelessly ill. These perceptions greatly contribute to stigma against those who work in or need help from psychiatry, and especially for those with mental illness, this stigma serves as a major barrier to recovery and community integration.

Historical perceptions

In prehistorical times, those suffering from mental disturbance were thought to be possessed by animal or natural spirits. Some communities shunned the mentally ill, while others may have carved out a shaman's role in honor of their unique characteristics. Ancient people formalized these constructs into more theistic conceptualizations; only with Hippocrates and his followers did spirituality cede to a more biomedical model as the explanation for mental illness.

This "progress" seemed to fade in medieval times, as society returned to spiritualistic explanations of illness—regarding people with mental illness either as witches or saints, possessed by Satan or God. Enlightenment-era thinkers may have shifted perceptions back to more rational and medical models, but the ironic outcome was increasing institutionalization and restraint—what Foucault called "the great confinement" of the Romantic period—at least until Pinel broke the chains at the Bicetre.

In the more modern eras from 1800 on, we have seen shifting models of psychological or neurobiological explanations and therapeutics for mental illness: the Tukes and Thomas Kirkbride giving way to Beard and Gall, who in turn gave way to Freud, who then yielded to Freeman and so forth, each "revolution" heralded by some cultural shift—muckraking, nihilism, antiscience, etc.

Throughout our history, perceptions have cycled between poles of understanding, depending on whether a particular era has been more focused on mind or body, custodialism or caring, science or religion, community or institution. These cycles play out similarly in media, film, and literature—reflecting and influencing public attitudes about psychiatry.

- For instance, in the United States, the 1950s was a golden age of psychiatry on film, with portrayals of heroic psychiatrists using psychological treatment to cure patients of a variety of illnesses—a perception of the field that grew out of successes during World War II, the rise and increasing popularity of outpatient psychiatry, and a reaction against institutional care.
- In 1957 alone, films like *Fear Strikes Out* and *The Three Faces of Eve* presented compassionate psychiatrists helping ill patients resolve inner conflicts that emerged as psychiatric symptoms.

- Of course, the golden age ended with the upheavals of the 1960s, the rise of the antipsychiatry movement, and anxiety about a disrupted social fabric: both the novel and film *One Flew over the Cuckoo's Nest* resonated with these viewpoints and even today serves as one of the more indelible images of psychiatry for many Americans.

Present perceptions of psychiatry

In recent times, new waves of antipsychiatry have been felt across the medical community.

- For example, groups affiliated with Scientology (a philosophy developed in the 1950's by science-fiction author L. Ron Hubbard) actively seek to disavow the field of psychiatry and the related treatments used by practitioners of psychiatry.
- Much of the criticism of psychiatry may be related to its relative youth within the medical community. For example, the pharmacological age of psychiatry only began in the mid-20th century. The progression of understanding and refining psychiatric diagnoses and treatments continually advances as our ability to comprehend the brain continually improves. However, this seemingly slow and steady pace has been the natural scientific progression of all medical fields, and potential risks and side-effects are associated with the advancement and administration of all medical treatments. As such, extreme groups that specifically target psychiatry within the medical field appear to be rooting their efforts in stigma as well as misunderstanding the needs of those who experience true psychiatric illness.

The field of psychiatry has come a long way from its early theoretical roots and is continually striving to ground all diagnoses and treatments on evidence-based studies as well as thoroughly researched protocols designed to improve the lives of patients who experience symptoms of psychiatric illness.

Advocacy groups and antistigma efforts undertaken by patients and professionals have had some effect on public perceptions. Yet illnesses like addiction are still seen as personal weakness, patients still suffer discrimination, and even medical students may choose nonpsychiatry specialties simply because of negative attitudes toward the field espoused by family, the community, or even physicians.

Those who work closely with psychiatric illness envision a major shift in public perceptions as a revolution in the broader society directs attention to the true suffering that can be associated with these often chronic and debilitating illnesses.

Stigma

Stigma is a Greek word meaning "mark," which originally referred to a sign branded onto criminals or traitors in order to publicly identify them. In its wider, modern sense, stigma refers to the sense of collective disapproval and group of negative perceptions attached to a particular people, trait, condition, or lifestyle.

How does stigma affect patients with mental illness?

Stigma affects those who suffer from mental illness in a number of ways. People may delay seeking treatment for fear that they may be perceived as "crazy," that they may lose their jobs, or that their friends or family will abandon them. Even when people enter treatment, they may have to pay more for treatment of their psychiatric illness than they would for treatment of a "medical illness."

This is just one example of how even our common language is reflective of stigma. Despite the evidence base for biologic underpinnings of psychiatric diseases, we speak of psychiatric illness as somehow separate from medical illness. This false dichotomy can potentially marginalize our patients. Another example of this has been the ease with which originally neutral descriptive terms for mental disorders have taken on a pejorative and disparaging meaning: cretin, maniac, spastic, imbecile, retarded, even neurotic. All have been abandoned in an attempt to free affected individuals from the approbation the name had acquired. Even something as subtle as saying a patient "is schizophrenic" rather than a patient "has schizophrenia" can be potentially stigmatizing. Identifying patients *as* a disease rather than people *with* an illness dehumanizes them, thus making it easier to treat them with less respect and to deny them basic rights and services.

Misunderstanding can maintain stigma

Misunderstanding of mental illness can perpetuate stigma. For instance, the portrayal of the mentally ill by the media reinforces the notion that people with mental illness are violent and unpredictable and that they should be feared or shunned. Movies from *Psycho* to *Silence of the Lambs* perpetuate the stereotype of the psycho-killer. Newspapers and television news shows often sensationalize crimes committed by the mentally ill. When not being accused of violence, the mentally ill are often laughed at. Again, the media play an important role—for instance, in July, 2002, *The Trentonian,* a paper widely read in New Jersey, reporting on a fire at a psychiatric hospital, ran the headline "Roasted Nuts."

Sometimes, those who would further stigmatize the mentally ill exploit the media for this purpose. Scientology actively recruits celebrities and media personnel, to further their message. Tom Cruise's antipsychiatry speech during a 2005 appearance on the *Today Show* is just one example of this. Beyond using the media to their advantage, celebrity Scientologists have tried to influence the law by giving testimony to state legislative bodies in support of antipsychiatry bills. The Scientologists recently took their antipsychiatry campaign a step further and opened an entire museum to showcase the "evils" of psychiatry.

However, other celebrities are willing to speak out about their own battles with mental illness, thus normalizing the experience, and letting people know that they are not alone in their suffering and that help is available and effective.

Stigma in the government

Despite huge strides forward, there is apparent stigma even at a governmental level. Despite more than a decade of efforts, true parity for mental health benefits remains elusive. The Mental Health Parity Act of 1996 which, by the end of 2006, had been extended five times and was set to expire barring another extension, prohibits discriminatory annual lifetime and dollar caps for mental health benefits compared to medical and surgical benefits. However, this is only the case if an insurer chooses to provide mental health coverage—and there is no such requirement in the Act. Legislation introduced in the U.S. House of Representatives would end cost-sharing and treatment limitations for mental health care as compared to other medical care. The bill, despite high support, is yet to see a vote. There is also no Senate companion to this bill (an amendment introduced by Senator Ted Kennedy (D-MA) failed in committee on a 10–10 tie). The high cost of providing mental health services is often cited by those who would oppose parity yet, based on data from the Federal Employee Health Benefit Program (which has offered full parity for mental health and substance abuse treatment since 2001), providing mental health benefits on par with other medical benefits does not appear to increase costs.

Institutionalized stigmatization exists in other forms as well. For instance, current Medicare law sets a 20% coinsurance rate for all Part B services except "with respect to expenses incurred . . . in connection with the treatment of mental, psychoneurotic, and personality disorders of any individual who is not an inpatient" (1833[c] of the Social Security Act). For those individuals seeking outpatient psychiatric services, the coinsurance rate is 50%. Emergency psychiatric care is also subject to discriminatory funding. In addition, the Emergency Medical and Labor Treatment Act (EMTALA) appropriately requires that psychiatric hospitals stabilize all patients in their emergency rooms regardless of their ability to pay, but Medicaid law prohibits payments to Institutions for Mental Disease (IMDs). So, while one federal law requires that patients receive treatment, another prohibits payment for that treatment.

As psychiatrists, we have a responsibility to our patients to fight against stigma. This can be done on many different levels:

- Educate patients and their families about the nature of their illness and the potential for treatment.
- Challenge the lack of knowledge about mental disorders often seen in our colleagues in other specialties.
- Avoid stigmatizing language.
- Write opinion editorials or letters to the editor of local and national newspapers challenging stigmatizing portrayals of the mentally ill in the news or other media outlets.
- Be politically active—write to your legislators, visit their offices, and vote for candidates who support equal treatment for mental illness.

Antipsychiatry

One view of medicine is that it is an applied science whose object of scientific curiosity is the understanding of the causes and processes of human illness and the study of methods of preventing or ameliorating them. In the scientific method, there are no absolute truths, only theories that fit the observed facts as they are currently known. All scientists must be open to the challenging of firmly established theories as new observations are made and new experiments reported.

All psychiatrists should retain this healthy scientific skepticism and be prepared to question their beliefs about the causes and cures of mental illness. Developments (and hence improvements in patient care) come from improvement in observation methods and trials of new treatment modalities. A result of this may be the enforced abandonment of cherished beliefs and favored treatments. Always remember that insulin coma therapy* was at one time believed to be an effective treatment for psychotic illnesses.

Although rigorous examination of the basic and clinical sciences of psychiatry is essential if the specialty is to progress, psychiatry as a medical specialty has, over the last 50 years, been subject to a more fundamental criticism—that the empirical approach and the medical model are unsuited to the understanding of mental disorder and that they cause harm to the individuals they purport to treat. This basic belief, known as "antipsychiatry," has been expressed by a variety of individuals over the years, reaching a peak in the late 1960s. Although the central arguments of the antipsychiatry movement have largely been discredited in the mainstream scientific literature, they have retained currency in some areas of the popular press, within some public organizations, and in certain religious cults such as the Church of Scientology. It is important to remember, however, that some of these ideas were, in part, the spur to the second renaissance of psychiatry as a medical specialty and thus should be reviewed.

Central antipsychiatry beliefs
- The mind is not a bodily organ and so cannot be diseased.
- The scientific method cannot explain the subjective abnormalities of mental disorder as no direct observation can take place.
- Mental disorder can best be explained by social, ethical, or political factors.
- The labeling of individuals as "ill" is an artificial device used by society to maintain its stability in the face of challenges.
- Medication and hospitalization are harmful to the individual so treated.

---

* In 1933 Manfred Sakel introduced insulin coma therapy for the treatment of schizophrenia. This involved the induction of a hypoglycemic coma using insulin; the rationale being that a period of decreased neuronal activity would allow for nerve cell regeneration. In the absence of alternative treatments, this was enthusiastically adopted by practitioners worldwide. However, with the advent of antipsychotics in the 1950s and the emergence of randomized controlled trials, it became clear that the treatment had no effect above placebo and it was subsequently abandoned.

The flaws of antipsychiatry

The antipsychiatry movement did raise some valid criticisms of then contemporary psychiatric practice; in particular:
- pointing out the negative effects of institutional living,
- criticizing stigma and labeling,
- alerting psychiatrists to the potential use of political change in improving patient care.

It was, however, fatally flawed by:
- a rejection of empiricism,
- an overreliance on single case reports,
- domination by a small number of personalities with incompatible and deeply held beliefs,
- associations with specific political rather than medical or scientific ideologies.

Prominent antipsychiatrists

- **Szasz** Rejected compulsory treatment. Author of *Pain and Pleasure* and *The Myth of Mental Illness*. Viewed disease as a bodily abnormality with an observable pathology to which, by its nature, the brain was immune. Saw mental illness as conflict between individuals and society. Rejected the insanity defense and committal to hospital. Accepted patients for voluntary treatment for drug-free analysis on payment of fee and acceptance of treatment contract.
- **Scheff** Worked in labeling theory. Wrote *Being Mentally Ill*. Hypothesized that mental illness was a form of social rule breaking. Labeling such individuals as mentally ill would stabilize society by sanctioning such temporary deviance.
- **Goffman** Wrote *Asylums*. Described the "total institution" observed as a result of an undercover study. Commented on the negative effects of institutions segregated from the rest of society and subject to different rules.
- **Laing** Author of *The Divided Self; Sanity, Madness and the Family*; and *The Politics of Experience*. Developed probably the most complete antipsychiatry theory. He saw the major mental illnesses as arising from early family experiences, in particular from hostile communication and the desire for "ontological security." He saw newborns as housing potential that was diminished by the forced conformity of the family and the wider society. Viewed normality as forced conformity and illness as "the reality which we have lost touch with."
- **Cooper** Revived antipsychiatry ideas. A committed Marxist, he saw schizophrenia as a form of social repression.
- **Busaglia** Wrote *The Deviant Majority*. Held that diagnosis didn't aid understanding of the patient's experience. Believed that social and economic factors were crucial. Successful in pressing for significant reform of the Italian mental health system.
- **Scull** Wrote *Museums of Madness*. Saw mental health systems as part of "the machinery of the capitalist system."
- **L. Ron Hubbard** founder of the, Church of Scientology, who view psychiatry as brutal, inhumane, and not a science. Published *Dianetics: the Modern Science of Mental Health,* which denies the biological basis of brain function. Hubbard later characterized mental health professionals as part of a conspiracy. The Church remains active and has some celebrity adherents in Hollywood.
- **Breggin** Modern advocate of antipsychiatry views. Author of *Toxic Psychiatry*, which views psychopharmacology as disabling normal brain function. Rejects results of systematic reviews.

A brief history of psychiatry

Ancient times ~4000 B.C. Sumerian records describe the euphoriant effect of the poppy plant. ~1700 B.C. First written record concerning the nervous system. 460–379 B.C. **Hippocrates** discusses epilepsy as a brain disturbance and hysteria as the "wandering uterus." 387 B.C. **Plato** teaches that the brain is the seat of mental processes. 280 B.C. **Erasistratus** notes divisions of the brain. 177 **Galen** lectures *On the Brain* and consolidated Hippocratic/Aristotelian ideas about mental illness (e.g., melancholia caused by excess black bile). ~1000 **Avicenna** was a Muslim physician who made early psychosomatic linkages.

Premodern 1486 **Kramer + Sprenger** wrote *Malleus Maleficarum* (*Witches' Hammer*) led to persecution of mentally ill "witches." 1520 **Paracelsus**, an Austrian who believed that psychiatric syndromes were natural diseases, not signs of spiritual possession. 1586 **Bright** writes *Treatise of Melancholia* the first English monograph on mental illness, depression either humoral or psychological. 1621 **Burton** writes *Anatomy of Melancholy* a classic text, consolidating medical and nonmedical literature on depression. 1649 **Descartes** describes the pineal as seat of mentation and dualist concepts of body and mind. 1656 **Bicêtre and Salpêtrière** asylums established by Louis XIV in France. 1755 **Perry** publishes *A Mechanical Account and Explication of the Hysteric Passion.* 1758 **Battie** publishes his *Treatise on Madness*, first recognized specialist in "madness." 1773 **Cheyne** publishes his book *English Malady,* launching the idea of "nervous illness." 1774 **Mesmer** introduces "animal magnetism" (later called hypnosis). 1793 **Pinel** is appointed to the Bicêtre and directs the removal of chains from the "madmen." 1794 **Chiarugi** publishes *On Insanity* specifying how a therapeutic asylum should be run.

1800–1850s 1808 **Reil** coins the term *psychiatry.* 1812 **Rush**, the Father of American Psychiatry, publishes *Medical Inquiries and Observations upon the Diseases of the Mind.* 1813 the **Tukes** were a Quaker family who founded York Retreat for care of mentally ill using moral treatment. 1813–1818 **Heinroth** links life circumstances to mental disorders in *Textbook of Mental Hygiene.* 1815 **Gall** began phrenology, the mapping of psychological "faculties" to the brain. 1817 **Parkinson** publishes *An Essay on the Shaking Palsy.* **Esquirol**, Pinel's student, lectures on psychiatry to medical students. 1825 **Bouillaud** presents cases of aphonia after frontal lesions. **Todd** discusses localization of brain functions. 1827 **Heinroth** appointed as the first professor of "psychological therapy" in Leipzig. 1832 **Chloral hydrate** discovered. 1838 **Esquirol** coined the term *hallucination,* and new classifications. **Ray** founder of American forensic psychiatry. 1843 **Braid** coins the term *hypnosis.* 1844 **APA** first U.S. specialty society formed (asylum "medical superintendants" initially), *Am J Psych* founded as *Am J Insanity* 1845 **Griesinger**, founder of neuropsychiatry, described psychiatric diseases as brain diseases, major synthetic text (*Mental Pathology*) 1848 **Phineas Gage** has his brain pierced by an iron rod with subsequent personality change, ushered in first golden age of neuroscience.

1850–1875 1854 **Falret, Ballenger** independently described "la folie circulaire" or "double forme," which **Kraepelin** later named manic-depression, 1854 **Kirkbride** set standards for hospital organization to care for the mentally ill. 1856 **Morel** describes "démence précoce"—deteriorating adolescent psychosis. 1863 **Kahlbaum** introduces the term *catatonia*. **Friedreich** describes progressive hereditary ataxia. 1864 **Hughlings Jackson** writes on aphonia after brain injury. 1866 **Down** describes "congenital idiots." 1868 **Griesinger** describes "primary insanity" and "unitary psychosis." 1869 **Galton** claims that intelligence is inherited in *Hereditary Genius*. 1871 **Hecker** describes "hebephrenia." 1872 **Huntington** describes symptoms of an hereditary chorea. 1874 **Wernicke** publishes *Der Aphasische Symptomenkomplex* on aphasias.

1875–1900 1876 **Ferrier** publishes *The Functions of the Brain*. **Galton** uses the term "nature and nurture" to describe heredity and environment. 1877 **Charcot**, a neurologist extremely influential to Freud and others, publishes *Lectures on the Diseases of the Nervous System*. 1880 **Beard** described neurasthenia, a uniquely American disease of mental/physical exhaustion. 1883 **Kraepelin** coins the terms "neuroses" and "psychoses." 1884 **Gilles de la Tourette** describes several movement disorders. 1885 **Lange** proposes use of lithium for excited states. 1887 **Korsakoff** describes characteristic symptoms in alcoholics. 1892 **American Psychological Association** formed. 1895 **Freud and Breuer** publish *Studies on Hysteria*, which lay the groundwork for psychoanalysis, use of hypnosis in psychiatry, defense mechanisms. 1896 **Kraepelin** describes dementia praecox. 1899 **Freud** publishes *The Interpretation of Dreams*, further exploring the unconscious.

1900–1910 1900 **Wernicke** publishes *Basic Psychiatry* in Leipzig. 1903 **Barbiturates** introduced. First volume of *Archives of Neurology and Psychiatry* published in United States. **Pavlov** coins the term "conditioned reflex." 1905 **Binet and Simon** develop their first IQ test. 1906 **Alzheimer** describes presenile degeneration. 1907 **Adler's** *Study of Organ Inferiority and Its Physical Compensation* published describing lifestyles and inferiority complex. Origins of **group therapy** in Pratt's work supporting TB patients in Boston. 1908 **Clifford Beers** wrote *A Mind That Found Itself*, a sensational book about asylum abuse, ushering in the mental hygiene movement 1909 **Brodmann** describes 52 cortical areas. **Cushing** electrically stimulates human sensory cortex. **Freud** publishes the case of Little Hans in Vienna.

1910s 1911 **Bleuler** publishes his textbook *Dementia Praecox or the Group of Schizophrenias*. 1913 **Jaspers** describes nonunderstandability in schizophrenia thinking. Syphilitic spirochaete established as cause of "generalized paresis of the insane" by **Noguchi** in the United States. **Jung** splits with Freud forming the school of "analytic psychology." **Goldmann** finds blood–brain barrier impermeable to large molecules. 1914 **Dale** isolates acetylcholine. The term **"shell shock"** is coined by British soldiers. 1916 **Henneberg** coins the term "cataplexy." 1917 **Epifanio** uses barbiturates to put patients with major illnesses into prolonged sleep. **Wagner-Jauregg** discovers malarial treatment, "fever therapy" for neurosyphilis, gets Nobel Prize for this in 1927.

1920s 1920 Moreno develops "psychodrama" to explore individual problems through reenactment. **Watson and Raynor** demonstrate the experimental induction of phobia in "Little Albert". **Crichton-Miller** found the Tavistock Clinic in London. **Klein** conceptualises development theory and the use of play therapy. **Freud's** *Beyond the Pleasure Principle* published. **1921 Rorschach** develops the inkblot projective test. **1922 Klaesi** publishes results of deep-sleep treatment, which is widely adopted. **1923 Freud** describes his "structural model of the mind," splitting it into id, ego and superego. **1924 Jones** uses the first example of systematic desensitisation to extinguish a phobia. **1927 Jacobi and Winkler** first apply pneumoencephalography to the study of schizophrenia. **Wagner-Jauregg** awarded the Nobel Prize for malarial treatment of neurosyphilis. **Cannon-Bard** describes his "theory of emotions." **1929 Berger** demonstrates first human electroencephalogram.

1930s 1930 First child psychiatry clinic established in Baltimore, headed by **Kanner**. **1931 Reserpine** introduced. **1932 Klein** publishes The *Psychoanalysis of Children*. **1933 Sakel** introduces "insulin coma treatment" for schizophrenia. **1934 Meduna** uses chemical (metrazol) convulsive therapy. **1935 Moniz and Lima** first carry out "prefrontal leucotomy." **Amphetamines** synthesized. **Dale and Loewi** share Nobel Prize for work on chemical nerve transmission. **1937 Klüver and Bucy** publish work on bilateral temporal lobectomies. **Papez** publishes work on limbic circuits and develops "visceral theory" of emotion. **1938 Cerletti and Bini** first use "electroconvulsive therapy." **Skinner** publishes The *Behaviour of Organisms* describing operant conditioning. **Hoffmann** synthesises **LSD**. **Kallman** publishes the *Genetic Theory of Schizophrenia* and founded the first full-time genetic department at a psychiatric institution in the United States. **1939 Schneider** defines his "first rank symptoms" of schizophrenia.

1940s 1942 Freeman and Watts publish *Psychosurgery* popularizing lobotomies in the United States. **1943 Antihistamines** used in schizophrenia and manic depression. **1946 Freeman** introduces "transorbital leucotomy." **Main** publishes *Therapeutic Communities*. **1948 Foulkes's** *Introduction to Group Analytical Psychotherapy* published. *International Classification of Diseases* (**ICD**) first published by WHO. **Jacobsen and Hald** discover the use of disulfiram. **Kinsey** reported on sexual behavior in males.

1949 National Institute of Mental Health (NIMH) is established. **Cade** introduces lithium for treatment of mania. **Penrose** publishes *The Biology of Mental Defect*. **Moniz** awarded Nobel Prize for treatment of psychosis with leucotomy. **Hess** receives Nobel Prize for work on the "interbrain." **Magoun** defines the reticular activating system. **Hebb** publishes *The Organization of Behaviour: A Neuropsychological Theory*.

1950s 1950 First World Congress of Psychiatry held at Paris. **Chlorpromazine** (compound 4560 RP) synthesized by **Charpentier**. **Roberts and Awapara** independently identify GABA in the brain. **Erikson** described developmental stages based on Freudian concepts. **1951 Papaire and Sigwald** report efficacy of chlorpromazine in psychosis. **1952** *Diagnostic* *and Statistical Manual* (**DSM-I**) introduced by the APA. **Eysenck** publishes *The Effects of Psychotherapy*. **Delay and Deniker** treat patients with psychological disturbance using chlorpromazine, ushering in the pharmacologic era and emptying asylums. **Delay, Laine, and Buisson** report isoniazid use in the treatment of depression. **1953 Lurie and Salzer** report the use of isoniazid as an antidepressant. **1954 Kline** reports that reserpine exerts a therapeutic benefit on both anxiety and obsessive-compulsive symptoms. **Delay and Deniker, Noce and Steck** report favorable effects of reserpine on mania. **1955 Clordiazepoxide**, the first benzodiazepine, synthesized by **Sternbach** for Roche. **Kelly** introduces his "personal construct therapy." **Shepherd and Davies** conduct the first prospective placebo-controlled, parallel-group randomized controlled trial in psychiatry, using reserpine in anxious-depressive out-patients. **1957 Meyer,** founder of modern American psychiatry, developed "psychobiology," influential pragmatist. **Imipramine** launched as an antidepressant. **Iproniazid** launched as an antidepressant. **Delay and Deniker** describe the characteristics of "neuroleptics." **1958 Carlsson** *et al* discover dopamine in brain tissues and identify it as a neurotransmitter, later winning Nobel Prize in 2000. Janssen develops **haloperidol,** the first butyrophenone neuroleptic. **Lehman** reports first (successful) trial of imipramine in the United States. **Diazepam** first synthesized by Roche.

1960s 1960 Merck, Roche, and Lundbeck all launch versions of **amitriptyline. 1961 Knight,** a London neurosurgeon, pioneers stereotactic subcaudate tractotomy. Founding of the **World Psychiatric Association.** Thomas **Szasz** publishes *The Myth of Mental Illness.* **1962 Ellis** introduces "rational emotive therapy." **United States Supreme Court** declares addiction to be a disease and not a crime. **1963 Beck** introduces his "cognitive behavioral therapy," as a short-term treatment for depression. **Carlsson** shows that "neuroleptics" have effects on cathecholamine systems. **1966 Gross and Langner** demonstrate effectiveness of **clozapine** in schizophrenia. **1968 Strömgren** describes "brief reactive psychosis." **Ayllon and Azrin** describe the use of "token economy" to improve social functioning. Publication of DSM-II and ICD-8. **1969 Bowlby** publishes first work on mother-infant attachment and how that relates to future mental illness.

1970s 1970 Laing and Esterson publish *Sanity, Madness and the Family.* **Rutter** publishes the landmark Isle of Wight study on the mental health of children. **Janov** publishes *Primal Scream.* **Maslow** describes his "hierarchy of needs." **Axelrod, Katz, and Svante von Euler** share Nobel Prize for work on neurotransmitters. **Carlsson, Corrodi** *et al.* develop zimeldine, the first of the SSRIs. **1972 Feighner** *et al.* describe operationalized St Louis criteria for diagnosis of schizophrenia, the forerunner of DSM-III. **1973 International Pilot Study of Schizophrenia** uses narrow criteria and finds similar incidence of schizophrenia across all countries studied. **1974 Hughes and Kosterlitz** discover enkephalin. **1975** Research diagnostic criteria (**RDC**) formulated by Spitzer *et al.* in the United States. **Clozapine** withdrawn following episodes of fatal agranulocytosis. **Kernberg** described narcissistic and borderline personality disorders **1976 Johnstone** uses CT to study schizophrenic brains **1977 Guillemin and Schally** share Nobel Prize for work on peptides in the brain. **Hobson** described neurophysiology of dreams, moving far away from Freudian conceptualizations. **1979 NAMI** founded as an advocacy organization for mentally ill patients and family members. **Russell** describes bulimia nervosa.

1980s 1980 DSM-III, developed by **Spitzer**, published by the APA, shifting nosology to descriptive, neo-Kraeplinian, categorical framework. **Crow** publishes his two-syndrome (type I and type II) hypothesis of schizophrenia. **1984 Klerman and Weissman** introduce "interpersonal psychotherapy." **Smith** *et al.* first use MRI to study cerebral structure in schizophrenia. **Andreasen** develops scales for the assessment of positive and negative symptoms in schizophrenia (SAPS and SANS). **1987 Liddle** describes a three-syndrome model for schizophrenia. **Fluvoxamine** introduced. **Mednick** publishes first prospective cohort study of schizophrenia using CT. **1988 Kane** *et al.* demonstrate efficacy of clozapine in treatment-resistant schizophrenia.

1990s 1990 Sertraline introduced. **Ryle** introduces "cognitive analytical therapy." **1991 Paroxetine** introduced. **1992 Moclobemide** introduced as first RIMA. The False Memory Syndrome Society Foundation formed in the U.S.A. Publication of **ICD-10**. **1993** **Huntington's disease** gene identified. Launch of **risperidone** as an "atypical" antipsychotic. **Linehan** first describes her "dialectical behaviour therapy," for the treatment of borderline personality disorder. **1994** Publication of **DSM-IV**. Launch of **olanzapine**. Gilman and Rodbell share the Nobel Prize for their discovery of G-protein coupled receptors and their role in signal transduction. **1995 Citalopram** (SSRI), **venlafaxine** (first SNRI) all introduced. **1997 Quetiapine** launched. **1999 Hodges** publishes first results from prospective Edinburgh High Risk (Schizophrenia) Study using MRI. **1996–1999 Laruelle** *et al* publish a series of papers clarifying the link between striatal dopamine release and positive psychotic symptoms in schizophrenia.

2000s 2000 Carlsson, Greengard, and Kandel share Nobel Prize for their work on neurotransmitters. **2001** launch of **Ziprasidone**. **2002, Mirtazapine** launched. **2003** launch of **Aripiprazole**, first commercially available dopamine partial agonist antipsychotic. **2005** publication of the first Clinical Antipsychotic Trials of Intervention Effectiveness (**CATIE**) trial sponsored by NIMH, the first noncommercial large scale trial comparing newer antipsychotics. **2006** publication of the Sequenced Treatment Alternatives to Relieve Depression (**STAR*D**) study, largest real-world study of treatment-resistant depression.

The future of psychiatric research and classification—endophenotypes

Classification of psychiatric illness remains dependent predominantly upon observational and self-report behavioral measures without reference to an underlying biological framework. Indeed, there are no well-established markers of abnormality in biological systems—"biomarkers"—for any of the major psychiatric disorders to aid diagnosis.

The recent research agenda for DSM-V has, therefore, emphasized a need to translate basic and clinical neuroscience research findings into a new classification system for all psychiatric disorders based upon underlying pathophysiologic and etiological processes.[1, 2] These pathophysiologic processes involve complex relationships between genetic variables, abnormalities in brain systems and related neuropsychological function and behavior, and may be represented as biomarkers of a disorder.[3]

Endophenotypes

Hasler and colleagues[4, 5] have further emphasized the importance of identifying psychiatric disease endophenotypes, a term previously used to describe an internal, intermediate marker of disease not clearly observable eye that links genetic variables associated with a specific disease with observable markers associated with the disease, e.g., the behavioral disturbances observed in many psychiatric illness.

They define an endophenotype as:
- associated with the illness.
- heritable.
- "state independent," i.e., present in an individual with the illness whether or not the illness is active.
- co-segregating with illness within families.
- present in unaffected relatives at a higher rate than in the general population.

Importantly, they also distinguish endophenotypes from diagnostic markers, at least for psychiatric illnesses, as the former may occur in one or more psychiatric diseases as currently defined because it cannot be assumed that our current definitions of psychiatric diseases are biologically valid.

Recommended further reading

1 Charney, D.S., Barlow, D.H., Botterton, K., Cohen, J.D., Goldman, D., Gur, R.E., Lin, K.-M., Lopez, J.F., Meador-Woodruff, J.H., Moldin, S.O., Nestler, E.J., Waton, S.J., Zalcman, S.J.: Neuro-science Research Agenda to Guide Development of a Pathophysi-ologically Based Classification System. In: *A Research Agenda for DSM-V* Kupfer, D.J., First, M.B., Regier, D.A. (Eds.) American Psychiatric Association, Washington DC, 2002.

2 Phillips, M.L., Frank, E. Redefining Bipolar Disorder—Toward DSM-V. *American Journal of Psychiatry*, **163**, 7, 2006.

3 Kraemer, H.C., Schultz, S.K., Arndt, S.: Biomarkers in psychiatry: methodological issues. *American Journal of Geriatric Psychiatry*, **10**, 653–659, 2002.

4 Hasler, G., Drevtets, W.C., Gould, T.D., Gottesman, I.I., Manji, H.K. Toward constructing an endophenotype strategy for bipolar disorders. *Biological Psychiatry*, in press, 2006.

5 Hasler, G., Drevets, W.C., Manji, H.K., Charney, D.S. Discovering endophenotypes for major depression. *Neuropsychopharmacology*, **29**, 1765–1781, 2004.

The future of psychiatric research and classification—biomarkers

Biomarkers

In the last decade, major advances in techniques such as neuroimaging and molecular genetics have facilitated the identification of biological abnormalities associated with different psychiatric illnesses. These findings may lead not only to the identification of biomarkers of psychiatric illnesses as currently defined to help increase diagnostic accuracy of these illnesses, but may also help with the development of a new classification system for psychiatric illness with reference to identified biologically relevant endophenotypes.

In schizophrenia, bipolar disorder, major depressive disorder and some anxiety disorders, there have been promising new developments which have demonstrated overlapping and distinct structural and functional regional brain abnormalities for these different psychiatric illnesses.

• For example, neuroimaging studies have linked functional abnormalities in prefrontal cortical regions during cognitive challenge tasks with many of these illnesses, while others have shown illness- and even symptom-specific patterns of functional abnormality in cortical and subcortical brain regions during cognitive and emotional challenge tasks.[1]

There are even emerging findings from neuroimaging studies identifying potential biomarkers predictive of treatment response and potential illness endophentypes.

Similarly, the development and employment of increasingly more sophisticated neurocognitive, endocrine, and pharmacological challenge paradigms in different psychiatric populations may also facilitate identification of biomarkers—and potential endophenotypes—in psychiatric illnesses. Although it could be argued that genetic linkage studies have met with limited success in identifying illness-specific associations in psychiatry, the rapidly developing fields of molecular genetics and functional genomics may lead to promising findings regarding relationships between genes, neural systems and behavior that help us understand more about the underlying pathophysiologic processes of all major psychiatric illnesses.

It is unlikely that identified biomarkers will be specific for one currently classified psychiatric illness. It will, therefore, become increasingly important to regard psychiatric illnesses within a series of domains and dimensions which will be defined biologically and etiologically. Clinically the domains could include arousal, attention and concentration, mood and emotional expression, perceptions, thought processing, intellectual/cognitive functions, personality and finally motor functions.[2] As biomarkers are identified that dimensionally define these domains both in terms of severity and duration we will develop an etiologically as well as clinically defined classification system, which is likely to be radically different from that which we currently use.

Conclusions

The challenge now for psychiatry is, therefore, to identify biomarkers and putative endophenotypes that will allow us to more accurately diagnose and classify psychiatric illness based on the biological factors that put individual patients at "adverse risk of consequences," (see 📖 p. 6, What is disease?). This reclassification will allow us to better understand and treat our patients. Ultimately the developments will help us to detect those at increased risk for developing psychiatric illnesses and intervene to reduce morbidity and mortality.

Recommended further reading

1 Phillips, M.L., Drevets, W.C., Rauch, S.L., Lane, R.D.: The neurobiology of emotion perception II: implications for understanding the neural basis of emotion per-ceptual abnormalities in schizophrenia and affective disorders. *Biological Psychiatry*, **54**, 515–528, 2003b.
2 Caine, E.D.: Etiologies, Environments and Genes – Challenges for Psychiatric Diagnosis During an Era of Scientific Transition. *Am. J. Geriatr. Psychiatry*, **15**, 12–16, 2007.

Psychiatric assessment

The clinical interview

In most branches of clinical medicine, diagnoses are made largely on the basis of the patient's history, with physical examination and investigation playing important complementary roles. In diagnosing primary psychiatric diseases, the physical examination and investigations may contribute less than in other medical specialities, whereas the clinical interview and keen observation of the longitudinal course of the illness play more major roles. For practical purposes, it is customary to bring these two skills together under the rubric of clinical interviewing. Clinical interviewing is, thus, a central skill of the psychiatrist and development of clinical interviewing skills is fundamental to psychiatric training. Developing clinical skills does not end with residency training. Though it is a critical period which can lay a strong foundation for learning sophisticated interviewing techniques throughout one's career.

The clinical interview includes both history taking and the mental status examination. In addition to its role in diagnosis, the clinical interview begins the development of a therapeutic relationship and is, in many cases, the beginning of treatment. The mental status examination is a systematic record of the patient's current psychopathology and cognitive functions.

Clinical interview skills cannot be learned from a textbook. This chapter is intended as a guide to the doctor or student developing skills in interviewing psychiatric patients. Trainees should also take the opportunity to observe experienced clinicians as they interview patients; to review video-taped consultations with a tutor; and most importantly, carry out many clinical interviews and present the results to supervisors. Skills in this area, as with all others, come with experience and practice.

This chapter describes a model for the assessment of general adult and geriatric psychiatry patients on the wards or in the outpatient clinic. For special patient populations, modifications or extensions to the standard interview are described in the appropriate chapter: substance use problems (📖 p. 615); forensic (📖 pp. 807–86); child and adolescent (📖 pp. 689–97); intellectual and developmental disabilities (mental retardation) (📖 p. 887); and psychotherapy (📖 p. 985).

The student or doctor coming to psychiatric interviewing for the first time is likely to be apprehensive. The symptoms that the patient describes may seem bizarre or incomprehensible, and the examiner may struggle for understanding and knowledge regarding which further questions to ask. Remember that the interviewer is not like a lawyer or policeman trying to "get at the truth" but rather an aid to the patient telling the story in their own words. Start by listening, prompting only when necessary, and aim to feel at the end of the interview that you really understand the patient's problems and their perception of them. It is important to maintain control of the interview and direct the flow of the interview toward the intended purpose. It is equally important to skillfully wrap up the interview within a reasonable timeframe.

The following pages describe the standard structure for a routine history, mental status examination, case summary and formulation. There are then pages devoted to the different symptom areas in adult psychiatry with suggested probe questions. These are intended as guides to the sort of questions to ask the patient (or to ask yourself about the patient) and may be rephrased in your own words.

Always consider your personal safety when interviewing

There is a risk of aggression or violence in only a minority of psychiatric patients. In the majority of patients, the only risk of violence is towards themselves. However, the fact that violence is rare can lead to doctors putting themselves at risk. To combat this, it is important to think about the risk of violence before every consultation with a new patient or with a familiar patient with new symptoms.

Before interviewing a patient, particularly for the first time, consider: **who** you are interviewing, **where** you are interviewing, and **with** whom. Ensure that the staff have this information.

- If possible, review the patient's records noting previous symptomatology and episodes of previous violence (the best predictor of future violence).
- A number of factors will increase the risk of violence including: previous history of violence, psychotic illness, intoxication with alcohol or drugs, frustration, feeling of threat (which may be delusional or relate to "real world" concerns).
- The ideal interview room has two doors that open both ways, one for you and one for the patient. If this is not available sit so that the patient is not between you and the door. Remove all potential weapons from the interview room.
- Familiarize yourself with the ward's panic alarm system *before you first need to use it*, alert the safety officers if you anticipate aggression or take a safety officer with you if know that the patient is aggressive.
- If your hospital organizes "break-away" or aggression management training courses, attend these regularly to keep your skills up-to-date.

Setting the scene

Introductions Observe the normal social etiquettes when meeting someone for the first time. Introduce yourself and any accompanying staff members by name and status. Ensure that you know the names and relationships of any people accompanying the patient (and ask the patient if they wish these persons to be present during the interview). It is best to introduce yourself by title and surname and refer to the patient by title and surname.

Seating The traditional consultation room with the patient facing the doctor across a desk is not optimal for psychiatry because it creates artificial barriers between the patient and clinician. To avoid this, use two or more comfortable chairs, of the same height, orientated to each other at an angle. This is less confrontational but allows direct eye contact as necessary. A clipboard will allow you to write notes as you go along. Before writing down the notes, explain to the patient the confidential nature and purpose of note taking.

Process Inform the patient of your status and specialty and explain the purpose of the interview. Explain the reasons for referral as you understand them and inform the patient of the information you have been told by the referrer. Patients often imagine you know more about them than you do. It is helpful to indicate to the patient how long the interview will last (including supervision time). This will allow both of you to plan your time, so as not to omit vital topics. Advise them that you may wish to obtain further information after the interview from other sources, and obtain their consent to talk to any informants accompanying them if this would add to your assessment. Check with your supervisor regarding required disclosure for evaluations that may result in completion of legal documents (e.g., involuntary commitment forms).

Termination Before terminating the interview, ask the patient whether you have covered all the areas and whether they have shared everything that they had wanted to when they arrived. Reassure them that you or your staff will be available if they remembered anything after the interview and that they may inform you in the subsequent sessions. In this way the patient comes to understand that the clinical interview is not a one-shot cross-sectional event but a longitudinal process.

Documentation For all clinical interviewing a written account is crucial, both as a way of recording and communicating information and as a medico-legal record. Preferred methods vary by institution. Typed or dictated notes are easiest to share with colleagues. For accuracy, it may be best to write up the account as you go along. This saves time afterwards and allows for a more accurate account of the patient's own words. All records should be legible, signed, and dated with exact time, and organized in a standard fashion. Initially you may find it helpful to write out the standard headings on sheets of paper beforehand. To protect confidentiality, it is important to properly delete or destroy any extra files or papers used to create the official medical record.

Interviewing patients with an interpreter When the doctor and the patient do not speak a common language, an interpreter is required. Even in situations where the patient appears to speak some English, sufficient for day-to-day conversation, an interpreter is still essential because idiomatic language and culturally specific interpretations of psychological phenomena may confuse understanding. Where possible the interpreter should share not only a language but also a cultural background with the patient, as many descriptions of psychiatric symptoms are culture specific. Do not use members of a patient's family as interpreters, except where unavoidable (e.g., in emergency situations). It is unethical to use children as interpreters except when absolutely necessary (e.g., in a life threatening situation).

Interviewing psychiatric patients

Interview structure

The exact internal structure of the interview will be decided by the nature of the presenting complaint. However, the interview will generally go through a number of more or less discrete phases:

Initiation Introduce yourself and explain the nature and purpose of the interview. Describe how long the interview will last and what you know about the patient already.

Patient led history Invite the patient to tell you about their presenting complaint. Use general open-ended questions and prompt for further elaboration. Let the patient do most of the talking: your role is to help them to tell the story in their own words. During this phase you should note down the major observations in the MSE. Having completed the history of the presenting complaints and the MSE you will be able to be more focused when taking the other aspects of the history.

Doctor-led history Clarify the details in the history, thus far, with appropriate questions. Clarify the nature of diagnostic symptoms (e.g., are these true hallucinations? Is there diurnal mood variation?) Explore significant areas not mentioned spontaneously by the patient.

Background history Complete the history by direct inquiry. This is similar to standard medical history taking, with the addition of a closer inquiry into the patient's personal history and environment.

Summing-up Recount the history as you have understood it back to the patient. Ensure there are no omissions or important areas uncovered. Indicate if you would like to obtain other third-party information, emphasizing that this would add to your understanding of the patient's problems and help you in your diagnosis.

Questioning techniques

Open v. closed questions An open question does not suggest the possible answers; a closed question expects a limited range of replies (e.g., "can you tell me how you are feeling?" and "is your mood up or down at the moment?"). In general, begin the interview with open questions, turning to more closed questions to clarify details or factual points. The point at which one switch from open ended to closed questions depends on the topic of interest, interview situation and the type of the patient. While evaluating personality domains, it may be useful to continue with the open ended questions whereas while evaluating risk in a guarded patient it could be useful to turn to more closed questions. With an over-inclusive patient, closed questions may help to keep the interview process focused. In an ER situation, it would make sense to switch to closed questions more quickly than in an inpatient situation.

Nondirective v. leading questions A leading question directs a patient towards a suggested answer (e.g., "is your mood usually worse in the mornings?" rather than "is your mood better or worse at any time of day?") Just as lawyers are reprimanded for "leading a witness" one should in general avoid leading patients to certain replies, as the desire to please the doctor can be a very powerful one.

Giving advice

Aim to leave at least the last quarter of the available interview time for discussion of the diagnosis, your explanation to the patient of your under-standing of the nature and cause of their symptoms, and the recommen-dations for treatment or further investigation or referral as indicated. The patient's confidence in your diagnosis will be improved by their belief that you really understand "what is going on" and spending time detailing exactly what you want them to do will pay dividends in increased adherence. A trainee may have to break at the end of the history-taking segment in order to present the case to your senior and obtain advice on management.

After the interview

The process of assessment certainly does not end with the initial clinical interview. In psychiatry, all diagnoses are to some extent provisional. You should follow your initial interview by gathering information from relatives, community contacts, other involved physicians or professionals, previous case records, as well as clarifying symptoms observed by other support staff. In the emergency situation a modification of this technique, focusing mainly on the acute problem, is more appropriate, with re-interviewing later to fill in the blanks if required. Informed, preferably signed, consent should be obtained for each individual prior to contact, regardless of their relationship to the patient or the provider.

Discussing management

In psychiatry, it is essential for successful management that the patient has a good understanding of their disorder and its treatment. There is no equivalent in psychiatry of the "simple fracture" when all that is required of the patient is to "lie back and take the medicine." The treatment of any psychiatric disorder begins at the initial interview, where in addition to the assessment, the doctor should aim to establish the therapeutic alliance, effectively communicate the management plan, instil a sense of hope in the patient, and encourage self-help strategies.

Establish a therapeutic relationship
- Aim to listen more than you speak (especially initially).
- Show respect for the patient as an individual (e.g., establish their preferred mode of address; ask permission for anyone else to be present at the interview).
- Explicitly make your actions for the benefit of the patient.
- Do not argue; agree to disagree if consensus cannot be reached.
- Accept that, in some patients, trust may take time to develop.

Communicate effectively
- **Be specific.** Explain what you think the diagnosis is and what the management should be.
- **Avoid jargon.** Use layman's language or explain specialist terms which you use.
- **Avoid ambiguity.** Clarify precisely what you mean and what your plans are. Be explicit in your statements to patients (e.g., say, "I will work with your case manager to help you with your housing" rather than "I'll arrange some community support for you").
- **Connect the advice to the patient.** Explain why you think what you do and what it is about the patient's symptoms that suggests the diagnosis to you.
- **Use repetition and recapitulation.** Restate the important information first and repeat it at the end.
- **Break up/write down.** Most of what is said to patients in medical interviews is rapidly forgotten or distorted. Make the information easier to remember by breaking it up into a numbered list. Consider providing personalized written information, in addition to any advice leaflets, etc. that you give the patient. This is imperative if the advice is complex and specific (e.g., dosage regimens for medication).

Instil hope
- Patients with mental health problems often feel extremely isolated and cut off from others They may feel that they are the only people ever to experience their symptoms. Reassure them that you recognize their symptoms as part of a pattern representing a treatable illness.
- Convey to the patient your belief that this illness is understandable and that there are prospects for recovery.

- Counteract unrealistic beliefs (e.g., fear of "losing my mind" or "being locked away forever").
- Where "cure" is not possible, emphasize that there is still much that can be done to manage the illness and ameliorate symptoms.

Encourage self-help

- Clarify for the patient what they can do to help themselves. For example, maintain treatment adherence (📖 *pp. 1046–7*), avoid exacerbating factors (e.g., drug or alcohol misuse), consider lifestyle changes (e.g., relocation, relationship counseling).
- Provide written self-help materials appropriate to the current disorder (📖 *p. 1143*).
- Where appropriate, encourage contact with/attendance at voluntary treatment organizations, self-help groups and patient organizations or recommend self-help books and patient manuals (📖 *pp. 1143–50*). Develop knowledge of, and links with, local resources and aim to have their contact numbers and location information available at the consultation.

History

Ideally, the history should be gathered in a standard order like the one presented here. This provides structure and logical coherence to the questioning, both for the doctor and the patient, and it is less likely that items will be omitted.

Basic information Name, age, and marital status. Current occupation. Route of referral. Current legal status (i.e., commitment under Mental Health Law).

Presenting complaints Number and brief description of presenting complaints. Which is the most troublesome symptom?

History of presenting complaints For each individual complaint record its nature (in the patient's own words as far as possible); chronology; severity; associated symptoms and associated life events occurring at or about the same time. Note precipitating, aggravating, and relieving factors. Note the evolution of the psychopathology based on these factors. Have these or similar symptoms occurred before? To what does the patient attribute the symptoms? It is important to conduct a symptom analysis to consider all psychiatric disorders in which a given symptom occurs, and either rule in or rule out each of them to a reasonable extent.

Past medical history Current medical conditions. Chronological list of episodes of medical or surgical illness.

Past psychiatric and medical history Previous psychiatric diagnoses. Chronological list of episodes of psychiatric inpatient, day hospital, and outpatient care. Episodes of symptoms for which no treatment was sought. Any illnesses treated by other physicians or clinicians. Detailed history of self-injurious behavior and suicide attempts.

Drug history List names and doses of current medication (have they been taking it?) Previous psychiatric drug treatments, with purpose, doses, and duration. History of adverse reactions or drug allergy. Any non-prescribed or alternative medications taken.

Family history Family tree (see opposite) detailing names, ages, relationship, and illnesses of first- and second-degree relatives. Detailed family history of mental illness, severity, drug history, and history of suicide attempts.

Personal history

Childhood Were there problems during their gestation or delivery? Did they reach development milestones normally? Was their childhood happy? Were there any abuses (emotional, physical or sexual)? In what sort of family were they raised?

   Education Which schools did they attend between childhood and leaving school or attending college? If more than one of each, why was this? Did they attend mainstream or specialized schools? Did they receive special support in school? How did they do academically? Did they enjoy school?—if not, why? Inquire about peer relationships and relationship with their teachers. At what age did they leave school and with what qualifications? Type of further education and qualifications attained. If they left higher education before completing the course of study—why was this?

Employment Chronological list of jobs. Which job did they hold for the longest period? Which job did they enjoy most? If the patient has had a series of jobs—why did they leave each? Account for periods of unemployment in the patient's history. Is the type of job undertaken consistent with the patient's level of educational attainment?

Relationships Sexual orientation. Chronological account of major relationships. History of (and reasons for) relationship breakdown. Are they currently in a relationship? Do they have any children from the current or previous relationships? With whom do the children live? What relationship does the patient have with them? What is their support system outside the family? Who do they talk to when they are having a bad day?

Forensic (📖 pp. 812–13) Have they been charged or convicted of any offences? What sentence did they receive? Do they have outstanding charges or convictions at the moment? Do they have any contact with the legal system (custody, probation, restraining orders).

Social history Current occupation. Are they working at the moment? If not, how long have they been off work and why? Current family/relationship situation. Alcohol and illicit drug use (📖 pp. 628–32). Main recreational activities.

Premorbid personality How would they describe themselves before becoming ill? How would others have described them? Has their level of functioning in any area changed?

Family tree diagram (genogram)

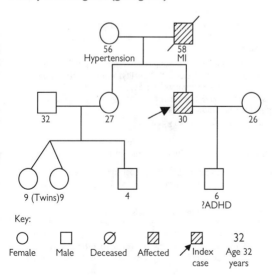

Key:

○	□	⊘	▨	↗▨	32
Female	Male	Deceased	Affected	Index case	Age 32 years

Mental status examination

The mental status examination (MSE) is an organized summary of the examining doctor's observations as to the patient's mental experiences and behavior at the time of interview. Its purpose is to suggest evidence for and against a diagnosis of psychiatric disorder, and if a disorder is present, to record the current type and severity of symptoms. The information contained should, together with the psychiatric history, enable a judgment to be made regarding the presence of and severity of any psychiatric disorder and the risk of harm to self or others. The findings of the MSE should always be viewed in light of the current or previous medical history and physical examination.

The required information can be obtained during the course of history taking or in a systematic fashion afterwards. The MSE should be recorded and presented in a standardized format, although the information contained may derive from material gained in different ways. It is helpful to record the patient's description of significant symptoms word for word.

Appearance (📖 pp. 52–3): Apparent age. Racial origin. Style of dress. Hygene and grooming. General physical condition. Abnormal involuntary movements including tics, grimaces stereotypies, dyskinetic movements, tremors etc.

Behavior (📖 pp. 52–3): Appropriateness of behavior. Level of motor activity. Apparent level of anxiety. Eye contact. Rapport. Abnormal movement or posture. Episodes of aggression. Distractibility.

Speech (📖 p. 54): Volume, rate, rhythm and tone. Spontaneity. Quantity and fluency. Abnormal associations, clanging and punning. Pressure of speech.

Affect (📖 p. 56): Objective, by observation. Note reactivity and range (i.e., full, labile, restricted, blunted, flat). Congruence (i.e., does it fit with what the patient is saying).

Mood (📖 pp. 56–9, p. 62): Subjective, symptoms from the patient. Mood evaluation should include the quality, range, depth, congruence, appropriateness and communicability; Stability and lability; Feelings of worthlessness, guilt and hopelessness. Feelings of guilt. Concentration and energy. Diurnal mood variation.

Anxiety and panic symptoms (📖 pp. 63–5).

Perception (📖 pp. 66–9): Hallucinations and pseudo-hallucinations. Depersonalisation and derealization. Illusions and imagery.

Thought process/form: Linearity, goal directedness, associational quality (i.e., loosening of associations), formal thought disorder and flight of ideas.

Thought content or Ideas and beliefs: delusions, over-valued ideas. Preoccupations (📖 pp. 70–73). Obsessive thoughts, ideas and impulses/compulsions (📖 pp. 63–64). Thoughts of suicide or deliberate self-harm (ideation) (📖 pp. 60–61). Thoughts of harm to others. Assess intent, lethality of intent, plan, and inimicality. Does the patient show any urge to act upon the plan?

Cognition: Attention and Concentration; Orientation to time, place and person; Level of comprehension. Short-term memory. (see Minimental status examination 📖, *pp. 82–3*).

Insight: Does the patient feel their experiences are as the result of illness? Will they accept medical advice and treatment?

Case summary

The written and oral presentation of the results of clinical interview should follow a standard format—history, MSE, results of physical examination, and case summary. The case summary can take a variety of forms, but the structure suggested here is suitable for most situations. You should include a brief synopsis of the case, a differential diagnosis with your favored working diagnoses, and a comment on etiological factors in this patient.

Synopsis This should be a short paragraph summarizing the salient points of the preceding information. Mention the basic personal information, previous psychiatric diagnosis, description of presentation, description of current symptoms, positive features on MSE, suicide risk, and attitude to illness.

Differential diagnosis This will usually be a short list of two or three possibilities. In an exam situation, mention other less likely possibilities you would consider in order to exclude. Your presentation should have directed you towards choosing one as your working diagnosis.

Formulation For general psychiatric patients the formulation should discussion on why this person has this illness at this time. You should identify the "three Ps"—predisposing, precipitating, and perpetuating factors for the current illness. Information for these factors should be considered for biological, psychological and social factors. This information will be important in guiding a suitable management plan. So, for example, in a patient with depressed mood following the birth of a baby: predisposing factors could be family history of depressive illness, female sex; precipitating factors could be the postpartum period, job loss, change of role, and feelings of inadequacy; and prolonging factors could be disturbed sleep, unsupportive partner.

Management plan Following the presentation of the history, MSE, physical examination, and formulation you would normally proceed to present or to document your initial management plan. This should include, where appropriate necessary investigations, (physical, psychological and social), initial drug treatment, instru-tions to support staff, outline the potential risks and level of care needed (outpatient, intensive outpatient, partial hospitalization, inpatient hospitalization, and voluntary or involuntary per local mental health laws).

Observations of appearance and behavior

The greater part of the MSE consists of empathic questioning about the patient's internal experiences. Nonetheless, important information regarding mental status can be obtained from careful observation of the patient's appearance, behavior, and manner, both during the interview and with other staff and patients. This is particularly important in some situations, for example with a patient who may be concealing the presence of psychotic symptoms, or where there is reason to doubt the patient's account. Also, observations such as dress or hygiene may provide subtle clues regarding the patient's improvement or deterioration.

Take time to observe the patient during the interview and ask yourself the following questions. If possible, ask support staff about observed behavior (e.g., does he have any abnormal movements or mannerisms; how does he interact with other patients; does he appear to be responding to unseen voices or commands?).

What is the patient's appearance? Describe the patient's physical appearance and racial origin. Compare what age they appear with their actual age (i.e., biological v. chronological age). What is their manner of dress and hygiene? Patients with manic illnesses may dress in an excessively formal, flamboyant, or sexually inappropriate manner. Patients with cognitive impairment may have mismatched or wrongly buttoned clothing.

What is the patient's behavior during the interview? Are there episodes of tearfulness? Do they attend to the interview or do they appear distracted? Do they maintain an appropriate level of eye contact? Do you feel that you have established rapport? Do they look hypervigilant (suggestive of paranoia)? Are they guarded (apprehensive or distrusting)?

What is the patient's level of activity during the interview? Does the patient appear restless or fidgety? Do they settle to a chair or pace during the interview? Is there a normal level of gesticulation during conversation?

Is there any evidence of self-neglect? Does the patient have lower than normal standards of self-care and personal hygiene? Are they malodorous, unshaven, or dishevelled? Are their clothes clean? Are there cigarette burns or food stains on their clothes?

Is the patient's behavior socially inappropriate? Is there embarrassing, overly familiar, or sexually forward behavior? All can be seen in the manic state or with cognitive impairment.

Is the patient's behavior threatening, aggressive, or violent? In manner or in speech does the patient appear hostile or threatening? Do you feel at risk? Is there aggressive or violent behavior on display during the interview? What prompts it?

Are there any abnormal movements? Does the patient have repetitive or rocking movements or bizarre posturing (stereotypies)? Do they perform voluntary, goal-directed activities in a bizarre way (mannerisms)? What is their explanation for this? For patients on antipsychotic medication, is there evidence of side-effects (e.g., stiffness, rigidity, tremor, akathisia)?

Is the patient distractible or do they appear to be responding to hallucinations? Does the patient appear to be attending to a voice other than yours? Are they looking around the room as if for the source of a voice? Are they mumbling, murmuring or mouthing soundlessly to themselves? Are there episodes of giggling, verbal outbursts, or other unexplained actions? Are the patients taking unnecessary interest in their surroundings? Are the patients picking up cues from the environment while they talk?

Speech

The content of the patient's speech (i.e., what they say) will be our major source of information for their history and mental status. The form of their speech (i.e., how they say it) can be abnormal in a number of mental disorders and should be observed and commented upon. See also Disorders of the form of thought, 📖 p. 76.

Is there any speech at all? A small number of patients are mute during interview. Here the doctor should aim to comment on; apparent level of comprehension. Does the patient appear to understand what is said? e.g., shakes or nods head appropriately; level of alternate communication. Can they write answers down, do they point or use gestures? and; level of structural impairment of the organs of speech. A patient who can cough on demand is demonstrably able to oppose both vocal cords normally.

What is the latency? This is the time taken by the patient to reply to your question. It is also called the reaction time. Does the patient tend to respond even before you complete the question? Alternatively, does the patient take more than usual time to respond?

What is the quantity of speech? Are answers unduly brief or monosyllabic? Conversely, are they inappropriately prolonged? Does the speech appear pressured? (e.g., there is copious, rapid speech, which is hard to interrupt?)

What is the rate of speech? There is a wide variation in normal rates of speech across the country. Rate of speech may vary with the age of the patient too. Is the patient's speech unusually slow or unusually rapid, given the expected rate? This may reflect acceleration or deceleration in the speed of thought in affective illnesses. How easy is it to interrupt the patient while he/she is talking? This reflects the pressure of speech.

What is the volume and quality of speech? Does the patient whisper? Or speak inappropriately loudly? Is there stuttering or slurring or speech?

What is the tone and rhythm of speech? Even in a non-tonal language like English, normal speech has a musical quality with the intonation of the voice and rhythm of the sentences conveying meaning (e.g., the rise in tone at the end of a question). Loss of this range of intonation and rhythmic pattern is seen in chronic psychotic illnesses.

How appropriate and coherent is the speech? Is the content of the speech appropriate to the situation? Does the patient answer questions appropriately? Are there inappropriate or pointless digressions? Can the meaning of the speech always be followed?

Is there abnormal use of language? Are there word-finding difficulties, which may suggest an expressive dysphasia? Are there neologisms (i.e., made up words), or metanyms (i.e., normal words used in an idiosyncratic manner)?

Abnormal mood

In describing disorders of mood, we draw a distinction between affect (the emotional state prevailing at a given moment) and mood (the emotional state over a longer period). To use a meteorological analogy, affect represents the weather, where mood is the climate. Consequently, mood requires a longitudinal history and may require collateral information. Assessment of pathological abnormality of affect involves assessing the severity, longevity, and ubiquity of the mood disturbance and its association with other pathological features suggestive of mood disorder.

The two central clinical features of depressive illness are (1) pervasively depressed and unreactive mood and (2) anhedonia—the loss of pleasure in previously pleasurable activities. The clinical symptoms of depression can be grouped into four categories, namely hedonic symptoms, vegetative symptoms, cognitive symptoms (often called together as neurovegetative symptoms), and cognitive distortions. In more severe cases, mood-congruent psychotic features may be observed. In addition to feeling depressed, many patients experience anxiety either associated with depression or as a prominent symptom. Depressed mood is the most common symptom of the mood disorders and in its milder forms has been experienced by most people at some point. Its experience is personal and is described in a variety of ways by different people: sometimes as a profound lowering of spirits, qualitatively different from normal unhappiness; sometimes as an unpleasant absence of emotions or emotional range; and sometimes as a more physical symptom of "weight" or "blackness" weighing down on the head or chest. Increasingly, severe forms of depressed mood are indicated by the patient's rating of greater severity as compared with previous experience, increased pervasiveness of the low mood to all situations, and decreased reactivity of mood (i.e., decreased ability of the mood to be lightened by pleasurable or encouraging events). The vegetative (biological) features include disturbance of sleep (particularly early morning waking and often difficulty getting to sleep, properly called "initial insomnia"), reduced appetite, changes in weight, and loss of libido. The cognitive symptoms include poor concentration, memory and retarded thought process as well as motor retardation, poor drive and motivation, and reduced energy levels. In addition, many patients may report cognitive distortions such as helplessness, hopelessness, unrealistic guilt and worthlessness. Eliciting these symptoms may have practical significance in predicting risk and in planning for psychotherapy. For example, hopelessness may predict risk for self-harm and cognitive behavior therapy may be offered if the cognitive distortions are prominent. Many depressed patients will have thoughts of deliberate self-harm or ending their lives as a way of ending their suffering. With increasingly severe depressed mood there are increasingly frequent and formed plans of suicide. The development of a sense of hopelessness towards the future is a worrying sign.

Mania and depression are often thought of as two extremes of illness with normality or euthymia in the middle. Morbid change in mood (either elevation or depression) can more accurately be considered as being on one side of a coin with normality on the other. Some patients display both manic and depressive features in a single episode—a "mixed affective state". Manic and depressive illnesses have, in common, increased lability (i.e., susceptibility to change) of mood, increased irritability, decreased sleep, and an increase in subjective anxiety.

The core clinical features of a manic episode are sustained and inappropriate elevation in mood (often described as feeling "on top of the world") and a distorted or inflated estimate of one's importance and abilities. The clinical picture also includes increased lability of mood, increased irritability, increased activity levels, disturbed sleep pattern with a sense of diminished need for sleep, and subjectively improved memory and concentration despite objective deterioration in these skills. With increasingly severe episodes of manic illness there is loss of judgment, an increase in inappropriate and risky behavior, and possibly the development of mood-congruent delusions.

Asking about depressed mood

Although these questions are designed to elicit the features of syndromal depression, it is important to look for the co-morbid conditions associated with depressed mood. This process keeps the interviewing broad-based and avoids premature conclusions about the nature of depression.

"How has your mood been lately?" Patients vary in their ability to introspect and assess their mood. Beginning with general questioning allows a more unbiased account of mood problems. Report any description of depression in the patient's own words. Ask the patient to assess the depth of depression (e.g., "on a scale of one to ten, where ten is normal and one is as depressed as you have ever felt, how would you rate your mood now?"). How long has the mood been as low as this? Inquire about any notable discrepancy between the patient's report of mood and objective signs of mood disturbance.

"Does you mood vary over the course of a day?" Clarify if the mood varies as the day goes on. If mood improves in the evening, does it return completely to normal? Does anything else change as the day goes on to account for the mood change (e.g., more company available in the evenings)?

"Can you still enjoy the things you used to enjoy?" By this point of the interview you should have some idea about the activities the patient formerly enjoyed. Depressed patients describe lack of interest in their previous pursuits, decreased participation in activities, and a sense of any participation being more of an effort.

"How are you sleeping?" Many patients will simply describe their sleep as "terrible". They should be asked further about time to bed, time falling asleep, wakefulness throughout the night, time of waking in the morning, quality of sleep (is it refreshing or not?), and any daytime napping. Any sleep-related phenomena, such as nightmares, sleep apnea?

"What is your appetite like at the moment?" Patients reporting a change in their appetite should be asked about reasons for this (loss of interest in food, loss of motivation to prepare food, or swallowing difficulties?) Has there been recent weight change (either loss or gain)? Do their clothes still fit? If the weight loss is observed, was the weight loss intentional? What was the reason for losing weight? How did you lose weight? Did you use any weight loss drugs? Was it prescribed or over the counter? Any binging or purging?

"How is your concentration?" Clarify any reported decline by asking about ability to perform standard tasks. Can they read a newspaper or watch a TV show? Ask about work performance.

"What is your memory like at the moment?" Again, clarify any reported decline. Clarify the nature of memory impairment; is there a problem in remembering recent events or recently learned information? Do they "misplace" their belongings? Do they remember when they are offered a clue?

"How is the sexual side of your relationship?" Potentially embarrassing topics are best approached in a professional and matter-of-fact way. It is important to inquire about this directly as the symptom of loss of libido can cause considerable suffering for both patient and partner and is less likely than other symptoms to be mentioned spontaneously. In addition to loss of libido, inquire regarding erectile dysfunction, premature ejaculation, vaginal discomfort or pain, or any anxieties related to sexual functioning. During treatment this symptom should again be explored as many psychotropic drugs negatively affect sexual performance.

"Tell me about any worries on your mind at the moment?" Characteristic of depressive illness is a tendency to preferentially dwell on negative issues.

"Tell me about any guilty feelings you may be experiencing at the moment" Patients with depressive illnesses often report feelings of guilt or remorse about current or historical events. In severe illnesses these feelings can become delusional. Aim to assess the presence and nature of guilty thoughts.

Asking about thoughts of self-harm

Completed suicide, unfortunately, may be an outcome in many psychiatric conditions. Thoughts of deliberate self-harm occur commonly and should always be inquired about. The majority of patients with illness of any severity will have had thoughts of deliberate self-harm at some stage. It should be emphasized that asking about deliberate self-harm does not "put the idea in their head", and indeed many patients will welcome the opportunity to discuss such worrying thoughts.

The assessment is not only of the presence of suicidal thoughts, but their severity and frequency and the likelihood of them being followed by suicidal action. One suggested method involves asking about behaviors and thoughts associated with increasing suicide risk. This tactful inquiry can be made in addition to an estimate of risk. The aim is not to trap the patient into an unwanted disclosure but to assess the severity of suicidal intent and hence the attendant risk of completed suicide.

"How do you feel about the future?" Many patients will remain optimistic of improvement despite current severe symptoms. A description of hopelessness towards the future and a feeling that things will never improve is worrying.

"Have you ever thought that life was not worth living?" A consequence of hopelessness may be the feeling that anything, even nothingness, would be better. They may feel their family would be better off without them.

"Have you ever wished you could go to bed and not wake up in the morning?" Passive thoughts of death (sometimes called "passive death wish" or "PDW") are common in mental illness and can also be found in normal elderly people towards the end of life, particularly after the deaths of spouses and peers.

"Have you had thoughts of ending your life?" If yes, inquire about the frequency and intensity of these thoughts—are they fleeting and rapidly dismissed; or more prolonged? Are they becoming more common?

"Have you thought about how you would do it?" Inquire about methods of suicide the patient has considered. Particularly worrying are violent methods that are likely to be successful (e.g., shooting, hanging, or jumping from a height).

"Have you made any preparations?" Aim to establish how far the patient's plans have progressed from ideas to action—have they considered a place, bought pills, carried out a final act (e.g., suicide note, or begun putting their affairs in order)?. What is the closest you have come to act upon these plans?

"Have you tried to take your own life?" Has there been a recent concealed attempt (e.g., overdose)? If so, consider whether current medical assessment is required.

Self-injurious behaviors Some patients report causing harm to themselves, sometimes repeatedly, without reporting a desire to die (e.g., lacerate their arms, legs, or abdomen; burn themselves with cigarettes). In these cases, inquire about the reasons for this behavior, which may be obscure even to the person concerned. In what circumstances do they harm themselves? What do they feel and think before harming themselves? How do they feel afterwards?

Asking about elevated mood

"How has your mood been lately?" As for inquiries about depressed mood, begin with a very general question. Report the patient's description of their mood in their own words. Clarify what the patient means by general statements such as "sad" or "on top of the world".

"Do you find your mood changes quickly?" Besides general elevation in mood, patients with mania often report lability of mood, with tearfulness and irritability, as well as elation. The pattern and type of mood variation should be noted if present.

"What is your thinking like at the moment?" Patients with mania often report a subjective increase in the speed and ease of thinking, with many ideas occurring to them, each with a wider variety of associated thoughts than normal. This experience, together with the nature of their ideas should be explored and described.

"Do you have any special gifts or talents?" A characteristic feature of frank mania is the belief that they have exceptional abilities of some kind (e.g., as great writers or painters) or that they have some particular insight to offer the world (e.g., the route to achieving world peace). These beliefs may become frankly delusional, with the patient believing they have special or magical powers. The nature of these beliefs and their implications and meaning for the patient should be described.

"How are you sleeping?" Manic patients describe finding sleep unnecessary or a distraction from their current plans. Inquire about the length and quality of sleep.

"What is your appetite like at the moment?" Appetite is variable in manic illnesses. Some patients describe having no time or patience for the preparation of food; others eat excessively and spend excessively on food and drink. Ask about recent weight gain or loss and about a recent typical day's food intake.

"How is your concentration?" Typically, manic patients have impaired concentration and may report this. In this case the complaint should be clarified by examples of impairment. Some manic patients overestimate their concentration, along with other subjective estimates of ability. Report on objective measures of concentration (e.g., attention to interview questioning or ability to retain interest in newspapers or TV, while on the ward).

"How is the sexual side of your relationship?" Again, this topic should be broached directly and straightforwardly. Manic patients sometimes report increased interest in sexual activity. Clarify the patient's estimate of his or her own sexual attractiveness and recent increase in sexual activity or promiscuity.

Anxiety symptoms

Anxiety symptoms are the most common type of symptoms seen in patients with psychiatric disorders. They are the core clinical features of the anxiety disorders in DSM-IV-TR and neurotic disorders in ICD-10. They are also prominent clinical features in psychotic illnesses, affective illness, organic disorders, and in drug and alcohol use and withdrawal.

Anxiety has two components: **psychic anxiety**—an unpleasant affect in which there is subjective tension, increased arousal, and fearful apprehension; and **somatic anxiety**—bodily sensations of palpitations, sweating, dyspnea, pallor, and abdominal discomfort. The sensations of anxiety are related to autonomic arousal and cognitive appraisal of threat which were adaptive primitive survival reactions.

Anxiety symptoms are part of normal healthy experience, particularly before novel, stressful, or potentially dangerous situations. Moderate amounts of anxiety can optimize performance (the so-called Yerkes-Dobson curve—plotting performance level against anxiety shows an inverse-U shape). They become pathological when they are abnormally severe, abnormally prolonged, or if they are present at a level out of keeping with the real threat of the situation.

Anxiety symptoms may be present at a more or less constant level as seen in **generalized anxiety**; or may occur only episodically as seen with **panic attacks**. Anxiety symptoms may or may not have an identifiable stimulus. Where a stimulus can be identified it may be very specific, as in a simple phobia (e.g., fear of cats or spiders); or may be more generalized, as in social phobia and agoraphobia. In phobias of all kinds there is avoidance of the feared situation. Because this avoidance is followed by a reduction in unpleasant symptoms it is reinforced and is liable to be repeated. Breaking this cycle is the basis of desensitization methods for treating phobias (📖 p. 1015).

The repetition of behaviors in order to achieve reduction in the experience of anxiety is also seen in the symptoms of **obsessions** and **compulsions**. Here, the patient regards the thoughts (obsessions) and/or actions (compulsions) as purposeless, but is unable to resist thinking about them or carrying them out. Resistance to their performance produces rising anxiety levels, which are diminished by repeating the resisted behavior.

Asking about anxiety symptoms

In inquiring about anxiety symptoms, aside from the nature, severity, and precipitants of the symptoms, it is important to establish, in all cases, the impact they are having on the person's life. Record what particular activities or situations are avoided because of their symptoms and, in the case of obsessional symptoms, note how much time the patient spends on them.

"Would you say you were an anxious person/a worrier?" There is a wide variation in the normal level of arousal and anxiety. Some people are inveterate "worriers", while others appear relaxed at all times. It can be challenging to convey the right meaning of the term "anxiety" to some patients. It would be useful to describe what you mean by anxiety. It is not uncommon for many patients to interpret the term as meaning panic attack, stress, paranoia, etc.

"Recently, have you been feeling particularly anxious/worried or on edge?" Ask the patient to describe when the symptoms began. Was there any particular precipitating event or trauma?

"What makes you anxious/worry?" It is useful to ask open ended questions such as this one and then seek answers for relatively more specific questions such as the one given below. Patients may be anxious for more than one thing. Always make it a point to elicit various situations that makes a patient anxious. This could provide valuable clues to simple phobia, agoraphobia, social phobia, PTSD, etc.

"Do any particular situations make you more anxious than others?" Inquire whether the patient feels anxious in anticipation of exposure to a situation. If the anticipatory anxiety is severe enough, they may totally avoid such situations and the reply to the question may be in the negative. Many patients may say "no" for fear of embarrassment. Reassure the patient regarding the non-judgmental nature of the interview. Establish whether the symptoms are constant or fluctuating. If the latter, inquire about those situations that cause worsening or improvement.

"Have you ever had a panic attack?" Ask the patient to describe to you what they mean by this. A classic panic attack is described as sudden in onset with gradual resolution over 30–60 minutes. There are physical symptoms of dyspnea, tachycardia, sweating, chest tightness/chest pain, and paresthesia (related to over-breathing); coupled with psychological symptoms of subjective tension and apprehension that "something terrible is going to happen" (p. 400).

"Do any thoughts or worries keep coming back to your mind, even though you try to push them away?"

"Do you ever find yourself spending a lot of time doing the same thing over and over—like checking things, or cleaning—even though you've already done it well enough?" Besides identifying the type of repetitive thought or action involved it is important to establish that the thoughts or impulses are recognized as the person's own (in contrast with thought insertion in psychotic illness) and that they are associated with resistance (although active resistance may diminish in chronic OCD). Patients with obsessional thoughts often worry that they are "losing their mind" or that they will act on a particular thought (e.g., a mother with an obsessional image of smothering her baby). Where the symptom is definitively that of an obsession, the patient can be reassured that they are not likely to carry it out.

Abnormal perceptions

Abnormal perceptual experiences form part of the clinical picture of many mental disorders. Equally, the range of normal perceptual experience is very wide. Patients vary in their ability to explain their subjective perceptual experiences.

The brain constantly receives large amounts of perceptual information via the five special senses of vision, hearing, touch, taste, and smell; the muscle, joint, and internal organ proprioceptors; and the vestibular apparatus. The majority of this information is processed unconsciously and only a minority reaches conscious awareness at any one time. An external object is represented internally by a sensory percept that combines with memory and experience to produce a meaningful internal percept in the conscious mind. In health, we can clearly distinguish between percepts which represent real objects and those which are the result of internal imagery or fantasy, which may be vividly experienced in the mind but are recognized as not real.

Abnormal perceptual experiences may be divided into two types:

- **Altered perceptions**—including sensory distortions and illusions—in which there is a distorted internal perception of a real external object.
- **False perceptions**—including hallucinations and pseudo-hallucinations—in which there is an internal perception without an external object.

Sensory distortions are changes in the perceived intensity or quality of a real external stimulus. They are associated with organic conditions and with drug ingestion or withdrawal. **Hyperacusis** (experiencing sounds as abnormally loud) and **micropsia** (perceiving objects as smaller and further away, as if looking through the wrong end of a telescope) are examples of sensory distortions.

Illusions are altered perceptions in which a real external object is combined with imagery to produce a false internal percept. Both lowered attention and heightened affect will predispose to experiencing illusions.

Affect illusions occur at times of heightened emotion (e.g., while walking through a dangerous area late at night, a person may see a tree blowing in the wind as an attacker lunging at them).

Completion illusions rely on our brain's tendency to "fill-in" presumed missing parts of an object to produce a meaningful percept and are the basis for many types of optical illusion. Both these types of illusions resolve on closer attention.

Pareidolic illusions are meaningful precepts produced when experiencing a poorly defined stimulus (e.g., seeing faces in a fire or in clouds).

Hallucinations A hallucination is defined as "a percept without an object" (Esquirol, 1838). As symptoms of major mental disorder, hallucinations are the most significant type of abnormal perception. It is important to appreciate that the subjective experience of hallucination is that of experiencing a normal percept in that modality of sensation. A true *hallucination* will be perceived as being in external space. It occurs in clear consciousness, appears clearly and vividly, outside conscious control, and patients usually lack insight. A *pseudo-hallucination* will lack one or all of these characteristics and be subjectively experienced as internal or "in my head". Hallucinating patients may accept that their experiences are not shared by others around them in the same way as a normal sensory experience.

Auditory hallucinations are most frequently seen in psychosis. Three experiences of auditory hallucinations are classically defined as Schniderian first-rank symptoms in schizophrenia (see Chapter 6 📖 *p. 207*). These are:

- Hearing a voice speak one's thoughts aloud (sometimes called thought echo).
- Hearing a voice narrating one's actions (often called a running commentary).
- Hearing two or more voices arguing.

Visual hallucinations are more frequently associated with medically related disorders of the brain or with drug and alcohol intoxication and withdrawal. They are very rarely seen in psychotic illness alone but are reported in association with dementias, cortical tumors, stimulant and hallucinogen ingestion, and, most commonly, in delirium tremens. The visual hallucinations seen in delirium tremens are characteristically "Lilliputian hallucinations" of miniature animals or people and sometimes insects.

Olfactory and gustatory hallucinations may be difficult to distinguish and occur in a wide range of mental disorders. Olfactory hallucinations are seen in epileptic auras, in depressive illnesses (where the smell is described as unpleasant or repulsive to others), and in schizophrenia. They may also occur in association with a persistent delusion of malodorousness. They may point to a non-psychiatric etiology, and should be carefully investigated.

Hypnagogic/hypnopompic hallucinations are transient false perceptions which occur while falling asleep (**hypnagogic**) or while waking (**hypnopompic**). They may have the characteristics of true or pseudo-hallucinations and are most commonly visual or auditory. While they are sometimes seen in narcolepsy and affective illnesses they are not indicative of ill health and are frequently reported by healthy people.

Elemental hallucinations are the hallucinatory experience of simple sensory elements, such as flashes of light or unstructured noises.

Extracampine hallucinations are those false perceptions where the hallucination is of an external object beyond the normal range of perception of the sensory organs (e.g., a patient living in Pittsburgh who says the can hear someone in New York, talking about them).

Functional hallucinations are hallucinations of any modality that are experienced simultaneously with a normal stimulus in that modality (e.g., a patient who only experiences auditory hallucinations when he hears the sound of the ward's air conditioning).

Reflex hallucinations are hallucinations in one modality of sensation experienced after experiencing a normal stimulus in another modality of sensation.

Asking about abnormal perceptions

Asking patients about their experience of abnormal perceptions and abnormal beliefs (e.g., hallucinations and delusions) presents a number of problems for the interviewer. Unlike symptoms such as anxiety, these symptoms are not part of normal experience, and so the interviewer may not have the same degree of empathic understanding. Patients will often fear the reaction of others to the revelation of psychotic symptoms (fear of being thought "crazy") and so hide them. When such symptoms are not present, patients may resent such questioning or regard it as strange or insulting.

As with most potentially embarrassing topics, the best approach is frankness, lack of embarrassment, and straightforwardness. If the interview, thus far, has not led to report of psychotic symptoms, the examiner should begin by saying something like:

"Now I want to ask you about some experiences which sometimes people have, but find difficult to talk about. These are questions I ask everyone." This makes clear that these questions are not as a result of suspicion in the examiner's mind or an indicator of how seriously he regards the patient's problems.

"Have you ever had the sensation that you were unreal—or that the world had become unreal?" The symptoms of depersonalization and derealization are non-specific symptoms in a variety of affective and psychotic conditions. Many patients find them difficult or impossible to explain clearly, commonly describing the experience as "like being in a play". Patients often worry about these experiences fearing they presage "going mad". They may therefore be reluctant to mention them spontaneously. It is important to differentiate this from epileptic aura. Therefore, past history of epileptic seizures, altered sensorium, automatisms, etc. should help in teasing apart the diagnostic dilemma. Sometimes, these symptoms may be the only distressing feature in the absence of other psychiatric diseases as is seen in depersonalization/derealization disorder.

"Have you ever had the experience of hearing noises or voices when there was nothing around to explain it?" If the patient agrees, then this experience should be further clarified: When did this occur? Was the patient fully awake? How often? Where did the sound appear to come from? If a voice was heard, what did it say? Did the patient recognize the voice? Was there more than one? How did the voice refer to the patient (e.g., as "you" or "him")? This is important because the former refers to second person auditory hallucinations and sometimes this can take the form of commanding or imperative auditory hallucination. In such cases, it is important to know the command and check how hard it is to resist these commands. The latter form refers to the third person auditory hallucination and could suggest strongly to the diagnosis of schizophrenia. Can the patient give examples of the sort of things the voice said?

"Do you ever see things that others don't seem to be able to see?" Again, clarify when and how often the experience occurred. What were the circumstances? Was the vision seen with the "mind's eye" or perceived as being in external space? Was it distinct from the surroundings or seen as part of the wallpaper or curtain pattern?

"Do you ever notice smells or tastes that other people aren't bothered by?" Again, clarify the details surrounding any positive response. Aim to distinguish olfactory hallucinations (where there is the experience of an abnormal odor) from a patient who has a delusion that he is malodorous. Olfactory and gustatory hallucinations can be part of epileptic aura. Other symptoms associated with these types of hallucinations need to be carefully explored. For example, the presence of loss of touch with the surroundings, automatisms, partial or full amnesia to the episode, headache, or exhaustion with or without full-blown generalized convulsions suggest complex partial seizures.

Abnormal beliefs

Examination of the patient's ideas and beliefs will form an important part of the MSE. Abnormal or false beliefs include primary and secondary delusions and over-valued ideas. More so than other symptoms of mental ill health, a patient with delusions fits the common preconceptions of "being crazy". Delusions are important symptoms in the diagnosis of the major psychoses.

Delusions

A delusion is a pathological belief which has the following characteristics:
- It is held with absolute subjective certainty and cannot be rationalized away.
- It requires no external proof and may be held in the face of contradictory evidence.
- It has personal significance and importance to the individual concerned.
- It is not a belief which can be easily understood as part of the subject's cultural or religious background.

Note: Although the content of the delusion is usually demonstrably false and bizarre in nature, this is not invariably so.

A **secondary delusion** is one whose development can be understood in the light of another abnormality in mental status or pre-existing psychopathology (e.g., the development of delusions of poverty in a severely depressed patient). A **primary delusion** cannot be understood in this way and must be presumed as arising directly from the primary pathological process. In other words, primary delusions arise de novo in the absence of pre-existing psychopathology. Delusions can be categorized by their content or by the manner in which they are perceived as having arisen (📖 p. 74).

Overvalued ideas

An overvalued idea is a nondelusional, nonobsessional abnormal belief that is held with a strong emotional valence. Here, the patient has a belief which is in itself acceptable and comprehensible but which is preoccupying and comes to dominate their thinking and behavior. The idea is not perceived as "external" or "senseless", but will, generally, have great significance to the patient. Over-valued ideas may have a variety of contents in different disorders (e.g., concern over physical appearance in dysmorphophobia; concern over weight and body shape in anorexia nervosa; concern over personal rights in paranoid personality disorder).

Asking about abnormal beliefs

Both at the initial interview and during subsequent treatment, professional staff dealing with a deluded patient should avoid colluding in the delusional belief system. The doctor should not be drawn into arguments about the truth of the delusion—by their nature delusions cannot be argued or rationalized away and arguments of this type will damage rapport. Nonetheless, the doctor should always make clear to the patient that he or she regards the delusional symptom as a symptom of mental ill health, albeit one which is very real and important to the patient concerned.

Delusional ideas vary in their degree of detail and in their intensity over the course of an illness episode. In evolving psychotic illness there will often be a perplexing sense of "something not being right" and ill-formed symptoms such as a vague sense that they are being spied upon or persecuted in some way. As the delusion becomes more fully formed it comes to dominate the person's thinking and becomes more **elaborated**—more detailed and with more "evidence" produced to support the belief. With treatment, the delusion will hopefully fade in importance and the person may come to appreciate the belief as false or, despite holding to its initial truth, will regard it as no longer important.

"Do you have any particular worries in your mind at the moment?" Beginning with a very general question like this offers the patient an opportunity to broach a topic which may have been concerning them but which they have been putting off mentioning.

"Do you ever feel that people are watching you or paying attention to what you are doing?" Ask the patient to describe this sensation and an episode of its occurrence. Distinguish normal self-consciousness or a patient's awareness of genuinely notable abnormality from referential delusions. A delusion will generally have further elaboration of the belief—there will be some "reason" why the reported events are happening. Elaboration may take the form of other beliefs about cameras, bugs, etc. It is critical to distinguish between referential or paranoid delusions from social phobia. An important distinguishing feature is the presence of fear of negative judgment by others, avoidance of social situation and feeling anxious in social phobia. It is also important to know the past legal/forensic history of the patient. Some patients who were involved in criminal activities in the past may be in a situation where they are being truly pursued by law enforcement authorities. Such a history does not rule out the presence of delusions but requires careful elicitation of morbidity of the feelings, temporal nature of such associations and stage of legal process in which they find themselves.

"When you watch the television, listen to a radio, or read the news, do you ever feel that the stories refer to you directly, or to things that you have been doing?" Invite the patient to elaborate further on a positive response. Again, probe for further elaboration of the belief and seek examples of when it has occurred.

"Do you ever feel that people are trying to harm you in any way?" Persecutory delusions are among the most common features of psychotic illness. There is potential for diagnostic confusion with paranoid personality traits, with suspicion and resentfulness towards medical and nursing staff and with genuine fears, understandable in the context of the patient's lifestyle (e.g., of retribution from drug dealers or money lenders). Explore the nature and basis of the beliefs and the supporting evidence that the patient provides.

"Do you feel that you are to blame for anything, that you are responsible for anything going wrong?" Delusions of guilt are seen in psychotic depression, in addition to the psychotic disorders. The affected individual may believe that they are responsible for a crime, occasionally one which has been prominently reported. On occasion these individuals may "turn themselves in" to the police rather than seeking medical help.

"Do you worry that there is anything wrong with your body or that you have a serious illness?" Hypochondriacal delusions show diagnostic overlap with normal health concerns, hypochondriacal overvalued ideas, and somatization disorder. Clarify this symptom by examining the patient's evidence for this belief and the firmness with which it is held.

Asking about the first-rank symptoms of schizophrenia

The first-rank symptoms are a group of symptoms which have special significance in the diagnosis of schizophrenia. There is no symptom that is pathognomonic of schizophrenia. The first-rank symptoms are useful because they occur reasonably often in schizophrenia and more rarely in other disorders and it is not too difficult to tell whether they are present or not. They can all be reported in other conditions (delirium, mood disorders). They do not give a guide to severity or prognosis of illness (e.g., a patient with many first-rank symptoms is not "worse" than one with few) and they may not occur at all in a patient who undoubtedly has schizophrenia. There are 11 first-rank symptoms, organized into four categories according to type.

Auditory hallucinations
- Voices discussing ("Voices heard arguing").
- Thought echo.
- Voices commenting ("Running commentary").

Delusions of thought interference
- Thought insertion.
- Thought withdrawal.
- Thought broadcasting.

Delusions of control
- Made affect (Passivity of affect).
- Made impulse (Passivity of impulse).
- Made act (Passivity of volitions).
- Somatic passivity.

Delusional perception
- A primary delusion of any content that is reported by the patient as having arisen following the experience of a normal perception.

"Do you ever hear voices commenting on what you are doing? Or discussing you between themselves? Or repeating your own thoughts back to you?" Start by asking how many voices they are hearing, do they talk directly to the patient or do they talk amongst themselves. For this symptom to be considered first-rank, the experience must be that of a true auditory hallucination where the hallucinatory voice refers to the patient in the third person (e.g., as "him" or "her" rather than "you"). Distinguish these experiences from internal monologues. Sometimes patients experience voices talking directly to them in second person (addressing the patient as "you") and at other times in third person. In such situations, ask the patient which one of them is more frequent and which one of them is more distressing. This can be of diagnostic importance because voices discussing and voices commenting alone is sufficient to meet criterion A of DSM-IV-TR schizophrenia or schizoaffective disorder.

"Do you ever get the feeling that someone is interfering with your thoughts?"—It may be that the patient does not understand this first open question, and you may have to supplement with: **"Do you feel that someone is putting thoughts into your head or taking them away? Or that your thoughts can be transmitted to others in some way?."** If the patient answers, "yes," they should be asked to elaborate (i.e., "tell me more about that?") It is the experience itself that renders this symptom first-rank. The patient may describe additional delusional elaboration (e.g., involving implanted transmitters or radio waves). The important point to clarify with the patient is that the experience is really that of thoughts being affected by an external agency and that it is not simple distraction or absentmindedness. For thought broadcasting, ensure that the patient is not simply referring to the fact that they are "easily read" or that they give away their emotions or thoughts by their actions. It is helpful to ask the patient to give examples of such experiences. Probe further to know how patients distinguish between their own thoughts as opposed to other peoples' thoughts that are inserted. In case of thought broadcasting, ask the patients as to what they do in order to stop their thoughts from being broadcast. If the symptom is distressing, patients may attempt to resolve the problem (e.g., calling the broadcasting networks to stop sending transmissions to them)

"Do you ever get the feeling that you are being controlled? That your thoughts or moods or actions are being forced on you by someone else?" Again, there may be delusional elaboration of this symptom but it is the experience itself, of an external controller affecting things which are normally experienced as totally under one's own control which makes this symptom first-rank. Clarify that the actions are truly perceived as controlled by an outside agency, rather than, for example, being directed by auditory hallucinations.

Delusional perception

This is an intriguing psychotic symptom. The important aspect of this symptom is that there is a normal perception followed by delusional explanation in the absence of pre-existing psychopathology. A psychotic symptom that is similar to this symptom is called delusional misinterpretation where a normal perception is interpreted based on pre-existing psychopathology. For example, a patient with a delusion that he is being tracked by the law enforcement officials or mafia could interpret the cars that pull over near their house to be those that belong to either the police or the mafia.

Disorders of the form of thought

In describing psychopathology, we draw a distinction between the content and the form of thought. Content describes the meaning and experience of belief, perception, and memory as described by the patients, while **form** describes the structure and process of thought. In addition to abnormalities of perception and belief, mental disorders can produce abnormality in the normal form of thought processes. This abnormality may be suggested by abnormalities in the form of speech, the only objective representation of the thoughts, or may be revealed by empathic questioning designed to elicit the patient's subjective experiences. Sometimes, when patients mutter to themselves, listen closely to see if it is comprehensible or not. If not easily comprehensible, this is usually indicative of a disorder of the form of thought.

Among the psychiatric symptoms which are outside normal experience, thought disorder is challenging to understand and perhaps the most difficult for the clinician to empathize. It may be helpful to consider a model of normal thought processes and use this to simplify discussions of abnormalities. In this model we visualize each thought, giving rise to a constellation of associations (i.e., a series of related thoughts). One of these is pursued, which in turn gives rise to a further constellation and so on. This sequence may proceed towards a specific goal driven by a *determining* tendency (colloquially the "train of thought") or may be undirected as in daydreaming ("letting one's mind wander"). Disturbances in the form of thought may affect the rate or the internal associations of thought as follows.

Accelerated tempo of thought is called **flight of ideas**. It may be reflected in the speech as **pressure of speech** or may be described by the patient. The sensation is of the thoughts proceeding more rapidly than can be articulated and of each thought giving rise to more associations than can be followed up. Flight of ideas may be a feature of a manic episode. In the majority of cases of fight of ideas, some form of association of each thought can be discerned. For example, it could be a superficial *clang association*, alliteration and punning that proceeds like the game of dominoes where the last move determines the next move. In milder forms, called *prolixity*, the rate is slow and eventually reaches the goal if allowed adequate time.

Decelerated tempo of thought, or psychic retardation, occurs in depressive illnesses. Here the subjective speed of thought and the range of associations are decreased. There may be decreased rate of speech and absence of spontaneous speech. In addition, the remaining thoughts sometimes involve gloomy themes. In both accelerated and decelerated thought there may be an increased likelihood for the determining tendency of thought to be lost (referred to as *increased distractibility*).

Disturbances of the associations between the thoughts are closely associated with schizophrenia and may be referred to as *schizophrenic* thought disorder. Four disturbances are classically described: snapping-off (entgleiten), fusion (verschmelzung), muddling (faseln), and derailment (entgleisen). In mild forms the determining tendency in the thoughts can be followed (increased follow-up of side associations is referred to as *circumstantiality*).

- **Thought blocking** or Snapping-off describes the subjective experience of the sudden and unintentional stop in a chain of thought. This may be unexplained by the patient or there may be delusional elaboration (e.g., explained as thought *withdrawal*).
- **Derailment** or *knight's move thinking* describes a total break in the chain of association between the meanings of thoughts.
- **Fusion** is when two or more related ideas from a group of associations come together to form one idea.

Assessing symptoms of thought disorder

Patients will rarely directly complain of the symptoms of thought disorder. In assessing the first-rank symptoms of schizophrenia the clinician will have inquired about delusions of thought control and about the passivity delusions. Both these symptom areas require the patient to introspect their thought processes; however, they will more rarely be aware of disorders which affect the form as opposed to the content of their thoughts. They can be asked directly about the symptoms of acceleration and deceleration of thought and these symptoms may be directly observable in acceleration or deceleration of speech. Observation and recording of examples of abnormal speech is the method by which formal thought disorder is assessed. Record examples of the patient's speech as verbatim quotes, particularly sentences where the meaning or the connection between ideas is not clear to you during the interview. Following recovery, patients can sometimes explain the underlying meaning behind examples of schizophrenic speech.

Abnormal cognitive function

All mental disorders affect cognition as expressed in affect, beliefs, and perceptions. The organic mental illnesses directly affect the higher cognitive functions of conscious level, clarity of thought, memory, and intelligence.

Level of consciousness This can range from full alertness to clouding of consciousness, stupor, and coma (**pathological unconsciousness**); or from full alertness to drowsiness, shallow sleep, and deep sleep (**physiological unconsciousness**).

Confusion Milder forms of brain insult are characterized by a combination of disorientation, misinterpretation of sensory input, impairment in memory, and loss of the normal clarity of thought—together referred to as confusion. It is the main clinical feature of delirium (📖 p. 978) and is also present during intoxication with psychotropic substances and occasionally as part of the clinical picture of acute psychotic illnesses.

- **Disorientation** An unimpaired individual is aware of who he is and has a constantly updated record of where he is and what time it is. With increasing impairment there is disorientation to time, then place, and lastly, with more severe confusion, disorientation to person.
- **Misinterpretation** With confusion there is impairment of the normal ability to perceive and attach meaning to sensory stimuli. In frank delirium there may be hallucinations, particularly visual, and secondary delusions, particularly of a persecutory nature.
- **Memory impairment** With confusion, there is impairment in both the registration of new memories and recall of established memories. Events occurring during the period of confusion may be unable to be recalled, or may be recalled in a distorted fashion, indicating a failure of registration.
- **Impaired clarity of thought** The layman's "confusion". A variable degree of impairment in the normal process of thought with disturbed linkages between meaning, subjective and objective slowing of thought, impaired comprehension, and bizarre content.

Memory Beyond the ephemeral contents of our minds, containing our current thoughts and current sensorium, our memory contains all records of our experience and personality.

- **Working memory** A very short-term, limited group of registers for information at the "front of the mind". Used for such purposes as holding a telephone number while dialing it. Most people have between 5 and 9 "spaces" or "chunks" available, with an average of 7 (the "magic number"). New information will enter at the expense of the old.
- **Short-term memory** Used to hold recent memories and experiences. Some short-term memory material may be transferred to long-term memory—a process taking time.
- **Long-term memory** Store for permanent memories with apparently unlimited capacity. There appear to be separate storage areas for information (**episodic memory**), learned skill (**procedural memory**), and emotional associations with people, places, or events (**emotional memory**), which can be differentially affected by a disease process.

Intelligence A person's intelligence refers to their ability to reason, solve problems, apply previous knowledge to new situations, learn new skills, think in an abstract way, and formulate solutions to problems by internal planning. It is stable through adult life, unless affected by a disease process. Intelligence is measured by the intelligence quotient (IQ), a unitary measure with a population mean of 100 and a normal distribution. There is a "hump" on the left-hand side of the population curve for IQ representing those individuals with congenital or acquired lowered IQ. No pathological process produces heightened IQ.

Acute v. chronic brain "failure" Despite its great complexity the brain tends to respond to insults, whatever their source, in a variety of stereotyped ways (e.g., delirium, seizure, coma, dementia). These present as clinically similar or identical whatever the underlying cause. Acute brain failure (delirium) and chronic brain failure (dementia) are two characteristic and stereotyped responses of the brain to injury. In common with other organ failure syndromes there is an "acute on chronic" effect, where patients with established chronic impairment are susceptible to developing acute impairment following an insult which would not cause impairment in a normal brain (e.g., the development of florid delirium in a woman with mild dementia who develops an infection).

Assessing cognitive function

Assessing level of consciousness The **Glasgow coma scale (GCS)** is a rapid, clinical measure of the level of conciousness (see opposite). In delirium both the level of conciousness and the level of confusion may vary rapidly on an hour-by-hour basis and may present as apparently "normal" on occasions. Patients with symptoms suggestive of delirium should therefore be re-examined regularly.

Assessing confusion Assess orientation by direct questioning. Some degree of uncertainty as to date and time can be expected in the hospitalized individual who is away from his normal routine. Directly inquire about episodes of perceptual disturbance and their nature. Document examples of confused speech and comment on the accompanying affect.

Assessing memory Working memory can be assessed by giving the patient a fictitious address containing six components, asking them to repeat it back to ensure registration, and asking for it after approximately five minutes. In assessing short-term memory by testing the patient's recall of recent events ensure you can verify that the patient's answers are in fact correct.

Mini mental status examination (MMSE) The MMSE (📖 p. 82) allows a standardized assessment of orientation, memory, concentration, and performance.

Level of intelligence In most cases formal IQ testing will not be used and the IQ is assessed clinically. Clinical assessment of IQ is by consideration of the highest level of educational achievement reached and by assessment of the patient's comprehension, vocabulary, and level of understanding in the course of the clinical interview. To some extent, this technique relies upon experience giving the clinician a suitable cohort of previous patients for comparison, and allowance should be made for apparent impairment that may be secondary to other abnormalities of the mental status. In any case, if there is significant doubt about the presence of mental impairment, more formal neuropsychological testing should be undertaken.

Glasgow coma score (GCS)[1]

The GCS is scored between 3 and 15, 3 being the worst (you cannot score 0), and 15 the best. It is composed of three parameters:

[E] Best eye response (maximum score − 4)
1. No eye opening
2. Eye opening to pain
3. Eye opening to verbal command
4. Eyes open spontaneously

[V] Best verbal response (maximum score − 5)
1. No verbal response
2. Incomprehensible sounds
3. Inappropriate words
4. Confused but converses
5. Orientated and converses

[M] Best motor response (maximum score − 6)
1. No motor response
2. Extension to pain
3. Flexion to pain
4. Withdrawal from pain
5. Localizing pain
6. Obeys commands

Notes:
- The phrase "GCS of 11" is essentially meaningless; the figure should be broken down into its components (e.g., E3 V3 M5 = GCS 11).

A GCS of 13 or more correlates with a mild brain injury; 9–12 with a moderate injury; and 8 or less, with a severe brain injury.

1 Teasdale G and Jennett B (1974). *Lancet* **2**, 81–4.

Mini mental status examination (MMSE)[1]

Orientation

"Which day of the week is it? What is the date? The month? The season? The year?" (*One point for each correct response*)

"What is the name of this building? What floor are we on? What town are we in? What county are we in? What State are we in?" (*One point for each correct response*)

Maximum 10 points

Registration/concentration/recall

"I am going to give you a list of 3 objects to remember. I want you to repeat them back to me and I will ask you to repeat them again later." [Say "apple," "penny," "table."] Repeat the list until the patient has learned all 3 words, up to a maximum of three tries. (*Score 1 point for each word learned after first repetition*)

"Spell the word "WORLD" backwards." (**D L R O W**) (Score 1 point for each letter in the correct place). Note: If the patient is a high school graduate or higher, "serial sevens" should be used instead. "Please subtract 7 from 100, and seven from that value until I tell you to stop." (100, 93, 86, 79, 72, 65) (*Score 1 point for each correct answer*)

"What were the 3 objects I asked you to remember a few moments ago?" (*Score 1 point for each object recalled*)

Maximum 11 points

Language/drawing

"I am going to show you an instruction. I want you to read it and do what it says." [Show card with **CLOSE YOUR EYES** written on it.] (*Score 1 point if the instruction is carried out.* If the patient reads the sentence aloud, prompt: "now do what it says.")

"Write a complete sentence on this piece of paper." [Offer pen and piece of paper.] (*Score 1 point if the patient writes a meaningful sentence with a verb.* Incorrect spelling and grammar do not matter.)

"Please make a copy of this drawing." [Show figure/drawing from 📖 p. 83.] (*Score 1 point if the patient draws two five-sided figures intersecting at a four-sided figure*)

"I am going to give you a sentence and I want you to repeat it back to me: No ifs ands or buts." (*Score 1 point if repeated correctly*)

"What are the names of these objects?" [Show a pen and a wristwatch]. (*Score 1 point for each object correctly named*)

"I am going to give you a piece of paper. When I do, take the paper in your right hand; fold the paper in half with both hands; and put the paper on your lap." [Offer piece of paper.] (*Score 1 point for each of the 3 actions*)

---

1 Folstein, M.F. *et al.* (1975). J *Psychiatr Res* **12**, 196–198.

Maximum 9 points
Note: *The test is scored out of a maximum of 30 points.*
A score of >27 is normal.
A score of <25 is suggestive of a diagnosis of dementia and should be further investigated.
Scoring may also be lowered by depressive illness or acute confusional state.

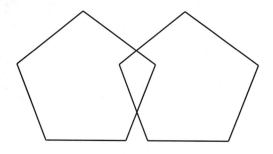

CLOSE YOUR
EYES

Supplementary tests of cerebral functioning

Where there is clinical suspicion of specific functional impairment, it is often useful to directly test the functioning of the different cerebral lobes. This provides more detailed supplementary information than the MMSE (which is essentially a screening test). More formal neuropsychological assessment may be required with additional, well-established psychological tests, although these will usually be administered by specially trained psychologists.

Frontal lobe functioning

Frontal assessment battery (FAB) A brief (10-minute) test of executive function (📖 p. 86), which essentially regroups tests often used when testing executive function at the bedside. These tests are associated with specific areas of the frontal lobes (i.e., conceptualization with dorsolateral areas; word generation with medial areas) and inhibitory control with orbital or medial areas. The maximum score is 18 and a cut-off score of 12 in patients with dementia has been shown to have a sensitivity of 79% for frontotemporal dementia v. Alzheimer's disease. However, any performance below 17 may indicate frontal lobe impairment.

The Wisconsin card sorting task The patient has to determine the rule for card allocation and allocate cards accordingly. When the rule changes, a patient with frontal lobe dysfunction is likely to make more errors (tests response inhibition and set shifting).

Digit span Short-term verbal memory is tested with progressively longer number sequences, first forwards (normal maximum digit span 6 ± 1) and, subsequently, in reverse order (normal maximum 5 ± 1).

Trail making test This is a "join the dots" test of visuomotor tracing testing conceptualization and set shifting. Test A is a simple number sequence; Test B is of alternating numbers and letters (more sensitive for frontal lobe dysfunction).

Cognitive estimate testing The patient is asked a question that requires abstract reasoning and cannot be answered by general knowledge alone (e.g., "How many camels are there in Pittsburgh?"). Although they are culture and educationally bound there are circumstances in which it may be useful to ask people to explain the meanings of common proverbs (i.e., "a rolling stone gathers no moss," "people in glass houses shouldn't through stones," etc.)

Parietal lobe functioning

Tests for dominant lesions

Finger agnosia Patient cannot state which finger is being touched with their eyes closed.

Astereoagnosia Patient unable to recognize the feel of common objects (e.g., coin, pen) with their eyes closed.

Dysgraphethesia Inability to recognize letters or numbers written on the hand.

(Note: Although of disputed clinical value, Gerstmann syndrome is classically described as: right-left disorientation, finger agnosia, dysgraphia, and dyscalculia; due to a lesion of the dominant (usually left) parietal lobe.)

Tests for nondominant lesions

Asomatognosia Patient does not recognize parts of their body (e.g., hand, fingers).

Constructional dyspraxia Inability to draw shapes or construct geometrical patterns.

Other problem areas
- **Visual fields** (as optic tracts run through the parietal lobe to reach the occipital lobe).
- **Speech**—alexia, receptive dysphasia (Wernicke area); conduction aphasia (cannot repeat a phrase, but does understand the meaning).
- **Reading/writing** (angular gyrus lesions).

Frontal assessment battery (FAB)

Domain	Instructions	Score
Similarities *(Concepts)*	"In what way are they alike?" A banana and an apple; A table and a chair; A tulip, a rose, and a daisy	Three correct: 3 Two correct: 2 One correct: 1 None correct: 0
Lexical fluency *(Mental flexibility)*	"Say as many words as you can beginning with the letter "S", except surnames or proper nouns" (If no response for 5 sec, say "for instance, snake"; do not count repetitions, variations)—time 60 sec	>9 words: 3 6–9 words: 2 3–5 words: 1 <3 words: 0
Motor series *(Programming)*	"Look carefully at what I'm doing." The examiner performs 3 times the fist-palm-edge series. "Now, with your right hand, do the same series, first with me, then alone."	6 correct consecutive series alone: 3 3 correct consecutive series alone: 2 3 correct consecutive series with the examiner: 1 <3 correct consecutive series with the examiner: 0
Conflicting instructions *(Sensitivity to interference)*	"Tap twice when I tap once". (Make 3 trials of 1–1–1 and 2–2–2 to make sure that patient has understood) Test series: 1–1–2–1–2–2–2–1–1–2	No error: 3 1–2 errors: 2 >2 errors: 1 4 consecutive errors: 0
Go/no go *(Inhibitory control)*	"Tap once when I tap once, do not tap when I tap twice." (a series of 3 trials is run with 1–1–1 and 2–2–2) Test series: 1–1–2–1–2–2–2–1–1–2	No error: 3 1–2 errors: 2 >2 errors: 1 4 consecutive errors: 0
Prehension behavior *(Environmental autonomy)*	"Do not take my hands." The examiner brings his hands close to the patient's hands (that are resting palms face upwards on his knees) and touches the palms of patient's hands. Repeat instructions and try again if patient takes the hands.	Does not take the examiner's hands: 3 Hesitates and asks what he has to do: 2 Takes the hands: 1 Takes the hands even after being told not to: 0

Frontal assessment battery (FAB), Dubois B *et al.* (2000). *Neurology* **55**, 1621–6.

Insight

The question of whether the patient has insight into the nature of their symptoms tends only to arise in psychiatric illnesses. In general, a patient with physical illness knows that their symptoms represent abnormality and seeks their diagnosis and appropriate treatment. In contrast, a variety of psychiatric illnesses are associated with impairment of insight and the development of alternative explanations by the patient as to the cause of their symptoms, for example:

- An elderly man with early dementia who is unable to recall where he leaves objects and attributes this to someone stealing them. He angrily accuses his son of the crime.
- An adolescent, with developing schizophrenia, who believes his auditory hallucinations and sense of being watched are caused by a neighbor who has planted cameras and loudspeakers into his home. He repeatedly calls the police and asks them to intervene.
- A middle-aged woman with worsening depression who develops the delusion that she is bankrupt and is shortly about to be evicted from her home in disgrace.

Impairment of insight is not specific to any one psychiatric condition and is not generally a diagnostically important symptom although it may be a crucial consideration in the management of a disorder. It tends to occur in psychotic and organic illnesses and in the more severe forms of depressive illness. Personality disorders are generally not associated with impairment of insight. Impairment of insight can give a crude measure of severity of psychotic symptoms and regaining of insight into the pathological nature of psychotic beliefs can give a similarly crude measure of improvement with treatment.

Insight can be defined succinctly as "the correct attitude to morbid change in oneself." It is a deceptively simple concept that includes a number of beliefs about the nature of the symptoms, their causation, and the most appropriate way of dealing with them. Insight is sometimes reported as an "all or nothing" measure—as something an individual patient either does or does not have. In fact, *insight is most usefully inquired about and reported as a series of health beliefs*:

- Does the patient believe that their abnormal experiences are symptoms of illness?
- Does the patient believe their symptoms are attributable to illness?
- Do they believe that the illness is psychiatric?
- Do they believe that psychiatric treatment might benefit them? Are they willing to weight the risks, benefits, and alternatives of treatment?
- Would they be willing to accept advice from a doctor regarding their treatment?

Beyond the simple question of whether the patient has impairment of insight or not, it is vital to understand how the patient views their symptoms, as this will tend to influence their compliance and future help-seeking behavior. It is important to emphasize that disagreement with the doctor as to the correct course of action does not necessarily indicate lack of insight. A patient may very well not agree to be admitted to hospital or to take a particular medication despite having full insight into the nature of their symptoms. In these cases the doctor should be sure to clarify that the patient has all the necessary information to make a suitable decision before considering the possible need for compulsory treatment.

Physical examination

Examination of the patient's physical condition is an integral part of a comprehensive psychiatric assessment. There are five main reasons why this is so:

- Physical symptoms may be a direct result of psychiatric illness (e.g., alcohol dependency—see 📖 p. 626; eating disorders—see 📖 p. 449; physical neglect in severe depression, schizophrenia, etc.)
- Psychiatric drugs may have physical side-effects (e.g., EPS (extra pyramidal side-effects) and antipsychotics, hypothyroidism and lithium, withdrawal syndromes—see 📖 p. 1074).
- Physical illnesses can cause or exacerbate mental symptoms.
- Occult physical illness may be present.
- In the case of later development of illness (or more rarely, medico-legal issues) it is helpful to have baseline physical findings documented.

Physical examination is all too often deferred and then not done, or not done as thoroughly as is indicated. It may well be acceptable to defer full examination on occasions (e.g., a distressed and paranoid man seen in the ER and well known to the team), but a full medical and psychiatric history with necessary medical investigation should be done and completed as the situation allows.

A routine physical examination has the aim of documenting the patient's baseline physical state, noting the presence or absence of abnormal signs which could be associated with mental or physical illness, and highlighting areas requiring further examination or investigation. Even if the patient refuses a physical examination you should write a note commenting on their general physical well-being and any signs or symptoms you can rule out by observation alone (e.g., jaundice, pallor (anemia), no obvious pain, no obvious respiratory distress, moving all four limbs equally, etc.). If you are able to conduct a physical examination you should note, at a minimum:

General condition Note height and weight. Does the patient look well or unwell? Are they underweight or are there signs of recent weight loss? Note bruising or other injuries and estimate their age.

Cardiovascular Radial pulse—rate, rhythm, and character. Blood pressure. Carotid bruits? Heart sounds. Pedal edema.

Respiratory Respiratory rate. Expansion. Percussion. Breath sounds to auscultation.

Abdominal Swelling or ascites. Masses. Bowel sounds. Hernias.

Neurological Pupilliary response, cranial nerve examination. Muscle wasting. Tone, strength. Sensation. Reflexes. Gait. Involuntary movements.

Some physical signs in psychiatric illness (and possible causes associations)

General examination

Parkinsonian facies	Antipsychotic drug treatment
	Psychomotor retardation (depression)
Abnormal pupil size	*Opiate/drug use*
Argyll-Robertson pupil	Neurosyphilis
Enlarged parotids	*Bulimia nervosa*
("hamster face")	*(secondary to vomiting)*
Hypersalivation	Clozapine treatment
Goiter	*Thyroid disease*
Multiple forearm scars	Borderline personality disorder
Multiple tattoos	*Antisocial personality disorder*
Needle tracks/phlebitis	IV drug use
Gynecomastia	*Antipsychotic drug treatment*
	Alcoholic liver disease
Russell's sign (knuckle callus)	Bulimia nervosa
	(secondary to inducing vomiting)
Lanugo hair	*Anorexia nervosa*
Piloerection ("goose flesh")	Opiate withdrawal
Excessive thinness	*Anorexia nervosa*

Cardiovascular

Rapid/irregular pulse	Anxiety disorder
	Drug/alcohol withdrawal
	Hyperthyroidism
	Hypothyroidism
Slow pulse	

Abdominal

Enlarged liver	Alcoholic liver disease
	Hepatitis
Multiple surgical scars	*Somatization disorder*
("checker-board" abdomen)	
Multiple self-inflicted scars	Borderline personality disorder

Neurological

Resting tremor	Increased sympathetic drive
	(anxiety, drug/alcohol misuse)
	Antipsychotic drug treatment
	Lithium treatment
	Antipsychotic drug treatment
	Tic disorder
	Huntington's/Sydenham's chorea
	Antipsychotic-induced dystonia
Involuntary movements	Catatonia
	Antipsychotic drug treatment
Abnormal posturing	Cerebellar disease (alcohol, lithium
Festinant (shuffling) gait	toxicity
road-based gait	

Clinical investigation

Clinical investigations, including blood testing, imaging techniques, and karyotyping, currently play a smaller role in psychiatric diagnosis than in other medical specialties. They are mainly carried out to **exclude medical conditions** which may be part of the differential diagnosis (such as hypothyroidism as a cause of lethargy and low mood) or as part of a research investigation. They should generally be carried out as a result of positive findings in the history or physical examination or in order to exclude serious and reversible occult disorders (such as syphilis as a cause of dementia).

"Routine" investigations may be carried out to assess general physical health, as well as provide a **baseline** measure prior to commencing medication known to have possible adverse effects (e.g., CBC and LFTs prior to starting antipsychotic medication; UA, creatinine clearance, TFTs prior to lithium therapy). Specific screening and monitoring tests are detailed in specific sections. It is good practice to screen new patients with some standard tests. The usual test battery will include: CBC (and differential), UA, LFTs, TFTs, glucose. Where there is suspicion of drug or alcohol misuse/dependency, MCV, B_{12}/folate, and toxicology screening may be added.

Other physical investigations are sometimes requested for baseline or pretreatment testing (e.g., EKG for patients on specific medications, or for younger or older patients) or for underlying (undiagnosed) physical disorder. Performance of a lumbar puncture, for example, is reserved for situations where there is clear evidence to suggest a neurological disorder presenting with psychiatric symptoms (e.g., suspected meningitis or encephalitis; multiple sclerosis) and, more often than not, in these circumstances a referral will be made for a neurological or internal medicine consultation.

Use of other tools, such as EEG, CT, or MRI (and SPECT or PET where available) require justification on the grounds of diagnostic need. EEGs may be used by psychiatrists; however, the results may be difficult to interpret as psychotropic medications may themselves produce specific or non-specific EEG changes. EEG may be useful where epilepsy is suspected (on clinical grounds), to monitor some acute (toxic) confusional states, to assess atypical patterns of cognitive impairment, to aid diagnosis in certain dementias (e.g., HIV), to evaluate particular sleep disorders, or as the gold standard for seizure monitoring during ECT. EEG should not be used as a general screening tool at this time.

Currently, brain imaging may not add to the *diagnosis* of primary psychiatric disorders, and should primarily be used where there is good evidence for possible neurological problems (e.g., history of significant head injury, epilepsy, multiple sclerosis, previous neurosurgery) or where history and clinical examination indicate the possibility of a space-occupying lesion (e.g., localizing neurological signs, unexplained fluctuating level of consciousness, severe headache, marked and unexplained acute behavioral change.) With the exception of organic disorders (e.g., the dementias—where diagnostic imaging techniques may add useful information to inform diagnosis, management, and prognosis), the sensitivity and specificity of imaging findings for most psychiatric conditions are still being established. Nevertheless, in many centers it has become routine to acquire a structural MRI scan from first episode psychosis patients, as increased lateral ventricular volume is a poor prognostic indicator.

As a general rule co-morbid or causative disorders will be suspected due to other symptoms and signs or by the atypical nature of the psychiatric picture, and the likelihood of revealing a totally unexpected diagnosis is small.

Common assessment instruments[1]

The diagnosis of psychiatric disorders is largely clinical, although assessment tools are increasingly used for both clinical and research purposes. A huge variety of assessment tools are available for the diagnosis of psychiatric disorders in general, for the diagnosis and assessment of severity of individual disorders, and for the monitoring of progress and treatment response in established cases. Their primary use is aiding in diagnosis and treatment response. Having said this, they should not be considered a primary means of diagnosis. Scales often have several versions, are either clinician, or patient, administered and vary in required skill and age of the administrator. Some are free by searching on the internet, while others are under copyright but are available for purchase from the manufacturer. A few examples of the more commonly found general and specific tests are given here.

General

General Health Questionnaire (**GHQ**) Self-rated questionnaire used as a screening instrument for the presence of psychiatric illness. Patient is asked to report the presence of a list of symptoms in the preceding weeks. Four versions are available using 12, 28, 30, and 60 items.

Primary Care Evaluation of Mental Disorders (**PRIME-MD**) One page patient completed questionnaire focusing on psychiatric illness commonly encountered in primary care. Has a corresponding Clinician Evaluation Guide. Copyright Pfizer, Inc.

Structured Clinical Interview for DSM-IV-TR (**SCID-I/SCID-II**) Clinician-administered semi-structured clinical interview for use with patients in whom a psychiatric diagnosis is suspected. Primarily used in research with trained interviewers to inform the operationalized diagnosis of Axis I and II disorders.

Diagnostic Interview Schedule (**DIS**) Can be used by non-clinicians to administer a fully-structured interview to diagnose a the major psychiatric illnesses for research purposes. Lengthy.

Global Assessment of Functioning Scale (**GAF**) 100-item, self-report rating scale measuring overall psychosocial functioning.

Quality of Life Interview (**QOLI**) Nonclinician administered fully-structured interview available in full and brief versions with 158 and 78 items respectively. Suitable for assessment of quality of life in those with enduring and severe mental illnesses.

Minnesota Multiphasic Personality Inventory (**MMPI**) Self-report questionnaire consisting of 567 questions covering eight areas of psychopathology, two additional areas of personality type, and three scales assessing truthfulness. Results are compared with normative data from non-clinical populations. Results generate information useful for a broad range of clinical applications.

---

1 Sajatovic, M. and Ramirez, L. (2003). *Rating Scales in Mental Health*, 2nd edition Hudson, OH: Lexi-Comp.

Mood disorders

Hamilton Rating Scale for Depression **(HAM-D)** Interviewer rated, 17-item rating scale for depressive illness. Not a diagnostic instrument; used to measure changes (e.g., as a result of drug treatment). 17 items scored according to severity, producing total score.

Montgomery-Asberg Depression Rating Scale **(MADRS)** 10-item observer-rated scale. Each item rated 0–6 with total score obtained.

Beck Depression Inventory **(BDI)** Self-rated questionnaire containing 21 statements with four possible responses for each. Total score is quoted with >17 indicating moderate and >30 indicating severe depression.

Mood Disorders Questionnaire **(MDQ)** Self-rated screen for bipolar disorder. 13 yes/no questions, and two others. Positive screen is "yes" 7/13, and "yes" to question 2, moderate/serious to question 3.

Young Mania Rating Scale **(YMRS)** Assesses mania symptoms and weighted severity over the past 48 hours.

Anxiety spectrum

Hamilton Anxiety Rating Scale **(HAM-A)** Clinician-administered rating scale for generalized anxiety disorder. 14 items each rated on a 5-point scale.

Yale-Brown Obsessive-Compulsive Scale **(Y-BOCS)** Clinician-administered semistructured interview allowing rating of severity in patients with a pre-existing diagnosis of OCD.

Schizophrenia

Positive and Negative Syndrome Scale **(PANSS)** Clinician-administered rating scale for assessment of severity and monitoring of change of symptoms in patients with a diagnosis of schizophrenia. Items covering positive symptoms, negative symptoms, and general psychopathology.

Scale for the Assessment of Positive/Negative Symptoms **(SAPS/ SANS)** Administered together, and completed from history and clinician observation. It breaks down into three divisions: psychoticism, negative symptoms and disorganization.

Brief Psychiatric Rating Scale **(BPRS)** Measures major psychotic and non-psychotic symptoms, primarily used for schizophrenia patients. Clinician-rated based on observation.

Involuntary Movement Scales Used to monitor potential movement side-effects of medication. Clinician-rated at baseline and on regular intervals. *Abnormal Involuntary Movement Scale* (AIMS), *Barnes Akathisia Scale* (BAS).

Substance Use (see chapter 15 for details)

CAGE (Cut Down? Annoyed? Guilty? Eye Opener?) Brief screening test for alcohol problems consisting of 4 yes/no questions, a score of 2 or more indicating the need for further assessment.

Alcohol Use Disorders Identification Test **(AUDIT)** Completed by skilled clinician to reveal if there is a need for further evaluation. Questions cover quantity and frequency of alcohol use, drinking behaviors, adverse psychological symptoms, and alcohol-related problems.

Assessment instruments specific to children

ADHD **(SNAP, Vanderbilt, Conners' Rating Scale)** Used to assess presence and severity of ADHD symptoms in multiple settings. Completed by adults who know the child well (parents, teachers). Also have subscales to measure other symptoms, such as disruptive behavior.

Anxiety **Screen for Child Anxiety Related Emotional Disorders (SCARED)** A self-report instrument designed to measure anxiety symptoms in children.

Autism Spectrum **Childhood Autism Rating Scale (CARS)** Ages 2 and up, scored by clinicians based on observation. **Gilliam Autism Rating Scale (GARS)** Ages 3 to 22, scored by teachers and parents as well as clinicians. **Autism Diagnostic Observation Schedule (ADOS)** A semi-structured and lengthy diagnostic interview given by specially trained clinicians. It uses standardized data to aid in the diagnosis of pervasive developmental disorders.

Depression **Children's Depression Inventory (CDI)** Self-report of depression symptoms for ages 7 to 17 (first-grade reading level).

Structured Interviews (Such as **K-SADS–PL**), are semistructured diagnostic interviews covering the spectrum of psychiatric illness in children, administered by trained clinicians only.

Older adults

Geriatric Depression Scale **(GDS)** Self-reported screen for depression using a series of Yes/No questions.

Instrumental Activities of Daily Living **(IADL)** Used to evaluate the day-to-day living skills in an older population. It can be used to evaluate treatment effectiveness or help identify placement needs of the individual.

Mini mental status examination **(MMSE)** Bedside interactive examination, clinician administered. Designed to test cognitive function at a point in time. While it is not diagnostic, it provides a screen that can also reveal changes over a period of time. The score is easily communicated to others for comparison. A score of 23–25 or less is considered impaired. (See chapter 2 📖 *pp. 82–3* for details).

Signs and symptoms of psychiatric illness

Symptoms of psychiatric illness

In general medicine, a *symptom* refers to an abnormality reported by the patient, whereas a *sign* refers to an abnormality detected by the doctor by observation or clinical examination. In psychiatry, the terms *symptom* and *sign* tend to be used synonymously because abnormalities of mental state are largely elicited by exploring, with the patient, their internal experiences.

Psychopathology is the study of abnormalities in mental state and is one of the core sciences in clinical psychiatry. **Descriptive psychopathology** includes close observation of the patient's behavior and empathic exploration of their subjective experience. The latter is called **phenomenology**. The following general terms are used as qualifiers for symptoms described in the following pages:

- *Subjective v. objective* Objective signs are those noted by an external observer; subjective signs are those reported by the patient.
- *Form v. content* A distinction is drawn between the *form and content of abnormal* internal experiences. For example, a patient may believe that he is continually under surveillance by agents of the FBI who are plotting to frame him for another's crimes. Here, the *content* of the symptom is the belief about the name and methods of the persecutor; the *form* is that of a persecutory delusion. *Content* is culture and experience related, whereas form is attributable to the type of underlying mental illness.
- *Primary v. secondary* Primary symptoms are considered as arising directly from the pathology of the mental illness; secondary symptoms arise as an understandable response to some aspect of the disordered mental state (e.g., a patient with severe depression developing a *secondary delusion* of being wicked and deserving punishment). Secondary symptoms can be understood in the light of knowledge of the patient's disordered mental state; primary symptoms can be empathized with but rarely fully understood.
- *Endogenous v. reactive* These terms have been largely made redundant by developments in understanding of mental disorders, but are still seen occasionally. It was formerly thought that some conditions arose in response to external events (e.g., depression arising after job loss) (*reactive*), while others arose spontaneously from within (*endogenous*).
- *Psychotic v. neurotic* in present classifications these terms are used purely descriptively to describe two common types of symptoms that may occur in a variety of mental disorders. Previously, they were used to distinguish those disorders characterized by impairment of insight, abnormal beliefs, and abnormal perceptual experiences (psychotic) from those where there was preserved insight but abnormal affect (neurotic).
- *Congruent v. incongruent* This is an observation made regarding the apparent appropriateness of a patient's affect toward their symptoms or their symptoms to their mood. A patient with apparent cheerfulness despite persecutory beliefs is described as having *incongruent* affect; a patient with profoundly depressed mood developing a delusion that they were mortally ill is described as possessing a *mood-congruent* delusion.

- *Structural v. functional* A distinction formerly made between those brain disorders with observable structural abnormalities on postmortem (e.g., Alzheimer's disease) and those without (e.g., schizophrenia). This usage has diminished since the discovery of definite observable brain changes in those disorders formerly called *functional psychoses*. Nowadays, the terms are more often used in neurology/neuropsychiatry to distinguish syndromes that generally have abnormal investigation findings (e.g., multiple sclerosis) (structural) from those without (e.g., conversion paralysis) (functional).

Glossary of psychiatric terms

Abnormal beliefs A category of disturbance that includes **delusions** and **overvalued ideas**.

Abnormal perceptions A category of disturbance that includes **sensory distortions** and **false perceptions**.

Abstract thinking Thinking characterized by the ability to use concepts or conceptual reasoning and to make and understand generalizations.

Acute confusional state See **delirium**.

Affect The external expressed emotional state observable in a patient at a particular moment and in response to a particular event or situation. Contrasted with **mood,** which is the prevailing emotional state of mind.

Affect illusion See **illusion**.

Agitated depression A combination of depressed **mood** and **psycho-motor agitation**, contrasting with the more common association of depressed mood with **psychomotor retardation**. A common presentation of depressive illness in the elderly.

Agitation See psychomotor agitation.

Agoraphobia A generalized **phobia** in which there is fear of places or social situations in which escape might be difficult or embarrassing, e.g., check-out lines, crowded areas, etc. Associated with **avoidance** of these stimuli.

Akathisia Subjective sense of an uncomfortable desire to move, relieved by repeated movement of the effected part (usually the legs). A side-effect of treatment with some antipsychotic drugs.

Alexithymia The inability to describe one's subjective emotional experiences verbally. May be a personality characteristic but is also associated with **somatization**.

Alogia Poverty of thoughts as observed by absence of spontaneous speech; the inability to speak. A **negative symptom** of schizophrenia and a symptom of depressive illness.

Ambitendency A **motor symptom of schizophrenia** in which there is an alternating mixture of **automatic obedience** and **opposition**.

Amnesia Loss of the ability to recall memories for a period of time. May be **global** (complete memory loss for the time period), or **partial** (patchy memory loss with "islands" of preserved memory).

Anergia The subjective feeling of lack of energy and sense of increased effort required to carry out tasks. Associated with depressive illness.

Anhedonia The feeling of absent or significantly diminished enjoyment of previously pleasurable activities. A core symptom of depressive illness, also a **negative symptom** of schizophrenia.

Anorexia Loss or lack of appetite for food. Seen in depressive illness and many general medical conditions. Interestingly, patients with anorexia nervosa often do not have anorexia as so defined. They commonly describe themselves as very hungry—controlling their desire for food by supreme effort in order to control their weight.

Anterograde amnesia The period of **amnesia** between an event (e.g., head injury) and the resumption of continuous memory. The length of anterograde amnesia is correlated with the extent of brain injury (see retrograde amnesia, 🕮 *p. 117*).

Anxiety A normal and adaptive response to stress and danger, which is pathological if prolonged, severe, or disproportional to with the real threat of the external situation. Anxiety has two components: *psychic* anxiety, which is an affect, characterized by increased arousal, apprehension, sense of vulnerability, and dysphoria; and *somatic/physiological* anxiety, in which there are bodily sensations of palpitations, sweating, dyspnea, pallor, and abdominal discomfort.

Aphonia Loss of the ability to vocalize. May occur with structural disease affecting the vocal cords directly, the 9th cranial nerve, or higher centers. May also occur in functional illness (e.g., conversion disorder) in which the underlying vocal cord function is normal. This can be demonstrated by asking the patient to cough—a normal cough demonstrates the ability of the vocal cords to oppose normally.

Asyndesis Synonym for **loosening of associations**.

Ataxia Loss of coordination of voluntary movement. Seen in drug and alcohol intoxication and organic disorders, particularly cerebellar.

Athetosis Sinuous, writhing involuntary movements.

Aura Episode of disturbed sensation occurring before a neurological condition (e.g., epileptic event). Wide range of manifestations although usually stereotyped for each individual.

Autistic thinking An abnormal absorption with the self, distinguished by interpersonal communication difficulties, a short attention span, and inability to relate to others as people.

Autochthonous delusion A primary **delusion** that appears to arise fully formed in the patient's mind without explanation (e.g., a patient suddenly becomes aware that he personally invented the Internet).

Automatic obedience A **motor symptom of schizophrenia** in which the patient obeys the examiner's instructions unquestioningly. This cooperation may be "excessive," with the patient going beyond what is asked (e.g., raising both arms and both legs when asked to raise an arm).

Automatism Behavior that is apparently conscious in nature but that occurs in the absence of full consciousness (e.g., during a temporal lobe seizure).

Autoscopy The experience of seeing a visual **hallucination** or **pseudo-hallucination** of oneself. Also known as "phantom mirror image." Uncommon symptom reported in schizophrenia and in temporal lobe epilepsy.

Autotopagnosia Condition in which one cannot identify or describe their own body parts. Individuals can dress and move appropriately, but cannot talk about their bodies.

Avoidance The action of not exposing oneself to situations that generate anxiety (e.g., a patient with **agoraphobia** remaining at home or a patient with PTSD following a car accident refusing to drive). Can be understood in terms of an operant conditioning model in which actions with reward—in this case reduction of anxiety—are repeated.

Belle indifference A surprising lack of concern for, or denial of, apparently severe functional disability. It is part of classical descriptions of hysteria and continues to be associated with operational descriptions of conversion disorder. It is also seen in medical illnesses (e.g., CVA) and is a rare and nonspecific symptom of no diagnostic value.

Biological features of depression Neurovegetative symptoms of moderate to severe depressive illness that reflect disturbance of core vegetative function. They are **depressive sleep disturbance, anorexia, loss of libido, anergia**, and impression of deterioration in memory and concentration.

Blunting of affect Loss of the normal degree of emotional sensitivity and sense of the appropriate emotional response to events. A **negative symptom** of schizophrenia.

Blocking Repeated and abrupt halt to speech as a result of losing one's train of thought.

Broca's aphasia A type of **expressive aphasia** due to damage to the posterior part of the inferior frontal gyrus of the dominant hemisphere (Broca's language area).

Bulimia Increased appetite and desire for food and/or excessive, impulsive eating of large quantities of usually high-calorie food. In Bulimia Nervosa, it includes behavior to control weight and overvalued ideas about body shape and weight.

Capgras syndrome ("l'illusion dessosies") A type of **delusional misidentification** in which the patient believes that a person known to them has been replaced by a "double," or imposter, who is to all external appearances identical, but is not the "real person."

Catalepsy Increased resting muscle tone that is not present on active or passive movement (in contrast to the rigidity associated with Parkinson's disease and **extrapyramidal side-effects**). A motor symptom of schizophrenia.

Cataplexy Symptom of narcolepsy in which there is sudden loss of muscle tone leading to collapse. Usually occurs following emotional stress.

Catastrophic reaction Response occasionally seen in patients with **dementia** who are asked to perform tasks beyond their, now impaired, performance level. There is sudden agitation, anger, and occasionally violence.

Catatonia Rare **motor symptoms of schizophrenia**. Describes a situation in which the patient's limbs can be passively moved to any posture that will then be held for a prolonged period of time. The associated rigidity is also known as **waxy flexibility** or **flexibilitas cerea**. See also **psychological pillow**.

Chorea Sudden and involuntary movement of several muscle groups with the resultant action appearing like part of a voluntary movement.

Circumstantial thinking A thought disorder in which irrelevant details and digressions overwhelm the direction of the verbal representation of the thought process. Eventually, the goal of the thought is reached. Can be normal, also seen in mania, thought disorders, and in obsessive-compulsive personality disorder.

Clang association An abnormality of speech in which the connection between words is their sound rather than their meaning. May occur during manic **flight of ideas**.

Claustrophobia Fear of being trapped in confined spaces.

Clouding of consciousness Conscious level between full consciousness and coma. Covers a range of increasingly severe loss of function with drowsiness and impairment of concentration and perception.

Coma vigil Vegetative state where persons can open their eyelids occasionally and demonstrate sleep-wake cycles. They are awake, but without conscious awareness.

Command hallucination An auditory hallucination of a commanding voice, instructing the patient toward a particular action. Also known as **teleological hallucination**.

Compulsion Repetitive ritualistic behavior or mental activity that is recognized by the patient as unnecessary and purposeless but that he/she cannot resist performing repeatedly (e.g., hand washing). The drive to perform the action is recognized by the patient as his or her own (e.g., there is no sense of possession or passivity) but it is associated with a subjective sense of need to perform the act, often in order to avoid the occurrence of an adverse event.

Concrete thinking The loss of the ability to understand abstract concepts and metaphorical ideas leading to a strictly literal form of speech and inability to comprehend allusive language. Seen in schizophrenia and in neurodegenerative illnesses.

Confabulation The process of describing plausible but imagined memories as facts for a period for which the patient has **amnesia**. Occurs in Korsakoff psychosis, dementia, and following alcoholic blackout.

Confusion The core symptom of delirium or acute confusional state. There is **disorientation**, **clouding of consciousness**, and deterioration in the ability to think rationally, lay down new memories, and to understand sensory input.

Conversion The development of features that are suggestive of physical illness but that are attributed to psychiatric illness or emotional disturbance rather than organic pathology. Originally described in terms of psychoanalytic theory in which the presumed mechanism was the "conversion" of unconscious distress to physical symptoms rather than allowing its expression in conscious thought.

Coprolalia A forced vocalization of obscene words or phrases. The symptom is largely involuntary but can be resisted for a time, at the expense of mounting **anxiety**. Seen in Tourette syndrome.

Cotard syndrome A presentation of psychotic depressive illness seen particularly in elderly people. There is a combination of severely depressed mood with **nihilistic delusions** and/or **hypochondriacal delusions**. The patient may state that he is already dead and should be buried, that his insides have stopped working and are rotting away, or that he has stopped existing altogether.

Couvade's syndrome A conversion symptom seen in partners of expectant mothers during their pregnancy. The symptoms vary but mimic pregnancy symptoms and so include nausea, vomiting, abdominal pain, and food cravings. It is not delusional in nature; the affected individual does not believe they are pregnant (compared to **pseudocyesis**). May be a cultural norm.

Craving A subjective sense of need to consume a particular substance (e.g., drugs or alcohol) for which there may be **dependence**.

Cultural bound syndromes Disorders occurring in particular localities/ethnic groups, often considered normal illnesses in that culture. The behavioral manifestations or subjective experiences particular to these disorders may or may not correspond to diagnostic categories in DSM-IV-TR or ICD-10. Refer to Chapter 22 for details.

Cyclothymia A mood disorder in which there is cyclical mood variation to a lesser degree than in bipolar disorder.

De Clérambault syndrome A form of **delusion of love**. The patient, usually female, believes that another, higher-status individual is in love with them. There may be an additional **persecutory delusional** component where the affected individual comes to believe that individuals are conspiring to keep them apart. The object may be an employer or doctor, or in some cases a prominent public figure or celebrity.

Déjà vu A sense that events being experienced for the first time have been experienced before. An everyday experience but also a nonspecific symptom of a number of disorders including temporal lobe epilepsy, schizophrenia, and anxiety disorders.

Delirium A clinical syndrome of **confusion** with a variable degree of **clouding of consciousness**, visual **illusions**, and/or visual **hallucinations**, lability of affect, and disorientation. The clinical features can vary markedly in severity hour by hour. Delirium is a stereotyped response by the brain to a variety of insults (📖 p. 978).

Delirium tremens The clinical picture of acute confusional state secondary to alcohol withdrawal. Comprises autonomic hyperactivity, **confusion**, **withdrawals**, visual hallucinations, and, occasionally, **persecutory delusions** and **Lilliputian hallucinations**.

Delusion An abnormal belief that is held with absolute subjective certainty (a false fixed belief), that requires no external proof, that may be held in the face of contradictory evidence, and that has personal significance and importance to the individual concerned. Cultural or religious beliefs are not included here, unless they are outside of the norm for that culture. Although the content is usually false and bizarre in nature, this is not invariably so.

Primary delusions are the direct result of psychopathology, whereas *secondary delusions* can be understood as having arisen in response to other primary psychiatric conditions (e.g., a patient with severely depressed mood developing delusions of poverty or a patient with progressive memory impairment developing a delusion that people are entering his house and stealing or moving items). Primary delusions can be subdivided by the method by which they are perceived as having arisen or into broad classes based on their content. If the patient is asked to recall the point at which they became aware of the delusion and its significance to them, they may report that the belief arose: "out of the blue" (*autochthonous delusion*); on seeing a normal perception (*delusional perception*); on recalling a memory (*delusional memory*); or on a background of anticipation, odd experiences, and increased awareness (*delusional mood*).

Twelve types of primary delusion are commonly recognized: persecutory delusions, grandiose delusions, delusions of control, delusions of thought interference, delusions of reference, delusions of guilt, delusional misidentification, hypochondriacal delusions, delusional jealousy, delusions of love, nihilistic delusions, and delusions of infestation.

Delusional elaboration Secondary delusions that arise in a manner that is understandable as the patient attempting to find explanations for primary psychopathological processes (e.g., a patient with persistent auditory hallucinations developing a belief that a transmitter has been placed in his or her ear).

Delusional jealousy A delusional belief that one's partner is being unfaithful. This can occur as part of a wider psychotic illness, secondary to organic brain damage (e.g., following the punch-drunk syndrome in boxers), associated with alcohol dependence, or as a monosymptomatic delusional disorder ("**Othello syndrome**"). Whatever the primary cause, there is a strong association with violence, usually toward the supposedly unfaithful partner. For this type of delusion, the content is not bizarre or inconceivable and the central belief may even be true. In general the evidence presented is flimsy at best and sometimes bizarre.

Delusional memory A primary **delusion** that is recalled as arising as a result of a memory (e.g., a patient who remembers his parents taking him to the hospital for an operation as a child becoming convinced that he had been implanted with control and monitoring devices that have become active in his adult life).

Delusional misidentification A delusional belief that certain individuals are not who they externally appear to be. The delusion may be that familiar people have been replaced with outwardly identical strangers (Capgras syndrome) or that strangers are really familiar people (Frégoli syndrome). A rare symptom of schizophrenia/ psychotic illnesses.

Delusional mood Period when there is an abnormal mood state characterized by anticipatory anxiety, a sense of something about to happen, and an increased sense of the significance of minor events. The development of a primary delusion may come as a relief to the patient in this situation.

Delusional perception A primary **delusion** that is recalled as having arisen as a result of a perception (e.g., a patient who, on seeing two white cars pull up in front of his house became convinced that he was, therefore, about to win a million-dollar sweepstakes). The perception is a real external object, not a hallucinatory experience.

Delusions of control A group of delusions that are also known as **passivity phenomena** or delusions of bodily passivity. They are considered **first-rank symptoms** of schizophrenia. The core feature is the delusional belief that one is no longer in sole control of one's own body. The individual delusions are that one is being forced by some external agent to feel emotions, to desire to do things, to perform actions, or to experience bodily sensations. Respectively, these delusions are called: **passivity of affect, passivity of impulse, passivity of volition, and somatic passivity.**

Delusions of guilt A delusional belief that one has committed a crime or other reprehensible act. A feature of psychotic depressive illness (e.g., an elderly woman with severe depressive illness who becomes convinced that her child, who died by accident many years before, was in fact murdered by her).

Delusions of infestation A delusional belief that one's skin is infested with multiple, tiny mite-like animals. It is also seen in acute confusional states (particularly secondary to drug or alcohol withdrawal), in schizophrenia, in neurodegenerative illnesses, and as **delusional elaboration** of tactile hallucinatory experiences.

Delusions of love A delusion in which the patient believes another individual is in love with them and that they are destined to be together. A rare symptom of schizophrenia and other psychotic illnesses, one particular subtype of this delusion is erotomania (a.k.a **de Clérambault syndrome**).

Delusions of reference A delusional belief that external events or situations have been arranged in such a way as to have particular significance for or to convey a message to the affected individual. The patient may believe that television news items are referring to him or that parts of the bible are about him directly.

Delusions of thought interference A group of delusions that are considered **first-rank symptoms** of schizophrenia. They are **thought insertion, thought withdrawal, and thought broadcasting.**

Dementia Chronic brain failure—in contrast with delirium (which is acute brain failure). In dementia, there is progressive and global loss of brain function. It is usually irreversible. Different dementing illnesses will show different patterns and rate of functional loss but, in general, there is impairment of memory, loss of higher cognitive function, perceptual abnormalities, **dyspraxia**, and disintegration of the personality.

Dependence The inability to control intake of a substance to which one is addicted. Dependence is characterized by primacy of drug-seeking behavior, inability to control intake of the substance once consumption has started, use of the substance to avoid **withdrawals**, increased tolerance to the intoxicating effects of the substance, and re-instigation of the pattern of use after a period of abstinence. Dependence has two components: **psychological dependence**, which is the subjective feeling of loss of control, cravings, and preoccupation with obtaining the substance; and **physiological dependence**, which is the physical consequences of withdrawal and is specific to each drug. For some drugs (e.g., alcohol) both psychological and physiological dependence occur; for others (e.g., LSD) there are no marked features of physiological dependence.

Depersonalization An unpleasant subjective experience in which the patient feels as if they have become "unreal." A nonspecific symptom occurring in many psychiatric disorders as well as in normal people.

Depressed mood The core feature of depressive illness. Milder forms of depressed mood are part of the human experience, but in its pathological form it is a subjective experience. Patients describe variously: an unremitting and pervasive unhappiness; a loss of the ability to experience the normal range of positive emotions (feeling of a lack of feeling); a sense of hopelessness and negative thoughts about themselves, their situation, and the future; somatic sensations of "a weight" pressing down on head and body; and a sort of "psychic pain" or wound.

Depressive sleep disturbance Characteristic pattern of sleep disturbance seen in depressive illness. It includes **initial insomnia** and **early morning waking**. In addition, sleep is described as more shallow, broken, and less refreshing. There is increased REM latency, where the patient enters REM sleep more rapidly than normal and REM sleep is concentrated in the beginning rather than the end of the sleep period.

Derailment A symptom of **schizophrenic thought disorder** in which there is a total break in the chain of association between the meaning of thoughts. The connection between the two sequential ideas is apparent neither to the patient nor to the examiner.

Derealization An unpleasant subjective experience in which the patient feels as if the world has become unreal. Like **depersonalization** it is a nonspecific symptom of a number of disorders.

Diogenes syndrome Extreme neglect of one's self, home, and/or environment, often with hoarding of objects, usually of no practical use. May be a behavioral manifestation of an organic disorder, schizophrenia, depressive disorder, or obsessive-compulsive disorder; or it may reflect a reaction late in life to stress in a certain type of personality.

Disinhibition Loss of the normal sense of which behaviors are appropriate in the current social setting; also loss of inhibition of inappropriate behaviors. Symptom of manic illnesses and occurs in the later stages of neurodegenerative illnesses and during intoxication with drugs or alcohol.

Disorientation Loss of the ability to recall and accurately update information about current time, place, and personal identity. Occurs in delirium and dementia. With increasing severity of illness, orientation for time is lost first, then orientation for place, with orientation for person usually preserved until dysfunction becomes very severe.

Dissociation The separation of unpleasant emotions and memories from consciousness awareness with subsequent disruption to the normal integrated function of consciousness and memory. **Conversion** and **dissociation** are related concepts. In **conversion** the emotional abnormality produces physical symptoms; whereas in **dissociation** there is impairment of mental functioning (e.g., in **dissociative fugue** and **dissociative amnesia**).

Distractibility Inability to maintain attention or the loss of vigilance on minimal distracting stimulation.

Diurnal variation A variation in the severity of a symptom depending on the time of day (e.g., depressed mood experienced as most severe in the morning and improving later in the day).

Double depression A combination of **dysthymia** and major depressive disorder. Used as a general term without diagnostic specificity.

Dysarthria Impairment in the ability to properly articulate speech. Caused by lesions in brain stem, cranial nerves, or pharynx. Distinguished from **dysphasia** in that there is no impairment of comprehension, writing, or higher language function.

Dyskinesia The impairment of voluntary motor activity by superimposed involuntary motor activity.

Dyslexia Impairment in one's ability to read, spell, and write words at the level normal for one's age or intelligence level.

Dysmorphophobia A type of **overvalued idea** in which the patient believes one aspect of his body is abnormal or conspicuously deformed.

Dysphasia Impairment in producing or understanding speech (**expressive dysphasia** and **receptive dysphasia**, respectively) related to cortical abnormality, in contrast with **dysarthria** in which the abnormality is in the organs of speech production or their neural substrate.

Dysphoria An emotional state experienced as unpleasant, unhappy, or unwell. Secondary to a number of symptoms (e.g., **depressed mood, withdrawals**).

Dyspraxia Impairment in ability to carry out complex motor tasks (e.g., dressing, eating) although the component motor movements are preserved.

Dysprosody Speech impairment characterized by a loss of control of intonation and rhythm.

Dysthymia Chronic, mildly depressed mood and diminished enjoyment, not severe enough to be considered a depressive disorder.

Early morning waking (EMW) Feature of **depressive sleep disturbance**. The patient wakes in the very early morning and is unable to return to sleep.

Echo de la pensée Synonym for **thought echo**.

Echolalia The repetition of phrases or sentences spoken by the examiner. Occurs in schizophrenia and mental retardation.

Echopraxia Motor symptom in which the patient imitates others' movements. This continues after being told to stop. This is often seen in schizophrenia.

Egomania Preoccupation with oneself.

Eidetic imagery The ability to retain and recall an accurate, detailed visual and/or auditory complex scene, which is popularly known as photographic memory. Not a **hallucination**.

Elation Severe and prolonged **elevation of mood**. A feature of manic illnesses.

Elemental hallucination A type of hallucination where the false perceptions are of very simple form (e.g., flashes of light or clicks and bangs). Associated with organic illness.

Elevation of mood The core feature of manic illnesses. The mood is preternaturally cheerful, the patient may describe feeling "high," and there is subjectively increased speed and ease of thinking.

Erotomania Synonym for **delusions of love**.

Euphoria Sustained and unwarranted cheerfulness. Associated with manic states and organic impairment.

Euthymia A "normal" mood state, neither depressed nor manic.

Expressive dysphasia Dysphasia affecting the production of speech. There is impairment of word-finding, sentence construction, and articulation. Speech is slow and "telegraphic," with substitutions, "null" words, and **perseveration**. The patient characteristically exhibits considerable frustration at his deficits. Writing is similarly affected. Basic comprehension is largely intact and emotional utterances and rote learned material may also be surprisingly preserved.

Extracampine hallucination A hallucination in which the perception appears to come from beyond the area usually covered by the senses (e.g., a patient in Pittsburgh "hearing" voices that seem to come from a house in Gettysburg).

Extrapyramidal symptoms (EPS) Symptoms of rigidity, tremor, and dyskinesia caused by the antidopaminergic effects of psychotropic drugs, particularly older and higher dose antipsychotics. Unlike in idiopathic Parkinson's disease, bradykinesia is less prominent.

False perceptions Internal perceptions that do not have a corresponding object in the external or "real" world. Includes **hallucinations** and **pseudo-hallucinations**.

First-rank symptoms (of schizophrenia) A group of symptoms originally described by Schneider, which are useful in the diagnosis of schizophrenia. They are neither pathognomic for, nor specific, to schizophrenia and are also seen in organic and affective psychoses. There are 11 symptoms in four categories:

Auditory hallucinations
- Voices heard arguing.
- Thought echo.
- Running commentary.

Delusions of thought interference
- Thought insertion.
- Thought withdrawal.
- Thought broadcasting.

Delusions of control
- Passivity of affect.
- Passivity of impulse.
- Passivity of volitions.
- Somatic passivity.

Delusional perception
- A primary delusion of any content that is reported by the patient as having arisen following the experience of a normal perception.

Fausse reconnaissance Delusional recognition of persons or places.

Flashbacks Exceptionally vivid and affect-laden re-experiencing of remembered experiences. Flashbacks of the initial traumatic event occur in PTSD and flashbacks to abnormal perceptual experiences initially experienced during LSD intoxication can occur many years after the event.

Flattening of affect Diminution of the normal range of emotional experience. A **negative symptom** of schizophrenia.

Flexibilitas cerea See **catalepsy**.

Flight of ideas Subjective experience of one's thoughts being more rapid than normal with each thought having a greater range of consequent thoughts than normal. Meaningful connections between thoughts are maintained. May also be an objective observation.

Folie à deux Describes a situation in which two people with a close relationship share a delusional belief. This arises as a result of a psychotic illness in one individual with development of a delusional belief, which comes to be shared by the second. The delusion resolves in the second person on separation, the first should be assessed and treated in the usual way.

Formal thought disorder A term that is confusingly used for three different groups of psychiatric symptoms:
- To refer to all pathological disturbances in the form of thought.
- As a synonym for **schizophrenic thought disorder**.
- To mean the group of **first-rank symptoms** that are delusions regarding thought interference (e.g., **thought insertion**, **thought withdrawal**, and **thought broadcasting**), although this is an incorrect use of the term.

Formication A form of tactile **hallucination** in which there is the sensation of numerous insects crawling over the surface of the body or under the skin. Can occur in alcohol or drug withdrawal, particularly from cocaine.

Free-floating anxiety **Anxiety** occurring without any identifiable external stimulus or threat.

Frégoli syndrome A rare type of **delusional misidentification** in which the patient believes different people are in fact one person (often a "persecutor") who changes appearance.

Functional hallucination A hallucination experienced only when experiencing a normal perception in that modality (e.g., hearing voices when the noise of an air conditioner is heard).

Fugue A **dissociative** reaction to unbearable stress. Following a severe external stressor (e.g., marital break-up) the affected individual develops global **amnesia** and may suddenly abandon a lifestyle and start a different one for a period of time. Consciousness is unimpaired. Following resolution, there is amnesia of the events that occurred during the fugue.

Fusion A symptom of **schizophrenic thought disorder** in which two or more unrelated concepts are brought together to form one compound idea.

Ganser syndrome The production of "approximate answers." Here the patient gives repeated wrong answers to questions that are nonetheless "in the right ballpark" (e.g., "What is the capital of Pennsylvania?"—"Pittsburgh"). Occasionally associated with organic brain illness, it is much more commonly seen as a form of **malingering** in those attempting to feign mental illness (e.g., in prisoners awaiting trial).

Garrulous Characterized by excessive and often trivial or rambling speech.

Global aphasia The loss of all ability to communicate.

Globus hystericus The sensation of a "lump in the throat" occurring without esophageal structural abnormality or motility problems. A symptom of anxiety and somatization disorders.

Glossolalia "Speaking in tongues." Production of nonspeech sounds as a substitute for speech. Seen in dissociative and neurotic disorders and accepted as a subcultural phenomenon in some religious groups.

Grandiose delusion A delusional belief that one has special powers, is unusually rich or powerful, or that one has an exceptional destiny (e.g., a man who requested admission to hospital because he had become convinced that God had granted him "the healing touch" and that coming into contact with him would cure others of mental illnesses). Occurs in all psychotic illnesses but particularly in manic illnesses.

Grandiosity An exaggerated sense of one's own importance or abilities. Seen classically in manic illnesses.

Hallucination An internal perception without a corresponding external object. The subjective experience of hallucination is that of experiencing a normal perception in that modality of sensation. A true hallucination will be perceived as in external space, distinct from imagined images, outside conscious control, and as possessing relative permanence. A **pseudo-hallucination** will lack one or all of these characteristics. Hallucinations are subdivided according to their modality of sensation and may be auditory, visual, gustatory, tactile, olfactory, or kinaesthetic. Auditory hallucinations, particularly of voices, are characteristic of psychotic illness, particularly schizophrenia, while visual hallucinations are characteristic of organic states.

Hemiballismus Involuntary, large-scale, "throwing" movements of one limb or one body side.

Hypersomnia Excessive sleepiness with increased length of nocturnal sleep and daytime napping. Occurs as core feature of narcolepsy and in atypical depressive states.

Hypnagogic hallucination A transient false perception experienced while on the verge of falling asleep (e.g., hearing a voice calling one's name which then startles you back to wakefulness to find no one there). The same phenomenon experienced while waking up is called **hypnopompic** hallucination. Frequently experienced by healthy people and not a symptom of mental illness.

Hypnopompic hallucination See **hypnagogic hallucination**.

Hypochondriacal delusions A delusional belief that one has a serious physical illness (e.g., cancer, AIDS). Most common in psychotic depressive illnesses.

Hypochondriasis The belief that one has a particular illness despite evidence to the contrary. Its form may be that of a primary **delusion**, an **overvalued idea**, **rumination**, or a **mood congruent** feature of depressive illness.

Hypomania Describes a mild degree of mania in which there is elevated mood.

Illusion A type of false perception in which the perception of a real world object is combined with internal imagery to produce a false internal perception. Three types are recognized: **affect**, **completion**, and **pareidolic illusions**. In **affect illusion** there is a combination of heightened emotion and misperception (e.g., while walking across a lonely park at night, briefly seeing a tree moving in the wind as an attacker). **Completion illusions** rely on our brain's tendency to "fill-in" presumed missing parts of an object to produce a meaningful perception and are the basis for many types of optical illusion. Both these types of illusions resolve on closer attention. **Pareidolic illusions** are meaningful perceptions produced when experiencing a poorly defined stimulus (e.g., seeing faces in a fire or clouds).

Imperative hallucination A form of **command hallucination** in which the hallucinatory instruction is experienced as irresistible, a combination of **command hallucination**, and **passivity of action**.

Impotence Loss of the ability to consummate sexual relationships. Refers to inability to achieve penile erection in men and lack of genital preparedness in women. It may have a primary medical cause, be related to psychological factors, or can be a side-effect of many psychotropic medications.

Incongruity of affect Refers to the objective impression that the displayed affect is not consistent with the current thoughts or actions (e.g., laughing while discussing traumatic experiences). Important in differentiating mood disorders with psychotic symptoms from schizophrenia.

Initial insomnia Difficulty getting off to sleep. Seen as a symptom of primary insomnia as well as in **depressive sleep disturbance** and in anxiety disorders.

Irritability Diminution in the stressor required to provoke anger or verbal or physical violence. Seen in manic illnesses, organic cognitive impairment, psychotic illnesses, and drug and alcohol intoxication. Can also be a feature of normal personality types and of personality disorder as well as depressive disorders.

Jamais vu The sensation that events or situations are unfamiliar, although they have been experienced before. An everyday experience but also a nonspecific symptom of a number of disorders including temporal lobe epilepsy, schizophrenia, and anxiety disorders.

Knight's move thinking Synonym for **derailment**.

Lability of mood Marked variability in the prevailing affect.

Lack of insight Loss of the ability to recognize that one's abnormal experiences are symptoms of psychiatric illness and that they require treatment.

Lilliputian hallucination A type of visual **hallucination** in which the subject sees miniature people or animals. Associated with organic states; particularly delirium tremens.

Logoclonia A repetition of words or parts of words. Often occurring in Alzheimer's disease or Parkinson's.

Logorrhoea Excess pressured speech or "verbal diarrhea." Symptom of mania.

Loosening of associations A symptom of **formal thought disorder** in which there is a lack of meaningful connection between sequential ideas.

Loss of libido Loss of the desire for sexual activity. Common in depressive illness and should be inquired about directly because it is usually not mentioned spontaneously. Should be distinguished from **impotence**.

Macropsia Seeing everything as larger than it really is.

Magical thinking A belief that certain actions and outcomes are connected although there is no rational basis for establishing a connection (e.g., "Step on a crack, break your mother's back"). Magical thinking is common in normal children and is the basis for most superstitions. A similar type of thinking is seen in psychotic patients and in schizotypal personality disorder.

Malingering Deliberately falsifying the symptoms of illness for a secondary gain (e.g., for compensation, to avoid military service, or to obtain an opiate prescription).

Mania A form of mood disorder initially characterized by **elevated mood, insomnia,** loss of appetite, increased libido, and **grandiosity**. More severe forms develop **elation** and **grandiose delusions**.

Mannerism Abnormal and occasionally bizarre performance of a voluntary, goal-directed activity (e.g., a conspicuously clenching of the jaw when stressed).

Mental retardation Diminished intelligence below the second standard deviation (IQ<70). Increasing severity of retardation is associated with decreased ability to learn, to solve problems, and to understand abstract concepts. Subdivided as mild: 50–55 to 70; moderate 35–40 to 50–55; severe 20–25 to 35–40; profound < 20–25.

Micrographia Small "spidery" handwriting seen in patients with Parkinson's disease; a consequence of being unable to control fine movements. This is most easily recognized by comparing their current signature with one from a number of years previously.

Micropsia Seeing everything as smaller than it really is.

Middle insomnia Wakefulness and inability to return to sleep occurring in the middle part of the night.

Mirror sign Lack of recognition of one's own mirror reflection with the perception that the reflection is another individual who is mimicking your actions. Seen in dementia.

Mood The subjective emotional state, in contrast to **affect,** which describes the expressed emotional state.

Mood congruent A secondary symptom that is understandable in the light of an abnormal mood state (e.g., a severely depressed patient developing a **delusion** that they are in severe debt, or a manic patient developing a **delusion** that they are exceptionally wealthy).

Morbid jealousy Synonym for **delusional jealousy**.

Motor aphasia A condition in which expression through speech or writing is impaired.

Motor symptoms of psychosis Schizophrenic illness is associated with a variety of soft neurological signs and motor abnormalities, which can also be seen with psychosis of other etiologies. In the modern era, many motor abnormalities will be attributed to the side-effects of antipsychotic drugs, but all were described in patients with schizophrenia prior to the introduction of these drugs in 1952. Recognized motor symptoms in schizophrenia/psychosis include: **catatonia, catalepsy, automatic obedience, negativism, ambitendency, mannerism, stereotypy, echopraxia,** and **psychological pillow**.

Multiple personality The finding of two or more distinct personalities in one individual. These personalities may answer to different names, exhibit markedly different behaviors, and describe amnesia for periods when other personalities were active. Also and more properly known as dissociative personality disorder.

Mutism Absence of speech without impairment of consciousness.

Negative symptoms (of psychosis) The symptoms of psychosis/ schizophrenia that reflect impairment of normal function. They are: lack of volition, lack of drive, apathy, **anhedonia, flattening of affect blunting of affect**, and **alogia**. Believed to be related to alterations in cortical networks and firing synchronicity.

Negativism A **motor symptom of psychosis** in which the patient resists carrying out the examiner's instructions and his attempts to move or direct the limbs.

Neologism A made-up word often used in an idiosyncratic way. Neologisms are found in schizophrenic speech and also in mania.

Nihilistic delusions A delusional belief that the patient has died or no longer exists or that the world has ended or is no longer real. Nothing matters any longer and continued effort is pointless. A feature of psychotic depressive illness.

Noesis The belief that one has a divine calling.

Nystagmus Involuntary rapid eye movements.

Obsession An idea, image, or impulse that is recognized by the patient as their own, but that is experienced as repetitive, intrusive, and distressing. The return of the obsession can be resisted for a time at the expense of mounting anxiety. In some situations the **anxiety** accompanying the obsessional thoughts can be relieved by associated **compulsion** (e.g., a patient with an obsession that his wife may have come to harm feeling compelled to phone her constantly during the day to check that she is still alive).

Othello syndrome A monosymptomatic delusional disorder in which the core delusion has the content of **delusional jealousy** (e.g., believing that their spouse or partner is unfaithful).

Overvalued ideas A form of **abnormal belief**. These are ideas that may be reasonable and understandable in themselves but that come to unreasonably dominate the patient's life; if more bizarre the patient can rationalize that they are not true.

Panic attack Paroxysmal, severe **anxiety**. May occur in response to a particular stimulus or occur without apparent stimulus.

Paranoid delusion Strictly speaking this describes most types of delusion. It is, however, more commonly used as a synonym for **persecutory delusion**.

Paraphasia The substitution of an unintended sound, word, or phrase. Occurs in organic lesions affecting speech.

Passivity phenomena Synonym for **delusions of control**.

Persecutory delusion A delusional belief that one's life is being interfered with in a harmful way.

Perseveration Continuing with a verbal response or action that was initially appropriate after it ceases to be appropriate (e.g., "Do you know where you are?"—"In the hospital"; "Do you know what day it is?"—"In the hospital"). Associated with organic brain disease and is occasionally seen in schizophrenia.

Phobia A particular stimulus, event, or situation which arouses **anxiety** in an individual and is therefore associated with **avoidance**. The concept of "biological preparedness" is that some fears (e.g., of snakes, fire, heights) had evolutionary advantage and so it is easier to develop phobias for these stimuli than other, more evolutionarily recent threats (e.g., of guns or electric shock).

Phantom mirror image Synonym for **autoscopy**.

Pica The eating of things that are not food such as ice, dirt, clay, starch.

Positive symptoms (of psychosis) The symptoms of psychosis/schizophrenia that are qualitatively different from normal experience (e.g., **delusions**, **hallucinations**, **schizophrenic thought disorder**). Believed to be related to neurochemical abnormalities as well as alterations in limbic and associated neural networks.

Posturing The maintenance of bizarre and uncomfortable limb and body positions. Associated with psychotic illnesses and may have **delusional** significance to the patient.

Poverty of content Speech that conveys little information because it is vague or sparse.

Poverty of speech Less speech than is normal.

Poverty of thought Thought that conveys little information because of vagueness, repetitions, or obscure phrases.

Pressured speech The speech is rapid, difficult to interrupt, and, with increasing severity of illness, the connection between sequential ideas may become increasingly hard to follow. Occurs in manic illness.

Priapism A sustained and painful penile erection, not associated with sexual arousal. A rare side-effect of antidepressant medication. If not relieved can cause permanent penile damage.

Pseudocyesis A false pregnancy. May be hysterical or delusional in nature and can occur in both sexes although more commonly in women. The belief in the false pregnancy may be accompanied by abdominal distension, lumbar lordosis, and amenorrhea.

Pseudodementia The concept that severe depression in the elderly may be associated with cognitive impairments that mimic dementia. It was traditionally suggested that cognition would improve as depression lifts, however, recent studies suggest that some degree of cognitive impairment usually remains.

Pseudo-hallucination A false perception that is perceived as occurring as part of one's internal experience, not as part of the external world. They may be described as having an "as if" quality or as being seen with the "mind's eye." Additionally, true hallucinations may become perceived as pseudo-hallucinations after recovery. They can occur in all modalities of sensation and are described in psychotic, organic, and drug-induced conditions as well as occasionally in normal individuals. (The hallucinations of deceased spouses commonly described by widows and widowers may have the form of a pseudo-hallucination.)

Pseudologica fantastica The production of convincing false accounts, often with apparent sincere conviction. There may be a grandiose or over-exaggerated flavor to the accounts produced. A feature of Munchausen's disease.

Psychic anxiety See **anxiety**.

Psychogenic polydipsia Excessive fluid intake without organic cause.

Psychological dependence See **dependence**.

Psychological pillow A **motor symptom of psychosis/schizophrenia**. The patient holds their head several inches above the bed while lying and can maintain this uncomfortable position for prolonged periods of time.

Psychomotor agitation A combination of **psychic anxiety** and excess and purposeless motor activity. A symptom common to many mental illnesses and found in normal individuals in response to stress.

Psychomotor retardation Decreased spontaneous movement and slowness in instigating and completing voluntary movement. Usually associated with subjective sense of actions being more of an effort and with subjective retardation of thought. Occurs in moderate to severe depressive illness.

Physiological dependence See **dependence**.

Racing thoughts The subjective experience of one's thoughts occurring rapidly, each thought being associated with a wider range of consequent ideas than normal and with inability to remain on one idea for any length of time. Occurs in manic episodes, sometimes referred to as "pressure of thought".

Receptive dysphasia **Dysphasia** affecting the understanding of speech. There is impairment in understanding spoken commands and repeating back speech. There are also significant abnormalities in spontaneous speech with word substitutions, defects in grammar, and syntax and **neologisms**. The abnormal speech so produced is however fluent (compared to **expressive dysphasia**). Patients may be unconcerned by their deficits.

Reflex hallucination The experience of a real stimulus in one sensory modality triggering a hallucination in another.

Retrograde amnesia The period of **amnesia** between an event (e.g., head injury) and the last continuous memory before the event.

Rumination A **compulsion** to engage in repetitive, nonproductive phrases or ideas, sometimes of a pseudo-philosophical nature. Often described in mood disorders and anxiety.

"Running commentary" A type of third-person auditory **hallucination** that is a **first-rank symptom** of schizophrenia. The patient hears one or more voices providing a narrative of their current actions, "he's getting up…now he's going toward the window."

Russell sign Skin abrasions, small lacerations, and calluses on the dorsum of the hand overlying the metacarpophalangeal and interphalangeal joints found in patients with symptoms of bulimia. Caused by repeated contact between the incisors and the skin of the hand during self-induced vomiting.

Schizophasia Synonym for **word salad**.

Schizophrenic speech disorder This includes the abnormalities in the form of speech consequent upon **schizophrenic thought disorder**, and those abnormalities in the use of language characteristic of schizophrenia such as use of **neologisms** and **stock words/phrases**.

Schizophrenic thought disorder A group of abnormalities in the subjective description of the form of thought which occur in schizophrenia. They include: **loosening of associations**, **derailment**, **thought blocking**, **and fusion**.

Sensory aphasia Impairment of the ability to understand spoken or written words and further characterized by fluent but meaningless speech.

Sensory distortions Changes in the perceived intensity or quality of a real external stimulus. Associated with organic conditions and with drug ingestion or withdrawals. Examples include: hyperacusis (hearing sounds as abnormally loud), micropsia ("wrong end of the telescope effect," perceiving objects which are close as small and far away).

Somatization The experience of bodily symptoms with no sufficient, physical cause for them, with presumed psychological causation.

Somnolence An excessively drowsy state.

Splitting of perception Loss of the ability to simultaneously process complementary information in two modalities of sensation (e.g., sound and pictures on television). Rare symptom of schizophrenia.

Stereotypy A repetitive movement that is not goal directed (in contrast to **mannerism**). The action may have delusional significance to the patient. Seen in psychosis and schizophrenia.

Stock phrases/stock words Feature of **schizophrenic speech disorder**. The use of particular words and phrases more frequently than in normal speech and with a wider variety of meanings than normal.

Stupor Reduction of responsiveness where there is no impairment of consciousness. Functional stupor occurs in a variety of psychiatric illnesses. Organic stupor is caused by lesions in the midbrain (the "locked-in" syndrome).

Synesthesia A stimulus in one sensory modality is perceived in a fashion characteristic of an experience in another sensory modality (e.g., "tasting" sounds or "hearing" colors). Occurs in hallucinogenic drug intoxication and in epileptic states.

Taciturn Not inclined to talk or give information.

Tangentiality Producing answers that are only very indirectly related to the question asked by the examiner.

Tardive dyskinesia A movement disorder associated with long-term treatment with antipsychotic drugs (although it was described in psychotic patients before the use of these drugs in clinical practice). There is continuous involuntary movement of the tongue and lower face. More severe cases involve the upper face and have choreoathetoid movements of the limbs.

Teleological hallucination Synonym for **command hallucination**.

Terminal insomnia Synonym for **early morning waking**.

Third-person auditory hallucinations Auditory hallucinations characteristic of schizophrenia in which voices are heard referring to the patient as "he" or "she," rather than "you." The **first-rank symptoms** of **"voices heard arguing"** and **"running commentary"** are of this type.

Thought blocking A symptom of **schizophrenic thought disorder**. The patient experiences a sudden break in the chain of thought. It may be explained as due to **thought withdrawal**. In the absence of such **delusional elaboration** it is not a **first-rank symptom**.

Thought broadcasting The delusional belief that one's thoughts are accessible directly to others. A **first-rank symptom** of schizophrenia.

Thought disorder See **formal thought disorder**.

Thought echo The experience of an auditory **hallucination** in which the content is the individual's current thoughts. A **first-rank symptom** of schizophrenia. Also known as **echo de la pensée**.

Thought insertion The delusional belief that thoughts are being placed in the patient's head from outside. A **first-rank symptom** of schizophrenia.

Thought withdrawal The delusional belief that thoughts are being removed from the patient's head by an outside agency. A **first-rank symptom** of schizophrenia.

Tic An Involuntary sudden twitch of a single muscle or muscle group.

Trichotillomania The **compulsion** to pull one's hair out.

Visual agnosia The inability to recognize common objects by sight. Most cases of visual agnosia are brought about through cerebral vascular accidents or traumatic brain injury to the right posterior parietal lobe.

"Voices heard arguing" A type of auditory **hallucination** that is a **first-rank symptom** of schizophrenia. The patient hears two or more voices debating with one another, sometimes about a matter over which the patient is agonizing (e.g., "He should take the medication; it's worked before," "No, not again, he won't take it this time").

Waxy flexibility See **catalepsy**.

Wernicke's aphasia/dysphasia A type of **receptive phasia** due to cortical lesions in or near the posterior portion of the left first temporal convolution (superior temporal gyrus)—known as the Wernicke area.

Withdrawals The physical sequela of abstinence from a drug to which one is **dependent**. These are individual to the drug concerned (e.g., sweating, tachycardia, and tremor for alcohol; dilated pupils, piloerection, abdominal pain, and diarrhea for opiates).

Word salad The most severe degree of **schizophrenic thought disorder** in which no connection of any kind is understandable between sequential words and phrases the patient uses. Sometimes called **schizophasia**.

Xenophobia irrational fear of strangers or foreigners.

Zoophobia Irrational fear of animals.

Evidence-based psychiatry

What is evidence-based medicine (EBM)?

EBM is the integration of the best research evidence with clinical experience and patient values.

- Best research evidence means the studies most likely to yield an accurate and unbiased answer to a question we have about a particular patient or patient group.
- Clinical experience means the skills we have learned during our medical training (e.g., history taking, bedside examination) and also our ability to elicit our patients' preferences and goals.

EBM in Practice

In order to practice EBM we need to first appreciate that we do not always know all the answers to our clinical questions. Once that fact has been appreciated, the following five skills need to be mastered:

- The ability to ask a clinical question in a way that captures the essence of the problem, is structured, and is most likely to yield an answer.
- The ability to search for an answer (the evidence) to our question in a way that is most efficient.
- The ability to critically appraise the evidence.
- The ability to apply the evidence to the patient.
- The ability to monitor our own progress.

Asking clinical questions

There are generally two types of question we ask about patients: those that we ask them (fact-finding questions) and questions about diagnosis, cause (or harm), treatment, and prognosis (clinical questions). Consider the following patient scenario:

A 29-year-old woman is admitted to your inpatient unit six weeks postpartum complaining of hearing voices commenting on her actions and thoughts that her baby is evil. She has never sought help for psychiatric reasons before, although her mother has long-standing bipolar disorder and has had many admissions to your hospital previously. She does not wish to be admitted to the hospital.

Examples of fact-finding questions include

- Does she have any wish to harm her baby?
- Is there anyone at home who could provide support?
- Does she have any symptoms of affective disorder?
- Is there a history of drug abuse?

Examples of clinical questions include

Diagnosis
What is the likelihood that the diagnosis will be schizophrenia given she describes a first-rank symptom of schizophrenia (e.g., running commentary)?

Cause/Risk
Does a family history of bipolar disorder increase the risk of postpartum psychosis?

Treatment
Is it likely that this woman would benefit rapidly from the administration of ECT?

Prognosis
What are the chances that the woman will harm her baby?

The ability to tactfully ask fact-finding questions is something taught to us as medical undergraduates and postgraduates. There is no underlying structure to these questions and searching the literature will not provide an answer to questions specific to each individual.

Structuring good clinical research questions

Clinical research questions, unlike fact-finding questions, can more easily follow a standard format that is likely to clarify the question in your own mind. They may also suggest a suitable study type to address the question. This approach is more likely to yield an answer when researching a topic. The general form of a research question is as follows (PICO format):

P: The patient **problem to be addressed**. A description of the main characteristics of the patient problem.

I: The **intervention** or maneuver being considered (e.g., the treatment or diagnostic test being contemplated), or an exposure (e.g., smoking, high stress levels).

C: The intervention (e.g., treatment) is usually **compared** to placebo or standard therapy; diagnostic tests are usually **compared** to a gold standard. The gold standard test in psychiatry is usually a structured clinical history and examination (e.g., the Structured Clinical Interview for DSM-IV-TR, see 📖 p. 94 Chapter 2).

O: The **outcome of interest** (e.g., improvement in symptoms, accurate diagnosis, side-effects, etc.).

Searching for the evidence

After formulating the structured clinical question, the next step is to decide upon the study type best able to answer the question. Taking the example of a therapy question, the study types most likely to answer a question in such a way that minimizes bias are ranked as follows:

Hierarchy of evidence

- A systematic review of two or more randomized controlled trials (RCTs).
- A single randomized controlled trial.
- A quasi-experimental study without randomization.
- Observational studies (e.g., cohort and case control).
- Case reports and series.
- Expert opinion.

Wherever possible, a systematic review of RCTs should be sought because it is less liable to bias than the other studies further down the hierarchy. Many people, when asked, "Where would you look for a study to answer your question?" will often suggest, "A textbook" or "Medline." However, textbooks are possibly out of date and many doctors have not been trained to use Medline to its greatest effect.

Searching Medline (www.PubMed.gov) Medline can be searched by referring to the PICO structure, and by thinking about the hierarchy of evidence. For example, if we wish to ask our question, "In women with postpartum psychosis, does ECT lead to a more rapid improvement in symptoms compared to antipsychotic drug treatment?," we would search:

1: Postpartum psychosis
2: ECT
Click on the History tab.
3: 1 AND 2
4: random$ (this line will identify most RCTs in any subject)
5: 3 AND 4

Organization of Database

Medline is organized by subject headings, but we do not need to know the subject heading to search. Medline will automatically look up a thesaurus and use more effective terms than the ones we specify.

A note on PubMed clinical queries

The PubMed Web site has a feature called "clinical queries," which searches for articles of a specific design. For example, if you search for "schizophrenia" AND "cognitive behavior therapy" in the clinical queries section of PubMed, you could specify that you are only interested in systematic reviews.

Limitations of Medline

Unfortunately, Medline does not cover all the psychiatric literature. Further training on Medline is available on the PubMed Web site and your local librarian.

www.Embase.com is another search engine similar to Medline, which includes book chapters, published abstracts, and additional nursing references.

Other resources

Fortunately, although Medline is a useful source of research evidence, there are many other resources that can be useful:

- The Cochrane Library consists of several sections including the database of systematic reviews and the register of controlled trials. The database of systematic reviews is probably the single most useful source of systematic reviews on the topic of therapy, although does not consider other areas of medical practice such as diagnosis, prognosis, etc. The database of controlled trials is also probably the single most useful source of individual RCTs and is easy to use. The Cochrane Library is available through Wiley InterScience http://www3.interscience.wiley.com and through Ovid, http://www.ovid.com, also usually available through your local medical library.
- ACP Journal Club is a synoptic journal provided by the American College of Physicians. It publishes article summaries from more than 200 peer-reviewed medical journals and can be accessed through Ovid.
- PsycINFO The American Psychological Association publishes an on-line database of abstracts of relevance to psychiatry and psychology. Many journals not indexed on either Medline or Embase can be found here. Available through Ovid.
- APA Practice Guidelines, published on line by the American Psychiatric Association at http://psych.org/psych_pract/treatg/pg/prac_guide.cfm, are intended to assist psychiatrists in making clinical decisions. They combine different levels of evidence with expert opinion. Watches, an additional feature, provides literature updates to published guidelines.
- Other resources: There are many other Web sites that provide either biomedical databases or pre-appraised evidence of relevance to practicing clinicians. The tendency for these links to become inactive has prevented us from printing a list of them here, although an up-to-date list is kept on the Centre for Evidence-Based Mental Health Web site at www.cebmh.com.

Critical appraisal

Critical appraisal can help us decide if a published report is likely to be valid (i.e., the results are likely to be true) or important (i.e., contain results important for clinical practice). The decision to use the published evidence also takes into account our patients' preferences and goals. When embarking on the critical appraisal of an article, many people consider this an invitation to condemn the article. This approach does little to inform our management of patients and should be replaced with a more considered judgment of validity:

• Is the study performed so badly that it can be of no use whatsoever?
• Is the study flawed and what effects are the flaws likely to have upon the published results?

The critical appraisal of an article addresses two main areas: validity and importance, irrespective of the study type. However, the questions we should ask ourselves in order to address these two areas depend on the study type.

Questions to assess the validity of a systematic review
(📖 p. 130)

• Does the review address a clearly focused question?
• Does the review apply suitable quality criteria?
• Does the review search for all relevant articles?
• Are the results consistent from study to study?

Questions to assess the validity of a RCT (📖 p. 132)

• Were patients randomized to two or more treatments and was the allocation of patients to treatment concealed?
• Were patients and investigators blind to the intervention received?
• Were patients treated equally apart from the intervention of interest?
• Was follow-up sufficiently long and complete?
• Were dropouts accounted for and included in the final results?

Questions to assess the validity of a risk/etiology study
(see Case-control studies 📖 p. 136)

• Was the exposure measured objectively?
• Was the outcome measured objectively and blind to exposure status?
• Was follow-up sufficiently long and complete?
• Did the investigators take into account any potential confounders?

Questions to assess the validity of a diagnostic study
(📖 p. 139)

• Were the study patients similar to those on whom the test would be used in clinical practice?
• Were the test and gold standard applied blind to the results of the other?
• Were the test and the gold standard applied independently, each without reference to the other?

Questions to assess the validity of a prognosis study
(see Cohort studies 📖 p. 136)

- Was a representative group of patients assembled at a common, preferably early, point in their illness?
- Were patients followed up prospectively for a sufficiently long period?
- Was the outcome assessed objectively?
- Did the investigators correct for the presence of confounding variables?

Systematic reviews (SRs) of RCTs[1]

Formulation of questions and protocol

Questions should be precise. The research designs, characteristics of participants/interventions, and outcomes should be prespecified. Research designs likely to yield biased results should be excluded (e.g., RCT with inadequate concealment), or at least noted and the effects examined in detail.

Search for relevant articles

Search should be comprehensive and repeatable. Should include more than Medline, because it is more likely to catalog English language, positive studies while ignoring foreign language, negative studies. Consider gray literature (e.g., abstracts, personal communications) and unpublished articles.

Review of abstracts and retrieval of full text

Potentially relevant abstracts should be reviewed by more than two reviewers with a mechanism for resolving disagreements. The same applies to retrieved articles. Prespecified criteria are likely to improve reliability and repeatability.

Summary of included/excluded studies

Reasons for exclusion and inclusion should be given to allow scrutiny/repeatability.

Meta-analysis (statistical summary)

Study results should be combined statistically, weighted for precision. Key terms:

• The finding of heterogeneity means that results vary from study to study more than expected by chance alone.
• Fixed-effects analysis assumes that the data come from normal populations who differ in their means, but not in the measurement errors. It answers the question of whether the studies included in the meta-analysis show that the treatment or exposure produced the effect on average.
• Random-effects analysis is more complex. It answers the question whether, on the basis of the studies that are examined, it is possible to comment that the treatment or the exposure will produce a result.
• If there is significant heterogeneity among the results of the included studies, random effects analysis will give wider confidence intervals than fixed effect analysis.
• Publication bias: the tendency for certain studies to be published according to their results. Usually, positive results are more likely to be published. Measured using a funnel plot (see Fig. 4.1 opposite).
• Common statistical tests: χ^2 and Q tests for heterogeneity; Z test for overall effect.

1 Moher, D., Cook, D.J., Eastwood, S., Olkin, I., Rennie, D., Stroup, D.F. Improving the quality of reports of meta-analyses of randomised controlled trials: the QUOROM statement. Quality Reporting of Meta-Analyses. *Lancet* 1999; **354**, 1896–900.

- Effect size (ES) measures the strength of relationship between treatment/exposure and the outcome. For dichotomous data ES is often expressed through odds ratios or relative risks. For continuous data, mean difference is used for several studies using the same scales; Standardized ES (mean difference/pooled standard deviation) can be used for several studies using different scales—rescales the results using standard deviation of each scale allowing them to be combined (e.g., "Cohen's d" and others).

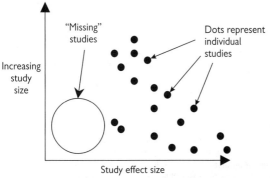

Fig. 4.1 Funnel plot showing how small negative studies appear "missing".

Randomized Controlled Trials[2]

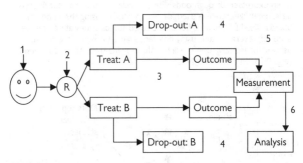

Fig. 4.2 Flow diagram of a RCT.

Appraisal criteria
Question
- What hypothesis was the trial designed to test?
- What were the primary and secondary outcome measures?

Selection of patients
- Generalizability/external validity: are the patients typical of those on whom the therapy will be used in practice?
- If not, should we expect that (a) the results will not apply at all or (b) there will be a smaller/greater effect in clinical practice?

Randomization
- Was the randomization method adequate? Computer-generated randomization by a third party at the point of entry into the trial is probably best.
- Would it be possible for patients/clinicians to guess, better than chance, the treatment to which they would eventually be allocated (allocation concealment)?
- Has randomization succeeded in forming two groups with similar baseline characteristics? Methods of ensuring this are: minimization (allocate patients to minimize overall differences on all prognostic factors) and stratification (stratify randomization by each important prognostic factor).

Interventions
- What interventions were intended for each group, and how and when were they actually administered?
- Were patients/clinicians/investigators/statisticians "blind" to the treatment. Note: There is no universally accepted meaning of *blind*; authors should explain what they mean.

2 Moher, D., Schulz, K.F., Altman, D. The CONSORT statement: revised recommendations for improving the quality of reports of parallel-group randomized trials. *JAMA*. Apr 18 2001; **285**(15), 1987–1991.

Participant flow

- How many patients were recruited, randomly assigned, received intended treatment, completed the study protocol, and were analyzed for the primary outcome? A flowchart should show these numbers.

Dropout

- Was the number of dropouts in both arms of the trial unequal (differential attrition) or greater than 10–20%? If so, even if the analysis takes this into account, the trial may be biased either toward or against the true effect size.

Analysis

- Were all patients analyzed in the groups to which they were randomized? (Intention-to-treat analysis.) If not, ignoring dropouts (completer only analysis) may overestimate effects of treatment. Methods of intention to treat include:
  - Last observation carried forward (assume no change in a score).
  - Worst-case scenario (assume dropouts in active arm have negative outcomes and dropouts in control arm have positive ones).
  - Mean imputation (assume dropout was average for this group).
  - Multiple imputations (model mean and variance, taking into account characteristics of the dropout).

Results

- If results (📖 p. 134) are presented as means, typically mean differences are shown, with a t-test or ANOVA and 95% confidence interval.
- If results are "time to an event", then a Kaplan-Maier curve (survival curve) may be shown with the results of a survival analysis (Log rank test, Cox proportional hazards).
- Often the results are shown as a proportion of people with a good or bad event in both groups (p1 and p2).

Effect Potency

- Is the effect large enough to be relevant in clinical practice? The number needed to treat (NNT) is given by $1/(p1-p2)$— 📖 p. 134.

Results of RCTs

Relative risk, absolute risk, and the number needed to treat

An important value to calculate from RCTs is the number needed to treat (NNT). The NNT arose because of limitations with the terms relative risk (RR) and absolute risk reduction (ARR).

Imagine you have an intervention for schizophrenia, Nopixol. You locate a trial in Medline, which finds the following results:

200 people with schizophrenia were randomized to placebo or Nopixol. Of the 120 people who received Nopixol, 30 relapsed by 6 weeks; of the 80 who were randomized to placebo, 60 relapsed over the same time. A 2x2 table helps to clarify the numbers:

	Relapse	No relapse	
Nopixol	30	90	120
Placebo	60	20	80

- The risk or probability of relapse in the Nopixol group is 30/120 or 0.25. This is called the experimental event rate (EER).
- The risk or probability of relapse in the placebo group is 60/80 or 0.75. This is called the control event rate (CER).
- The relative risk (RR) is the EER/CER = 0.25/0.75, which is 0.33. This means the risk of relapse on Nopixol is 0.33 times the risk on placebo. Another way of saying this would be to say that the relative risk of relapse is reduced by 67% on Nopixol. It is sometimes called the relative risk reduction (RRR). This is usually not a good measure of clinical usefulness because if relapse was 100 times less common in both groups, the RR and RRR would stay the same. This would not reflect the fact that clinically the treatment effect had diminished considerably.
- The absolute risk reduction (ARR) is the CER − EER = 0.75−0.25, which is 0.5. This means that for every person treated with Nopixol, the risk of relapse is reduced by about 50%.
- If the risk for each person is reduced by 50% by Nopixol instead of placebo, then it's intuitive that we need to treat two people to prevent, on average, one relapse. This is called the NNT. More generally, the NNT is equal to 1/ARR, or 1/0.5. In this case, the NNT = 2.

Moderators

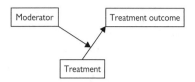

Moderators specify for whom or under what conditions the treatment works. For example, the magnitude of benefit from long-term antidepressant treatment is less in older depressed patients with more severe concomitant medical illnesses. Thus, medical illness is a moderator of the antidepressant treatment effect. This is different from a simple risk factor, which leads to poorer outcomes with both active treatment and control.

Mediators

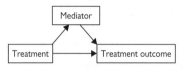

Mediators are possible mechanisms through which a treatment might achieve its effects. For example, CBT for panic disorder succeeds by eliminating catastrophic cognitions concerning the bodily changes.

Recommended further reading

For an easy-to-read guide to risk factor research, see Kraemer HC, Lowe KK, Kupfer DJ *To your health. How to understand what research tells us about risk.* Oxford University Press, 2005.

Cohort studies[1]

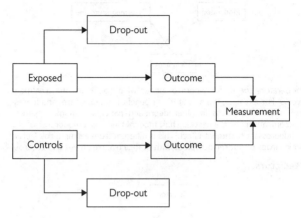

Fig. 4.3 Flow diagram of a cohort study.

Appraisal criteria
Exposure1
The exposure should be clearly defined and may be stratified into levels of increasing "dose." The controls should not be exposed but should be similar to the exposed group. Bias will be introduced if controls differ in many ways apart from the exposure (e.g., drug users differ from non-drug users in many respects: employment, criminal record, etc.).

Drop-out
Drop-outs are virtually inevitable. The effects may bias the results, especially if dropouts are over 20% or if they are unequal. Some studies minimize attrition by consulting several sources, sending reminders, consulting government statistics (e.g., records of hospital admissions), and other methods of tracking people.

Measurement
Measurement should be conducted objectively and blind to exposure status. In practice this is sometimes difficult.

Retrospective/prospective
Exposure may be ascertained from case notes (retrospectively) or at interview (prospectively). Cohort studies often have retrospective and prospective components.

Analysis
$P_{a,b}$—proportion in group a or b who have the outcome, then
P_a-P_b = absolute risk, p_a/p_b = relative risk, NNT = 1/absolute risk If results are "time to an event," then a survival analysis may be conducted.

Correction for confounding variables is usually accomplished using ANCOVA, linear regression (outcomes measured on a scale), or logistic regression (where the outcome is an event).

Recommended further reading

1 Fleiss JL: The Design and Analysis of Clinical Experiments. New York, NY. John Wiley & Sons, Inc, 1999.

Comparing ways of measuring the importance of an intervention

There are many ways in which the benefit of an intervention can be measured. Cynically, one might expect the authors of an article to present the method that shows their intervention in the best light, so the reader will need to be aware of the main methods by which the utility of an intervention can be measured and their consequent strengths and limitations.

Method	Explanation	Advantages	Disadvantages
Treatment benefit			
P-value	Gives the probability that the observed difference between the treatments is due to chance.	Provides a clear test of an investigator's hypothesis and is provided with all major statistical packages.	Clinically insignificant treatments may still be statistically significant. Gives little indication of precision.
Relative risk	Gives the risk of an event in one group divided by the risk in the other group.	Provides a clear indication of how many times better or worse a treatment is compared to another.	May mislead when outcomes are rare. (e.g., a relative risk of 10 would be unimpressive if the event occurred only once in 10,000 patients)
Absolute risk	Gives the risk of an event in one group minus the risk in the other group.	Provides a clearer indication of clinical significance.	The figure in itself may not seem very meaningful either to clinicians or patients. Takes appropriate account of baseline risk.
Number needed to treat (NNT)	States the number of patients required to be treated with the experimental intervention in order to prevent one additional adverse outcome	Relatively intuitive. Provides a clear indication of how much therapeutic effort is required to bring about one additional "good" outcome.	In spite of obvious advantages, has not come into universal use. NNTs published in meta-analyses may be misleading unless the patients included in the primary studies are very like your own.

Note: Confidence intervals are a welcome addition to any published figure about treatment benefit because they convey information about precision and statistical significance.

Diagnostic studies[1]

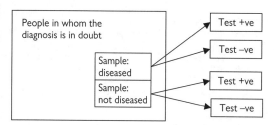

Fig. 4.4 Flow diagram of a diagnostic study.

Appraisal criteria

Sample
- Did the sample consist of people in whom the diagnosis was in doubt and in whom the test would be used in practice?

Gold standard
- Was a suitable gold standard applied regardless of the test results?

Test
- Was the test applied blindly without knowledge of the results of the gold standard and vice versa?

Reliability
- Could the diagnostic test be applied reliably over time or between raters?

Diagnostic test performance
- What are the sensitivity and specificity? They are less useful clinically than the positive and negative predictive values (PPV and NPV). See 📖 p. 140.
- What are the PPV and NPV? These are useful when you have a test result and you want to know its meaning. See 📖 p. 140.

Recommended further reading
1 Fleiss, J.L. The Design and Analysis of Clinical Experiments. New York: John Wiley & Sons, Inc, 1999.

Ways of measuring diagnostic utility

Ways of measuring diagnostic utility

Method	Explanation	Advantages	Disadvantages
Sensitivity	Measures the proportion of people with a disorder correctly classified by a test. When sensitivity is very high, a negative test will tend to rule out the disorder (SnNOut).	Easily calculated and intuitive. Usually supplied in published papers. Does not depend on prevalence.	Not very useful in clinical practice unless very high.
Specificity	Measures the proportion of people *without* a disorder correctly classified by a test. When specificity is very high, a positive test will tend to *rule in* the disorder (SpPIn).	Easily calculated and intuitive. Usually supplied in published papers. Does not depend on prevalence	Not very useful in clinical practice unless very high.
Positive predictive value	Measures the proportion of people with a positive test result who actually have the disorder	Clinically useful. Easy to understand and communicate to colleagues and patients.	Tend to fall as the prevalence of the disorder falls. May mislead if the prevalence of the disorder in your practice is lower than that of the study
Likelihood ratio for a positive test	A ratio of the probability of a positive test coming from someone with the disorder compared to one without the disorder.	Does not depend on the prevalence. Can be adapted to a variety of other situations	More difficult to calculate than the above. May not seen intuitively very meaningful

Calculating useful values:
Diagnostic test
Target disorder

	Present	Absent
positive	a	b
negative	c	d

Sensitivity = a/(a + c)   Positive predictive value (PPV) = a/(a + c)
Specificity = d/(b + d)   Negative predictive value (NPV) = d/(c + d)
Likelihood ratio for a positive test = Sensitivity/(1 − Specificity)
Likelihood ratio for a negative test = (1 − Sensitivity)/Specificity

Note: Further details on how to calculate these values are provided in several texts[1] and on a number of Web sites[2]

Recommended further reading

1 Lawrie, S.M., McIntosh, A.M., Rao, S. (2000). Critical Appraisal for Psychiatry. Churchill Livingstone.
2 www.cebm.net.

Qualitative studies[1]

Purpose

Qualitative studies are usually used to measure beliefs or attitudes in situations in which quantitative research would be less meaningful or impractical. Results are usually presented as text without numbers or figures in a way that is intended to preserve the richness of the data in its rightful context. For example, the question, "What are the attitudes of patients with borderline personality disorder to their diagnosis?" might be answered better by describing what the patients actually said than by performing a survey and summarizing attitudes on a scale with medians and interquartile ranges.

Appraisal criteria

Clear question

Like all studies, the research should address a clear topic or question. Unlike quantitative research, hypotheses may emerge in the course of the study and be tested out.

Patient selection

Unlike quantitative research, which should address a representative sample, qualitative researchers often purposely sample patients in order to obtain typical or exemplar cases.

Information gathering

The gathering and analysis of information is not standardized. Therefore, the study should describe exactly how this was performed.

Material engagement

- Did investigators make contact with their subject material?
- Did they check reactions?
- Did investigators seek non-confirming data?

Iteration

- Did investigators cyclically develop hypotheses and then test them with their sample?

Grounding

- Were there systematic ways of linking observations with interpretations?

Disclosure of investigators' prejudice

- Did investigators examine their own attitudes/beliefs/values/ preconceptions as they embarked on the study?

Coherence

- Are the results coherent?
- Was the interpretation internally consistent?

Testimonial validity

- Did the study subjects agree with the investigator's interpretations?

Reflexive validity
- Did the observations change the investigator's understanding of theory?

Catalytic validity
- Did the investigator reorient, focus, and energize participants?

Triangulation
- Was there an attempt to confirm the investigators using another method (e.g., by obtaining another sample or by observation of the same sample using a different method)?

Recommended further reading

1 Taylor, Steven J. and Bogden, Robert. *Introduction to Qualitative Research Methods*, New York: Wiley, 1998.

Economic studies

Types of studies
Cost analysis
Costs only.

Effectiveness analysis
Consequences only.

Economic analyses
Costs and consequences of ≥2 interventions.

Types of analyses
Consequences equal
Cost minimization analysis (find cheapest intervention).

Consequences unequal
Outcomes measured in same natural units (e.g., rating scales or admission/readmissions) = cost effectiveness analysis.

If consequences unequal, and benefits measured in different units (e.g., comparing CBT for schizophrenia with ECT for depression) then convert consequences:
• to monetary units = cost-benefit analysis, or
• to patient preferences = cost-utility analysis.

Costs and perspective
Costs should be considered from a broad perspective. Interventions, which appear to be less expensive and equally effective at a hospital level, may shift costs to other areas (e.g., social work, criminal justice system), which were not apparent because of too narrow a perspective.

Direct costs
Salaries, drugs, buildings, etc.

Indirect costs
Gains/losses in productivity.

Intangible costs
E.g., cost of improved health.

Incremental cost
Cost of each additional unit of production.

Opportunity cost
Benefits forgone by using capital to provide one intervention over another (a concept of economic analyses rather than an actual cost).

Discounting
In order to take into account (1) the preference to pay for things later rather than sooner and (2) the devaluation in currency over time, future costs should be discounted so they appear at current prices. Occasionally economists argue that future consequences should also be discounted.

Consequences

The consequences of an intervention should be measured alongside the study used to measure costs (usually a clinical trial). The more rigorous the study design (SRs > RCTs > CTs) and the more valid, the more likely the results of the economic analysis are to be true.

Dominance

If one intervention is more effective and cheaper than an alternative, then choice is easy. In all other situations, consider the incremental cost-effectiveness ratio:

Incremental cost-effectiveness ratio:

$$(ICER) = \frac{\text{Differences in costs}}{\text{Differences in consequences}}$$

For example, an intervention causing 2 extra remissions in schizophrenia at an extra cost of $100,000 has an ICER of $50,000 per additional remission. ICER gives a measure of the extra cost for each additional unit of benefit. There's no cutoff; the ICER should help compare different interventions and come to a decision. Nonparametric statistics are used to give p-values and 95% confidence intervals for the ICER (randomization tests, Monte-Carlo analyses).

Sensitivity analysis

Economic analyses make assumptions about costs and consequences of different treatments. To test the robustness of an economic analysis, estimated benefits and costs can be varied one at a time or simultaneously to see if they alter the results of the analysis:

- One-way (one variable at a time).
- Extreme case (alter a variable to the extremes of its plausible range).
- Multiway (vary 2 or more variables simultaneously).
- Monte-Carlo analyses are a way of varying several parameters simultaneously without assuming normality.

Applying the evidence to patients

Having found valid and important new evidence about a particular problem, a couple of further question need to be asked:

- What is the likely benefit for my patient?
- Does my patient actually want it?

Treatment

Chronic intractable conditions and mild and very benign conditions may fail to show the benefits of therapy demonstrated in clinical trials because the patient's baseline risk differs from those patients initially randomized.

In either situation, it is possible simply to guess what the likely benefit for your patient will be, or one of several numerical methods may be used instead. The simplest numerical method involves an educated guess about how likely your patient is to benefit compared to the average patient in the trial. If your patient is half as likely to benefit, then the NNT from the trial is doubled. Other techniques are available that are both more accurate and more time consuming.[1]

Finally, the decision to start a new treatment depends on other things apart from efficacy. Firstly, and most importantly, your patient may actually not want it because of undue side-effects or perhaps the regime (e.g., thrice-daily dosing) may be excessively inconvenient for them.

As well as potential harms, the decision to adopt a treatment or service at a health service level may also take account of economic evaluations.
Note: Guard against drug company information!

Although drug representatives will extol the virtues of their medication over the competition, often on the basis of efficacy, little evidence exists to suggest, for example, that one antipsychotic is more effective than another.[2,3] Although doctors do not feel pharmaceutical representatives influence them, this is in contradiction to the best available evidence on the subject.

Diagnosis

Diagnostic tests shown to be effective in a research setting may be of little utility in your clinical practice for two main reasons.

Firstly, the prevalence of the condition may be different in your setting. If the prevalence of the condition is lower in your setting, the PPV will be lower, although negative result will actually be more likely to indicate an absence of the condition.

Secondly, the test itself may be too costly in terms of the financial, staff, and training resources required to administer it. Patients' values and expectations may also be very important in the context of a disease for which there is no effective intervention (e.g., Huntington's disease) or where the diagnostic test is itself harmful or unpleasant.

1 Lawrie, S.M., McIntosh, A.M., Rao, S. *Critical Appraisal for Psychiatry.* Edinburgh: Churchill Livingstone, 2000.
2 Geddes, J., Freemantle, N., Harrison, P., Bebbington, P. (2000). Atypical antipsychotics in the treatment of schizophrenia: systematic overview and meta-regression analysis. *BMJ* **321**, 1371–1376.
3 Stroup, T.S., Lieberman, J.A., McEvoy, J.P. *et al.* (2006). Effectiveness of olanzapine, quetiapine, risperidone and ziprasidone in patients with chronic schizophrenia following discontinuation of a previous atypical antipsychotic. *Am J Psychiatry* **163**(4): 611–22.

Objections to EBM

Case against EBM	Answer to criticism
It denigrates clinical experience.	EBM is the integration of the best available evidence with clinical expertise and patient values. Both are necessary for EBM.
It is "cookbook" medicine.	EBM takes into account our individual patient's likely risk/benefit, goals, and preferences.
It is a cost-cutting tool.	EBM has been used by governments and other organizations to cut costs/ resources. In most cases this has nothing to do with the original meaning of EBM, which can result in increased costs as well as efficiency savings.
It is based on patients in clinical trials who are very unlike patients in practice.	This is true of published clinical research in general. This should prompt us to conduct pragmatic, large trials that mirror actual clinical practice more closely than ever.[3]
Evidence-based mental health (EBMH) often attracts an additional criticism: Psychiatric patients are unique and their problems cannot be reduced into neat categories.	The truth is all people are unique and we must separate those characteristics patients share with other patients (i.e., diagnoses) from those that are common to all patients and those that are unique to an individual. Medicine, and psychiatry, can learn nothing without imposing an organization (e.g., diagnoses or dimensions). However, the practice of psychiatry must take into account individual preferences/goals as much as any other field of medicine.

Organic illness in psychiatry

Presentations of organic illness

All psychiatric illnesses are by their nature "organic"—that is, they involve abnormalities of normal brain structure or function. The term "organic illness" in modern psychiatric classification, however, refers to those conditions with demonstrable etiology in CNS pathology. Organic disorders related to substance misuse are dealt with in Chapter 15 📖 p. 615. This chapter deals with those disorders that are caused by traumatic, inflammatory, degenerative, infective, and metabolic conditions.

Many psychiatric syndromes can have an organic etiology. For this reason, every patient who presents with psychiatric symptomatology requires a thorough physical examination (in most cases including neurological examination and special investigations) before a somatoform disorder diagnosis is made. Although psychiatrists do not have to be expert neurologists, a sound knowledge of those conditions that bridge neurology and psychiatry is essential. Historically, these disciplines have not always been separated and, in this era of biological psychiatry, they are once again converging as increasing evidence emerges of brain dysfunction underlying most psychiatric disorders. Having said this, it is important to remember that biological, psychological, and social factors interact in a dynamic process in the generation of psychiatric symptoms.

Below are listed common organic causes of psychiatric syndromes (delirium, dementia, and amnestic disorders are discussed later).

Organic causes of psychosis

- Neurological (epilepsy; head injury; brain tumor; dementia; encephalitis e.g., herepes simplex virus [HSV], human immunodeficiency virus [HIV]; neurosyphilis; brain abscess; cerebrovascular accident [CVA]; Wilson's Disease).
- Endocrine (hyper/hypothyroidism; Cushing's; hyperparathyroidism; Addison's disease).
- Metabolic (uremia; sodium imbalance; porphyria).
- Systemic lupus erythematosus (SLE; "lupus psychosis").
- Medications (steroids; L-dopa; isoniazid [INH]; anticholinergics; antihypertensives; anticonvulsants; stimulants).
- Drugs of abuse (cocaine; lysergic acid diethylamide [LSD]; cannabis; phencyclidine [PCP]; amphetamines; opioids; ecstasy, mescaline, psilocybin).
- Toxins.

Organic causes of depression

- Neurological (CVA; epilepsy; Parkinson's disease; brain tumor; dementia; multiple sclerosis [MS]; Huntington's disease; head injury).
- Infectious (HIV; Epstein-Barr virus [EBV]/infectious mononucleosis; brucellosis).
- Endocrine and metabolic (hypothyroidism; Cushing's; Addison's disease; parathyroid disease; vitamin deficiency [B_{12} and folate]; porphyria).
- Cardiac disease (myocardial infarction [MI]; chronic heart failure [CHF]).
- Autoimmune disorders (SLE; Rheumatoid arthritis).

- Cancer.
- Medications (alpha-interferon; isotretinoin; estrogen/progesterone; statins; H2 receptor antagonists, e.g., cimetidine; analgesics, especially narcotics; antihypertensives; L-dopa; anticonvulsants, especially barbiturates; antibiotics e.g., cycloserine; acyclovir; metronidazole; steroids; oral contraceptive pills [OCP]; metoclopramide; salbutamol; disulfiram; cytotoxins).
- Drugs of abuse (alcohol; benzodiazepines; cannabis; cocaine; opioids; ecstasy).
- Toxins.

Organic causes of mania

- Neurological (CVA; epilepsy; brain tumor; head injury; MS).
- Endocrine (hyperthyroidism).
- Medications (isoniazid; levodopa; anticholinergics; cyclosproin; levothyroxine; cimetidine; yohimbine; steroids; antidepressants; mefloquine; cytotoxics).
- Drugs of abuse (cannabis; cocaine; amphetamines).
- Toxins.

Organic causes of anxiety

- Neurological (epilepsy; dementia; head injury; CVA; brain tumor; MS; Parkinson's disease).
- Endocrine (hyperthyroidism, hypercortisolemia, pheochromocytoma).
- Pulmonary (chronic obstructive pulmonary disease [COPD]).
- Cardiac (arrhythmias; CHF; angina; mitral valve prolapse).
- Infections (pediatric autoimmune neuropsychiatric disorders associated with streptococcal infections (PANDAS)).
- Medications (levodopa; theophylline; albuterol, salmetrol; caffeine; decongestants (e.g., phenylphrine); levothyroxine; steroids; antidepressants; antihypertensives; flumazenil; yohimbine; fenfluramine).
- Drugs of abuse (alcohol; benzodiazepines; caffeine; cannabis; cocaine; LSD; ecstasy; amphetamines; ecstasy).

Dementia—general overview

Dementia is a syndrome of irreversible, global cognitive deficit. The DSM-IV-TR criteria for dementia are modeled after "cortical dementia" (e.g., Alzheimer's disease) in which memory impairment (especially short-term memory) is the earliest and most prominent cognitive deficit with subsequent appearance of impairment in other cognitive domains.

However, this definition may not describe all dementias (e.g., "subcortical" dementias, such as Parkinson's Dementia, where memory impairment is a later symptom). Although many dementias are progressive, this is not an essential element of the diagnosis (e.g., cognitive deficits can be stable in dementia due to traumatic brain injury). For a diagnosis of dementia to be made, there must be significant and new impairment of normal functioning. Other possible diagnoses (see differential diagnosis below), particularly delirium or depression, must be excluded. The goal of the diagnostic assessment is to identify potential etiologies and treatments for the dementia, and correct any "reversible" causes of dementia.

The various etiologies of dementia are still being researched, but are commonly listed as follows:

- Alzheimer's disease (55%),
- vascular dementia (20%),
- general medical condition + substance-induced persisting disorders (10%),
- reversible causes (15%), including subdural hematoma; NPH; vitamin B_{12} deficiency; metabolic causes; hypothyroidism.

Expanded etiology of dementia

Parenchymal/degenerative
Alzheimer's disease; Pick's disease; Parkinson's disease; Huntington's disease; Wilson's disease; MS; motor neurone disease [MND]; Lewy Body disease; progressive supranuclear palsy.

Intracranial
Tumor; head trauma; subdural hematoma; CVA; normal pressure hydrocephalus (NPH).

Infection
Creutzfeldt-Jakob disease (prion disease); neurosyphilis; HIV-associated dementia; tuberculosis [TB].

Endocrine
Hypothyroidism; hyperparathyroidism; Cushing's and Addison's diseases.

Vitamin deficiency
B_{12}, folate, pellagra (niacin), thiamine.

Toxins
Alcohol; heavy metal poisoning (e.g., mercury).

Non-cognitive clinical features (see Clinical syndromes, 📖 p. 154)
- Personality change, social withdrawal, apathy, lability of affect, disinhibition, "silliness," diminished self-care, fatigue.
- Hallucinations and delusions often paranoid (20–40%) and poorly systematized.
- Anxiety and/or depression in 50%.
- Neurological features (e.g., seizures, focal deficits, primitive reflexes, pseudobulbar palsy, long-tract signs).
- See Catastrophic reaction, 📖 p. 178.
- Pseudobulbar palsy (emotional incontinence).
- Sundowning—increased confusion and agitation as evening approaches.
- Agitation and aggression.

Differential diagnosis includes
- Delirium.
- Depression (pseudodementia 📖 p. 586).
- Amnestic syndromes (📖 p. 174).
- Mental retardation.
- Psychotic disorders.
- Normal ageing (📖 p. 578).

Medical work up may include: CBC; lytes; calcium; magnesium; phosphate; BUN/Creatinine; glucose; LFT; UA; ESR; TSH; RPR; HIV; vitamin B_{12} and folate; blood culture; LP; EEG; CXR; ECG; CT; MRI; SPECT.

Principles of management

Assessment
To make diagnosis and to address functional and social issues.

Cognitive enhancement
Acetylcholinesterase inhibitors; NMDA-receptor partial antagonist.

Treat psychosis/agitation
Antipsychotics (low dose atypical agents preferable).

Treat depression/insomnia
SSRIs; hypnotics.

Treat medical illness and address cerebrovascular risk factors

Avoid medications that may increase confusion
For example; benzodiazepines, anticholinergic medications.

Psychological support and illness education for caregivers

Functional management
Maximize mobility; encourage independence with self-care, toilet, and feeding; assist with communication.

Social management
Supportive housing; activities; financial matters; legal matters (power of attorney, wills, and guardianship).

Clinical syndromes of dementia

Clinical syndromes of dementia

Dementias may be classified in terms of primary site of pathology. Since site of pathology in the brain correlates with cognitive impairments and, to some extent neuropsychiatric symptomatology, this is a useful system of classification.

1. Cortical dementias involve primarily the cortex and are divided into:

- Frontotemporal dementia/ Pick's disease (20%) (📖 p. 168); NPH and motor neurone disorders (MND) (70%) (📖 p. 176). Characterized by prominent personality change, which may manifest as a frontal lobe syndrome. A common cause of early-onset dementia, it is often undiagnosed. Language impairments tend to involve reduction in content (semantic anomia). CT shows frontotemporal (FT) atrophy and SPECT shows decreased FT metabolism.
- Posterior-parietal Alzheimer's disease (📖 p. 157). Characterized by early memory loss and focal cognitive deficits. Personality changes are later manifestations. Language impairments initially involve problems with word-finding (lexical anomia).

2. Subcortical dementias Parkinson's disease (📖 p. 198); Huntington's disease (📖 p. 200); Wilson's disease (📖 p. 201); Binswanger encephalopathy (📖 p. 170); PSNP (📖 p. 196); HIV-associated dementia (📖 p. 186); NPH (📖 p. 176). Clinical features: gross psychomotor slowing; depressed mood; movement disorders; impairment in executive function and attention/working memory >> amnesia; personality changes.

3. Cortical-subcortical dementias e.g., Lewy Body dementia (📖 p. 164). Clinical features: mixed cortical and subcortical symptoms.

4. Multifocal dementias e.g., CJD (📖 p. 172). Clinical features: rapid onset and course; involves cerebellum and subcortical structures.

Alzheimer's disease (1)

Also termed "dementia of the Alzheimer type" (AD),[1] this is the most common cause (70%) of dementia in older people. It is a degenerative disease of the brain with prominent cognitive and behavioral impairment that is sufficiently severe to interfere significantly with social and occupational function. It affects approximately 4.5 million people in the United States and more than 30 million worldwide. As the percentage of the total population aged over 65 is increasing in the developed world, the burden of AD-related health care is likely to increase.

Epidemiology

Lifetime risk for general population is 10–15%. 10% of cases have onset <60 years old. Risk factors for early onset include genetics (presenilin 1 and 2, APP) and Down syndrome. 90% of cases have onset ≥60 years old. Risk of AD increases with age: 1% at age 60 years; doubles every 5 years; ~50% of those aged 85 years. Risk factors for late onset include:

- apolipoprotein E4 (APOE4) gene,
- previous head injury,
- hypothyroidism,
- family or personal history of Down syndrome,
- Parkinson's disease, or AD.

Possible protective factors include NSAIDs, higher level of premorbid education.

Pathophysiology

Amyloid plaques

Insoluble β-amyloid peptide deposits as senile plaques or "β-pleated sheets" in the hippocampus, amygdala, and cerebral cortex. Increased density with advanced disease.

Neurofibrillary tangles (NFTs)

Consist of phosphorylated Tau protein and are found in the cortex, hippocampus, and substantia nigra. (NFTs also found in normal aging, Down syndrome, dementia pugilistica, and progressive supranuclear palsy). However, even low densities of NFTs in the cortices of the medial temporal lobes should be considered abnormal.

The co-occurrence of amyloid plaques and NFTs was described by Alois Alzheimer in his original description of the disorder and now is accepted universally as a hallmark of the disease.

Up to 50% loss of neurons and synapses in the cortex and hippocampus

Genetics

40% have a positive family history of AD (especially early onset).

Early Onset Illness associated genes: Responsible for 10% of cases

- Chromosome 21—the gene for amyloid precursor protein (APP) is found on the long arm. Also implicated in Down syndrome.
- Chromosome 14—codes for presenilin 1 (implicated in β-amyloid peptide).
- Chromosome 1—codes for presenilin 2 (implicated in β-amyloid peptide).

Late Onset Illness associated genes
- Chromosome 19—codes for APOE4. Confers risk of disease and earlier age of onset. One E4 allele increases risk of AD by 3x; two E4 alleles by 9x. However, 60% of cases with no E4 alleles.

Cholinergic hypothesis
The pathological changes lead to degeneration of cholinergic nuclei in the basal forebrain (nucleus basalis of Meynert). This results in reduced cortical acetylcholine (ACh).

Recommended further reading

1 Kuljis, R.O. (2002). www.emedicine.com

Alzheimer's disease (2)

Clinical features

Profile of cognitive impairment is reflected in the DSM-IV-TR. The diagnostic work group of the National Institute of Neurological and Communication Disorders and Stroke (NINCIDS) have elaborated more specific criteria. Symptoms are insidious in onset; patient and families usually do not seek evaluation until a notable events occurs (e.g., patient cannot find car in a parking lot, patient becomes a victim of elder abuse).

- Earliest cognitive impairment is impaired short-term memory secondary to impaired encoding of information. Over time, retrieval is also affected and patient loses long-term memory.
- Aphasia follows later and typically involves both receptive and expressive problems. The patient may exhibit lexical anomia (word-finding difficulty) early in disease course.
- Disorientation is common, especially for time.
- Other focal cognitive deficits include apraxia (inability to carry out motor functions despite intact motor system, e.g., does not know how to dress, use stove, tie shoes); and agnosia (inability to recognize objects despite intact sensory function, e.g., no longer can recognize objects). Occasionally, a patient may present with Gerstmann syndrome, indicating right parietal disease, characterized by finger agnosia, R/L disorientation, acalculia, and dysgraphia.
- Impaired visuospatial skills and executive function are common.
- Spastic paraparesis is an unusual feature in late onset disease.
- Neuropsychiatric symptoms: Predict more rapid cognitive decline; leads to greater burden on the caregiver.
  - Delusions usually of a paranoid nature; 20% in mild AD, >40% in severe disease.
  - Auditory and/or visual hallucinations (which may be simple misidentification); ~20% in mild/moderate AD; >40% in severe AD.
  - Depression affects 30% patients across all stages.
  - Anxiety present in >20%.
  - Apathy affects ~20% in mild AD, ~40% in severe AD.
  - Other behavioral disturbances include aggression, wandering (20–40%), irritable (>30%), disinhibition (>30%), incontinence, excessive eating, and searching behavior.
  - Personality change often reflects an exaggeration of premorbid traits with coarsening of affect and egocentricity.

Clinical Stages

- Predementia phase referred to as "mild cognitive impairment."
- Mild AD characterized by mild short-term memory loss; word finding difficulties; repetitive questioning; loss of hobbies, other interests; impaired ADLs (e.g., managing finances).
- Moderate AD involves progression of cognitive impairment; aphasia; dysexecutive syndrome; impaired basic ADLs (e.g., bathing); patient requires assistance and supervision.
- Severe AD characterized by agitation; altered sleep patterns; major assistance required for basic ADLs.

- Profound/Very Severe AD is characterized by bedbound state; no speech: incontinent; loss of basic psychomotor skills.
- Average 8 years (range 1–20 years) from diagnosis to death.

DSM-IV-TR Criteria for Dementia of the Alzheimer's Type[1]

- Memory Impairment.
- At least one additional cognitive impairment: Aphasia; Apraxia; Agnosia, Executive Functioning.
- Cognitive impairments lead to significant impairment in social or occupational functioning AND represent a decline from previous level of functioning.
- Typically gradual onset with progressive cognitive decline.
- Other causes (medical and neurological disorders or substance abuse) are not present.
- Not better accounted for by delirium or other psychiatric disorder.

Investigations

Diagnosis is based on clinical presentation and the exclusion of other causes of dementia.

- Mental state examination: Search for evidence supporting dementia versus another diagnosis (e.g., delirium, symptoms of depression, psychosis, etc.).
- Cognitive testing is essential and may begin with a mini mental state examination (MMSE) (p. 82), but later involve specific neuropsychological testing.
- Physical examination: Examine for evidence supporting vascular etiology (focal signs, reflexes, and plantar responses), Parkinson's disease, or other medical etiology.
- Blood tests (📖 p. 153).
- EEG useful to exclude delirium, CJD, etc.
- Brain imaging: Structural imaging studies have nonspecific finding and are mainly useful to exclude other etiology. CT—cortical atrophy, especially over parietal and temporal lobes and ventricular enlargement. MRI—atrophy of grey matter (hippocampus, amygdala, and medial temporal lobe). Functional imaging studies are more specific. SPECT—reduced rCBF in temporal and posterior parietal lobes (also frontal lobes in advanced disease). PET—20–30% reduction in oxygen and glucose metabolism in temporal and posterior parietal lobes. MRS—↓N-acetylaspartate.

National Institute of Neurological and Communicative Disorders and Stroke (NINCDS) and Alzheimer's Disease and Related Disorders Association (ADRDA) criteria[2,3]

Probable Alzheimer's disease
- *Criteria include*: the presence of dementia, deficits in at least two areas of cognition, progressive deterioration, no clouding of consciousness, age between 40 and 90, absence of systemic disorders.
- *Diagnosis is supported by*: progressive deterioration of individual cognitive function, impaired activities of daily living, family history of dementia, normal lumbar puncture, electroencephalogram, and evidence of atrophy (or progression) on CT scan.
- *Features not consistent with the diagnosis*: plateaus in the course of the disease, associated psychiatric symptoms, neurological signs, seizures, normal CT scan.
- *Diagnosis unlikely if*: sudden onset, focal neurological signs, seizures or gait disturbance early in the disease.

Possible Alzheimer's disease
- Diagnosis can be made in the presence of atypical features; in the presence of a systemic disease (not considered to be the cause of dementia); in the presence of a single progressive cognitive deficit.

Definite Alzheimer's disease
- Criteria are the clinical criteria for probable Alzheimer's disease plus histological evidence of the disorder.

Recommended further reading

1 Kuljis, R.O. (2002). www.emedicine.com
2 McKhann, G., Drachman, D., Folstein, M., *et al.* (1984). Clinical diagnosis of Alzheimer's disease: report of the NINCDS-ADRDA Work Group under the auspices of Department of Health and Human Services Task Force on Alzheimer's Disease. *Neurology* **34**, 939–44.
3 Husain, M.M., Garrett, R. Clinical diagnosis and management of Alzheimer's disease. Neuroimaging Clin N Am. 2005 Nov; **15**(4), 767–77.

Alzheimer's disease (3)— pharmacological treatments[1]

Acetylcholinesterase inhibitors (AChEIs), the first drugs to be licensed for the treatment of AD, act by increasing the level of ACh at cholinergic synapses in the CNS by inhibiting the breakdown of ACh. Acetylcholinesterase inhibitors:

* slow the progression of the disease (e.g., slow loss of cognitive function),
* lead to preserved functional ability,
* delay the need for supervised living accommodations.

Medications do not delay death. Hence, it is important to start these medications early in the disease course; however, they should also be initiated in the patient who is diagnosed at a later stage as well. Approximately 30% of patients may experience a transient improvement in cognitive and functional ability with initiation of medication. Failure to detect an improvement in cognition/function with initiation is NOT a reason to stop this medication. Controversy exists regarding how long treatment should continue (until death v. at some meaningful endpoint e.g., nursing home placement). They also have beneficial effects on behavioral symptoms of the disease and are recommended as first-line agents in the management of psychiatric complications of AD.

First-generation AChEIs

* Tacrine (Cognex): Developed in the 1980s. No longer used due to significant GI side-effects; hepatotoxicity; 4x daily dosage.

Second-generation AChEIs

FDA approved for mild to moderate AD; donepezil is also FDA approved for severe AD. Switching between agents is acceptable. All associated with GI side-effects; bradycardia; GI bleed (rare); use with caution in severe asthma.

* Donepezil (Aricept): Piperidine derivative; GI absorbed with liver metabolism; long half-life (70hrs); highly selective (acts centrally only) ↓side-effects; linear and predictable kinetics; no liver toxicity; narrow dose range; Dose once a day; starting dose 5mg/d; titrate to 10mg/d maximum.
* Rivastigmine (Exelon): Short half-life (12hrs); inhibits AChE and butyrylcholinesterase in CNS. Dose 2x day; starting dose 1.5–3mg bid; titrated to 6mg bid maximum dose.
* Galantamine (Razadyne/Reminyl): Selectively inhibits AChE and acts as an allosteric ligand at nicotinic ACh receptors; metabolized in liver; short half-life (5hrs); selective. Dose 2x day; starting dose 4mg bid; titrate to 24mg/day maximum.

NMDA-receptor partial antagonist

The NMDA receptor binds excitatory glutamate in the CNS and has a role in LTP and learning/memory function. Memantine (Namenda) is a noncompetitive, PCP-site, NMDA partial antagonist that may protect neurons from glutamate-mediated excitotoxicity. FDA approved as an augmenting agent to second-generation AChE in moderate to severe AD.

Other (possible) treatment strategies

Some evidence supports other approaches to AD: β-amyloid peptide vaccination; cholesterol-lowering drugs; red wine; and anti-platelet agents (such as low-dose aspirin) in patients with co-morbid cerebrovascular disease.

Recommended further reading

1 Lyketsos, C., Colenda, C., Beck, C., et al. (2006). Position statement of the American Association for Geriatric Psychiatry regarding principles of care for patients with dementia resulting from Alzheimer disease. Am J Geriatr Psychiatry **14**(7), 561–72.

Dementia with Lewy bodies (DLB)

DLB is a common form of senile dementia (~15–20% of cases in hospital[1] and community-based samples[2]) that shares clinical and pathological features of both AD and Parkinson's disease.

Epidemiology

Age of onset: 50–83yr. Age at death: 68–92yr, M>F.

Clinical features

In DSM-IV-TR nosology, DLB is coded as Dementia Due to Other General Medical Condition. Consensus diagnostic criteria are presented below.[3] Cognitive impairment predominately affects attention, executive function and visuospatial ability. Memory impairment (retrieval deficits) appears later. Attention and alertness fluctuate. Language is preserved until late. DLB is suspected to occur in about 70% of patients with parkinsonism (especially limb rigidity, gait disorder). 20–50% have a resting tremor. Essential to diagnosis is that onset of cognitive impairment predates or is concurrent with onset of motor disturbance. The mean survival time/rate of cognitive decline is similar to Alzheimer's disease (but rapid deterioration over 1–2yr does occur). Worsening of Parkinsonism is similar in rate to Parkinson's disease (10% decline per year.)

Pathological features

Typically mixed picture.[2] Lewy bodies eosinophilic intracytoplasmic neuronal inclusions of abnormally phosphorylated neurofilament proteins aggregated with ubiquitin and alpha-synuclein, found in brain-stem nuclei (especially basal ganglia), paralimbic, and neocortical structures. Associated with neuronal loss (especially brain-stem and basal forebrain cholinergic projection neurons—with associated reduction in ACh transmission in neocortex). The neurites have a distinctive pattern of ubiquitin and alpha-synuclein immunoreactive neuritic degeneration—in substantia nigra, hippocampal region (CA2/3), dorsal vagal nucleus, basal nucleus basilis of Meynert, and transtentorial cortex (may be more relevant to neuropsychiatric symptom formation than cortical Lewy bodies). Alzheimer-type changes and senile plaques present in a similar density and distribution, but with fewer neurofibrillary tangles and less tau pathology. Vascular disease occurs in ~30% with unknown clinical significance.

Differential diagnosis

Differential diagnosis includes dementia syndromes (e.g., AD, Parkinson's disease dementia), delirium, other neurological diseases (e.g., Parkinson's disease, progressive supranuclear palsy, multisystem atrophy, CJD), psychiatric disorders. In AD, parkinsonism usually presents late whereas memory and language impairment present early. In Parkinson's, disease dementia, the cognitive impairment starts after parkinsonism onset; language is preserved early although hypophonia/dysarthria may interfere with communication.

Assessment

Diagnosis is based on clinical evaluation. Some tests can be supportive of diagnosis. (See consensus criteria).

Pharmacologic Management

- AChEIs: (see Alzheimers disease section for drug details) Not yet FDA approved specifically for DLB, but evidence supports effectiveness in some DLB cases (increase in cognitive function). May also decrease neuropsychiatric symptoms (e.g., apathy/ psychosis /agitation) and are recommended as first line therapy.[3]
- Antipsychotics: Avoid or use with great caution: severe sensitivity reactions (40–50%)—e.g., irreversible parkinsonism, impairment of consciousness, NMS-like autonomic disturbances—with 2–3-foldincrease in mortality.
- Levodopa: Start at low dose and titrate slowly to treatment motor symptoms to reduce risk of exacerbating psychotic symptoms. Paired with carbidopa in Sinemet.

Consensus criteria for the clinical diagnosis of probable and possible dementia with Lewy bodies[3]

- The central diagnostic feature is progressive cognitive decline that interferes with social or occupational function. Prominent or persistent memory impairment may not necessarily occur in the early stages but is usually evident with progression. Deficits on tests of attention and of executive function and visuospatial ability may be especially prominent.
- Two of the following core features are essential for a diagnosis of probable DLB; one is essential for possible DLB.
  - Fluctuating cognition with pronounced variations in attention and alertness.
  - Recurrent visual hallucinations, which are typically well formed and detailed.
  - Spontaneous motor features of parkinsonism.
- Suggestive features (the diagnosis of probable DLB can be based on the presence of one core plus one suggestive feature): REM sleep disturbance; severe neuroleptic sensitivity; low dopamine transporter reuptake in the basal ganglia based on SPECT or PET studies.
- Other commonly seen features: Repeated falls; syncope; transient loss of consciousness; severe autonomic dysfunction; depression; systematized delusions; hallucinations in other modalities; relative preservation of medial temporal lobe structures on CT/MR; generalized low uptake on SPECT/PET with reduced occipital activity; low uptake MIBG scintigraphy; prominent slow wave activity on EEG with temporal lobe transient sharp waves.
- Cognitive decline is not better accounted for by another cause of dementia.
- In DLB, dementia starts before or concurrently with parkinsonism (if present). A diagnosis of Parkinson's disease dementia (PDD) is more appropriate if dementia occurs during well-established Parkinson's disease.

Recommended further reading

1 Weiner, M. (1999). Dementia associated with Lewy bodies: dilemmas and directions. *Archives of Neurology* **56**, 1441.
2 Holmes, C., Cairns, N., Lantos, P., Mann, A. (1999). Validity of current clinical criteria for Alzheimer's disease, vascular dementia and dementia with Lewy bodies. *Br J Psych* **174**, 45–50.
3 McKeith, I.G., Dickson, D.W., Lowe, J., et al. (2005). Diagnosis and management of dementia with Lewy bodies: Third report of the DLB consortium. *Neurology* **65**, 1863–1872.

Frontotemporal dementia (FTD)[1]

An umbrella term used to describe neurodegenerative dementias characterized by preferential atrophy of fronto-temporal regions, with usually
early onset (accounts for ~20% of presenile cases). FTD has several subsumed
diagnoses including:

- Pick's disease,
- corticobasal degeneration,
- progressive supranuclear palsy,
- neurofibrillary dementia,
- frontotemporal lobar degeneration,
- frontotemporal dementia with parkinsonism.

FTD may also be seen in motor neurone diseases (MND). Pathophysiology
is poorly understood and does not clearly correlate with the specific
diagnosis. Hence, an NIH workgroup has recommended that diagnosis be
based on phenotypic presentation (as described below).

Epidemiology

Age of onset: 35–75 years old. 20-40% of patients have a clear family
history.

Clinical features and subtypes

The most common presentation involves profound alteration in character/
social conduct, with relative preservation of cognition. Patients may demonstrate lack of inhibition leading to impulse and inappropriate behavior
(e.g., breaches of etiquette, tactlessness, disregard for personal safety,
increased/inappropriate sexual behavior); apathy; impaired insight and
indifference for one's actions; dietary changes (e.g., overeating, food fads);
compulsive and repetitive behaviors (e.g., drinking from an empty cup,
echolalia, perseveration, verbal stereotypies).

The less common presentation involves loss of language function with
relative preservation of other cognitive functions and normal behavior.
(Behavioral disturbances can develop later in the disease course). Language
impairment involves either isolated loss of expressive language (initially
spoken, followed by reading and writing) or loss of both expressive and
receptive language abilities.

Cognitive symptoms

Cognitive symptoms can include frontal lobe dysfunction, such as impaired
attention, ineffective retrieval strategies, poor organization, and lack of
self-monitoring.

Neurological

No early signs; primitive reflexes and parkinsonism (with progression);
MND signs (muscle weakness and wasting, rigidity) present in a minority
of patients.

Pathological features

Macroscopic

Of frontal and anterior temporal lobes, degeneration of the striatum.

Microscopic
Brain pathology at autopsy is variable and poorly correlates with clinical presentation: tau-positive inclusions with associated neuron loss and gliosis; insoluble tau with variable microtubule binding repeats; MND inclusions.

Differential diagnosis
AD, cerebrovascular dementia, Huntington's disease, Parkinson's disease. Depression, mania, psychotic disorders, substance abuse.

Investigations
Neuropsychology: Impaired frontal lobe function. EEG: usually normal. CT/MRI: bilateral (asymmetrical) abnormalities of frontal/temporal lobes. SPECT: frontal and/or temporal lobe abnormalities.

Management
Currently, no specific pharmacological treatments.

NIH Work Group Recommended Clinical Criteria for FTD[1]

- Development of behavioral or cognitive deficits manifested by either:
  - early and progressive change in personality, characterized by difficulty in modulating behavior, often resulting in inappropriate responses or activities; or
  - early and progressive change in language, characterized by problems in expression or severe naming difficulty and problems with word meaning.
- Behavioral or cognitive deficits lead to significant impairment in social or occupational functioning AND represent a decline from previous level of functioning.
- Course is characterized by gradual onset and continuous decline in function.
- Behavioral or cognitive deficits are not better accounted for by another neurological, medical or psychiatric disorder or substance abuse, and do not occur exclusively during a delirium.

Recommended further reading

1 McKhann, G.M., Albert, M.S., Grossman, M., *et al.* (2001). Clinical and pathological diagnosis of frontotemporal dementia: Report of the Work Group on Frontotemporal Dementia and Pick's Disease. *Neurology* **51**, 1546–1554.

Vascular dementia

Vascular dementia is the second most common cause of dementia after AD, accounting for 20% of cases and results from thromboembolic or hypertensive infarction of small- and medium-size vessels. It can coexist with AD. The variability in its presentation is not adequately captured by the DSM-IV-TR definition, which is consistent with a vascular dementia with prominent cortical involvement. Presentations include:

Cognitive deficits following a single "strategic" stroke
Not all strokes result in cognitive impairment, but when they do the deficits depend upon the site of the infarct. Cognitive deficits tend to be particularly severe with certain midbrain and thalamic strokes. Some recovery of cognitive deficits during poststroke rehabilitation may occur.

Multi-infarct dementia (MID)
Multiple strokes leading to stepwise deterioration in cognitive function. Between strokes there are periods of relative stability. Risk factors for cardiovascular disease are usually present. MID is reflected in the DSM-IV-TR criteria for vascular dementia.

Progressive small-vessel disease (Binswanger disease)
Multiple microvascular infarcts of perforating vessels leading to progressive lacunae formation and white-matter disease/leukoariosis on MRI. This is a subcortical dementia with a clinical course characterized by gradual intellectual decline, generalized slowing, and motor problems (e.g., gait disturbance and dysarthria). Depression, apathy, and pseudobulbar palsy are common.

Cerebral Autosomal Dominant Arteriopathy with Subcortical Infarcts and Leukoencephalopathy (CADASIL)
The first known genetic form of vascular dementia, is associated with Notch-3 gene mutations on chromosome 19, which leads to progressive degeneration of the smooth muscle cells in blood vessels, primarily the small arteries that innervate the white matter and the basal ganglia. Symptoms (stroke, dementia, migraine with aura and mood disorders) appear from mid-20s to mid-40s; death typical by age 65. Characteristic MRI finding is hyperintensities in the subcortical white matter and basal ganglia on T2-weighted images. CADASIL is also known by other names, including hereditary multi-infarct dementia and Familial Binswanger's disease

Epidemiology of vascular dementia
With the exception of CASASIL, vascular dementia is most common in the 60–75-year-old age group. Risk factors include:
- family or personal history of cardiovascular disease.
- smoking.
- diabetes mellitus.
- hypertension.
- hyperlipidemia.
- polycythemia.

- coagulopathies.
- hyperhomocysteinemia.
- sickle cell anemia.
- valvular disease.
- atrial fibrillation.
- atrial myxoma.
- carotid artery disease.

Clinical features[1]

Determined by site of ischemic lesion (cortical v. subcortical). Course can be stepwise or gradually progressive. Cognitive deficits can be variable and are determined by location of ischemic lesions. Depression, anxiety, apathy, psychomotor slowing, affective lability, and personality changes are common. Physical signs include features of atherosclerotic disease along with neurological impairments (e.g., rigidity, akinesia, brisk reflexes, and pseudobulbar palsy). Ten percent have seizures at some point. Cause of death is usually ischemic heart disease, CVA, or renal failure.

Investigations

- Routine dementia screen (📖 p. 153).
- Serum cholesterol, clotting screen, vasculitis screen (ESR; CRP; complement; ANF; rheumatoid factor; anti-DNA antibodies; antiphospholipid antibodies; etc.), syphilis serology, homocysteine levels, testing for Notch-3 mutations (if age appropriate).
- ECG, CXR, CT, and MRI are essential.
- Other investigations may include: echocardiogram (for cardiac/valvular defects or disease); carotid artery Doppler ultrasound.

Management of vascular dementia

- Establish causative factors.
- Aggressive treatment of cerebrovascular risk factors including general health interventions (changing diet, stopping smoking, managing hypertension, optimizing diabetic control, and increasing exercise).
- AchE may support cognitive function, although these drugs are not FDA approved for vascular dementia.[2]

Recommended further reading

1 Bowler, J.V. and Hachinski, V. (eds): *Vascular Cognitive Impairment: Preventable Dementia.* Oxford University Press, 2003.

2 Roman, G.C., Wilkinson, D.G., Dood,y R.S., *et al.*: Donepezil in vascular dementia: combined analysis of two large-scale clinical trials. *Dement Geriatr Cogn Disord.* (2005) **20**(6), 338–344.

Prion diseases[1]

Prion diseases are rapid, aggressive, dementing illnesses caused by deposits of prion proteins throughout the brain. They are rare and are best considered as "slow virus infections." Prions spread throughout the brain by causing irreversible change in neighboring tissue. The typical pathological finding is a "spongy encephalopathy," and in terms of the nosology of the dementias, prion disease is considered a "multifocal dementia." Although prion diseases tend to respect the species barrier (e.g., "scrapie" is a prion disease limited to sheep), there is emerging evidence that this is not always the case (e.g., vCJD). Three diseases are recognized in humans.

Creutzfeldt-Jakob disease (CJD)

A rare disease of 50–70 year-olds with equal sex distribution. 85% of cases are spontaneous or sporadic; 10% result from genetic mutation; 5% result from iatrogenic transmission during transplant surgery of dura, corneal grafts, and pituitary growth hormone. The clinical picture is one of rapidly deteriorating dementia, with early neurological signs (cerebellar and extrapyramidal signs, myoclonus). Death within 4–5 months. EEG shows "periodic triphasic complexes." CT indicates atrophy of cortex and cerebellum.

New variant CJD (vCJD)

The rise of vCJD followed an epidemic of bovine spongiform encephalopathy (BSE) in cattle. BSE is a prion disease of cows that is thought to have been caused by cattle feeds that contained CNS material from infected cows. The disease in humans affects mainly young men in their 20s and is characterized by early anxiety and depressive symptoms, followed by onset of extrapyramidal symptoms, myoclonus and a progressive dementia. Notable dysesthesia, paresthesia. Lack of "periodic triphasic complexes" on EEG. Seven percent of cases with "pulvinar sign" on MR imaging (increased symmetrical signal intensity in posterior thalamus). Typical course is 1 yr until death.

Kuru

This was a rare disease of New Guinea cannibals who ate the brains of their deceased relatives. The incubation period was prolonged—up to 40 yrs before disease onset, which was then rapid and fatal.

Protective genotype for prion diseases?

Researchers at University College London have recently suggested that cannibalism was common and widespread in human ancestors. They analyzed DNA from 30 elderly Fore women from Papua New Guinea who had participated in many cannibalistic feasts before they were banned by the Australian government in the 1950s. It was the practice of the Fore for women and children to consume the brains of dead kin in the belief that this act would recycle the spirit of the dead within the living. At the peak of the epidemic (1920–1950) Kuru killed 1% of the population annually. Most of the women survivors tested by researchers had a particular genotype that was much less common in the younger population, indicating that it conferred substantial protection against the disease. Interestingly, none of the patients who have to date contracted new variant CJD in Britain carry the protective genotype. This suggests that this genotype is protective against prion diseases in humans. The researchers then examined DNA from various ethnic groups around the world and found that all, except the Japanese, carried the protective genotype to a similar degree. Genetic tests showed that this gene could not be there by chance, but was a result of natural selection. This implies that ancestral human populations were exposed to some form of prion disease. They conclude that frequent epidemics of prion disease caused by cannibalism in human ancestors would explain the worldwide existence of the protective genotype in modern humans.

From Mead, S., Stumpf, M.P., Whitfield, J., et al. (2003). Balancing selection at the prion protein gene consistent with prehistoric kuru-like epidemics.
Science **300**, 640–643.

Recommended further reading

1 Belay, E.D., Schonberger, L.B. (2005). *Annu Rev Public Health* **26**, 191–212.

Amnestic disorders

The amnestic disorders are syndromes characterized by memory impairment (anterograde and/or retrograde amnesia), which are caused by a general medical condition or substance use, and where delirium and dementia have been excluded as causative of the amnesia. Amnestic disorders may be transient or chronic (< or >1month). Amnestic conditions usually involve some or all of the following neuroanatomical structures: frontal cortex; hippocampus and amygdala; dorsomedial thalamus; mamillary bodies; and the periaqueductal grey matter (PAG). In terms of neurochemistry, glutamate transmission at the NMDA receptor is often implicated in amnesia, mainly due to its role in memory storage in the limbic system (via long term potentiation, LTP). A number of amnestic disorders are recognized:

Wernicke's encephalopathy (📖 p. 634)

An acute syndrome, with a classic tetrad of symptoms (ataxia, ophthalmoplegia, nystagmus, and acute confusional state), caused by thiamine depletion, usually related to alcohol abuse, and associated with pathological lesions in the mamillary bodies, PAG, thalamic nuclei, and the walls of the third ventricle.

Korsakoff syndrome (📖 p. 634)

Amnesia and confabulation associated with atrophy of the mamillary bodies, usually following Wernicke's encephalopathy (rarer causes include: head injury; hypoxia brain injury; basal/temporal lobe encephalitis; and vascular insult).

Vascular disease

Insults to the hippocampus (especially involving the posterior cerebral artery or basilar artery) may result in an amnestic disorder. Other regions implicated include: parietal-occipital junction; bilateral medio-dorsal thalamus; basal forebrain nuclei (e.g., aneurysm of the anterior communicating artery).

Head injury

An open or closed head injury involving acceleration or deceleration forces may result in injury to the anterior temporal poles (as this structure collides with the temporal bone). Anterograde or post-traumatic amnesia (PTA) is prominent with retrograde amnesia relatively absent. Prognosis is related to length of PTA—better prognosis associated with PTA of less than 1 week.

Herpes simplex virus (HSV) encephalitis

Affects medial temporal lobes and results in deficits in short term memory (STM) storage.

Temporal lobe surgery

Bilateral damage or surgery to the medial temporal lobes results in an inability to store new short-term memories (e.g., "patient HM") (see box 📖 p. 175).

Hypoxic brain damage

Hypoxia following asphyxia from CO poisoning, near drowning, etc, may damage sensitive CA1 and CA3 neurons in the hippocampus. This results in problems with STM storage.

Multiple sclerosis (MS)

40% of patients have some amnesia due to plaques in the temporal lobes and diencephalon resulting in difficulty with recall.

Alcohol blackouts

Significant alcohol intoxication may lead to amnesia for the period of intoxication. This usually only occurs in the context of chronic alcohol misuse.

ECT

There may be a period of mild anterograde and/or retrograde amnesia for several hours following administration of ECT. More rarely there may be ongoing patchy memory loss for up to 6–9 months.

Transient global amnesia (TGA)

This is a syndrome of amnesia lasting 6–24 hrs caused by transient ischemia of the temporal lobes and/or diencephalon. It is more common in patients over 50 yrs of age and may occur in the context of hypertension or migraine. Differential diagnosis includes dissociative disorders and malingering, and diagnosis is often unclear.

Other causes of amnesia

Substances (benzodiazepines, anticholinergics); space occupying lesions (e.g., tumors); hypoglycemia.

"Patient HM"

On 23 August 1953, patient HM underwent a bilateral medial temporal lobe resection in an attempt to control his epileptic seizures. This resulted in a severe anterograde memory impairment that has made HM one of the most studied patients in the history of cognitive psychology.

HM's syndrome is surprisingly isolated, with impairment mostly limited to his inability to register new facts into long-term memory, despite immediate memory being preserved for both verbal and nonverbal tasks. Although his operation was performed when he was 27, his memories are intact until age 16, with an 11-year retrograde amnesia.

His IQ is above average, with almost normal language production and comprehension—he can understand and produce complex verbal material (but is impaired on tests of semantic and symbolic verbal fluency). His perceptual abilities are normal except for his sense of smell (2° to damage of the olfactory tracts). Despite the fact that some of his spatial abilities are compromised, he does not have any attentional deficit.

Normal pressure hydrocephalus[1]

Normal pressure hydrocephalus (NPH) is a syndrome in which there is dilatation of cerebral ventricles (especially third ventricle) and normal CSF pressure at lumbar puncture. It typically presents insidiously with progressive deterioration. The classical triad of symptoms include gait ataxia, dementia, and urinary incontinence; all three symptoms are not necessary for diagnosis. Importantly, the dementia is potentially reversible if NPH is treated promptly.

Etiology

Fifty percent of cases are idiopathic. 50% are secondary to mechanical obstruction of CSF flow across the meninges (e.g., meningitis; subarachnoid hemorrhage; trauma; radiotherapy).

Clinical features

Progressive slowing of cognitive and motor functioning consistent with a pattern of subcortical dementia. Ataxia is due to pyramidal upper motor neuron paraparesis. Urinary incontinence may be a late symptom.

Investigations

CT scan shows ↑ size of the lateral ventricles and thinning of the cortex. 24-hour intracranial pressure monitoring.

Treatment

NPH due to mechanical obstruction is more responsive to ventriculo-peritoneal shunt than idiopathic NPH, where response is variable.

Recommended further reading

1 Marmarou, A., Bergsneider, M., Relkin, N., *et al.* Diagnosing idiopathic normal-pressure hydro-cephalus. *Neurosurgery* (2005). Sep; **57**(3 Suppl), S4–16.

Chronic subdural hematoma[1]

A chronic subdural hematoma (SDH) results from rupture of the bridging veins between the dura and arachnoid mater and tends to occur over the frontal and/or parietal cortices. Bilateral SDH is present in <30% of cases. SDH produces pressure on the brain with subsequent loss of function in the affected area. SDH should be suspected when there is a changing pattern in cognitive function, especially if risk factors for SDH exist: post trauma; elderly after a fall; infancy; cerebral atrophy (e.g., chronic alcoholism, AD); clotting disorders; anticoagulant therapy; arachnoid cysts (in patients < 40 years old).

Clinical features

SDH develop insidiously over days to weeks and may become clinically evidence only months later. There may be no history of recent trauma. Headache, altered level of consciousness, cognitive impairment (including possible memory impairment) may all occur, often with fluctuations in severity. Focal signs are sometimes detected including hemiparesis, hemiopsia, papilledema, CN III dysfunction, asymmetric reflexes. The general trend is toward a dementia picture, which is characteristically of a subcortical nature.

Investigations

CT scan during the first three weeks may not show the SDH as it is isodense during the early phase. Therefore, contrast should be used. Later on, as the SDH liquefies, a low-density convexity may be detected over the fronto-parietal cortex.

Treatment

No treatment indicated in absence of mass effect or neurological symptoms/signs; SDH may resolve. If needed, surgical drainage of SDH via burr holes or via craniotomy.

Recommended further reading

1 Sinson, G., Reiter, G.T. (2002). www.emedicine.com.

Psychiatric sequelae of CVA[1]

A range of psychiatric problems may occur following stroke/cerebro-vascular accident (CVA), including:

Cognitive disorders
- Vascular dementia (📖 p. 170).
- Subcortical dementia (📖 p. 164).
- Amnestic disorder (📖 p. 174).

Personality changes
These tend to involve a constriction in the range of interests and a loss of intellectual flexibility. Irritability is common and "catastrophic reactions" may occur in response to stress or change in routine. Emotional flexibility may be reduced and affective responses often become shallow and stereotyped.

Pathological laughing or crying (emotional incontinence)
Presentation involves outbursts of emotion, stereotypically either crying or laughing, which is perceived by the patient to be outside of his/her control and occurring in situations that would not normally trigger the affective response. Affects 20–25% within first six months after stroke. Onset may be within hours of stroke. Responsive to both SSRI and TCA antidepressants; response notable within first 1–2 days of treatment.

Poststroke depression
Major depression after stroke is extremely common (up to 35% of cases); up to 70% of cases with significant depressive features. Its onset is usually between 3 and 24 months following the stroke. Coded as mood disorder due to general medical condition in DSM-IV-TR nosology.

Etiology
- Biological risk factors—direct physiological effects of the brain injury, with location (e.g., left anterior frontal), large size, increased age, and female gender.
- Psychological risk factors—sudden dependency; disability; premorbid personality traits (especially neurotic or highly independent individuals).
- Social risk factors—being alone; lack of social support; financial worries.
- Treatment (antidepressants): SSRIs and mirtazapine are considered safe following stroke but some evidence suggests that nortriptyline may be more efficacious.

Psychoses
Manic, hypomanic, and paranoid psychoses may result from a CVA, especially rignst hemisphere infarcts. "Peduncular hallucinosis" is an uncommon psychosis characterized by visual and auditory hallucinations and is associated with infarcts involving the pons and midbrain.

Korsakoff syndrome (📖 p. 634)
A rare chronic complication of subarachnoid hemorrhage.

Recommended further reading

1 Sinson, G., Reiter, G.T. (2002). www.emedicine.com Psychiatric sequelae of CUA.

Psychiatric aspects of head injury (1)[1]

Head injuries are unfortunately common in a world characterized by use of motor vehicles, drug and alcohol abuse, and falls. The peak incidence of head injury is between the ages of 15 and 24 years, although, with an aging population, the number of elderly with brain injuries is rapidly growing. Improved prehospital and acute medical care has resulted in large numbers of individuals surviving with neuropsychiatric consequences. Most head injury survivors who present to psychiatric services have emotional symptoms and personality changes ranging from subtle to severe. A smaller number manifest serious and lasting cognitive sequelae, such as apathy, disinhibition, and amnesia. There are also important acute psychiatric effects of head injury.

Severity of brain injury

Defined by initial Glasgow Coma Scores (p. 81)
- 3–8 Severe brain injury.
- 9–12 Moderate brain injury.
- 12–15 Mild brain injury (concussion), or if radiological findings are present, mild-complicated brain injury.

Acute psychological effects of head injury

Most significant head injuries are closed and involve a period of loss of consciousness (which may extend from brief concussion to prolonged coma). On recovery of consciousness there are often memory deficits. Amnesia is classified in terms of the following:

Post-traumatic amnesia (PTA)

Includes the period of injury and the period following injury (until normal memory resumes). Often associated with post-traumatic delirium. A state that may follow severe head injury and occurs as the individual begins to regain consciousness. This is characterized by prolonged and variable confusion, with or without behavioral symptoms, anxiety, affective lability, paranoia, delusional misinterpretation, and hallucinations.

Retrograde amnesia (RA)

Includes the period between the last clearly recalled memory prior to the injury and the injury itself. It is usually a dense amnesia that can be quite variable depending on the severity of the injury, lasting anywhere from seconds months, and shrinks with time, although it is common for patients to have a permanent loss of memory surrounding the time of the injury.

Factors associated with increased psychiatric morbidity following head injury
- Increased duration of loss of consciousness.
- Increased duration of PTA.
- Increased age, arteriosclerosis, and alcoholism.
- Increased area of damage.
- Increased neurological sequelae (focal deficits, epilepsy, etc.).
- Dominant or bilateral hemisphere involvement.
- Premorbid psychiatric disease.

Recommended further reading

1 Rao, V. and Lyketsos, C. (2000). Neuropsychiatric sequelae of traumatic brain injury. *Psychosomatics* **41**, 95–103.

Psychiatric aspects of head injury (2)

Chronic psychiatric syndromes following head injury

A number of chronic syndromes are recognized following head injury:

Cognitive impairment

There may be focal cognitive deficits such as amnesia, or diffuse problems including slowing, apathy, affective blunting, decreased concentration, executive difficulties, and short-term memory impairment. Emotional liability, such as pathological laughing or crying may occur. If symptoms are severe, it is particularly important to exclude NPH, SDH, or coexisting AD. Treatment: SSRI, antipsychotics; neurostimulants.

Personality/behavioral changes

Personality changes are most likely after head injury to the orbito-frontal lobe or anterior temporal lobe. "Frontal lobe syndrome" is characterized by disinhibition, impulsivity, irritability, and aggressive outbursts. Treatment may include neurostimulants (methylphenidate or amantadine) or mood stabilizing medications (valproic acid or carbamazepine).

Sleep cycle dysregulation

May exacerbate underlying delirium, confusion, or depression. Treatment with trazodone has been shown to be quite efficacious; avoid benzodiazepines if possible as it may worsen memory disturbance.

Psychoses

A schizophrenia-like psychosis with prominent paranoia is associated with left temporal injury, while affective psychoses (especially mania in 9% of patients) are associated with right temporal or orbito-frontal injury. There is also an increased prevalence of schizophrenia post head injury (>2.5% develop the disorder). Treatment: Cautious use of antipsychotics (risk of seizure), anticonvulsants.

Other psychiatric disorders

Depressive illness is most common but anxiety states (including PTSD) are common sequelae. Persistent depression and anxiety occur in roughly 1/3 of head-injury survivors. Suicide risk is also higher post head injury. Treatment: SSRIs.

Postconcussional syndrome

This is a common phenomenon after mild head injury. The main symptoms are: headache; dizziness; insomnia; irritability; emotional lability; headaches and myofascial pain; increased sensitivity to noise, light, etc; fatigue; poor concentration; anxiety; and depression and poor sleep regulation. Treatment is mainly focused on specific symptoms.

Medications and head injury

As a general rule, persons with head injury are much more sensitive to medications, and caution should be used particularly with sedating drugs. Medications with high D2 receptor activity (i.e., typical antipsychotics, metoclopramide) have been associated with slowed motor recovery and should be avoided if possible in this population.

Factors influencing psychiatric disability and prognosis

- Mental constitution—i.e., vulnerability due to genetics, temperament (premorbid personality: increased risk in histrionic, hypochondriacal, and dependent personalities), IQ ("cerebral reserve"), age.
- Emotional impact of injury—i.e., extent of psychological trauma.
- Setting, circumstances, and repercussions of injury.
- Iatrogenic factors.
- Home and social environment (including secondary gain issues).
- Compensation and litigation issues (including secondary gain issues).
- Post-traumatic epilepsy (PTE)—occurs in 13.8 % of all persons with brain injury; groups with higher rates include those with biparietal contusions (66%) and dural penetration with bone or metal fragments (62.5%).
- Size and location of brain damage: frontal, temporal, dominant side worse.

Sequelae in children

In children, there is usually less psychopathology after head injury due to increased brain plasticity. Recovery may continue for up to five years after injury (as opposed to two years in adults). Problems are generally behavioral in nature and include aggression, delinquency, and ADHD-like symptoms.

Psychiatric aspects of epilepsy

The lifetime prevalence of experiencing a seizure is approximately 5%, whereas the prevalence of epilepsy (recurrent seizures) is 0.5–1%. Most (~60%) cases of epilepsy have unknown etiology. Seizures may be *generalized* or *focal*. Generalized seizures involve the whole cortex and lead to loss of consciousness (LOC). Focal seizures begin in one area of the cortex and may become secondarily generalized. Focal seizures are subclassified as simple partial (i.e., localized motor/sensory features without LOC or memory loss); complex partial (i.e., associated changes in conscious level, with or without aura/automatism). Between 10% and 50% of patients with epilepsy have psychiatric symptoms.

Psychiatric aspects of epilepsy may be related to:
- Psychosocial consequences of diagnosis (e.g., unemployment, stigma and ostracism, restricted activities, dependency).
- Psychiatric syndromes directly attributed to epilepsy.
- Neuropsychiatric effects of medication.

Psychiatric syndromes attributed to epilepsy are best considered by their temporal relationship to seizures (preictal, ictal, postictal, interictal).

Preictal
- Patients may experience a variety of vague symptoms during the days and hours leading up to the seizure. These are termed prodromal symptoms and include feelings of tension and insomnia.
- Preictal depression[1]. Periods of depression and irritability can precede a seizure by hours to days; frequently relieved by the seizure. Affects 10–20% of patients with epilepsy. Patient frequently do not meet traditional DSM criteria for major depression.
- An aura may occur immediately prior to seizure onset. This is most common in complex partial seizures (CPSs)—temporal lobe epilepsy (TLE) or extratemporal epilepsy (e.g., frontal CPSs). Auras are typically stereotyped e.g., autonomic or visceral aura (epigastric sensation); derealization and depersonalization experiences; cognitive symptoms ("forced thinking," ideomotor aura, déjà vu, jamais vu, fugue and twilight states); affective symptoms (anxiety, euphoria); perceptual experiences (auditory, visual, sensory, and olfactory hallucinations or illusions).

Ictal
- Automatisms commonly accompany complex partial seizures. They are quasi-purposeful simple or complex stereotyped behaviors that are repeated inappropriately or that are inappropriate for the situation. The individual seems out of touch during the automatism and will subsequently be amnesic of this behavior. Suggest a focal origin for the seizure such as the medial temporal lobe. Automatisms may be the basis of twilight and fugue states (EEG may aid differential diagnosis.)
- Epilepsia Partialis Continua (EPC): A condition of prolonged CPSs, lasting hours to days (may be confused with delirium or psychosis) (e.g., temporal, frontal, or cingulate seizures). There are variable behavioral, cognitive, and perceptual symptoms and periods of amnesia.

- Bizarre aggressive behavior.
- Ictal depression:[1]
- Classically with sudden onset; seen in CPS; reported to occur in up to 10% of TLE patients. Symptoms range from mild to severe; ictal suicides have been reported.

Postictal

- Postictal delirium: A very common (10%) confusional state following a seizure with disorientation, inattention, variable levels of consciousness, and sometimes paranoia. Can last hours to days and shows a trend toward improvement and normal consciousness. If prolonged, suspect EPC.
- Postictal psychosis:[2] Usually follows a cluster of seizures or an increase in the frequency of seizures; may follow withdrawal of anticonvulsant therapy. Thought to result from sub-threshold kindling activity. It usually only occurs in individuals with epilepsy for >10 yrs (particularly associated with a left temporal lobe focus). Clinically, there is an initial nonpsychotic interval (lasting hours to weeks) following a seizure. Thereafter, the individual develops a brief psychotic episode with variable psychotic and affective symptoms. The episode resolves after a period of days to one month. It may recur two or three times in a year. EEG shows marked changes during the psychotic episode.
- Postictal depression:[2] May last hours to days; more common in CPS originating in right temporal structures or bilateral limbic areas. Patients with postictal depression usually suffer from other epilepsy related depressions as well.

Interictal[3]

- Brief interictal psychosis occurs unrelated to a seizure, when there is good control of epilepsy. In this way seizures are antagonistic to the psychosis in that the EEG normalizes during the psychosis. This is called "forced normalization." A seizure may end the psychotic episode. This form of psychosis has been termed "alternating psychosis" (i.e., there is an inverse relationship between severity of epilepsy and severity of psychosis). There may be premonitory symptoms such as anxiety and insomnia while the psychosis is characterized by hallucinations and paranoia. Notably, the antagonistic relationship between seizures and psychosis is demonstrated where anticonvulsants may aggravate psychosis, and where antipsychotics may reduce the seizure threshold.
- Chronic interictal schizophrenia-like psychosis. A chronic schizophrenia-like psychotic illness is 6–12 times more common in epileptics than in the general population. It is particularly associated with left TLE and is more common in early onset severe epilepsy and in women with epilepsy. There is often a period of 10–15 years that elapses between diagnosis of epilepsy and onset of the psychotic illness. Clinically the illness is very similar to idiopathic schizophrenia although there tends to be a prominent affective component. The chronic course is likewise similar. There is typically no family history of schizophrenia and an absence of premorbid schizotypal traits. Pathologically, it may represent

the cumulative effects of chronic kindling due to a temporal lobe focus (e.g., in TLE).
- Interictal dysphoric disorder:[1] Typically involves episodes of short duration (hours to 2–3 days) involving various combinations of the following symptoms: depressed mood, anergia, pain, insomnia, fear, anxiety, paroxysmal irritability, euphoria. Seen in refractory epilepsy, especially TLE.

Other presentations

Cognitive deterioration

Cognitive deterioration is a common outcome of chronic epilepsy and is related to a number of factors including repeated seizures with cerebral hypoxia and the neurological effects of chronic anticonvulsant therapy.

Conversion disorders

Patients with epilepsy at increased risk, especially for pseudoseizures.

Mania

Flor-Henry first described the association between right-side TLE and manic illness.

Epileptic personality syndrome

Also known as Waxman-Geshwind syndrome, this is a controversial phenomenon traditionally associated with chronic TLE. The classic traits include: religiosity; hyposexuality; hypergraphia; and "viscosity of personality."

Violence

A controversial issue. There does seem to be an increased risk of violence and aggression in people with TLE or frontal-lobe epilepsy. "Episodic dyscontrol" is believed to be the result of subthreshold kindling in these regions of the brain and anticonvulsants are often effective in reducing aggressive outbursts.

The ecstatic seizures of Prince Myshkin

He was thinking, incidentally, that there was a moment or two in his epileptic condition almost before the fit itself (if it occurred in waking hours) when suddenly amid the sadness, spiritual darkness and depression, his brain seemed to catch fire at brief moments. . . His sensation of being alive and his awareness increased tenfold at those moments which flashed by like lightning. His mind and heart were flooded by a dazzling light. All his agitation, doubts and worries, seemed composed in a twinkling, culminating in a great calm, full of understanding . . . but these moments, these glimmerings were still but a premonition of that final second (never more than a second) with which the seizure itself began. That second was, of course, unbearable.

Dostoevsky: *The Idiot*

Recommended further reading

1 Seethalakshimi, R., Ennapadam, S., Krishnamoorthy, S. (2007). Depression in epilepsy: phenomenology, diagnosis and management. *Epileptic Disord* **9**(1), 1–10.

2 Sachdev, P. (1998). Schizophrenia-like psychosis and epilepsy: the status of the association. *AJP* **155**, 325–336.

3 Lishman, W.A. *Organic Psychiatry*. 2nd ed. United Kingdom:Blackwell Science 1997.

HIV/AIDS and psychiatry

The HIV/AIDS epidemic means that, increasingly, psychiatrists are encountering individuals with psychological and neuropsychiatric complications of HIV infection. In some developing countries, rates of infection are as high as 38% (with rates in hospitals as high as 70–80%). Both diagnosis with the disease and the mortality associated with it has major consequences for the psychological and social functioning of individuals and their communities. In areas in which large numbers of young adults are dying from the disease, there are even larger numbers of children becoming orphans, with all the developmental, emotional, and social problems associated with the loss of parental care and support. In other communities, people with HIV/AIDS are subject to stresses related to their lifestyle choices (e.g., prejudice related to sexual orientation or directed at those with addictions). Stigma also contributes to the psychological burden of infected individuals and their families.

Improved outcome for patients on antiretroviral therapy brings additional stresses related to living with uncertainty about the future. The responsibility of caregivers working with patients with HIV/AIDS goes far beyond treating immediate physical problems. Holistic practice requires the health care professional to adopt a true biopsychosocial approach with appreciation of the emotional state of the patient as well as the host of social, economic, spiritual, and ethical challenges accompanying diagnosis with the disease.

Contexts in which psychiatric problems may arise

There are a number of contexts in which psychiatric problems may arise in relation to HIV/AIDS:

- The "worried well" (i.e., HIV-ve people may be concerned about being infected due to contact with HIV+ve sources/individuals).
- Pretest anxiety.
- Posttest stress may precipitate a psychiatric illness such as adjustment disorder, major depressive episode, and suicidality.
- Living with HIV/AIDS often results in stressful life events (e.g., losing a job, becoming economically disadvantaged, and experiencing social alienation).
- Individuals with psychiatric needs (e.g., victims of abuse; MR patients) may be more vulnerable to becoming infected with the virus.
- Direct HIV infection of CNS causing neuropsychiatric symptoms.
- Opportunistic infections and/or tumors of the CNS, which may manifest as neuropsychiatric symptoms.
- Antiretroviral medications may cause psychiatric symptoms (e.g., AZT (zidovudine) is associated major depressive episode, whereas isoniazid prophylaxis may precipitate a psychotic illness).

Counseling HIV/AIDS patients

- Pretest counseling: consider meaning of a positive result; what actions the individual will take; confidentiality issues; fears of individual; high risk behaviors; reactions to stress; social and other implications of positive result.

- Posttest counseling: clarify distortions; assess emotions; decide who to tell; discuss prevention of transmission; offer support to individual and family.

Ethical issues
- HIV testing: issues of informed consent. Consent must be obtained before testing blood for HIV status.
- Confidentiality: encourage individual to tell sexual partner(s) and other medical personnel; if individual refuses, check your local health department rules on result reporting.
- Resource allocation: e.g., availability and affordability of antiretroviral drugs.

HIV/AIDS and psychiatry—clinical presentations[1,2]

Psychiatric symptoms seen in HIV infection may represent HIV penetration of the brain but may also be secondary to opportunistic CNS infections (toxoplasmosis, papovavirus, cytomegalovirus [CMV], HSV), tumors (non-Hodgkin's lymphoma, and Kaposi), systemic disease, and adverse effects of medications. Any patient with acute onset of psychiatric symptoms in the absence of prior psychiatry history should undergo a complete medical and neuropsychiatric evaluation to rule out potentially reversible medical causes. HIV testing is an essential part of such an evaluation.

Depression

Many HIV +ve individuals experience depression at some point during their illness. The estimated point prevalence of major depression is 9.4%, which represents an approximately 2x greater prevalence than HIV –ve controls.[1] Depression in this context may have multiple causes, including potential side-effects from highly active antiretroviral treatment (HAART) regimens. Treatment: (1) For depressions that start soon after HAART initiated, recommendation is to wait one to two weeks before beginning depression treatment because symptoms may spontaneously resolve. If no resolution, treat depression aggressively; if unsuccessful, consider change in HAART regimen to exclude CNS active agents (e.g., zidovudine, efavirenz). (2) If patient with history of severe depression or serious suicide attempt, consider prophylactic antidepressant treatment prior to initiating HAART. (3) For patients who develop depression while receiving HAART, treat aggressively; change HAART regimen only if psychopharmacology fails. Medications: SSRIs are well tolerated. Review drug-drug interactions with HAART agents.

Suicide

There is a 30x increased risk of suicide in individuals who are HIV +ve. High-risk times include: at diagnosis; at the death of an HIV +ve friend; as the individual experiences deterioration in physical health.

Mania

Manic symptoms may develop in the context of HIV psychosis or as a result of treatment with antiretroviral agents. Treatment: Lithium is preferable (beware risk of toxicity) because there is some evidence suggesting that sodium valproate may increase viral replication.

Anxiety

Infection with the virus is associated with increased risk of GAD, panic disorder, PTSD, and OCD.

Chronic pain

Up to 80% of patients experience chronic pain at some point, in particular chronic headache. This may lead some individuals to self-medicate, putting them at risk of substance dependence.

Psychosis

New-onset psychosis occurs in 0.5–15% of HIV +ve patients. HIV infection may also exacerbate pre-existing psychiatric conditions, Psychosis typically characterized by fluctuating symptoms that may alter over hours to days. Atypical bizarre psychotic symptoms may give way to prominent mixed affective symptoms, which in turn may change to a withdrawn apathetic state. Treatment includes low-dose haloperidol or preferably an atypical (e.g., olanzapine, quetiapine) due to increased sensitivity to extrapyramidal side-effects. CNS penetrating antiretroviral agents may also reduce psychotic symptoms.

HIV-associated cognitive changes

Epidemiology

90% of AIDS patients have CNS changes postmortem. Seventy to eighty % develop a cognitive disorder. 30% develop HIV-associated dementia (HAD).

Pathology

Direct CNS infection: HIV is neurotropic, entering the brain through endothelial gaps; the virus attaches to group 120 on CD4 +ve sites of microglial cells; a cascade opens calcium channels leading to glutamate and nitrous oxide excitotoxicity; this results in neuronal death and increased apoptosis. Sites include basal ganglia and subcortical and limbic white matter.

Clinical presentation

Minor cognitive-motor disorder

Asymptomatic HIV+ve patients can have very early CNS infection. Symptoms include abstract reasoning, learning difficulties, slowed information processing, and mild motor slowing. Even mild cognitive impairment can be disabling and lead to unemployment.

HIV-associated dementia (HAD)

Previously termed "AIDS dementia."

- A progressive subcortical dementia with prominent psychomotor slowing; impairment of memory and language is less prominent. More common in advanced HIV disease (estimated prevalence of 15%). Prior to the development of antiretroviral therapies, HAD was uniformly fatal with a mean survival after diagnosis of six months.
- Of note, in the HAART era, more patients with cognitive impairment are surviving longer; hence, the overall prevalence of cognitive disorders in HIV is increasing.

Assessment

Rule out potential reversible causes such as opportunistic infection via imaging and lumbar puncture. HAD has nonspecific findings including on CT/MRI (atrophy, ↑ T2 signal) and EEG (generalized slowing). Neuropsychiatric testing is often appropriate: MMSE is not sensitive; consider alternative testing batteries such as HIV Dementia Scale.

Treatment

Antiretroviral therapies.

Recommended further reading

1 Glenn, J., Treismana, B., Adam, I., et al. (2002). Neurologic and psychiatric complications of antiretroviral agents *AIDS* **16**(9), 1201–1215.
2 Wojna, V., Nath, A. (2006). Challenges to the Diagnosis and Management of HIV Dementia *AIDS Reader* **16**(11), 615.

Neuropsychiatric aspects of CNS infections

Viral encephalitis

- Mumps, varicella-zoster, arbovirus, rubella—may result in behavioral problems, learning difficulties, and ADHD-like symptoms in children.
- HSV 1—Involves inferior frontal and anterior temporal lobes. Acute phase: delirium, hallucinations, and TLE. Chronic sequelae: Korsakoff's psychosis, dementia, and Kluver-Bucy syndrome. EEG: slowing with bursts of increased slow-wave in the temporal region.
- Influenza—a rare chronic outcome is Encephalitis Lethargica, characterized by parkinsonism, oculogyric crises, and psychosis.
- Ebstein-Barr virus/infectious mononucleosis—may result in myalgic encephalitis or chronic fatigue syndrome.
- Measles—rarely leads to subacute sclerosing panencephalitis, a chronic persisting CNS infection. Onset 2–10 years after initial measles infection. Progressive deterioration; 95% die within 1–3 years of onset. Features include: behavioral problems, deteriorating intellectual function, movement disorders (ataxia, myoclonus), seizures, and, finally, dementia in a child. Pathology: white and grey matter changes to occipital, cerebellum and basal ganglia. EEG: "periodic complexes".

Tuberculosis

- TB meningitis—especially in children and young adults; caseating exudate covers the base of the skull leading to vascular infarcts and hydrocephalus; cranial nerves may become involved. Psychiatric symptoms include: apathy; withdrawal; insidious personality changes; delirium; hallucinations; chronic behavioral problems.
- Tuberculoma—presents with focal signs, seizures, raised ICP.

Neurosyphilis

Historically known as "General Paresis of the Insane" or "Cupid's disease", neurosyphilis is a chronic outcome of direct spirochetal infection of the brain parenchyma. It manifests more commonly in men in their 40s–50s, roughly 15–20 years after primary infection. The spirochetes have a predilection for frontal and parietal lobes and the disease typically presents as a progressive frontal dementia.

Classic symptoms

Grandiosity, euphoria, and mania with mood-congruent delusions. Disinhibition, personality change, and memory impairment are also common.

Neurological features

Argyll-Robinson pupils; "trombone tongue"; tremor; ataxia; dysarthria; myoclonus; hyperreflexia; spasticity; and extrapyramidal signs.

PANDAS

Afflicted children (age 3 years to puberty) experience an abrupt onset of obsessive-compulsive disorder and/or a tic disorder in association with group A Beta-hemolytic streptococcal infection (a positive throat culture for strep. or history of Scarlet Fever.) Symptoms fluctuate and there are association neurological abnormalities (motoric hyperactivity, or adventitious movements, such as choreiform movements). Additional symptoms can include ADHD symptoms, separation anxiety, mood changes, sleep disturbance, night- time bed wetting and/or day-time urinary frequency, fine/gross motor changes, and joint pains.

"Megalomania in General Paralysis"

Gentlemen,—You have before you today a merchant, aged forty-three, who sits down with a polite greeting, and answers questions fluently and easily . . . His illness began about two years ago. He became absent-minded and forgetful, to such an extent at last that he was dismissed by the firm for whom he had worked. Then, a year ago, he became excited, made extensive purchases and plans, weeping now and then in the deepest despair, so that he had to be taken into the hospital. On admission, he felt full of energy . . . and intended to write verses here, where he was particularly comfortable. He could write better than Goethe, Schiller, and Heine. The most fabulous megalomania quickly developed. He proposed to invent an enormous number of new machines, rebuild the hospital, build a cathedral higher than that at Cologne, and put a glass case over the asylum. He was a genius, spoke all the languages in the world, would cast a church of cast-steel, get us the highest order of merit from the Emperor, find a means of taming the madmen, and present the asylum library with 1000 volumes, principally philosophical works. He had quite godly thoughts . . . When at its height, the disease may present a great resemblance to maniacal states, but the physical examination and proof of the defective memory will save us from confusing it with them. So also will the senseless nature of the plans and the possibility of influencing them, and the feebleness and yielding character of the manifestations of the will, which are all greater in general paralysis.

Kraepelin E (1913). *Lectures on Clinical Psychiatry*,
3rd English Ed. Bailliére, Tindall and Cox: London.

Autoimmune disorders and psychiatry

Systemic lupus erythematosus (SLE)

This multi-system autoimmune vasculitis is most common in women; onset in their 30s. Psychiatric symptoms occur in 60% of cases. The CNS neuronal injury is related to antineuronal antibodies and microvasculopathy (with infarction, inflammation, and coagulopathy) mediated by antiphospholipid antibodies. Seizures, cranial nerve palsies, peripheral neuropathy, "spinal stroke", and other focal signs may occur in addition to dermatological, rheumatological, hematological, and cardiovascular complications. Drugs used to treat the condition may have psychiatric side-effects (e.g., steroids; isoniazid; hydralazine). Treatment can include corticoid steroids. Psychiatric syndromes include:

- Cognitive impairment is the most common SLE associated neuropsychiatric syndrome, affecting up to 80% of cases.
- Depression—up to 50% of SLE patients experience clinically significant depressive illness.
- Psychosis—transient psychotic episodes with a recurrent and fluctuating course. Symptoms are variable with auditory and visual hallucinations as well as paranoia, affective instability, and disturbed sensorium.
- Schizophrenia-like psychosis—a rare finding in SLE.

Polyarteritis nodosa (PAN)

A rare immune-mediated necrotizing vasculitis that is characterized by saccular aneurysms and infarction and is more common in young men. Neuropsychiatric findings include: stroke; focal signs; seizures; "spinal stroke"; delirium; auditory and visual hallucinations.

Movement disorders in psychiatry

Movement disorders occur in three contexts within psychiatry:
- Extrapyramidal diseases with psychiatric symptoms (e.g., Parkinson's disease).
- Psychiatric disorders with abnormal movements (e.g., stereotypies; tics).
- Medication-induced movement disorders (e.g., EPS).

Tics[1]

Tics are spontaneous, stereotyped movements that can be motor and/or vocal and usually involve abnormal levels of dopamine (DA) in the basal ganglia. Tics can be related to genetic, infectious, and other causes.
- Tourette syndrome, Transient tic disorder, and Chronic motor or vocal tic disorder is spectrum of tic disorders with genetic overlap with each other and with ADHD and OCD (📖 pp. 700, 740).
- Tics are part of several infection-associated neuropsychiatric syndromes including CJD; Sydenham's chorea; PANDAS, encephalitis
- Tics can be seen after drug exposure (L-dopa; ritalin; cocaine; amphetamines) and brain injury (CO poisoning, CVA, head trauma).

Tremor
- Exaggerated physiological tremor—(8–12Hz); occurs at rest and with action. Causes include stress; anxiety; caffeine; medications.
- Essential tremor—(6–12Hz); occurs at rest, with action and postural; most noticeable symmetrically in upper limbs. Familiar.
- Extrapyramidal tremor—(4Hz); resting tremor; e.g., parkinsonism.
- Cerebellar, midbrain, or red nucleus—(4–6Hz); intention tremor; causes include trauma; vascular; MS; neoplasia; etc.

Catatonia (📖 p. 1104)

A motor syndrome that has several causes and is diagnosed (DSM-IV) by the presence of 2 or more of the following:
- Motor immobility—catalepsy ("waxy flexibility"); stupor.
- Motor excitement.
- Negativism or mutism.
- Posturing, stereotypies, or mannerisms.
- Echolalia or echopraxia.

Recommended further reading
1 Black, K.J., Webb, H. (2006). www.emedicine.com.

Extrapyramidal symptoms

Pathophysiology

Movement disorders commonly involve a disequilibrium of neurotransmitters such as dopamine (DA), acetylcholine (ACh), and GABA within the circuits of the basal ganglia. Levels of DA and ACh tend to be inversely related. For example, in parkinsonism, there is decrease in DA with an increase in ACh; conversely, chorea is characterized by an increase in DA and a decrease in ACh.

Core symptoms in extrapyramidal disease:

- Negative symptoms—bradykinesia, postural abnormalities, etc.
- Positive symptoms—rigidity and involuntary movements (resting tremor, chorea, athetosis, hemiballismus, dystonia).

"Parkinsonism"

A syndrome characterized by four core symptoms:
- slow "pill-rolling" tremor (4Hz).
- rigidity.
- bradykinesia.
- postural abnormalities.

Etiology

- Degenerative diseases idiopathic Parkinson's disease (PD) (85% cases); progressive supranuclear palsy (PSNP); multiple system atrophy (MSA); corticobasal degeneration (CBD); ALS-dementia-Parkinson complex of Guam (ADPG).
- Medication neuroleptics; antidepressants.
- Toxins cobalt; manganese; magnesium; organophosphates.
- Infections: Encephalitis lethargica (postinfluenza); CJD.
- Miscellaneous: CVA of the basal ganglia; trauma of the basal ganglia; NPH; neoplasia of the basal ganglia; dementia pugilistica ("punch drunk" syndrome); Lewy body dementia.

Multiple system atrophy (MSA)

Three syndromes

Striatonigral degeneration; Shy-Drager syndrome; olivopontocerebellar degeneration.

Characterized by

Parkinsonism; ataxia; vertical gaze palsies; pyramidal signs; autonomic abnormalities.

Progressive supranuclear palsy (PSNP)

Also known as Steele-Richardson-Olzewski syndrome, PSNP has its onset in the 50s and 60s age range and is characterized by a tetrad of clinical findings: subcortical dementia; pseudobulbar palsy; supranuclear palsy; dystonia (of the head and neck).

Encephalitis lethargica

Roughly 20 years after the great influenza epidemic of the late 1910s, large numbers of patients who had suffered influenza encephalitis during the epidemic, developed this disorder (also called "postencephalitic parkinsonism"). Clinical findings were: parkinsonism, oculogyric crises, pupillary abnormalities, psychosis).[1] The disorder was the subject of the book (and film) by Oliver Sacks entitled Awakenings.

Recommended further reading

1 Recent examination of archived brain material from the epidemic has failed to demonstrate influenza RNA. It is now thought to be autoimmune mediated—see Dale, R.C., Church, A.J., Surtees, R.A., et al. (2004). Brain **127**, 21–33.

Parkinson's disease (PD) and psychiatric illness

500,000 to 750,000 Americans currently diagnosed with Parkinson's Disease (PD). Parkinson's disease results in progressive impairment of voluntary initiation of movement, associated with a dementia of variable severity, as well as psychiatric morbidity. It is caused by gradual loss of dopaminergic neurons in the substantia nigra (pars compacta). This results in reduced DA and increased ACh in the basal ganglia. The remaining cells of the substantia nigra contain Lewy bodies.

Epidemiology

Occurs in 20:100,000 people; typically has its onset in the 50s and peaks during the 70s; M:F = 3:2; 5% of cases are familial; 25% patients are disabled or die within 5 years and ~60% within 10 years; rare survival ~20 years.

Symptoms and signs of PD

- Tremor—resting, "pill-rolling" tremor of 4Hz; this is an early sign that may start unilaterally and may be asymmetrical in intensity; tremor increases with excitement or fatigue and diminishes during sleep.
- Rigidity—"lead-pipe" or "cog-wheel" rigidity, especially in flexor muscles.
- Bradykinesia—slowness; difficulty initiating movement; reduced facial expression and blinking; "mask facies"; reduced arm swing; "festinating gait"; reduced voluntary speech; micrographia; "freezing" episodes.
- Postural abnormalities—flexed posture; postural instability with frequent falls.
- Autonomic instability—postural hypotension; constipation; urinary retention; sweaty, greasy, seborrheic skin; hypersalivation with drooling.
- Fatigability.
- Positive glabellar tap.
- "Air pillow sign."

Parkinson's disease dementia (PDD)

Epidemiology

30% of PD patients develop dementia.

Clinical presentation

- Early stages characterized by difficulties in attention, working memory, and executive functioning.
- Memory impairments are mild early and mainly involve difficulty in retrieval.
- Later stages are characterized with severe cognitive impairment, visual hallucinations, delusions and agitation.
- By convention, onset of dementia occurs at least two years after diagnosis of Parkinson's disease. If less than two years, consider DLB.
- DSM-IV-TR criteria for dementia due to general medical condition does not reflect the subcortical nature of PDD.
- Pathology due to reduced DA in the frontal lobes; overlap with both DLB and AD.

Treatment

Rivastigmine is the only drug FDA approved for PDD. It slows cognitive deterioration without significant adverse effect on motor symptoms.

Depression in PD

40–70% of PD patients are affected with depression. The depressive illness may be due to the actual disease process itself as well as a reaction to the stress of the illness. Reduced levels of monoamines (DA, NA, and 5HT) may lead to depression. Mood fluctuations are often noted in association with changes in plasma DA levels. Depression in PD is more common in women and in left-sided disease and is often atypical in nature.

Treatment

Poor response to SSRIs; generally good response with ECT (improves both the depressive illness and motor symptoms but can precipitate delirium).

Psychosis in PD

Visual hallucinations common. May affect up to 40% of cases with late disease and likely represents an affect of the underlying disease. Earlier psychosis less common and may be more likely related to medications used to treat PD including anticholingeric medications, L-Dopa, and DA agonists. Treatment: Use "atypical" antipsychotics with a lower risk of worsening motor symptoms.

Huntington's disease (HD)

A genetic disease characterized by a combination of progressive dementia and worsening chorea. There is autosomal dominant inheritance with 100% penetrance; thus 50% of a patient's offspring will be affected. Onset of symptoms and diagnosis is usually in adulthood, often after the patient has reproduced. A diagnostic test has become available, which allows presymptomatic diagnosis, but because no treatment is available, there are major ethical issues surrounding screening.

Pathology

The Huntington's gene is located on the short arm of chromosome 4 (4p16.3). Under normal conditions, this gene produces a 348 kDa cytoplasmic protein called huntingtin (Htt). A genetic defect in number of the trinucleotide repeat (CAG) leads to the disease state; specifically, the presence of 37 or more CAG repeats produces a mutated form of Htt (mHtt). The greater the number of CAG repeats, the earlier the onset of symptoms and increasing severity of symptoms (a phenomenon known as genetic anticipation). It is unclear how mHtt leads to disease. Other findings include greatly decreased GABA neurons in the basal ganglia, which leads to increased stimulation of the thalamus and cortex by the globus pallidus. Also increase in DA transmission.

Clinical features

Classic triad of chorea, dementia, and a family history of HD. Chorea is a movement disorder characterized by initial jerks, tics, gross involuntary movements of all parts of the body, grimacing, and dysarthria. There is increased tone with rigidity and stiffness, positive primitive reflexes, and abnormal eye movements. Clinical course: onset usually during 30s and 40s; a small number of "juvenile onset" cases; deteriorating course to death within 10–12 years.

Psychiatric syndromes

Occur in 60–75% of patients with HD.
- Anxiety and depression are common.
- Psychosis occurs early and paranoia is common and sometimes schizophrenia-like.
- Aggression and violence.
- Subcortical dementia—slowing, apathy and amnesia.

Investigations

EEG: slowing. CT/MRI: atrophy of basal ganglia with "boxing" of the caudate and dilation of ventricles. PET: decreased metabolism in the basal ganglia.

Treatment

No treatment arrests the course of the disease. However, haloperidol (or other antipsychotics) may help reduce abnormal movements.

Wilson's disease (WD)

Wilson's disease (WD) is a rare genetic disease mapped to the long arm of chromosome 13 (13q14.3) that involves an abnormality of copper metabolism. Copper deposits in the liver cause cirrhosis and in the basal ganglia, resulting in degeneration of the lentiform nucleus ("hepato-lenticular degeneration").

Clinical features

Onset in childhood/adolescence or early adulthood. Liver cirrhosis. E/P signs include: tremor; dystonia; increased tone; "flapping tremor" of wrists; "wing-beating tremor" of shoulders; "risus sardonicus" of face (facial spasm also seen in tetanus); bulbar signs (dysphagia, dysarthria); Kayser-Fleischer rings on slit lamp examination (green-brown corneal deposits in Descemet's membrane).

Psychiatric syndromes

Approximately 30% of cases affected
- Mood disturbances—common.
- Subcortical dementia—25%.
- Psychosis—rare.

Investigations

Increase in serum/24 hour urine copper; ↓ serum ceruloplasmin.

Treatment

Halts disease progression. Usually involves zinc salts to block copper absorption; D-penicillamine (Cuprimine) or Trientine Hcl (Syprine) to increase urinary excretion of copper; and low copper diets. There are also maintenance treatments, such as Zinc Acetate (Galzin). Follow Cu levels and liver function.

Schizophrenia and related psychoses

Introduction

Schizophrenia is a devastating, lifetime psychiatric illness that affects 1% of the population worldwide. Schizophrenia most frequently develops in the late second to third decade of life, with the average age of onset earlier in males than females. The life course of schizophrenia is variable, but frequently involves repeated episodes throughout life with increasing impairment. The relative early age of onset and chronic nature of the illness, coupled with direct costs of medical treatment and the indirect costs of lost productivity due to social and occupational dysfunction, result in a tremendous financial burden to society. Prognosis is considered better with later onset in life, acute rather than insidious onset, high premorbid social and occupational functioning, the presence of co-morbid mood symptoms, positive rather than negative symptoms, and strong social supports.

The clinical presentation of schizophrenia involves a diverse range of signs and symptoms that can be classified into three groups.

Positive symptoms

Positive symptoms are also called psychotic symptoms, which include disturbances in sensory processes such as hallucinations (which are most commonly auditory), delusions (which are most commonly persecutory), and disorganization of thought processes (see Schneider's "symptoms of first rank", 📖 p. 207).

Negative symptoms

Negative symptoms include reduced or inappropriate expression of emotions, loss of the normal level of motivation or drive (anhedonia and avolition), loss of awareness of socially appropriate behavior, flattening of affect, poverty of speech, and difficulty in abstract thinking (see Bleuler's four As 📖 p. 206).

Cognitive symptoms

Cognitive symptoms include impairments in attention, memory, and executive function.

Other symptoms

Other symptoms include formal thought disorder (a loss of the normal flow of thinking usually apparent in the subject's speech or writing, derailment, incoherence), agitation, depression, poor concentration, poor sleep, and "soft" nonlocalizing neurological signs.

Why are there so few famous people with schizophrenia?

Often there is a history of declining social and educational function, which precludes significant achievements (sometimes in spite of early promise). The chronic course of the condition and the major disruptions caused by periods of more severe symptoms also makes it less likely that a person with schizophrenia will achieve as much as their peers. Until relatively recently, there have been few specific treatments for the disorder, and even today, prognosis is at best guarded (p. 223).

Nonetheless, there are notable exceptions to the rule: people who have battled with the disorder and achieved greatness in their chosen fields—in the arts, Vaslav Fomich Nijinsky (1891–1950), the "God of the Dance," whose personal account is found in his autobiography *The Diary of Vaslav Nijinksy*; in sport, Lionel Aldridge (1941–1998), a member of Vince Lombardi's legendary Green Bay Packers of the 1960s, who played in two Super Bowls, and, until his death, gave inspirational talks on his battle against paranoid schizophrenia; and, in popular music, Roger (Syd) Barrett (1946–2006) of Pink Floyd and Peter Green (1946–) of Fleetwood Mac. Perhaps the most famous, due to a recent academy award-winning dramatization of his life, is the mathematician John Forbes Nash Jr. (1928–), who was awarded (jointly with Harsanyi and Selten) the 1994 Nobel Prize in Economic Science for his work on game theory. His life story (upon which the film was based) is recorded by Sylvia Nasar in the book *A Beautiful Mind*.

Important historical perspectives on schizophrenia

Benedict Morel (1809–1873)
Benedict Morel coined the term "démentia précoce" to describe the deteriorating course of an illness that began in adolescence.

Emil Kraeplin (1856–1926)
Emil Kraeplin used the term "dementia praecox" to describe a chronic, progressive disease with an early age of onset and prominent cognitive and psychotic symptoms. He distinguished dementia praecox from manic-depressive psychosis and its associated periods of full remission.

Eugen Bleuler (1857–1939)
Eugen Bleuler first used the term "schizophrenia" to describe the split between thought, emotion, and behavior found in the illness. Bleuler noted that schizophrenia is not always associated with a deteriorating course. He described what is now known as the four As of schizophrenia: loose Associations, incongruent Affect, Autism, and Ambivalence. He considered hallucinations and delusions to be accessory symptoms.

Kurt Schneider (1887–1967)
Kurt Schneider provided a clinically useful description of the positive symptoms of schizophrenia (termed "first-rank symptoms" or "symptoms of first rank").

Schneider's "symptoms of first rank" (1959)

- Auditory hallucinations taking the form of one of the following:
  - Voices repeating the subject's thoughts aloud ("dankenlautwerden," "écho de la pensée") or anticipating their thoughts.
  - Two or more hallucinatory voices discussing the subject or arguing about him or her in the third person.
  - Voices commenting on the subject's thoughts or behavior, often in the form of a running commentary.
- The sensation of alien thoughts being put into the subject's mind by some external agency (thought insertion) or of his or her own thoughts being taken away (thought withdrawal).
- The sensation that the subject's thinking is no longer confined to his/her own mind, but is instead shared by, or accessible to others (thought broadcasting).
- The sensation of feelings, impulses, or acts being experienced are carried out under external control, so that the subject feels as if he or she were being hypnotized or had become a robot (passivity of affect, impulse, or volition).
- The experience of being a passive and reluctant recipient of bodily sensations imposed by some external agency (somatic passivity).
- A delusional perception, i.e., a delusion arising fully on the basis of a genuine perception that others would regard as commonplace and unrelated.

Pathophysiology of schizophrenia

The dopamine hypothesis

Simply stated, the original dopamine (DA) hypothesis posits that schizophrenia results from excessive activity of the DA system and is based on two observations.

- First, the mechanism of antipsychotic medications involves the blockade of DA receptors.
- Second, agents that effectively increase DA activity, such amphetamine-induced release of DA from presynaptic vesicles, have been found to induce and exacerbate psychotic symptoms in normal controls and in patients with schizophrenia, respectively.
- Additional evidence from imaging studies have found that amphetamine induces a greater displacement of radiolabeled-ligand bound to D_2 receptors in the striatum (suggesting a predisposition to release larger amounts of DA) in never-treated schizophrenia patients.

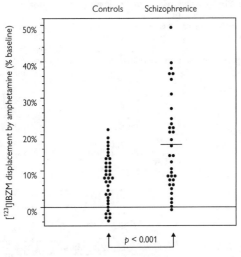

Fig. 6.1 This graph illustrates the effect of amphetamine (0.3mg/kg) on [^{123}I]IBZM binding in healthy control subjects and untreated patients with schizophrenia using single photon emission tomography (SPET). The y-axis shows the percentage decrease in [^{123}I]IBZM binding potential induced by amphetamine, which is a measure of the increased occupancy of D_2 receptors by dopamine following the challenge. Thus these results indicate that, when challenged with amphetamine, patients with schizophrenia release more dopamine than healthy controls. This effect is only seen in patients with schizophrenia when they are acutely psychotic. (From Laruelle, M., Abi-Dargham, A., Gil, R., Kegeles, L., Innis, R. Increased dopamine transmission in schizophrenia: relationship to illness phases. (1999). *Biological Psychiatry* **46**(1): 56–72).

- More recently, the DA hypothesis has undergone some revision to suggest that excessive subcortical DA activity is associated with the positive symptoms of schizophrenia, whereas deficient cortical DA activity is associated with the negative and cognitive symptoms of schizophrenia.
  - For example, lesions of the DA system in the prefrontal cortex of monkeys have been reported to result in some cognitive dysfunction.

However, several lines of evidence suggest that the pathophysiology of schizophrenia is significantly more complicated than the DA hypothesis.

- For example, postmortem studies have, in general, revealed limited evidence of abnormalities in markers of the DA system in schizophrenia.
- In addition, the extended period of exposure required for full clinical response to antipsychotic medications suggests that their efficacy may involve more downstream effects on neural circuitry than just the immediate blockade of DA receptors.
- Also, clozapine, considered the most efficacious of antipsychotic medications, has a relatively lower affinity for D_2 receptors.
- Furthermore, antipsychotic medications have limited utility in the treatment of the negative and cognitive symptoms of schizophrenia.
- Finally, the DA system is a remarkably complicated neurotransmitter system that modulates, and is modulated by, other neurotransmitter systems from different brain regions. Thus, the DA system may be more involved as a downstream consequence of other, more primary, lesions in the brain in schizophrenia.

The NMDA receptor hypofunction hypothesis

Multiple lines of clinical evidence suggest that glutamatergic neurotransmission may be deficient in schizophrenia. For example, phenylcyclidine (PCP) and ketamine, which are antagonists of the NMDA subtype of glutamate receptor, may induce schizophrenia-like symptoms in control subjects and exacerbate these symptoms in subjects with schizophrenia. Furthermore, NMDA receptor antagonists can induce positive, negative, and some cognitive symptoms, in contrast to DA agonists (see above), which induce predominantly psychotic symptoms.

These NMDA receptor antagonists induce symptoms in adults, but only rarely in children, which mimics the delayed age of onset of schizophrenia. Conversely, agents that facilitate NMDA receptor function, such as glycine, which binds to a modulatory site on NMDA receptors, and D-cycloserine, which is a selective partial agonist at the glycine modulatory site, have been reported to improve some positive and negative symptoms and cognitive dysfunction in schizophrenia. These clinical studies suggest that NMDA receptors may be hypofunctional in schizophrenia.

However, genetic studies have failed to find evidence of linkage of the NMDAR1 subunit to schizophrenia. Furthermore, radiolabeled-ligand binding studies and analyses of mRNA expression have not consistently reported decreased NMDA receptor levels in schizophrenia. Thus, although predominantly clinical observations suggest that DA and glutamate neurotransmission appear to be involved in the pathophysiology of schizophrenia, abnormalities in these neurotransmitter systems do not appear to fully account for the illness.

Diagnosis (1)—symptoms and categories

The diagnosis of schizophrenia is made on the basis of symptoms as outlined in the DSM-IV-TR. There is no single sign or symptom that is pathognomonic for schizophrenia. The symptoms of schizophrenia are conventionally divided into positive (new symptoms or signs) and negative (loss of a previous function). See previous 🕮 p. 204.

Key points in diagnosing pathological delusions

Clinical judgment is necessary to distinguish delusions from overvalued ideas, particularly when the ideas expressed are not necessarily bizarre or culturally abnormal (and may actually have some basis in reality). Such judgments may be informed by:
• the degree of plausibility.
• evidence of systemization, complexity, and persistence.
• the impact of the beliefs on behavior.
• allowing for the possibility that they might be culturally sanctioned beliefs different from one's own.
• informants from the same sociocultural background as the patient.
• observation of associated characteristics, including hallucinations.
• history of "morbid change."

Diagnosis (2)—DSM-IV-TR criteria

Characteristic symptoms

Two (or more) of the following, each present for a significant portion of time during a one-month period (or less if successfully treated):

- delusions.
- hallucinations.
- disorganized speech.
- grossly disorganized or catatonic behavior.
- negative symptoms, i.e., affective flattening, alogia, or avolition.

Note: Only one Criterion A symptom is required if delusions are bizarre or hallucinations consist of a voice that keeps up a running commentary on the person's behavior or thoughts, or two or more voices conversing with each other.

Social/occupational dysfunction

For a significant proportion of the time since the onset of the disturbance, one or more major areas of functioning such as work, interpersonal relations, or self-care are markedly below the level achieved prior to the onset (or when the onset is in childhood or adolescence, failure to achieve expected level of interpersonal, academic, or occupational achievement).

Duration

Continuous signs of the disturbance persist for at least six months. This six-month period must include at least one month of symptoms (or less if successfully treated) that meet Criterion A (i.e., active-phase symptoms) and may include periods of prodromal or residual symptoms. During these prodromal or residual periods, the signs of the disturbance may be manifested by only negative symptoms or two or more symptoms listed in Criterion A present in an attenuated form (e.g., odd beliefs, unusual perceptual experiences).

Schizoaffective and mood disorder exclusion

Schizoaffective disorder and mood disorder with psychotic features have been ruled out because either:

- no major depressive, manic, or mixed episodes have occurred concurrently with the active-phase symptoms; or
- if mood episodes have occurred during active-phase symptoms, their total duration has been brief relative to the duration of the active and residual periods.

Substance/general medical condition exclusion

The disturbance is not due to the direct physiological effects of a substance (e.g., a drug of abuse, a medication) or a general medical condition.

Relationship to a pervasive developmental disorder

If there is a history of autistic disorder or another pervasive developmental disorder, the additional diagnosis of schizophrenia is made only if prominent delusions or hallucinations are also present for at least a month (or less if successfully treated).

DSM-IV-TR also allows for course specifiers: for example, "episodic," with or without interepisodic residual symptoms (each episode meets Criteria A for schizophrenia); "continuous"; "single episode in partial remission," (some clinically significant residual symptoms remain); "single episode in full remission"; "other or unspecified pattern." Note that if residual symptoms include "prominent negative symptoms," this may also be included as a specifier, e.g., "continuous with prominent negative symptoms".

ICD-10 schizophrenia

At least one of the following:
- Thought echo, insertion, withdrawal, or broadcasting.
- Delusions of control, influence, or passivity; clearly referred to body or limb movements or specific thoughts, actions, or sensations; and delusional perception.
- Hallucinatory voices giving a running commentary on the patient's behavior or discussing him/her between themselves, or other types of hallucinatory voices coming from some part of the body.
- Persistent delusions of other kinds that are culturally inappropriate or implausible (e.g., religious/political identity, superhuman powers and ability).

Or, at least two of the following:
- persistent hallucinations in any modality, when accompanied by fleeting or half-formed delusions without clear affective content, persistent overvalued ideas, or occurring every day for weeks or months on end.
- breaks of interpolations in the train of thought, resulting in incoherence or irrelevant speech or neologisms.
- catatonic behavior such as excitement, posturing, or waxy flexibility, negativism, mutism, and stupor.
- negative symptoms such as marked apathy, paucity of speech, and blunting or incongruity of emotional responses.
- a significant and consistent change in the overall quality of some aspects of personal behavior, manifested as loss of interest, aimlessness, idleness, a self-absorbed attitude, and social withdrawal.

Duration of ≥1 month.

Categories

DSM-IV-TR	ICD-10	Key symptoms
Paranoid type	Paranoid schizophrenia	Delusions and hallucinations
Disorganized type	Hebephrenic schizophrenia	Disorganized speech and behavior (often silly/shallow) and flat or inappropriate affect
Catatonic type	Catatonic schizophrenia	Psychomotor disturbance (see 📖 pp. 217, 1104)
Undifferentiated type	Undifferentiated schizophrenia	Meeting general criteria, but no specific symptom subtype predominates
	Postschizophrenic depression	Some residual symptoms, but depressive picture predominates
	Residual schizophrenia	Previous positive symptoms less marked; prominent negative symptoms
	Simple schizophrenia	No delusions or hallucinations—a "defect state" (negative symptoms) gradually arises usually without an acute episode.

Differential diagnosis of psychosis

Substance-induced psychotic disorder

Induced by, for example, alcohol, stimulants, hallucinogens, steroids, antihistamines, sympathomimetics. Careful history taking may reveal onset, persistence, and cessation of symptoms to be related to drug use.

Psychotic disorder due to a general medical condition

Focused history, examination, and investigations should help exclude other disorders (e.g., head injury, CNS infection, CNS tumor).

Mood disorders with psychotic features

Mood and related biological symptoms are usually more severe and precede psychosis.

Brief psychotic disorder and schizophreniform disorder

Diagnosed only after the psychotic symptoms have resolved based on the time course.

Delusional disorder

Presence of at least one nonbizarre delusion with a lack of thought disorder, prominent hallucinations, mood disorder, and flattening of affect.

Schizophrenia

Presence of psychotic symptoms other than relatively circumscribed delusions, greater functional impairment.

Dementia and delirium

Evidence of cognitive impairment or altered/fluctuating level of consciousness, respectively. Delirium, characteristically has a waxing and waning course. Note: also consider "late paraphrenia," which, although not included in DSM-IV-TR, has an extensive literature and is thought to be distinct from delusional disorder and schizophrenia, associated with social isolation, aging, medical problems/treatments, and sensory loss.

Body dysmorphic disorder

Significant overlap with delusional disorder, few significant differentiating factors exist.

Post-traumatic stress disorder

Evidence of a past, life-threatening trauma.

Pervasive developmental disorder

Evidence of impairment in functioning from the preschool years.

Obsessive-compulsive disorder
Significant overlap with delusional disorder and, if reality testing regarding obsessions or compulsions is lost, delusional disorder is often diagnosed.

Hypochondriasis
Health concerns generally are more amenable to reality testing and are less fixed than in delusional disorder.

Paranoid personality disorder
Absence of clearly circumscribed delusions, presence of a pervasive, stable pattern of suspiciousness or distrust.

Schizotypal personality disorder
Odd or eccentric behavior, absence of clearly circumscribed delusions.

Misidentification syndromes
Easily confused with delusional disorder, may be associated with other CNS abnormalities.

Induced/shared psychotic disorder
Evidence that relatives or close friends share similar delusional beliefs.

A note on formulation

Even in the absence of a specific cause, the etiology of schizophrenia is predominantly influenced by factors affecting the brain. However, the following areas might be considered as a guide to the assessment of predisposing, precipitating, and perpetuating factors:
- Biological: consider family history of psychiatric illness, recent substance abuse, drug noncompliance, history of obstetric complications, brain injury, and co-morbid medical illness.
- Psychosocial: consider recent stressful life events, family cohesion or friction, living conditions, attitude regarding and knowledge of illness.

Other clinical presentations
For the most part, patients with schizophrenia will present with the symptoms outlined above and a decrease in social functioning and self care. There are, however, other more rare presentations such as:
- **Catatonia**—once part of a subtype of schizophrenia these, mainly motor, symptoms may occur in any form of schizophrenia and include.
  - Ambitendence—the alternation between opposite movements.
  - Echopraxia—automatic imitation of another persons movements even when asked not to.
  - Stereotypies—repeated regular fixed parts of movement (or speech) that are not goal directed, e.g., moving the arm backward and outward repeatedly while saying, "But not for me."
  - Negativism—motiveless resistance to instructions and attempts to be moved, or doing the opposite of what is asked.
  - Posturing—adoption of inappropriate or bizarre bodily posture continuously for a substantial period of time.

- Waxy flexibility—the patient's limbs can be "moulded" into a position and remain fixed for long periods of time.

ECT may have a specific benefit for the catatonic symptoms in schizophrenia, although this is by no means proven.

Water intoxication

This involves the patient drinking sometime gallons of liquid a day (usually water) leading to severe electrolyte disturbances and sometimes death.

The cause is sometimes delusional in origin but water intoxication is often associated with syndrome of inappropriate antidiuretic hormone secretion (SIADH). SIADH is associated with schizophrenia but may also be caused by psychotropic medications such as antipsychotics and lithium.

Treatment is fluid restriction and, if SIADH is thought to be secondary to medication, then the medication should be stopped or reduced.

Epidemiological factors and the pathophysiology of schizophrenia

Multiple genetic and environmental factors appear to be involved in the etiology of schizophrenia. For example, the risk of developing schizophrenia in relatives increases with the proportion of shared genes. See table below.

Schizophrenia liability based on affected relatives	
Family member(s) affected	**Risk (approximate)**
Identical twin	46%
One sibling/fraternal twin	12–15%
Both parents	40%
One parent	12–15%
One grandparent	6%
No relatives affected	0.5–1%

The genetic contribution to schizophrenia overall is between 70 and 80%.

Although there is a high degree of heritability in schizophrenia, genetic liability alone is not sufficient for the clinical appearance of the disorder. Indeed, although many potentially susceptible genes have been discovered, the degree of risk conferred by each gene is relatively small, and the biological consequences are mostly unknown. In addition, pre- and perinatal environmental factors such as severe maternal malnutrition, maternal influenza, obstetrical complications, and urban birth are also associated with increased risk for schizophrenia.

Furthermore, the presence of some cognitive and behavioral signs during the premorbid and prodromal stages of the illness, as well as the delayed appearance of full clinical symptoms until around adolescence and early adulthood, suggests that schizophrenia represents a neurodevelopmental illness. Interestingly, the use of cannabis during adolescence, but not adulthood, has been reported to increase the risk for schizophrenia later in life. Thus, the etiology of schizophrenia is thought to involve the interaction between genetic susceptibility, environmental risk factors, and neurodevelopmental processes that lead to the eventual clinical appearance of the illness.

Physical examination

A thorough medical history, including a review of systems (ROS), is the basis for a comprehensive patient assessment.

ROS key features

- HEENT—headache, head injury, abnormal movements of the mouth or tongue (see AIMS exam, 📖 p. 242), diplopia, hearing impairment (delusional disorder is more common in the hearing impaired).
- Respiratory—dyspnea, orthopnea.
- Cardiovascular—chest pain, palpitations.
- Gastrointestinal—constipation (can be side-effect of anticholinergic psychotropic drugs), nausea, vomiting.
- Genitourinary—urinary hesitancy (retention in men caused by anticholinergic drugs); in women, a menstrual history.
- Neurologic—history of seizures or stroke.

Physical exam

Inpatient psychiatric patients require a full physical examination. Although the need for a complete physical examination of an outpatient is based on presenting complaints, it cannot be overemphasized that psychiatric patients frequently have systemic co-morbidities, which can be missed without a thorough physical examination.

A full neurological examination may be the most important investigation, and may focus on gait inspection; examination of the extremities for weakness and/or altered sensation; examination of hand-eye coordination; examination of smooth ocular pursuit; and examination of the cranial nerves. The abnormal involuntary movement scale (AIMS, see 📖 p. 242) is used to examine potential movement side-effects of certain medications.

Mental status exam

Be sure to check orientation, attention, concentration, and antero-grade/retrograde memory at a minimum. Consider underlying neurological condition when disorientation is present or if memory problems are severe or persistent in spite of adequate treatment.

Course and prognosis

There is usually a large degree of uncertainty regarding the course and prognosis in first-episode patients, regardless of their presenting symptoms or demographic and personal history.

Approximate guide to course and prognosis at 13 years' follow-up[1]

- Approximately 15–20% of first episodes will not recur.
- Few people will remain employed.
- 52% are without psychotic symptoms for at least two years.
- 52% are without negative symptoms.
- 55% show good/fair social functioning.

Prognostic factors in schizophrenia

Poor prognostic indicators include:
- Poor premorbid adjustment.
- Insidious onset.
- Onset in childhood or adolescence.
- Cognitive impairment.
- Enlarged ventricles.
- Symptoms fulfilling multiple criteria in DSM-IV-TR for diagnosis.

Good prognostic factors include:
- Marked mood disturbance, especially elation, during initial presentation.
- Family history of affective disorder.
- Female sex.
- Living in a developing country.

Recommended further reading

1 Mason, P., Harrison, G., Glazebrook, C., et al. (1995). Characteristics of outcome in schizophrenia at 13 years. *BJP* **167**, 596–603.

Relapse, response, remission, and recovery

"The four Rs" of schizophrenia outcome

As is common with many other psychiatric disorders, schizophrenia is generally described as a relapsing and remitting condition. Until recently, however, there has been no general consensus on measuring or defining "the four Rs" for the individual schizophrenia patient or for schizophrenia treatment and outcome studies. This has hampered comparison of outcomes between studies and across time.

Relapse

Relapse may be broadly defined as a deterioration in clinical presentation such than an additional intervention is required. The intervention could vary from a change in psychosocial support through an adjustment or change in medication up to admission to hospital, depending on the severity of the relapse. There are, as yet, no widely accepted operationalized guidelines for quantitatively assessing a relapse in schizophrenia. This is despite the fact that "relapse prevention" is currently one of the primary aims of schizophrenia treatment and is a frequent primary outcome measure in long-term clinical trials of both medication and psychosocial treatments.

Response

Response to treatment is also often broadly defined. In treatment trials response rates are usually quoted as the percentage of a treatment cohort who has a specific percentage reduction in score on one of the standard rating scales.

For example, for a given intervention, 70% of the treatment cohort had a 20% reduction in the rating scale whereas 50% of the treatment cohort had a 40% reduction.

Thus, 70% of people treated responded at the 20% level and 50% at the 40% level. Although this type of response description may have face validity regarding treatment trial outcomes, it has been criticized as inadequate. This is particularly the case for people who are severely ill at initiation of treatment, who may achieve a 40% reduction in a rating scale with treatment, but who still may be markedly impaired and unable to function normally in the community.

Remission and Recovery

Remission and recovery are linked constructs but currently poorly defined.

A recent working party, following on from previous work to define remission criteria for mood and anxiety disorders, has attempted to address the issue of remission in schizophrenia. They suggest that while for schizophrenia, "complete recovery implies the ability to function in the community, socially and vocationally, as well as being relatively free of disease-related psychopathology," remission might be considered a less demanding and more readily achieved goal. They further argue that an operationalized definition of remission will serve to emphasize outcomes that are relevant to patients, carergivers, and clinicians, and thus maximize functional improvement.

This is in contrast with the current treatment perspective that is focused on relapse prevention. This may narrow the therapeutic view to the extent that the wider functional and quality-of-life disabilities in schizophrenia may be neglected. Using a dimensional approach and the three groups of characteristic symptoms, psychoticism, disorganization and negative symptoms, the proposed definition remission is, "a state in which patients have experienced an improvement in core signs and symptoms to the extent that any remaining symptoms are of such low intensity that they no longer interfere significantly with behavior and are below the threshold typically utilized in justifying an initial diagnosis of schizophrenia".

Clinical management of schizophrenia

The 2004 APA Treatment Recommendations for Patients with Schizophrenia divide the treatment of schizophrenia into three treatment phases:
- Acute Phase (initial presentation).
- Stabilization Phase (early symptom remission).
- Stable Phase (maintenance treatment).

Correctly identifying the phase of illness helps practitioners identify the goals of therapy. Briefly, the goals of acute phase treatment are to ensure patient safety, to perform a comprehensive physical and psychiatric assessment to identify underlying etiology or contributing factors to the psychotic episode as well as provide prompt treatment of psychotic symptoms, and to establish a therapeutic alliance with the patient and the patient's family. Acute phase treatment may involve psychiatric hospitalization if patient safety or compliance cannot be ensured in a less restrictive setting.

During the stabilization phase, the patient's psychotic symptoms are in early remission or substantially reduced or in early remission. The goals of this phase are to provide sustained symptom remission, minimize patient stress, and coordinate a successful transition to the community, including arranging for enhanced family and community supports.

During the stable phase of illness, the goals of treatment are to manage medication side-effects, to monitor medication adherence, and to teach the patient to engage in psychiatric self-monitoring. Furthermore, the focus of care includes general medical care, the involvement of family and other community supports, and the identification and reduction of factors likely to contribute to relapse.

Acute phase

Initial psychiatric assessment

1. *Physical assessment and evaluation of general medical health*
- Vital signs and body weight (including waist circumference).
- Identification of substance intoxication/withdrawal syndromes including urine or serum toxicology screen.
- Pregnancy test for women of childbearing age.
- EKG (and documentation of pretreatment QTc).
- CBC, electrolytes, liver function testing, metabolic panel.
- Brain imaging for first break (MRI preferred over CT), in the setting of focal neurologic signs or atypical presentations.
- EEG if symptoms suggest seizure activity.

2. *Psychiatric assessment*
- Safety assessment
  - Imminent danger to self or others may require acute hospitalization. Specifically, practitioners should elicit and document:
    — History or presence of suicide attempt or suicidal ideation (including means and intensity.)
    — Prominent mood symptoms.
    — Command hallucinations, hopelessness, anxiety, EPS, substance use disorders.

- — History of aggression or violence during current or past psychotic episodes.
- — Whenever possible elicit information from collateral informants.
- Environmental Adaptations
  - Establish rapport with patient, minimize the use of multiple interviewers whenever possible.
  - If possible, perform the assessment in a structured, simple environment with minimal extraneous noise and stimuli.
  - Employ clear, simple communication.
  - Employ restraints only when necessary to prevent aggressive behavior toward self and others.
  - With acutely agitated patients, assessments should be conducted with the interviewer closest to the door, to reduce risk that the interviewer will become cornered or unable to leave the interview promptly if safety is in jeopardy.

3. Pharmacotherapy

- Management of acute psychosis in schizophrenia will almost always involve the use of an antipsychotic agent (either a newer "atypical" or older "typical" antipsychotic). Frequently, treatment augmentation with benzodiazepines can be helpful in controlling severely distressed patients. Of note, in acute psychotic episodes resulting from alcohol or benzodiazepine withdrawal, benzodiazepines should be the primary agent used (📖 p. 230).
- Medication should be administered promptly.
  - Assess whether the patient is too cognitively impaired to engage in a discussion of risks and benefits of treatment, or represents an imminent safety risk to self or others.
  - If possible, administration of any medication should follow a doctor-patient discussion of the risks, benefits, and alternative treatments.
  - When this is not feasible, state regulations allowing for emergency involuntary treatments should be followed.
  - Whenever possible, a baseline laboratory evaluation (see Physical assessment, above) should be completed prior to the initiation of pharmacotherapy, or as soon as possible thereafter.

Antipsychotic medications in the acute phase

Selection of an antipsychotic medication is guided by the patient's past history with antipsychotics (i.e., history of prior symptom remission, side-effects, patient preference). A review of antipsychotic medication is provided in other sections. Atypical ("second-generation") antipsychotics are the agents of choice in the treatment of schizophrenia due to decreased risks of EPS (extrapyramidal symptoms) and tardive dyskinesia. However, practitioners may consider typical (first generation), antipsychotics in patients with a history of successful treatment with first generation antipsychotics, preference for a first generation antipsychotic, or in patients who have failed two or several trials of second-generation antipsychotics, but are unwilling or unable to receive clozapine.

- The goal of pharmacotherapy treatment is to optimize therapeutic benefit while minimizing side-effects.
- Educate patients about common side-effects of antipsychotics to improve the reporting of short-term side-effects (see 📖 p. 238).
- Side-effects such as nausea, sedation, dystonias, and postural hypotension may be more likely to resolve early in treatment, while EPS and akathisia are more likely to persist.
- With the exception of clozapine, there is no convincing evidence that one atypical antipsychotic is more efficacious than another. Clozapine is indicated for use in treatment resistant schizophrenia, and is discussed later 📖 p. 246.
- Use of orally disintegrating tablets (risperidone, olanzapine) or short-acting intramuscular preparations (olanzapine IM, ziprasidone IM) may be indicated when compliance is in question (i.e., suspicion of diverting or "cheeking" medication).
- While the acute tranquilizing effects of antipsychotic medication may occur within 30–60 minutes of administration, the full therapeutic response can take 2–4 weeks, with maximal effects not fully realized for up to 6 months. Prudence is necessary, because titrating doses too high or too quickly in the acute treatment phase can result in more side-effects without increased therapeutic benefit, and a greater risk that the patient will be noncompliant later in therapy.
- The practice of "Rapid Neuroleptization" (using antipsychotic doses well in excess of 1,000mg chlorpromazine equivalents in the first 24 hours of treatment) has not been demonstrated to provide more complete or immediate tranquilization, but it does lead to an increased side-effect burden.
- Due to their potent D_2 receptor blocking properties, EPS are common with high potency typical antipsychotic medications. They also occur with the atypical antipsychotics with less frequency and severity. Adjunctive medications commonly used to treat these extrapyramidal side-effects include:
    - benztropine 0.5–1mg po t.i.d.
    - diphenhydramine 25–50mg po t.i.d.

- Acute dystonia (an abrupt, painful contraction of one or more skeletal muscle groups) is a side-effect distinct from EPS, and is believed to be an idiosyncratic reaction to the dopamine blocking effects of antipsychotic medications. Prompt administration of benztropine 1–2mg po/IM or diphenhydramine 50–100mg po/IM can reverse dystonia. IM administration may result in more rapid reversal of dystonia than oral administration.

Emergent pharmacotherapy in the acute phase

Although oral administration is optimal to minimize patient distress, and most patients prefer oral medications, intramuscular agents may be necessary to reduce acute agitation and psychosis in patients who are unable or unwilling to comply with oral medication. Commonly used agents include:

- olanzapine 5–10mg IM.
- ziprasidone 20mg IM (black box warning for QTc prolongation).
- haloperidol 5–10mg IM (consider co-administration with benztropine 1–2mg IM to reduce risk of EPS or acute dystonic reaction).
- consider adjunctive use of lorazepam 1–2mg IM for severe agitation or aggression.

If the patient is willing to take oral medication, but adherence is in question, use of orally disintegrating tablets (risperidone M-Tab; olanzapine zydis) or liquid (risperidone, aripiprazole) is recommended. Liquid and orally disintegrating formulations do not provide more rapid tranquilization than traditional oral medication formulations.

Adjunctive medications in the treatment of acute psychosis

Benzodiazepines

- Benzodiazepines are the primary agent for acute psychosis due to alcohol or benzodiazepine withdrawal. Please refer to section on alcohol intoxication and withdrawal for dosing strategies 📖 p. 644.
- While benzodiazepines are not indicated as monotherapy in schizophrenia, they are commonly used in conjunction with an antipsychotic in the treatment of acute anxiety, agitation, or catatonia.
- Benzodiazepines may be administered in oral and parenteral form.
- Lorazepam 1–2mg IM/po/IV for acute distress or agitation.
- Diazepam 5–10mg IM/po.

Antidepressants, mood stabilizers

- Depressive syndromes are common during all phases of schizophrenia, and can increase the risk of suicidal behavior.
- Antidepressants are frequently employed to treat depressive symptoms.
- Antidepressants that inhibit dopamine reuptake (MAOIs; bupropion) should be avoided or used with caution.

Electroconvulsive Therapy (ECT)

- ECT has been employed in treatment-resistant patients who have failed to benefit from clozapine, particularly when co-morbid mood symptoms are present, or in the setting of catatonia unresponsive to antipsychotics and benzodiazepines.
- In general, antipsychotic medications that have provided partial response prior to ECT are continued during the course of ECT.
- ECT is also used in the presence of severe co-morbid mood symptoms (depression, mania) which are unresponsive to medications, psychotherapy, or require more rapid symptom remission than can be expected with antidepressant medication.

Stabilization phase

The goals of the stabilization phase (early remission or significant reduction in psychotic symptoms) include:

- Sustained symptom remission.
- Adherence to medication and therapy appointments.
- Minimization of stress.
- Successful transition and continued support in the community.
- Establishment of a long-term treatment plan.
- Medication doses that resulted in acute symptom remission should be sustained for at least six months unless they are intolerable.
- Monitor for common side-effects (EPS, sedation, weight gain).
- At each appointment, body weight, waist circumference, pulse, and blood pressure should be recorded to screen for early signs of metabolic syndrome.
- Educate patient and family about the illness and contributing factors to relapse, including medication nonadherence and substance use. If possible, and with the patient's consent, identify one or more community informants that can contact the treatment team if signs of psychosis reemerge.
- Educate and engage patient in symptom monitoring.
- Arrange follow-up with outpatient mental health providers prior to hospital discharge.

Stable phase

The goals of stable phase treatment are continued symptom remission, prevention of psychotic relapse, social rehabilitation, and improvement in overall quality of life.

Antipsychotic pharmacotherapy—reduction of relapse risk

- The importance of continuing antipsychotic medications even after symptom remission in schizophrenia has been well established.
- One-year relapse rates among patients taking placebo is approximately 70%, compared to roughly 30%, or lower, relapse rate among patients taking antipsychotic medication.
- APA treatment guidelines recommend that first-episode patients continue maintenance antipsychotics for no less than one to two years following their psychotic episode. Even then, relapse rates after medication discontinuation can be as high as 75%.
- Patients with recurrent episodes should be maintained on medications for a minimum of five years of stability before a discontinuation trial is considered.
- Patients with recurrent, severe psychotic episodes (severe functional impairment, violent behavior) should be maintained indefinitely.
- Despite the known benefits of maintenance antipsychotic treatments, data from the Clinical Antipsychotic Trials of Intervention Effectiveness (CATIE) trial indicate that patient discontinuation of antipsychotic medications is common, due to perceived ineffectiveness of the medication, intolerable side-effects, or both. Of the 1,432 patients with schizophrenia randomized to receive an atypical antipsychotic, 74% discontinued the medication prior to the conclusion of the 18-month trial.

General approach to prescribing

Brief history and introduction

Although no efficacious treatments are presently available for either the negative or cognitive symptoms of schizophrenia, effective treatments do exist for the positive, or psychotic, symptoms (i.e., hallucinations, delusions, and disorganization).

Chlorpromazine, considered the first antipsychotic or "neuroleptic" medication, was first discovered in the 1950s. The antipsychotic effects of chlorpromazine were later determined to involve blockade of dopamine (D_2) receptors, leading to the "dopamine hypothesis" of schizophrenia. Treatments of psychosis developed subsequently involving medications with a variable but often high affinity for D_2 receptors had a narrow therapeutic range and are now termed "typicals." However, these D_2 receptor antagonists can yield Parkinsonian-like side-effects or extrapyramidal symptoms (EPS).

The newest class of antipsychotics, the "atypicals," also act as D_2 receptor antagonists; however, they have additional pharmacodynamic profiles, including antagonism of the 5-HT_{2A} receptor, have a wider therapeutic range and have a lower likelihood of causing EPS. Typicals and atypicals are generally considered to be equally effective in the treatment of schizophrenia, with the notable exception of clozapine. However, side-effect profiles of these two classes of medications differ significantly. Unfortunately, a large percentage of patients with schizophrenia (up to three-quarters in the recent CATIE study) eventually discontinue treatment due to inefficacy, side-effects, or choice.

Typical antipsychotics

In general, typical antipsychotics have a wide range of affinities for the D_2 receptor, when compared relative to chlorpromazine. Chlorpromazine has a relatively low affinity for the D_2 receptor, whereas haloperidol and fluphenazine have relatively high affinities for the D_2 receptor.

As a rule of thumb, typicals with a high affinity for D_2 receptors have lower anticholinergic side-effects and this is actually similar for atypicals. Some evidence suggests that the degree of occupancy of D_2 receptors may correlate with clinical outcome. For example, 65–70% occupancy of striatal D_2 receptors may yield antipsychotic efficacy, while 80% receptor occupancy increases the risk of EPS.

Interestingly, older practice methods involved dosing with typicals until EPS occurred, then reducing the dose slightly. Although atypical antipsychotic medications have largely overtaken typical antipsychotic medications as the first choice in treatment of psychotic symptoms, typicals remain valuable tools in part due to their;

- Equality in efficacy.
- Lower risk of metabolic side-effects.
- Availability in long-acting injectable depot formulations (haloperidol and fluphenazine).

The newer, "atypical," antipsychotics (1)

These antipsychotics are not a separate class as such. Each of these drugs has a slightly different pharmacological profile but share in common a wider therapeutic range than the older, "typical" antipsychotics.

Aripiprazole (Abilify®)

Pharmacology

- D_2 receptor partial agonist; partial agonist at 5-HT_{1A} receptors; high-affinity antagonist at 5-HT_{2A} receptors; low-/moderate-affinity antagonist at H_1 and α_1 receptors; no anticholinergic effect.

Dosages and preparations

- 2, 5, 10, 15, 20 and 30mg tablets.
- 10, 15, 20 and 30mg oral disintegrating tablet.
- 1mg/ml oral solution.
- Dosage 10–30mg once daily.
- Optimum dose 10–20mg once daily.

Side-effects

- Low EPS similar to placebo at all doses (initial akathisia-like symtoms can occur in the first two to three weeks of treatment).
- Does not increase plasma prolactin levels (and may decrease levels).
- Less weight gain than olanzapine.

Olanzapine (Zyprexa®)

Pharmacology

- Receptor antagonism: $5\text{-HT}_{2A} = H_1 = M_1 > 5\text{-HT}_{2C} > D_2 > \alpha_1 > D_1$.

Dosages and preparations

- 2.5, 5, 7.5, 10, 15, and 20mg tablets.
- Zydis (disintegrating tablet) 5, 10, 15 and 20mg.
- Short acting intramuscular 10mg.
- Optimum dose 10–20mg per day, occasionally up to 30mg per day.

Side-effects

- EPS similar to placebo in clinical doses.
- Sedation; weight gain; dizziness; dry mouth; constipation.
- Less increase in prolactin than haloperidol or risperidone.
- Possibly glucose dysregulation.

Paliperidone (INVEGA®)

Metabilite of risperidone (9-OH-risperidone)

Phamacology

- Receptor antagonism: similar profile to risperidone, but lower D_2 affinity, similar D_3 lower 5-HT_{2A}, similar 5-HT_{2C}, similar H_1, lower α_{1A} but higher α_{2A} affinity.

Quetiapine (Seroquel®)

Pharmacology

- Receptor antagonism: $H_1 > a_1 > 5\text{-HT}_2 > \alpha_2 > D_2$.

Dosages and preparations

- 25, 50, 100, 200, 300 and 400mg tablets.
- Dose range is 300mg to 800mg in divided doses, optimal dose may be.
- 500mg–800mg per day or higher.

Side-effects

- EPS = placebo.
- No increase in prolactin; sedation; dizziness (postural hypotension); constipation.
- Infrequent—dry mouth, weight gain.
- Consider ophthalmologic examination for cataracts.

Risperidone (Risperdal®)

Pharmacology

- Receptor antagonism: $5\text{-}HT_2 > D_2 = \alpha_1 = \alpha_2$; little histamine H_1 affinity; minimal D_1, $5\text{-}HT_1$ affinity.

Dosages and preparations

- 0.25, 0.5, 1, 2, 3, 4mg tablets.
- 1mg/ml liquid.
- M-tab 0.5, 1, 2, 3 and 4mg (disintegrating tablet).
- Intramuscular extended release 25, 37.5, 50mg.
- Dosage 3–6mg daily given in 1–2 doses.

Side-effects

- Markedly less pseudoparkinsonism than typical antipsychotics at lower doses, but dystonias and akathisia can occur; tachycardia; some weight gain; raised serum prolactin.

Ziprasidone (Geodon®)

Pharmacology

- Receptor antagonism: $5\text{-}HT_{2A} > D_2 > 5\text{-}HT_{1A} > \alpha_1 > H_{1};$.
  No anticholinergic effect; Weak 5-HT and NE reuptake inhibition.

Dosages and preparations

- 20, 40, 60 and 80mg tablets.
- 40mg to 160mg, 80mg probably minimal effective dose.

Side-effects

- EPS = placebo. No appreciable weight gain; No appreciable cholinergic side-effects; Appears to reduce prolactin relative to placebo.
- Concerns over tendency to increase QTc., therefore, specific monitoring: EKG at baseline with subsequent dose titration to evaluate QTc.
- Headache, nausea, and insomnia most common side-effects (but occur in <10% of patients).
- Insomnia, pharyngitis, rash, and tremor more common than with placebo.

The newer, "atypical," antipsychotics (2)

Soon to be available in the United States

Bifeprunox

Pharmacology
- D_2 receptor partial agonist.
- Partial agonist activity at $5-HT_{1A}$ receptors.
- High-affinity antagonist at $5-HT_{2A}$ receptors.
- Low/moderate affinity antagonist at H_1 and α_1 receptors.
- No anticholinergic effect.
- Little hepatic metabolism, may have fewer side-effects than risperidone.

The following are currently not available in the United States, but they used in other countries

Amisulpride

Pharmacology
- Selective and equipotent antagonism for D_2 and D_3.
- Limbic selective.
- Negligible affinity for other receptors.

Efficacy
- As efficacious as haloperidol for acute and chronic schizophrenia.
- Optimum dose 400–800mg per day.
- At 50–300mg effective for patients with mainly negative symptoms.

Side-effects
- Low EPS similar to placebo at lower doses.
- Less weight gain compared with risperidone or olanzapine.
- Dose-dependent EPS and prolactinemia at higher doses.

Sertindole

Withdrawn due to concerns about increase in QTc. Limited reintroduction in 2002 in Europe under strict monitoring.

Pharmacology
- D_2, $5-HT_2$, and α_1 antagonist.
- D_2 limbic selectivity.

Efficacy
- Effective against positive and negative symptoms of schizophrenia.

Side-effects
- EPS = placebo.
- Minimal short-term increase in prolactin.
- Increase in QTc—needs EKG monitoring.
- Nasal congestion, decreased ejaculatory volume, postural hypotension, and dry mouth.
- Occasionally raised liver enzymes.

Zotepine

Pharmacology
- High affinity for D_1 and D_2 receptors, also 5-HT$_2$, 5-HT$_6$, and 5-HT$_7$ receptors.
- Inhibits NA reuptake.

Efficacy
- Effective against positive and negative symptoms of schizophrenia but controlled trial data limited.

Side-effects
- EPS less than typical antipsychotics.
- Seizures at higher doses (above 300mg).
- Weight gain.
- Sedation.
- Constipation, asthenia, dry mouth, akathisia.
- Raised hepatic enzymes.

Side-effect profiles of newer antipsychotics

Extrapyramidal side-effects

EPS appear to result from blockade of D_2 receptors and include akathisia (severe restlessness), dystonias (involuntary muscle contractions with severe forms including opisthotonus [back spasm] and oculogyric crisis), and Parkinsonian symptoms (coarse resting tremor, cogwheel rigidity, shuffling gait). EPS can be treated with anticholinergic medications (e.g., benztropine), antihistamines (e.g., diphenhydramine), benzodiazepines, and beta-blockers. EPS are commonly associated with typicals and less often with atypicals. See 📖 p. 1056.

Tardive dyskinesia

TD is a potentially irreversible syndrome of abnormal movements, most commonly orobuccolingual in origin (such as lip smacking and tongue protrusions), that occur months after onset of antipsychotic treatment. The incidence of TD increases proportionally to the length of exposure to antipsychotic medication, and the elderly are at highest risk of developing TD. TD may actually worsen after cessation of treatment with antipsychotic medications. Atypicals are less likely to cause TD than typicals. There are no treatments for TD that are widely considered to be effective. See 📖 p. 1062.

Neuroleptic malignant syndrome (NMS)

NMS is a potentially deadly syndrome that can occur with antipsychotic treatment. NMS is more common with typicals, particularly within the first 2 weeks of treatment initiation; however, NMS can potentially occur at anytime with any antipsychotic medication. NMS is characterized by initial appearance of mental status changes, followed by muscle rigidity, rhabdomyolysis resulting in myoglobinuria and subsequent kidney failure, fever, leukocytosis, autonomic instability, and remarkably elevated creatinine kinase (1000–100,000 IU/L). Treatment includes urgent transfer to an intensive care unit, cessation of antipsychotic medication, benzodiazepines, and dantrolene. See 📖 p. 1066.

Hyperprolactinemia

Hyperprolactinemia is associated with blockade of D_2 receptors in the tuberoinfundibular dopamine system and results in hypogonadism, infertility, amenorrhea, galactorrhea and gynecomastia. Hyperprolactinemia is more common with typicals and risperidone. See 📖 p. 1051.

Anticholinergic side-effects

Anticholinergic side-effects include blurred vision, dry mouth, urinary retention, constipation, sinus tachycardia, and memory problems and are more commonly seen with low potency typicals (i.e., chlorpromazine), olanzapine, and quetiapine.

Antiepinephric side-effects

Antiepinephric side-effects include primarily orthostatic hypotension and occur mostly commonly with quetiapine and clozapine.

Weight gain and increased risk of diabetes

These are associated primarily with atypical medications including clozapine, olanzapine, quetiapine, and risperidone. APA guidelines recommend baseline metabolic screening including a lipid panel, HgbA1C or fasting blood sugar, and monitoring for weight gain. See 📖 *p. 1048*.

QTc prolongation (QTc >500 milliseconds)

QTc prolongation has been reported to occur for all antipsychotic medications. Present APA guidelines suggest obtaining a baseline EKG in patients with a cardiac history who will be starting ziprasidone. See 📖 *p. 1078*.

Elevated seizure risk

Elevated seizure risk is primarily seen with higher doses of clozapine and chlorpromazine.

Pharmacotherapy of schizophrenia

Antipsychotic medications (from APA Guidelines)

Drug	Trade name	Typical Dose (mg/day)	Chlorpromazine equivalent	$t_{1/2}$ (hr)
Typicals				
Haloperidol	Haldol®	5–20	2	21
Fluphenazine	Prolixin®	5–20	2	33
Thiothixene	Navane®	15–50	5	34
Perphenazine	Trilafon®	16–64	10	10
Chlorpromazine	Thorazine®	300–1000	100	6
Atypicals				
Aripiprazole	Abilify®	10–30		75
Clozapine	Clozaril®	150–600		12
Olanzapine	Zyprexa®	10–30		33
Risperidone	Risperdal®	2–8		24
Quetiapine	Seroquel®	300–800		6
Ziprasidone	Geodon®	40–160		7

Side-effect profile (from APA Guidelines)

Table 6.1 Selected side-effects of commonly used antipsychotic medications[a]

Medication	EPS/TD	Prolactin elevation	Weight gain	Glucose abnormalities	Lipid abnormalities	QTc prolongation	Sedation	Hypotension	Anticholinergic side-effects
Thioridazine	+	++	+	+?	+?	+++	++	++	++
Perphenazine	++	++	+	+?	+?	0	+	+	0
Haloperidol	+++	+++	+	0	0	0	++	0	0
Clozapine[b]	0[c]	0	+++	+++	+++	0	+++	+++	+++
Risperidine	+	+++	++	++	++	+	+	+	0
Olanzapine	0[c]	0	+++	+++	+++	0	+	+	++
Quetiapine[d]	0[c]	0	++	++	++	0	++	++	0
Ziprasidine	0[c]	+	0	0	0	++	0	0	0
Aripiprazole[e]	0[c]	0	0	0	0	0	+	0	0

[a] 0 = No risk or rarely causes effects at therapeutic dose. +Mild or occasionally causes side-effects at the therapeutic dose. ++ Sometimes causes side-effects at therapeutic dose. +++ Frequently cause side-effects at the the therapeutic dose.? Data too limited to rate with confidence. Table adapted from Tandon, R. (1998). Antipsychotic agents, in Quitkin, F.M., et al.(eds.), Current psychotherapeutic Drugs, 2nd ed., Philadelphia: Current Medicine, ☐ pp. 120–154, permission sought.
[b] Also causes agranulocytosis, seizures, and myocarditis.
[c] Possible exception of akathisia.
[d] Also carries warning about potential development of cataracts.
[e] Also causes nausea and headache.

Examining for abnormal involuntary movements

The abnormal involuntary movement scale (AIMS)[1] is a useful tool for examining and monitoring the occurrence of EPS in patients on antipsychotic medication. It can be utilized in different patient populations including adults, children and adolescents. Total scores are generally not reported. Changes in global and individual area scores are observed over time. Administer AIMS before starting an antipsychotic for a baseline measure, and at least every 6 months thereafter.

AIMS—examination procedure
- Either before or after completing the examination procedure, observe the patient unobtrusively at rest (e.g., in the waiting room).
- The chair to be used in this examination should be a hard, firm one without arms.
  - Ask the patient whether there is anything in his or her mouth (such as gum or candy) and, if so, to remove it.
  - Ask about the current condition of the patient's teeth. Ask if he or she wears dentures. Ask whether teeth or dentures bother the patient now.
  - Ask whether the patient notices any movements in his or her mouth, face, hands, or feet. If yes, ask the patient to describe them and to indicate to what extent they currently bother the patient or interfere with activities.
  - Have the patient sit in a chair with hands on knees, legs slightly apart, and feet flat on floor. (Look at the entire body for movements while the patient is in this position.)
  - Ask the patient to sit with hands hanging unsupported—if male, between his legs; if female and wearing a dress, hanging over her knees. (Observe hands and other body areas.)
  - Ask the patient to open his or her mouth. (Observe the tongue at rest within the mouth.) Do this twice.
  - Ask the patient to protrude his or her tongue. (Observe abnormalities of tongue movement.) Do this twice.
  - Ask the patient to tap his or her thumb with each finger as rapidly as possible for 10 to 15 seconds, first with right hand, then with left hand. (Observe facial and leg movements.)
  - Flex and extend the patient's left and right arms, one at a time. Note any rigidity.
  - Ask the patient to stand up. (Observe the patient in profile. Observe all body areas again, hips included.)

1 AIMS was originally described by Ecdeu, G.W. (1976) in the Assessment Manual for Psychopharmacology, revised ed. (Washington, DC, U.S. Department of Health, Education, and Welfare). A more recent discussion can be found in: Munetz, M.R. and Benjamin, S. (1988). How to examine patients using the Abnormal Involuntary Movement Scale. *Hospital and Community Psychiatry* **39**, 1172–7.

- Ask the patient to extend both arms out in front, palms down. (Observe trunk, legs, and mouth.)
- Have the patient walk a few paces, turn, and walk back to the chair. (Observe hands and gait.) Do this twice.

AIMS—scoring procedure

- Complete the examination procedure before making ratings.
- For the movement ratings (the first 3 categories below), rate the highest severity observed: 0 = none; 1 = minimal (may be extreme normal); 2 = mild; 3 = moderate; 4 = severe.
- According to the original AIMS instructions, one point is subtracted if movements are seen only on activation, but not all investigators follow that convention.

Facial and oral movements

- Muscles of facial expression (e.g., movements of forehead, eyebrows, periorbital area, cheeks. Include frowning, blinking, smiling, grimacing).
- Lips and perioral area (e.g., puckering, pouting, smacking).
- Jaw (e.g., biting, clenching, chewing, mouth opening, lateral movement).
- Tongue. Rate only increase in movement both in and out of mouth, not inability to sustain movement.

Extremity movements

- Upper (arms, wrists, hands, fingers). Include movements that are choreic (rapid, objectively purposeless, irregular, spontaneous) or athetoid (slow, irregular, complex, serpentine). Do not include tremor (repetitive, regular, rhythmic movements).
- Lower (legs, knees, ankles, toes). May include lateral knee movement, foot tapping, heel dropping, foot squirming, inversion and eversion of foot.

Trunk movements

- Neck, shoulders, hips (e.g., rocking, twisting, squirming, pelvic gyrations). Include diaphragmatic movements.

Global judgments

- Severity of abnormal movements. 0,1,2,3,4 (based on the highest single score on the above items). This may be better if it said 0–4 instead of 0,1,2,3,4.
- Incapacitation due to abnormal movements. 0 = none, normal; 1 = minimal; 2 = mild; 3 = moderate; 4 = severe.
- Patient's awareness of abnormal movements. 0 = no awareness; 1 = aware, no distress; 2 = aware, mild distress; 3 = aware, moderate distress; 4 = aware, severe distress.

Dental Status

- Current problems with teeth and/or dentures. 0 = no; 1 = yes.
- Does patient usually wear dentures? 0 = no; 1 = yes.

Clozapine (Clozaril®) (1)—guidelines

Clozapine (Overview)

Clozapine, an atypical antipsychotic drug, is a tricyclic dibenzodiazepine derivative. Like other atypical antipsychotics, clozapine is a dopamine receptor antagonist and a $5HT_{2A}$ receptor antagonist. Clozapine exhibits relatively strong blockade of D_1 and D_4 receptors, and its effects on D_2 receptors are relatively weak when compared to traditional antipsychotics. The lower affinity of clozapine for D_2 receptors may partially explain the infrequency of EPS and hyperprolactinemia with clozapine. Clozapine has significant anticholinergic, antihistaminic, and antiadrenergic activity, accounting for the common side-effects of somnolence, weight gain, constipation, and orthostasis, among others.

Clozapine is known to be an effective antipsychotic, especially in patients with a history of treatment-resistant schizophrenia. However, due to the significant risks of agranulocytosis (rarely observed with other atypical antipsychotics) and increased risk of seizure, clozapine is not recommended as a first-line agent in the treatment of schizophrenia. It should be used only in patients who have failed to demonstrate adequate response to one or more trials of first-line antipsychotic therapy, or in the treatment of severe, recurrent, suicidal behaviors in patients with schizophrenia and schizoaffective disorder.

Due to the agranulocytosis risk, physicians must register themselves and their patients with The Clozaril (Clozapine) National Registry maintained by Novartis Pharmaceuticals (contact information at the end of this section). Patients must receive weekly to monthly monitoring of complete blood counts for the duration of clozapine therapy.

Clozapine has two FDA indications

Treatment-resistant schizophrenia

- The effectiveness of clozapine in the treatment-resistant schizophrenia population was established in a 6-week trial comparing clozapine with chlorpromazine.
- In the Clozapine Collaborative Trial[1] (1988), clozapine was found to be statistically superior to chlorpromazine in reducing Brief Psychiatric Rating Scale (BPRS) scores in a group of patients who had failed to show significant improvement with open-label haloperidol (30% of clozapine patients met criteria for response at 6 weeks, compared to 7% of chlorpromazine treated patients).
- Chakos et al.[2] (2001) performed a meta-analysis of seven controlled trials comparing first-generation antipsychotics to clozapine. They found clozapine superior in both clinical response rates and tolerability.
- In the CATIE trial[3], 99 patients who failed to improve on atypical antipsychotics were randomized to receive either clozapine (n = 49) or another atypical antipsychotic (either quetiapine, olanzapine, or risperidone; N = 50). Clozapine-treated patients had lower positive and negative symptom scores on measures of positive and negative symptoms of schizophrenia at 3 months, and had a roughly three-times longer time to discontinuation of pharmacotherapy for any reason (10.5 months versus approximately 3 months) (McEvoy, 2006[3]).

Risk reduction of recurrent suicidal behavior

- The effectiveness of clozapine in the treatment of recurrent suicidal behavior in patients with schizophrenia and schizoaffective disorder was demonstrated in a 2-year prospective, randomized comparison of clozapine and olanzapine (the International Suicide Prevention Trial, or InterSePT[4]).
- The study enrolled patients with a history of recent suicide attempt (within 3 years), hospitalization for suicidal ideation (SI), moderate-to-severe SI with depressive symptoms, or moderate-to-severe SI with command auditory hallucinations.
- Only one quarter of these patients met criteria for treatment-resistance.
- Patients were permitted to take other psychotropic medications (including antipsychotic medications) during the trial.
- Patients received 200mg–900mg of clozapine daily, or 5–20mg of olanzapine.
- The primary efficacy measure was time to a significant suicide attempt or completed suicide, hospitalization due to SI, or worsening in baseline suicidality (assessed by blinded raters using a validated instrument).
- The risk for the primary efficacy measure at 2 years was 24% for the clozapine-treated group, and 32% for the olanzapine-treated group (95% CI for the actual between-group difference was between 2% and 14%).

Contraindications to clozapine therapy

- Previous or current neutropenia or other blood dyscrasias, previous myocarditis, pericarditis, cardiomyopathy, severe renal or cardiac disorders, active liver disease, progressive liver disease, and hepatic failure. Patients with known seizure disorders should not be started on clozapine therapy.

Recommended further reading

1 Kane, J., *et al.* (1998). Clozapine for the treatment-resistant schizophrenic. A double-blind comparison with chlorpromazine. *Archives of General Psychiatry*, **45**(9): 789–96.

2 Chakos, M., *et al.* (2001). Effectiveness of second-generation antipsychotics in patients with treatment-resistant schizophrenia: a review and meta-analysis of randomized trials. *Am J Psych.* **158**(4): 518–26.

3 McEvoy, J.P., *et al.* (2006). CATIE Investigators. Effectiveness of clozapine versus olanzapine, quetiapine, and risperidone in patients with chronic schizophrenia who did not respond to prior atypical antipsychotic treatment. *Am J Psych*, **163**(4): 600–610.

4 Meltzer, H.Y., *et al.* (2003). Clozapine treatment for suicidality in schizophrenia: International Suicide Prevention Trial (InterSePT). [Erratum appears in *Arch Gen Psych*, **60**(7): 735.] *Archives of General Psychiatry*, **60**(1): 82–91.

Clozapine (2)

Clozapine dosing guidelines

Day	Morning dose (mg)	Night-time dose (mg)
1	—	12.5
2	12.5	12.5
3	25	25
4	25	25
5	25	50
6	25	50
7	50	50
8	50	75
9	75	75
10	75	100
11	100	100
12	100	125
13	125	125
14	125	150
15	150	150
18	150	200
21	200	200
28	200	250

- Gradually increase[*] by 50–100mg/wk (max dose should not exceed 900mg/day).
- If adverse effects are noted, reduce dose until side-effects settle, then increase again more slowly.
- Lower doses may be required for elderly, female, or non-smoking patients, and if the patient is on other medication that may affect the metabolism of clozapine.
- When there has been a break in treatment for more than 48 hours, treatment should be reinitiated with 12.5mg once or twice on the first day, and re-titrated.

[*] Routine blood level monitoring is not recommended; however, increasing dose until plasma level of 350mcg/L is achieved is sometimes recommended.

Clozapine (3)—adverse reactions

Major adverse reactions

Agranulocytosis

- Agranulocytosis is defined as an absolute neutrophil count (ANC) below 500/mm^3. It is potentially fatal if not detected early.
- Signs of agranulocytosis include high fever, lethargy, pharyngitis, and ulcerations of the oral and anal mucosa. Patients on clozapine should be instructed to report these symptoms to their doctors immediately.
- The risk of agranulocytosis for patients taking clozapine is 1.6% in the first month of therapy. The risk peaks in the third month of therapy, and then drops sharply. However, it never reaches zero.
- For this reason, patients must have CBC monitored weekly for the first six months of clozapine treatment, twice monthly for the second 6 months, and monthly thereafter (assuming there are no hematologic abnormalities).
- Clozapine should be discontinued immediately if agranulocytosis is detected. In the event of a below normal value on CBC monitoring (that does not meet criteria for angranulocytosis), clozapine should either be stopped or CBC's monitored more frequently.
- Patients whose WBC and ANC counts do not fall below 2000/mm^3 and 1000/mm^3, respectively, can be re-challenged with clozapine. However, this is to be done with extreme care, with full consideration of the risks and benefits.
- Patients with a history of moderate leukopenia have a 12-fold increased risk of developing agranulocytosis on re-challenge (compared to all patients receiving clozapine).

Seizure

- The 1-year incidence of seizure with clozapine therapy is approximately 5%.
- The risk appears to be dose-dependent (greater risk at higher doses).
- Patients with a history of epilepsy, head trauma with loss of consciousness, or other risks for seizure may be at increased risk.
- Other medications that are well known to decrease seizure threshold (e.g., bupropion, clomipramine) should be avoided or used with extreme caution.

Myocarditis

- Post-marketing surveillance data in the United States, Canada, the U.K., and Australia revealed myocarditis rates with clozapine range between 5.0 and 96.6 cases per 100,000 patient-years of therapy.
- The possibility of myocarditis should be considered in patients complaining of chest pain, shortness of breath, fever, palpitations, other symptoms of heart failure, or abnormal EKG findings.

Other adverse reactions

- Eosinophilia (1%); cardiomyopathy (very rare); pulmonary embolism; hepatitis; neuroleptic malignant syndrome, and tardive dyskinesia (case reports only).

- Weight gain and metabolic syndrome are risks associated with atypical antipsychotics but to widely varying degrees. These are discussed elsewhere.
- Clozapine is not FDA-approved in the treatment of elderly patients with dementia-related psychosis. Such patients are at increased risk of death when treated with antipsychotic medications.

Common side-effects

- The most common side-effects of clozapine tend to be anticholinergic (constipation, somnolence, dry mouth, blurred vision, difficulty passing urine) and antiadrenergic (orthostatic hypotension, sexual dysfunction).
- Weight gain and salivary hypersecretion are also very commonly reported.
- Tachycardia was observed in up to 25% of patients taking clozapine during pre-marketing clinical trials (with an average increase in heart rate of 10–15 beats/minute). This tachycardia is found in all positions monitored, and does not reflect reflex tachycardia in response to orthostasis.
- Fever (temperatures above 38C) has been observed in patients on clozapine, most commonly in the first three weeks of therapy.
- A list of the most commonly reported side-effects among subjects in the InterSePT trial is presented in Clozapine (4)–managing side-effects 📖 p. 250.

Drug Interactions

- Clozapine is metabolized primarily via CYP450 1A2, 2D6, and 3A4 isoenzymes.
- Thus, medications that affect the efficiency of these enzymes can theoretically alter the metabolism of clozapine.
- CYP450 enzyme inducers such as carbamazepine, rifampin, phenytoin, and nicotine may reduce plasma clozapine levels.
- CYP450 enzyme inhibitors such as caffeine, citalopram, ciprofloxacin, erythromycin, and cimetidine may increase plasma levels.
- Use of clozapine with other drugs primarily metabolized by isoenzyme 2D6 (certain antidepressants such as paroxetine, fluoxetine, fluvoxamine, and sertraline as well as phenothiazine antipsychotics) may result in elevated levels of clozapine or the other drug. These drugs should be used with caution.

Clozapine (4)—managing side-effects

Dealing with clozapine side-effects

Problem	Possible solution
Constipation	Encourage high-fiber diet, adequate fluid intake, use of stool-softeners and/or laxative if persistent
Fever	Symptomatic relief, check CBC and look for sources of infection
Hypersalivation	Consider use of hyoscine hydrobromide (up to 300mcg tid), pirenzepine (up to 50mg tid)
Hypertension	Monitor closely, slow rate or halt dose increase, if persistent consider use of hypotensive agent (e.g., atenolol)
Hypotension	Advise caution when getting up quickly, monitor closely, slow or halt dose increase
Nausea	Consider use of anti-emetic (avoid metoclopramide and prochlorperazine if previous problems with EPS)
Neutropenia/agranulocytosis	Stop clozapine, if outpatient admit to hospital
Nocturnal enuresis	Avoid fluids in the evening, alter dose scheduling, if severe consider use of desmopressin
Sedation	Reschedule dosing to give smaller morning or total dose
Seizures	Withhold clozapine for 24 hrs, resume at lower dose, consider prophylactic anticonvulsant (e.g., valproate)
Weight gain	Dietary and exercise counseling (see 📖 p. 1048)

Clozapine (5)—initiation and monitoring

Initiation and monitoring of clozapine

- The normal therapeutic dose range for clozapine is 300–600mg daily.
- In some cases, patients require up to 900mg daily to achieve stability.
- Split dosing is generally more tolerable, however patients stable in the lower dose range may prefer qhs dosing.
- Patients should be started on 12.5mg qd or bid initially, and then increasing by an average of 12.5mg daily for the first week (or 25mg every-other-day), and by 25mg daily in the second week.
- Thus, after 2 weeks of titration, a patient should be at approximately 300mg total daily dose.
- Thereafter, an increase of 50mg weekly is reasonable, to a maximum dose of 900mg. If patients experience significant side-effects, the titration should be slower.
- If there has been a break in treatment in excess of 48 hours, it is recommended that the patient be re-initiated at 12.5mg bid and titrated back to the therapeutic dose as outlined above.

For more information, or to become a clozapine provider

- Becoming a clozapine provider is fast and easy provided you have a DEA license.
- You will need a baseline WBC and ANC on any patient you wish to start on clozapine and will need to register them with the Clozaril National Registry.
- You will need to submit the WBC and ANC counts to the pharmacy providing clozapine to the patient.
- To register, call The Clozaril National Registry at 1-800-448-5938 or download up-to-date prescribing information at https://www.clozarilcare.com.

Clozapine interactions

Effect	Examples
Increased drowsiness, sedation, dizziness, and the possibility of respiratory depression	Ethanol, H1-blockers, opiate agonists, anxiolytics, sedatives/hypnotics, tramadol, and TCAs
Increased possibility of developing myelosuppressive effects	Concomitant use of clozapine with other drugs known to cause bone marrow depression (e.g., chemotherapy agents and carbamazepine)
Drugs known to induce CYP1A2 activity may reduce clozapine efficacy	Carbamazepine, phenobarbital, phenytoin, rifabutin, and rifampin
Drugs known to inhibit the activity of CYP1A2 may increase clozapine serum levels	Cimetidine, clarithromycin, ciprofloxacin, diltiazem, enoxacin, erythromycin, or fluvoxamine
Drugs known to inhibit the activity of CYP2D6 may increase clozapine serum levels	Amiodarone, cimetidine, clomipramine, desipramine, fluoxetine, fluphenazine, haloperidol, paroxetine, quinidine, ritonavir, sertraline, and thioridazine
Highly protein-bound drugs may increase clozapine serum concentrations	Digoxin, heparin, phenytoin, or warfarin
Worsening of anticholinergic effects	H₁-blockers; phenothiazines; TCAs; and other drugs with antimuscarinic properties
Increased risk of hypotension	Antihypertensive agents

Other specific interactions

- Lithium can increase the risk of developing seizures, confusion, dyskinesia and possibly, NMS.
- May interfere with the action of AChEIs (e.g., donepezil and tacrine).
- Smoking cigarettes (tobacco) increases the clearance of clozapine and may result in a substantial reduction in clozapine plasma concentrations (higher doses of clozapine may be necessary).
- Because the plasma concentration of clozapine is increased by caffeine intake and decreased by nearly 50% following a 5-day caffeine-free period, dosage changes of clozapine may be necessary when there is a change in a patient's caffeine-drinking habit.

Antipsychotic depot injections

Antipsychotic drugs may be given as a long-acting depot preparation (the active drug in an oily suspension) injected into a large muscle (usually gluteus maximus), allowing for sustained release over 1–4 weeks. Previously, only conventional antipsychotics were available, but now a number of atypical preparations, with a variety of slow-release systems, are in development and will find their place in clinical practice. At the moment, only risperidone, of the newer drugs, has been approved as a long acting injection. Dose for dose, the efficacy of these preparations is not greater than oral medication, but they do increase the likelihood of compliance.

Indications

Poor compliance with oral treatment, failure to respond to oral medication, memory problems or other factors interfering with ability to take medication regularly, clinical need to ensure patient compliance (e.g., if the patients are subject to compulsory treatment legislation).

Administration

Patients should first be given a small test dose as undesirable side-effects can be prolonged. In general not more than 2–3mL of oily injection should be administered at any one site; correct injection technique (including the use of z-track technique) and rotation of injection sites are essential. If the dose needs to be reduced to alleviate side-effects, it is important to recognize that the plasma-drug concentration may not fall for some time after reducing the dose, therefore it may be a month or longer before side-effects subside.

Dosing schedules

(see opposite).

Specific side-effects

Pain/swelling at injection site, rarely abscesses, nerve palsies. Side-effects as for oral medication but may take 2–3 days to emerge and may persist for weeks after discontinuation. The older depot injections may be more likely to cause EPS, although good evidence for this is lacking.

Cautions

As for oral antipsychotic medication. Also, previous neuroleptic malignant syndrome or any condition where the drug may need to be withdrawn rapidly.

Generic name	Trade name	Test dose	Interval between test and treatment	Usual starting dose	Between dose interval	Dose range
Risperidone	Risperdal Consta	25mg	2 weeks	25–37.5mg (max 50mg /2 weeks)	2 weeks	25–50 mg/2 weeks
Fluphenazine decanoate	Modecate	12.5mg	4–7 days	12.5–100mg	14–35 days	
Haloperidol decanoate	Haldol	50mg	4 weeks	50–300mg (max 300 mg/4 weeks)	4 weeks	50–300 mg/4 weeks

Dose equivalents

These equivalents are intended only as an approximate guide; individual dosage instructions should also be checked; patients should be carefully monitored after any change in medication.

Do not extrapolate beyond the maximum dose for the drug

Flupenthixol decanoate 40mg/2 wks
    = Fluphenazine decanoate 25mg/2 wks
    = Haloperidol decanoate 100mg/4 wks
    = Pipothiazine palmitate 50mg/4 wks
    = Zuclopenthixol decanoate 200mg/2 wks
Risperidone 25mg/2 wks DEPOT is equivalent to approximately.
3–4mg/d ORAL.

Schizoaffective disorder

This disorder has features of both schizophrenia and a mood disorder with the patient meeting Criterion A for schizophrenia concurrently with meeting criteria for either a major depressive episode, a manic episode, or a mixed episode (meet both major depression and manic criteria every day for a week). There are varying theories on whether schizoaffective disorder is a type of schizophrenia, a type of mood disorder, or a distinct third type of psychosis.

Epidemiology

Lifetime prevalence is 0.5–0.8%. There are limited data on gender and age differences.

Etiology

Unknown.

DSM-IV-TR

- An uninterrupted period of illness during which, at some time, there is either a major depressive episode, a manic episode, or a mixed episode concurrent with symptoms that meet Criterion A for schizophrenia. Note: The major depressive episode must include Criterion A1: depressed mood.
- During the same period of illness, there have been delusions or hallucinations for at least 2 weeks in the absence of prominent mood symptoms.
- Symptoms that meet criteria for a mood episode are present for a substantial portion of the total duration of the active and residual periods of the illness.
- The disturbance is not due to the direct physiological effects of a substance (e.g., a drug of abuse, a medication) or a general medical condition.

Specify type

Bipolar type

If the disturbance includes a manic or a mixed episode (or a manic or a mixed episode and major depressive episodes).

Depressive type

If the disturbance only includes major depressive episodes.

Differential diagnosis

See differential for psychosis.

Course and prognosis

Overall, patients have a better prognosis than patients with schizophrenia and a worse prognosis than patients with a mood disorder. They also tend to have a non-deteriorating course.

Treatment

Mood stabilizers (typically lithium or carbamazepine) for bipolar type, SSRIs for depressive type, and antipsychotics for the psychotic symptoms.

ICD-10

- Schizophrenic and affective symptoms simultaneously present and both are equally prominent.
- Excludes patients with separate episodes of schizophrenia and affective disorders.

Schizophreniform disorder

This is similar to schizophrenia; however, the symptoms last at least one month but less than 6 months.

Epidemiology

Most common in adolescence and young adults, much less common than schizophrenia. Lifetime prevalence is 0.2%.

Etiology

Unknown but probably similar to schizophrenia.

DSM-IV-TR

- Criteria A, D, and E of schizophrenia are met.
- An episode of the disorder (including prodromal, active, and residual phases) lasts at least 1 month but less than 6 months. (When the diagnosis must be made without waiting for recovery, it should be qualified as "Provisional").

Specify if

With good prognostic features

As evidenced by two (or more) of the following:

- Onset of prominent psychotic symptoms within 4 weeks of the first noticeable change in usual behavior or functioning.
- Confusion or perplexity at the height of the psychotic episode.
- Good premorbid social and occupational functioning.
- Absence of blunted or flat affect.

Without good prognostic features

If fewer than two of the above features are present.

Differential diagnosis

See differential for psychosis, 📖 p. 216.

Course and prognosis

As above, psychosis lasting for more than 1 month but less than 6 months. Patients return to baseline functioning once the disorder has resolved. Progression to schizophrenia is estimated to be between 60–80 percent. Some patients have 2 or 3 recurrent episodes.

Treatment

Antipsychotics ± a mood stabilizer and psychotherapy.

Schizoid and schizotypal disorders are considered personality disorders, not psychotic disorders. See page 📖 p. 542–552 for details.

Delusional disorder (1)

Key features
Delusional disorder is an uncommon condition in which patients present with circumscribed symptoms of non-bizarre delusions, but with absence of prominent hallucinations and no thought disorder, mood disorder, or significant flattening of affect. Symptoms should have been present for at least 1 month. (ICD-10 specifies at least 3 months for delusional disorder but, if it less than this, allows diagnosis under other persistent delusional disorder). DSM-IV-TR specifies particular subtypes (see below).

Points to note
- Patients rarely present directly to psychiatrists. More often they may be seen by other physicians due to somatic complaints, lawyers due to paranoid ideas, or the police when they act on, or complain about their delusions.
- Careful assessment and diagnosis is vital, because delusions are the final common pathway of many illnesses. When delusional disorder is discovered, treatment can be fraught with difficulty because of the reticent nature of such patients. With persistence, a combination of biopsychosocial treatments can be effective.
- Delusional disorders represent a heterogeneous group of conditions that appear distinct from mood disorders and schizophrenia, although there is significant diagnostic (and genetic) overlap with paranoid personality traits/disorder. Data suggest that among patients diagnosed with delusional disorder, less than 3–22% are later reclassified as schizophrenic and less than 10% are later diagnosed with a mood disorder.

Clinical features
- Level of consciousness is unimpaired.
- Observed behavior, speech, and mood may be affected by the emotional tone of delusional content (e.g., hyperalertness with persecutory delusions).
- Thought process is generally unimpaired, but thought content reflects preoccupation with circumscribed (usually a single theme), non-bizarre delusions (determination of bizarreness is useful in differentiating from schizophrenia).
- Hallucinations may occur, but generally are not prominent and reflect delusional ideas (more commonly olfactory/tactile than visual/auditory).
- Cognition and memory are generally intact.
- Insight and judgment are impaired to the degree that the delusions influence thought and behavior; risk should be formally assessed (e.g., potential for violence to self and others and past history of previous behaviors influenced by delusions).
- Persistent anger and fear are risk factors for aggressive "acting-out" behaviors.

DSM-IV-TR subtypes

- Erotomanic (de Clerambault syndrome). Patients present with the belief that some important person is secretly in love with them. Clinical samples are often female and forensic samples contain a preponderance of males. Patients may make efforts to contact this person, and some cases are associated with dangerous or assaultative behavior.
- Grandiose. Patients believe they fill some special role, have some special relationship, or possess some special ability. They may be involved with social or religious organizations.
- Jealous[2] (Othello syndrome). Patients possess the belief that their spouse or partner has been unfaithful. Often patients try to collect evidence and/or attempt to restrict their partners' activities. This type of delusional disorder has been associated with forensic cases involving murder.
- Persecutory. This is the most common presentation of delusional disorder. Patients are convinced that others are attempting to do them harm. Often they attempt to obtain legal recourse, and they sometimes may resort to violence.
- Somatic. Varying presentation, from those who have repeat contact with physicians requesting various forms of medical or surgical treatment, to patients who are concerned with bodily infestation, deformity, or odor.
- Mixed. Presence of one or more of the above themes; no single theme predominating.
- Unspecified. The theme cannot be determined or does not fit the listed categories.

Delusional disorder (2)

Epidemiology

Relatively uncommon, but not rare. Prevalence is estimated at 0.025–0.03% (may account for 1–2% of hospital admissions) with an age range of 18–90 yrs (mean 40–49 yrs). Persecutory type is most common; but delusional jealousy is more common in men and erotomania is more common in women. Fifty percent of patients are employed and 80% are married.

Risk factors

Advanced age, social isolation, group delusions, low socio-economic status, premorbid personality disorder, sensory impairment (particularly deafness), recent immigration, family history, and history of head injury or substance use disorders.

Course and prognosis

Onset may be acute or insidious. Course is very variable even with treatment: remission (33–50%), improvement (10%), persisting symptoms (33–50%). Course is less chronic and functioning is better preserved than in schizophrenia. Better prognosis for those who are female, married, with acute onset, where stress is a factor, and for jealous or persecutory subtypes. Jealous subtype may have a better prognosis than the persecutory subtype. If symptoms have persisted for more than 6 months and there is a co-morbid diagnosis of depression, outcome is worse.

Differential diagnosis

See differential diagnosis for psychosis, 🕮 *p. 216*.
- Substance-induced delusional disorders (e.g., alcohol, stimulants, hallucinogens, steroids, antihistamines, sympathomimetics). Careful history taking may reveal onset, persistence, and cessation of symptoms to be related to drug use.
- Other physical disorders. Focused history, examination, and investigations should help exclude other disorders (e.g., head injury, CNS infection, epilepsy).
- Late paraphrenia. Thought to be distinct from delusional disorder and schizophrenia associated with aging, social isolation, medical problems and treatments, and sensory loss.
- Dysmorphophobia/body dysmorphic disorder (🕮 *p. 966*). Significant overlap with delusional disorder, and few significant differentiating factors exist.
- Obsessive-compulsive disorder (🕮 *p. 420*). Significant overlap with delusional disorder and, if reality testing regarding obsessions or compulsions is lost, delusional disorder often is diagnosed.

- Hypochondriasis (📖 p. 960). Health concerns generally are more amenable to reality testing and are less fixed than in delusional disorder.
- Paranoid personality disorder (📖 pp. 538–548). Absence of clearly circumscribed delusions presence of a pervasive, stable pattern of suspiciousness or distrust.
- Misidentification syndromes (📖 p. 269). Easily confused with delusional disorder, may be associated with other CNS abnormalities.
- Induced/shared psychotic disorder (aka, "folie-a-deux"; 📖 p. 268). Evidence that relatives or close friends share similar delusional beliefs.

Etiology of delusional disorder

Biological
- Delusions can be a feature of a number of biological conditions, suggesting possible biologic underpinnings for the disorder.
- Most commonly, neurological lesions associated with the temporal lobe, limbic system, and basal ganglia are implicated in delusional syndromes.
- Neurological observations indicate that delusional content is influenced by the extent and location of brain injury.
- Prominent cortical damage often leads to simple, poorly formed, persecutory delusions.
- Lesions of the basal ganglia elicit less cognitive disturbance and more complex delusional content.
- Excessive dopaminergic and reduced acetylcholinergic activity have been linked to the formation of delusional symptoms.

Psychodynamic/psychological
- Freud proposed that delusions served a defensive function, protecting the patient from intrapsychically unacceptable impulses through reaction formation, projection, and denial.
- Cognitive Theory: Delusions are seen as the result of cognitive defects, where patients accept ideas with too little evidence for their conclusions; delusions are the result of attempting to find a rational basis for abnormal perceptual experiences.

Social/Other
Certain social situations may increase the chances of developing delusional disorder. For example:
- social isolation,
- jealousy,
- lowered self-esteem,
- people seeing their own defects in others,
- rumination over meaning and motivation.

Management
Typical obstacles to the treatment of delusional disorder:
- The patient's denial of the illness which causes difficulties in establishing a therapeutic alliance,
- The patient's experiences of significant social and interpersonal problems (which may confirm his/her firmly held beliefs),
- Antipsychotic medication is often of limited efficacy.

Hospital admission should be considered if there is a clear risk of harm to self or violence toward others. Otherwise, outpatient treatment is preferred. Approaches to management include:
- Separation from source or focus of delusional ideas (if possible).
- Pharmacological
  - Data for pharmacotherapy are limited to case reports or small open-label interventions.
  - Given the symptomatic overlap with psychotic disorders, antipsychotics (typical and atypical) have some utility.

There was a widely-held anecdotal view supporting the preferential use of pimozide. However, although there are no full scale clinical trials, what evidence there is suggests that no antispsychotic is preferentially effectve; that response rates are around 50%, with 90% of patients seeing some improvement; and that somatic delusions are the most likely to respond.[1]
- Other sources favor the use of SSRIs[2] given the overlap with obsessive-compulsive disorder, body dysmorphic disorder, and mood disorder.
- Benzodiazepines may be useful when there are marked anxiety symptoms.
- Data for the use of anticonvulsant agents and mood stabilizers are even more limited.
- Psychological/psychotherapeutic.
  - Individual therapy requires persistence in establishing a therapeutic alliance without validating or overtly confronting the patient's delusional system.
  - Supportive therapy may help with isolation and distress stemming from the delusional beliefs (reframing problems due to delusional beliefs as symptoms).
  - Cognitive techniques, such as reality testing and reframing.
  - Insight-orientated therapy in order to develop a sense of "creative doubt" in the internal perception of the world through empathy with the patient's defensive position.
  - Educational and social interventions such as social skills training (e.g., not discussing delusional beliefs in social settings) and minimizing risk factors (e.g., sensory impairment, isolation, stress, and precipitants of violence) to reduce the impact of the delusional belief system.

Recommended further reading

1 Manschreck TC, Khan NL: Recent advances in the treatment of delusional disorder. Can J Psychiatry 2006. 51, 114–119.
2 Manschreck TC (1996). Delusional disorder: the recognition and management of paranoia. J Clin Psychiatry 57, Suppl. 3,32–8.

Brief psychotic disorder

Clinical features (Acute and Transient Psychotic disorders—ICD-10)

Sudden onset, variable presentation (including perplexity, inattention, formal thought disorder, delusions or hallucinations, disorganized or catatonic behavior), usually resolving within less than 1 month (DSM-IV-TR) or 3 months (ICD-10). Remission is complete and the individual returns to premorbid functioning.

Etiology

Sometimes these disorders occur in the context of an acute stressor (both DSM-IV-TR and ICD-10 allow for specifying "with or without" marked stressor(s)/acute stress); for example, bereavement, marriage, unemployment, imprisonment, accident, childbirth, or migration and social isolation (due to language and cultural factors). Psychodynamic theories suggest deficient ego strength as the possible mechanism.

Epidemiology

Development of brief psychotic disorder is associated with certain personality types (e.g., paranoid, borderline, histrionic). It is more prevalent in developing nations where there is a strong emphasis on traditional values (may demonstrate "culture-specific" features—see 🕮 p. 1031). Age of onset is later in industrialized nations in comparison to developing countries. It is more common in women.

Differential diagnosis

- Organic disorders—dementia/delirium.
- Bipolar/depression—delusions of guilt and persecution.
- Substance use disorders.
- Personality disorder—paranoid, borderline, histrionic.
- Culture specific disorders (see 🕮 p. 1031).
- Factitious disorder or malingering.
- Schizophreniform disorder (if it continues for more than 1 month).

Management

- Assessment is vital to make the appropriate diagnosis.
- Lab work including complete blood count, basic metabolic panel, TSH, vitamin B_{12}, and brain imaging such as CT/MRI may help rule out medical causes.
- Short-term admission may be necessary to provide support, nursing care, and specific assistance with psychosocial stressors.
- Short-term use of antipsychotics or benzodiazepines may be helpful.
- Antidepressants and/or mood stabilizers may be useful to prevent further episodes.

Course and prognosis

- By definition, these disorders are brief and resolve within days, weeks, or, more rarely, months.

- Prognosis is better if there is a short interval between onset and full-blown symptoms (DSM-IV-TR: within 4 weeks). Prognosis is also improved if patient has confusion and perplexity, good premorbid social and occupational functioning, and absence of blunted or flat affect.
- Outcome is better than schizophrenia (both socially and symptomatically).
- Relapse is common, with increased mortality and suicide rates compared to the general population.

ICD-10 subtypes

ICD-10 allows for these disorders to occur with or without the presence of an acute stressor, and outlines the following subtypes:
- Acute polymorphic psychotic disorder with or without symptoms of schizophrenia.
    - Variable and changeable psychotic symptoms (from day to day, or hour to hour) with frequent intense emotional turmoil.
    - Includes Perris' (1974) "cycloid psychosis" after Karl Leonard's description for which the treatment of choice is lithium (Perris, 1978).
    - Also "bouffee delirante" (Magnan), the concept which was reviewed by Allodi (1982) who stressed the avoidance of long-term medication, highlighting socio-cultural factors, especially migration and language.
- Acute schizophrenia-like psychotic disorder, which is also referred to as "brief schizophreniform psychosis" or "schizophrenic reaction."
- The psychotic symptoms are relatively stable but do not last more than a month (ICD-10, DSM-IV-TR brief psychotic disorder), or last between 1 and 6 months (DSM-IV-TR schizophreniform disorder).
- Other acute predominantly delusional psychotic disorder.
    - Onset is acute (2 weeks or less), delusions or hallucinations are present most of the time. If delusions persist for longer than 3 months, the diagnosis should be changed to persistent delusional disorder (see 📖 p. 260).
    - Includes the Scandinavian concept of "psychogenic/reactive psychosis" for which the prognosis is good and the treatment of choice is supportive psychotherapy and the short-term use of medication (Stromgren, 1989).
    - "Hysterical psychosis" (Hirsch and Hollander, 1969) which includes three subtypes: culturally sanctioned behavior (like culture specific disorders); appropriation of psychotic behavior (conversion process); true psychosis ("failure of repression when faced with acute stress in a vulnerable ego", as in histrionic personality.
    - "Ganser syndrome" (📖 p. 111) which is characterized by approximate answers, disorientation, clouding of consciousness, hallucinations, motor disturbance, anxiety or apathy, normal ADLs, and sudden resolution with amnesia for the period of illness. Proposed mechanisms are similar to the differential diagnosis for acute and transient psychotic disorders (see opposite): hysterical conversion, organic confusion, psychosis, or malingering.

Shared delusional disorder

Also known as "folie à deux" (or even "folie à trois" or "folie à famille"!), this disorder was recognized and described by Harvey as early as 1651, and was more recently reviewed as a concept by Howard in 1994. It is classified under Induced delusional disorder in ICD-10. It is rare in clinical settings. Silveira and Seeman (1995) also reviewed the literature and found an equal sex ratio; a broad range of ages; 90% are couples, siblings, or parent/child; and social isolation is a factor in 2/3 of cases. The disorder is co-morbid with depression, dementia, and mental retardation; and there is a common association with hallucinations. Without intervention the course is usually chronic.

Subtypes
- Folie imposée—the delusions of one with primary psychotic illness are adopted by an individual who is healthy. Separation of the two usually cures the normally healthy individual.
- Folie simultanée—identical delusions arising in two people at the same time.
- Folie communiquée—the delusions of the person with primary psychotic illness are adopted by a healthy individual after a period of resistance. The normally healthy individual is not cured by separation alone.
- Folie induite—there is pre-existing primary psychosis in both patients, and one patient adopts fellow patient's delusions.

Etiology
Psychodynamic theories
These include the fear of losing important relationships in an otherwise isolated individual with little scope for reality testing; or the passive acceptor has repressed oedipal fantasies that are released by the psychotic partner causing identification of the dominant partner with a parent.

Learning theory
Learning theory suggests that psychotic thinking is learned through "observational learning".

Social isolation
Factors secondary to language, geographical barriers, and personality may also be responsible for the illness.

Management
- Separation—may lead to complete remission in up to 40% of cases.
- Psychological—aimed at giving up delusional beliefs (equivalent to rejecting a close relationship).
- Pharmacological—for the active, not the passive, partner, as for delusional disorder.

Recommended further reading
1 Howard, R. (1994). Induced psychosis. *British Journal of Hospital Medicine*, **51**(6): 304–307.
2 Silveria, J.M., Seeman, M.V. (1995). Shared psychotic disorder: a critical review of the literature. *Canadian Journal of Psyhiatry/Revue Canadienne de Psychiatrie*, **40**(7): 389–395.

Delusional misidentification syndromes

Usually manifesting as symptoms of an underlying disorder (e.g., schizophrenia, mood disorder, delusional disorder, organic disorder), these syndromes rarely occur in isolation. Recently, interest has been focused on these rare (and bizarre) symptoms because of the insight they may give into the normal functioning of the brain (a "lesion" paradigm). Examples include:

- Capgras syndrome (l'illusion dessosies; 📖 p. 102)—the patient believes others have been replaced by identical or near identical imposters. Can apply to animals and other objects, and is often associated with aggressive behavior.
- Frégoli syndrome (l'illusion de Frégoli; 📖 p. 111)—an individual, most often unknown to the patient, is actually someone they know "in disguise". Usually the individual is thought to be pursuing or persecuting the patient in some way.
- Intermetamorphosis delusion—the patient believes he/she can see others change (usually temporarily) into someone else (both external appearance and internal personality).
- Subjective doubles delusion—the patient believes he or she has a double ("doppelgänger") who exists and functions independently.
- Autoscopic syndrome—the patient sees a double of him or herself projected onto other people or objects nearby.
- Reverse subjective double syndrome—the patient believes that he or she is an imposter in the process of being physically and psychologically replaced.
- Reverse Frégoli syndrome—the patient believes others have completely misidentified him/her.

Etiology

Psychodynamic

Views include seeing these syndromes as the extremes of normal misidentification due to intense focusing on particular details; the effects of beliefs and emotions on perception; the effects of vivid imagination in a person experiencing a disorder of mood, judgment, and coenaesthesia (sense of wholeness); manifestations of the defense mechanisms of projection, splitting, or regression with loss of identity and flawed reconstruction.

Biological

There may be evidence of underlying right hemisphere dysfunction, anterior cortical atrophy, temporal lobe pathology, bifrontal disconnectivity, with resultant impaired facial recognition and/or information processing.

Management

- Full physical and psychiatric assessment.
- Interventions should be directed toward any underlying problem.

Depressive disorders

Introduction

Depressive disorders are common, with a lifetime prevalence of up to 20% in primary care settings. They rank fourth as causes of disability worldwide, and it has been projected that they may rank second by the year 2020. The prevalence of depressive symptoms may be as high as 30% in the general population with women being twice as likely to be affected as men.

Although effective treatments are available, depression often goes undiagnosed and undertreated. Depressive symptoms are often regarded by both patients and physicians as understandable given current social circumstances and/or background. Although in many cases this may be true, patients should not be denied interventions that may help relieve some of the disabling symptoms of depression, thereby allowing them to cope better with any current social problems.

Moreover, it should always be remembered that depressive disorders have significant potential morbidity and mortality. Around 2/3 of all depressed patients contemplate suicide at some point, and the lifetime rate of depressed patients actually committing suicide may be as high as 15%. In persons aged 20—35yrs, suicide is the second leading cause of death, and depressive disorders are a major factor in up to 70% of these deaths. Aside from suicide, deaths can result from accidents due to impaired attention and concentration or due to illnesses that can be seen as sequelae of depressive disorders, such as substance dependence. In terms of overall morbidity, depressive disorders are comparable to advanced coronary artery disease, and their impact on personal relationships, social functioning and occupational productivity can be devastating. Depressive disorders also contribute to higher morbidity and mortality when associated with other physical disorders (e.g., myocardial infarction, stroke, diabetes, obesity), and their successful diagnosis and treatment has been shown to improve both medical and surgical outcomes. In short, these are potentially deadly and debilitating disorders that deserve serious and sustained clinical care.

Most depressed patients initially present to their primary care provider and often with problems other than low mood, such as fatigue, loss of energy, decreased libido, insomnia, or general malaise. Physicians ought to remain alert to the possibility of depressive illness in such patients, as early and effective interventions may be critical in the prevention of major morbidity and co-morbidity.

Unfortunately, there remains a reluctance on the part of some patients to consider pharmacological interventions for what are perceived as primarily emotional problems, despite overwhelming evidence of efficacy. While medication is not the only possible treatment for mild to moderate depression, when antidepressants are prescribed the onus is on the physician to give a therapeutic dose for an adequate length of time. Treatment failure is often due to patient nonadherence, particularly when the patient feels that their problems have not been taken seriously or when insufficient psycho-education regarding these disorders and their treatment has been provided. In a group of patients who generally have feelings of low self-worth or guilt, it is critical that they understand the rationale behind any treatment, and that their response to and tolerance of such treatment is regularly reviewed, at least in the early stages.

Depression among the famous

As depression is relatively common, it is not surprising that many famous people have had a depressive illness. However, there still remains a stigma attached to psychiatric illness, and it is only recently that people have become more willing to publicly discuss their illnesses. One study examined the lives of almost 300 world famous men and found that over 40% had experienced some type of depression during their lives[1]. Highest rates (72%) were found in writers, but the incidence was also high in:
- Artists (42%).
- Politicians (41%).
- Intellectuals (36%).
- Composers (35%).
- Scientists (33%).

Famous people who have publicly stated they have had a depressive illness include

Alanis Morissette, musician
Anne Rice, writer
Anthony Hopkins, actor
Barbara Bush, former First Lady
Amy Tan, writer
Billy Joel, musician, composer
Courtney Love, musician, actor
Billy Corgan, musician
Ellen DeGeneres, comedienne
Terry Bradshaw, quarterback
Elton John, musician

Halle Berry, actress
Harrison Ford, actor
Janet Jackson, musician
Jessica Lange, actress
Jim Carrey, actor, comedian
Joan Rivers, comedienne, TV host
John Cleese, comedian, actor
William Styron, writer

Leonard Cohen, musician, writer
Lou Reed, musician
Dick Clark, TV host
Marlon Brando, actor
Monica Seles, athlete (tennis)
Ozzy Osbourne, musician
Trent Reznor, musician
Mike Wallace, TV journalist

Paul Simon, composer, musician
Roseanne Barr, comedienne
Brooke Shields, actress
Sheryl Crow, musician
Sinead O'Connor, musician
S.P. Morrissey, musician
Stephen Hawking, scientist
Drew Barrymore, actress
Winona Ryder, actress
Yves Saint Laurent, designer
Greg Louganis, Olympic diver

Other famous people (deceased) known to have had a depressive illness

Samuel Becket, Menachem Begin, David Bohm, Kurt Cobain, Rodney Dangerfield, Charles Dickens, William Faulkner, Michel Foucault, Judy Garland, Ernest Hemingway, Audrey Hepburn, William James, Franz Kafka, John Keats, Claude Monet, Richard Nixon, Georgia O'Keeffe, Laurence Olivier, Wilfred Owen, George Patton, Sylvia Plath, Jackson Pollock, Cole Porter, Mark Rothko, Dmitri Shostakovich, Tennessee Williams.

Recommended further reading

1 Post, F. (1994). Creativity and psychopathology. A study of 291 world-famous men. *BJP* **165**, 22–34.

Historical perspective

The changing face of depression

Our current ideas of what constitutes depression date from the mid-eighteenth century. Before this, old notions of "melancholia," steeped in classical humoral theories (derived from the Greek *melaina kole,* black bile), reflected "intensity of idea" (J. Haslam, 1809)—the presence of few, rather than many, delusions. Sadness and low mood were not considered primary symptoms. The "melancholic" symptoms we regard today as part of depressive disorder would have been called "vapours," "hypochondria," or "neuroses." *Depression,* a term referring to "reduced functioning" in other medical disciplines, eventually became associated with mental depression. It was adopted because it implied a physiological change, and was defined as "a condition characterized by a sinking of the spirits, lack of courage or initiative, and a tendency to gloomy thoughts" (Joseph Jastrow, 1901).

This concept was enlarged and legitimized by Emil Kraepelin (1921) who used the term "depressive states" in his description of the unitary concept of "manic-depressive illness," encompassing melancholia simplex and gravis, stupor, fantastical melancholia, delirious melancholia, and involutional melancholia. A number of assumptions surrounded the affective disorders at that time: they involved primary pathology of affect, had stable psychopathology, had brain pathology, were periodic in nature, had a genetic basis, occurred in persons with certain personality traits, and were "endogenous" (not related to precipitants).

In 1917 Sigmund Freud published *Mourning and Melancholia,* influencing more than a generation in emphasizing cognitive and intrapsychic factors in the etiology of depressive disorders, conceptualized as the uneasy feeling of guilt in reaction to aggressive impulses directed against an ambivalently loved internalized object. With the rise of psychoanalytic theory, clinical descriptions shifted in focus from objective behavioral signs to subjective symptoms.

Over the intervening years there has been much debate about whether a "biological" type of depression exists separate from a "neurotic" type. Terminology has fluctuated around "endogenous," "vital," "autonomous," "endomorphic," and "melancholic" depression, characterized by distinctive symptoms and signs, a genetic basis, and running a course unrelated to psychosocial factors. In contrast, "neurotic" or "reactive" depression was thought to be capable of manifesting in multiple forms, show responsiveness to environmental situations, and, therefore, run a more variable course.

Although electroconvulsive therapy (ECT) was widely accepted as a treatment for "vital" depression, the received wisdom regarding the "reactive" depressive disorders was that their deep-seated psychological basis required a different kind of treatment entirely, a therapy consisting of sustained psychological investigation and exploration. The advent of anti-depressant drug therapy in the 1950s, however, rendered these distinctions less readily apparent, and ushered in an era of further inquiry into the biological complexities of depressive disorders.

Depressive disorders in the DSM-IV-

DSM-IV-TR provides a categorical classification of unipolar de
disorders by dividing them into types based on criteria sets with
features. Basic to this classification scheme is the concept of th
depressive episode as defined by a specified criteria set of de
symptoms (see 📖 p. 282). Although all unipolar depressive disor
defined by the absence of any previous manic, hypomanic, or mi
sodes, they are divided into the following types by the number, c
and etiology (if known) of the depressive symptoms present:

Major depressive disorder (📖 p. 284)
Prominent depressive symptoms that have, at least once, met th
fied criteria set for a major depressive episode.

Dysthymic disorder (📖 p. 286)
Prominent depressed mood + at least two additional depressiv
toms, lasting for at least two years, with no symptom-free period
than two months in a row, but no major depressive episode in
two years of the symptoms.

Substance-induced mood disorder with depressive feat
Prominent depressive symptoms arising during or within one m
substance intoxication or withdrawal or otherwise etiologically re
medication use.

Mood disorder due to a general medical condition with
depressive features
Prominent depressive symptoms arising as a direct physiological
quence of a medical condition as evident from labwork, physical e
history.

Adjustment disorder with depressed mood
Prominent depressive symptoms, not meeting the criteria for a
depressive episode, arising in response to an identifiable stre
occurring within three months of the onset of the stressor(s), and re
within six months after the stressor (or its consequences) has end

Depressive disorder not otherwise specified
Prominent depressive symptoms that do not clearly meet the crite
any of the aforementioned depressive disorders or that have an in
minable etiology. DSM-IV-TR also includes premenstrual dys
disorder, postpsychotic depressive disorder, and major depressive ep
superimposed on primary psychotic disorders within this category.

The antidepressants and beyond
The antidepressant era was inadvertently born in the early 1950s when
investigators, seeking to improve antituberculosis drug therapy, synthesized a derivative from isoniazid. This new agent, iproniazid, had the
unexpected action of psychostimulation in tuberculosis (TB) patients. It
was soon found to be an inhibitor of monoamine oxidase and capable of
reversing the depressogenic properties of reserpine. Iproniazid was subsequently promoted as a "psychic energizer" for "nervous" conditions. Its
efficacy in treating anxious-depressed patients was clearly established by
1955, although its usefulness was limited by its potential hepatotoxicity
and production of hypertensive crises.

A similar incidental discovery occurred when investigators, seeking to
enhance the range of available tranquilizing medications for psychotic
patients, began synthesizing agents from chlorpromazine. One such agent,
obtained by substituting an ethylene linkage for sulfur, was found to be
ineffective in calming agitated patients but did alleviate depressive symptoms. This agent was imipramine, which was soon marketed worldwide
as an antidepressant in 1958, closely followed by amitriptyline in 1960.

Around the same time new "anxiolytics" were also emerging, with mepr-
obamate in 1955, and the first benzodiazepine, chlordiazepoxide, in 1960.
The search for agents with greater anxiolytic and less sedating properties led
to the introduction of diazepam in 1963. One negative consequence of this
newly developed psychopharmacology was the overprescription in the
1960s and 1970s of these agents to help with problems of living and emerging evidence of potential physiologic dependence, particularly in the case of
the benzodiazepines. Partly as a result, nonpharmacological treatments flour-
ished, in the form of various rebranded psychotherapies.

As the neuropharmacologic action of the tricyclic antidepressants
(TCAs) and monoamine oxidase inhibitors (MAOIs) gradually became
more understood, biological psychiatrists and psychopharmacologists
developed monoamine theories of depression. These theories would
lead to the development of specific monoamine selective antidepressants—in the first instance, the selective serotonin reuptake inhibitors
(SSRIs), with zimelidine patented in 1971, indalpine launched in 1978, and
fluoxetine, patented in 1974 and launched in 1988.

The emphasis on safety and side-effect issues when comparing the
SSRIs to the TCAs, and the fall from grace of the benzodiazepines,
opened the floodgates in the 1980s and 1990s for the promotion of SSRIs
not only in the treatment of depression, but also for anxiety disorders.
Advances in monoamine theories also allowed for the development of
dual-action agents (e.g., serotonin and norepinephrine reuptake inhibitors
[SNRIs]—venlafaxine noradrenergic and specific serotonergic antidepressants; [NaSSAs]—nefazodone/mirtazepine; noradrenergic and dopaminergic-
uptake inhibitors [NDRIs]—bupropion) and other selective agents (e.g.,
noradrenaline reuptake inhibitors [NARIs]—reboxetine [not available in the
United States]).

Current theories of depression attempt to integrate biological models
of stress (and the involvement of the hypothalamic-pituitary-adrenal
[HPA] axis) with evidence from neuropharmacology, biological psychology, genetics, and functional neuropathology. In this way, a multifactorial

"biopsychosocial model" (see 📖 *p. 292*) emerges, which may help unite the apparently divergent ideas of depression. Clinical symptoms and signs are seen as the final common pathway in a complex interaction between genes and the environment in determining predisposition biological vulnerability, which may (or may not) subsequently lead biological variations in functioning necessary for behavioral and emotion change. This may be due to further psychosocial stressors or genetica predetermined factors that give rise to alterations in brain functionir Research into these interdependent factors may well lead to great understanding of the etiology of depressive disorders, as well as allowi the development of diagnostic tests and individualized treatments.

Diagnosis (1)—depressive episode symptoms

DSM-IV-TR lists the specific diagnostic criteria set for a major depressive episode and includes additional criteria/descriptors to allow the clinician to further qualify the current or most recent episode.

DSM-IV-TR criteria for major depressive episode

- **Five** (or more) of the following symptoms have been present during the same **two-week** period and represent a change from previous functioning; **at least one** of the symptoms is either (1) depressed mood or (2) loss of interest or pleasure. Note: Do not include symptoms that are clearly due to a general medical condition, or mood-incongruent delusions or hallucinations.
  - Depressed mood most of the day nearly every day, as indicated by either subjective report (e.g., feels sad or empty) or observation made by others (e.g., appears tearful). Note: In children and adolescents, can be irritable mood.
  - Markedly diminished interest or pleasure in all, or almost all, activities most of the day, nearly every day (as indicated by either subjective account or observation made by others).
  - Significant weight loss when not dieting or weight gain (e.g., a change of more than 5% of body weight in a month), or decrease or increase in appetite nearly every day. Note: In children, consider failure to make expected weight gains.
  - Insomnia or hypersomnia nearly every day.
  - Psychomotor agitation or retardation nearly every day (observable by others, not merely subjective feelings of restlessness or being slowed down).
  - Fatigue or loss of energy nearly every day.
  - Feelings of worthlessness or excessive or inappropriate guilt (which may be delusional) nearly every day (not merely self-reproach or guilt about being sick).
  - Diminished ability to think or concentrate, or indecisiveness, nearly every day (either by subjective account or as observed by others).
  - Recurrent thoughts of death (not just fear of dying), recurrent suicidal ideation without a specific plan, or a suicide attempt or a specific plan for committing suicide.
- The symptoms do not meet criteria for a mixed episode (see 📖 p. 348).
- The symptoms cause clinically significant distress or impairment in social, occupational, or other important areas of functioning.
- The symptoms are not due to the direct physiological effects of a substance (e.g., a drug of abuse, a medication) or a general medical condition (e.g., hypothyroidism).
- The symptoms are not better accounted for by Bereavement, i.e., after the loss of a loved one, the symptoms persist for longer than two months or are characterized by marked functional impairment, morbid preoccupation with worthlessness, suicidal ideation, psychotic symptoms, or psychomotor retardation.

DSM-IV-TR criteria for severity/psychotic/remission specifiers for current (or most recent) major depressive episode

- **Mild**—Few, if any, symptoms in excess of those required to make the diagnosis and symptoms result in only minor impairment in occupational functioning or in usual social activities or relationships with others.
- **Moderate**—Symptoms or functional impairment between mild and severe.
- **Severe without psychotic features**—Several symptoms in excess of those required to make the diagnosis, and symptoms markedly interfere with occupational functioning or with usual social activities or relationships with others.
- **Severe with psychotic features**—Delusions or hallucinations, if possible, specify whether the psychotic features are mood-congruent or mood-incongruent.
- **Mood-congruent psychotic features**—Delusions or hallucinations whose content is entirely consistent with the typical depressive themes or personal inadequacy, guilt, disease, death, nihilism, or deserved punishment.
- **Mood-incongruent psychotic features**—Delusions or hallucinations whose content does not involve typical depressive themes or personal inadequacy, guilt, disease, death, nihilism, or deserved punishment. Included are such symptoms as persecutory delusions (not directly related to depressive themes), thought insertion, thought broadcasting, and delusions of control.
- **In partial remission**—Symptoms of a major depressive episode are present but full criteria are not met, or there is a period without any significant symptoms of a major depressive episode lasting less than two months following the end of the major depressive episode. (If the major depressive episode was superimposed on dysthymic disorder, the diagnosis of dysthymic disorder alone is given once the full criteria for a major depressive episode are no longer met).
- **In full remission**—During the past two months, no significant signs or symptoms of the disturbance were present.

Diagnosis (2)—major depressive disorder

DSM-IV-TR then specifies the diagnostic criteria for major depressive disorder, on the basis of the previously or currently categorized major depressive episode(s) and exclusion through history-taking and/or review of systems of other previous mood episodes or psychiatric disorders.

DSM-IV-TR diagnostic criteria for major depressive disorder

- Presence of one or more major depressive episode(s). Note: To be considered separate episodes, there must be an interval of at least two consecutive months in which criteria are not met for a major depressive episode.
  - Single episode—Presence of a single major depressive episode.
  - Recurrent—Presence of two or more major depressive episodes.
- The major depressive episode(s) is not better accounted for by schizoaffective disorder and is not superimposed on schizophrenia, schizophreniform disorder, delusional disorder, or psychotic disorder not otherwise specified.
- There has never been a manic episode, a mixed episode, or a hypomanic episode. Note: This exclusion does not apply if all of the manic-like, mixed-like, or hypomanic-like episodes are substance induced or treatment induced or are due to the direct physiological effects of a general medical condition.

Finally, DSM-IV-TR specifies additional symptom features that can be used to further describe and/or subtype patients with major depressive disorder, thereby improving clinical specificity and helping guide initial treatment and subsequent management considerations. These include: melancholic features, catatonic features, atypical features, postpartum onset, and seasonal pattern.

DSM-IV-TR criteria for melancholic features specifier

- Either of the following, occurring during the most severe period of the current episode:
  - Loss of pleasure in all, or almost all, activities.
  - Lack of reactivity to usually pleasurable stimuli (does not feel much better, even temporarily, when something good happens).
- Three (or more) of the following:
  - Distinct quality of depressed mood (i.e., the depressed mood is experienced as distinctly different from the kind of feeling experienced after the death of a loved one).
  - Depression regularly worse in the morning.
  - Early morning awakening (at least two hours before usual time of awakening).
  - Marked psychomotor retardation or agitation.
  - Significant anorexia or weight loss.
  - Excessive or inappropriate guilt.

DSM-IV-TR criteria for catatonic features specifier

The clinical picture is dominated by at least two of the following:
- Motoric immobility as evidenced by catalepsy (including waxy flexibility) or stupor.
- Excessive motor activity (that is apparently purposeless and not influenced by external stimuli).
- Extreme negativism (an apparently motiveless resistance to all instructions or maintenance of a rigid posture against attempts to be moved) or mutism.
- Peculiarities of voluntary movement as evidenced by posturing (voluntary assumption of inappropriate or bizarre postures), stereotyped movements, prominent mannerisms, or prominent grimacing.
- Echolalia or echopraxia.

DSM-IV-TR criteria for atypical features specifier

- Mood reactivity (e.g., mood brightens in response to actual or potential positive events).
- Two (or more) of the following features:
  - Significant weight gain or increase in appetite.
  - Hypersomnia.
  - Leaden paralysis (i.e., heavy, leaden feelings in arms or legs).
  - Long-standing pattern of interpersonal rejection sensitivity (not limited to episodes of mood disturbance) that results in a significant social or occupational impairment.
- Criteria are not met for melancholic features or catatonic features during the same episode.

DSM-IV-TR criteria for postpartum onset specifier

Onset of episode within four weeks postpartum.

DSM-IV-TR criteria for seasonal pattern specifier

- There has been a regular temporal relationship between the onset of major depressive episodes in bipolar I or bipolar II disorder or major depressive disorder, recurrent, and a particular time of the year (e.g., regular appearance of the major depressive episode in the fall or winter). Note: Do not include cases in which there is an obvious effect of seasonal-related psychosocial stressors (e.g., regularly being unemployed every winter).
- Full remissions (or a change from depression to mania or hypomania) also occur at a characteristic time of the year (e.g., depression disappears in the spring).
- In the last two years, two major depressive episodes have occurred that demonstrate the temporal seasonal relationship defined in Criteria A and B, and no nonseasonal major depressive episodes have occurred during that same period.
- Seasonal major depressive episodes (as described earlier) substantially outnumber the nonseasonal major depressive episodes that may have occurred over the individual's lifetime.

Diagnosis (3)—dysthymic disorder

DSM-IV-TR diagnostic criteria for dysthymic disorder

- Depressed mood for most of the day, for more days than not, as indicated either by subjective account or observations by others, for at **least two years**. Note: In children and adolescents, mood can be irritable and duration must be at least **one year**.
- Presence, while depressed, of **two (or more)** of the following:
  - Poor appetite or overeating.
  - Insomnia or hypersomnia.
  - Low energy or fatigue.
  - Low self-esteem.
  - Poor concentration or difficulty making decisions.
  - Feelings of hopelessness.
- During the two-year period (one year for children or adolescents) of the disturbance, the person has never been without the symptoms above for more than two months at a time.
- No major depressive episode has been present during the first two years of the disturbance (one year for children and adolescents); i.e., the disturbance is not better accounted for by chronic major depressive disorder, or major depressive disorder, in partial remission. Note: There may have been a previous major depressive episode provided there was a full remission (no significant signs or symptoms for two months) before development of the dysthymic disorder. In addition, after the initial two years (one year in children and adolescents) of dysthymic disorder, there may be superimposed episodes of major depressive disorder, in which case both diagnoses may be given when the criteria are met for a major depressive episode.
- There has never been a manic episode, a mixed episode, or a hypomanic episode, and criteria have never been met for cyclothymic disorder.
- The disturbance does not occur exlusively during the course of a chronic psychotic disorder, such as schizophrenia or delusional disorder.
- The symptoms are not due to the direct physiological effects of a substance (e.g., a drug or abuse, a medication) or a general medical condition (e.g., hypothyroidism).
- The symptoms cause clinically significant distress or impairment in social, occupational, or other important areas of functioning.

As a description of the experience of the symptoms of depression, the following has never been bettered

I have of late but wherefore I know not lost all my mirth, forgone all custom of exercises; and indeed it goes so heavily with my disposition that this goodly frame, the earth, seems to me a sterile promontory, this most excellent canopy, the air, look you, this brave o'erhanging firmament, this majestical roof fretted with golden fire, why, it appears no other thing to me than a foul and pestilent congregation of vapours. What a piece of work is a man! how noble in reason! How infinite in faculty! in form and moving how express and admirable! In action how like an angel! in apprehension how like a god! the beauty of the world! the paragon of animals! And yet, to me, what is this quintessence of dust? Man delights not me: no, nor woman neither.

Shakespeare: *Hamlet* (Act II Scene 2)

Epidemiology of depression

Current prevalence
2–5% from multiple sources for the general population.

Lifetime prevalence
10–25% in females, variable across populations; 5–12% in males, variable across populations.

Risk factors
Genetic
Two to four times increased risk for those with a first-degree relative with recurrent major depressive disorder.

Childhood experiences
Loss of a parent (especially before age 11), lack of parental care, parental alcoholism or antisocial traits, childhood sexual abuse.

Personality traits
Neuroticism/anxiety, impulsivity, obsessionality.

Marital status
In males, low rates associated with marriage, high rates with separation or divorce; in females, rates are similar, but less clear.

Adverse life events
Especially "loss" events (with increased risk two to three months after event) in vulnerable individuals.

Social stressors
Brown and Harris[1] found that, for women, having three or more children under the age of 11, lack of paid employment, and lack of a confiding relationship were associated with increased risk of depression. Recent studies support only the lack of a confiding relationship, not the other factors.

Physical illness
Especially if chronic, severe, or painful. Neurological disorders, including Parkinson's disease, MS, stroke, and epilepsy appear to have a higher risk, perhaps due to shared neuropathology. Higher rates are also noted in post-MI, diabetic, and cancer patients, although family and personal history of depression are important determinants of occurrence. In individuals with two or more chronic physical illnesses, the prevalence of severe major depression is four times higher than that of individuals without the conditions.

Co-morbidity
About two-thirds of patients will also meet criteria for another psychiatric disorder (e.g., anxiety disorders, substance misuse, alcohol dependency, personality disorders).

1 Brown, G.W. and Harris, T.O. *Social Origins of Depression: A Study of Psychiatric Disorders in Women.* London: Tavistock Publications (1978).

Etiology of depression

The etiology of depression has yet to be fully understood. However, it is likely to be due to the interplay of biological, psychological, and social factors in the lifespan of an individual. Psychosocial stressors may play a role as both precipitants and perpetuating factors, increasing the risk of chronicity and recurrence, whereas individuals with an established depressive disorder are at higher risk of further stressors of many kinds. One attempt to integrate these factors is the biopsychosocial model (see 📖 p. 292).

Neurobiological factors

Structural brain changes

Reduced volumes have been found in the left hippocampus, caudate nucleus, left parietal cortex, and frontal association cortices of patients with chronic depressive disorders.

Functional brain changes

Decreased metabolism in frontal, temporal, and parietal areas, possibly more pronounced on the left side (especially in older patients); increased metabolism in limbic and paralimbic regions such as the subgenual cingulate (especially in younger patients with severe depression, reversible with active and effective treatment).

Neurotransmitter abnormalities

The discoveries that amine depletion (by reserpine) and tryptophan (5HT-precursor) depletion produce depression, and that agents that increase the concentration of monoamines (e.g., 5HT, NE, DA) at the synaptic cleft are effective antidepressants, suggested that reduced monoamine function caused depression. Although disturbances in monoaminergic systems are unquestionably involved in the pathophysiology of depression, the exact role of these systems as neuromodulatory circuits and their complex interactions with pre- and postsynaptic receptor expression, second messengers, neurokinins, and transcription factors continue to be elucidated.

Endocrine changes

Studies in depressed patients have described blunted prolactin and growth hormone (GH) responses to 5HT agonists, blunted GH responses to clonidine (NE system) and apomorphine (DA system), and an increased GH response to physostigmine (ACh system), thereby suggesting neuroendocrine disturbances in depression possibly related to reduced monoamine functioning and increased cholinergic functioning. Elevated cortisol levels are seen in ~50% of depressed patients (especially with melancholic or psychotic features) and as many as ~50% of depressed patients do not suppress cortisol in response to a single dose of dexamethasone, a synthetic cortisol analogue. (This finding, however, is of little diagnostic utility, as many other psychiatric conditions show a similar response.)

Changes in sleep pattern

Reduction of total deep (slow wave, non-rapid eye movement [REM]) sleep and an overall increase in nocturnal arousal are commonly seen in depressed patients and are reflected in delayed sleep onset, increased nocturnal awakenings, reduced REM latency, and a longer first REM period.

Genetic factors

Appear to influence the risk of depression by altering individual sensitivity to the effects of life stressors. Linkage analysis suggests an association between the genes 5HTT (encoding the serotonin transporter) and CREB1 (encoding cyclic AMP response element binding protein) and depression, treatment response, and, possibly, suicidal behavior. Other studies have implicated polymorphisms in the genes HTR2A (encoding the 5HT2A receptor), GRIK4 (encoding the KA1 kainate-type glutamate receptor), and BCL2 (encoding a protective mitochondrial membrane protein) in antidepressant response.

Psychological and social factors

Personality/temperament

These are enduring traits with a biological basis, influenced over the lifespan by inherited factors, experience, and maturation. They mediate the level and nature of response to sensory experience, are regulated by context, and manifest as subjective emotions and objective behaviors. Certain temperaments (e.g., "neuroticism") may increase vulnerability to depression, perhaps due to the presence of autonomic hyperarousal (heightened responses to emotional stimuli) or lability (unpredictable responses to emotional stimuli).

Adversity

Disruption of normal social, marital, parental, or familial relationships is correlated with high rates of depression and is a risk factor to recurrence. An etiological role has yet to be demonstrated, but adverse childhood experiences and chronic stressors throughout childhood may influence the sensitivity of individuals to later stressful events. Low self-esteem (negative view of self, the past, current events, and the future) has been proposed as a vulnerability factor, although it remains debatable whether this is a causal factor or merely a symptom of depression.

Gender

Although the increased prevalence of depression in women is a robust finding, explanations of this finding are varied. These have included: restricted social and occupational roles, being over- or underoccupied, ruminative response styles, and endocrine factors (suggested by the increased risk of depression in the premenstrual and postpartum periods). There is, however, little supportive evidence for these theories. One popular hypothesis is that women may more readily acknowledge their depressive symptoms and seek treatment for depression, whereas men may not and instead may tend to express their symptoms differently (e.g., through alcohol abuse or antisocial behavior).

Social factors

In explaining why people of low socioeconomic status (i.e., low levels of income, employment, and education) are at demonstrably higher risk for depression, two main arguments exist: social causation—the stress associated with such problems leads to depression (i.e., an "environmental" argument); and social selection—predisposed individuals drift down to lower social positions or fail to rise from them (i.e., a "genetic" argument). There is perhaps stronger evidence for the social causation argument, as social isolation (living alone, lacking a social network, infrequent social interactions) has been shown to be a major risk factor.

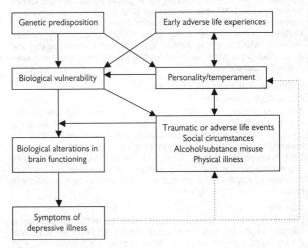

Fig. 7.1 The biopsychosocial model of depression.

Differential diagnosis

Other psychiatric disorders

Inherent to the DSM-IV-TR diagnostic classification of unipolar depressive disorders is the effective "ruling-out" of the bipolar affective disorders, through the absence of any previous manic, hypomanic, or mixed episodes. In practice, this is a major clinical challenge, as patients with bipolar disorders can have poor memory for such episodes or may not have yet experienced them. This means the clinician should be fully aware of the clinical features that may be broad indicators of a potential underlying bipolar disorder (see 🕮 p. 352).

Aside from the bipolar disorders, there are many other psychiatric disorders and conditions that share some of the clinical affective and/or neurovegetative features of depressive disorders:

- ADHD.
- Anxiety disorders.
- Alcohol use disorders.
- Bereavement.
- Conduct disorder.
- Dementias.
- Depersonalization disorder.
- Eating disorders.
- Impulse control disorders.
- Normal periods of human sadness.
- Personality disorders (borderline, avoidant, dependent).
- Schizoaffective disorders.
- Schizophrenia and other psychotic disorders.
- Sleep disorders.
- Sexual disorders (hypoactive sexual desire disorder, orgasmic disorder, male erectile disorder, sexual arousal disorder, sexual aversion disorder).
- Somatoform disorders (body dysmorphic disorder, hypochondriasis, pain disorder, somatization disorder, undifferentiated somatoform disorder).
- Substance use disorders.

General medical conditions

Many patients who have depressive symptoms also have one or more general medical conditions, and it can at times be difficult to discern how much to attribute these symptoms (especially neurovegetative) to a primary depressive disorder or to the medical condition. A temporal association (onset, exacerbation, remission) between the condition and the depressive symptoms can help guide the clinician, especially if the condition is known to have a direct association with the development of such symptoms (see Table 7.1).

Pharmacological causes of depressive symptoms

Finally, many substances (prescribed for a medical condition, used recreationally, or through environmental exposure) can induce depressive symptoms. A listing of such pharmacological agents is given in Table 7.2.

Table 7.1 General medical conditions with depressive features

Cardiopulmonary

Cardiomyopathy	Congestive heart failure
Cerebral ischemia/stroke	Postmyocardial infarction
Chronic obstructive pulmonary disease (COPD)	Restrictive lung disease

Endocrine

Hypothyroidism	Hyperthyroidism
Cushing's disease	Addison's disease
Hyperparathyroidism	Hypoparathyroidism
Hypoglycemia	Hypopituitarism
Pheochromocytoma	Carcinoid
Ovarian failure	Testicular failure
Perimenstrual syndromes	Menopausal symptoms
Prolactinoma	

Infectious/Inflammatory

Influenza	Tertiary syphilis
Mononucleosis	Hepatitis
HIV/AIDS	Tuberculosis
Encephalitis	Lyme disease
Systemic lupus erythematosis	Rheumatoid arthritis
Toxoplasmosis	Viral pneumonia

Neoplastic

Pancreatic adenocarcinoma	Lung neoplasms
Leukemias	Lymphomas

Neurological

Multiple sclerosis	Parkinson's disease
Head trauma	Brain tumors
Wilson's disease	Huntington's disease
Epilepsy	

Nutritional deficiencies/Metabolic deficiencies

Folate deficiency	B_{12} deficiency
Pyridoxine (B_6) deficiency	Riboflavin (B_2) deficiency
Thiamine (B_1) deficiency	Iron deficiency

Table 7.2 Pharmacological causes of depressive symptoms

Analgesics and anti-inflammatory agents		
Fenoprofen	Ibuprofen	Indomethacin
Opiates	Phenacetin	Phenylbutazone
Benzydamine		

Antibacterial and antifungal agents		
Ampicillin	Clotrimazole	Cycloserine
Ethionamide	Dapsone	Griseofulvin
Metronidazole	Nitrofurantoin	Nalidixic acid
Sulfonamides	Streptomycin	Tetracyclines
Thiocarbanilide		

Anticholinesterases		
Cimetidine	Diphenoxylate	Lysergide
Mebeverine	Metoclopramide	Salbutamol

Antineoplastic agents		
C-Asparaginase	Bleomycin	Mithramycin
Trimethoprim	Vincristine	Zidovudine
6-Azauridine		

Cardiac and antihypertensive agents		
Bethanidine	Clonidine	Digitalis
Guanethidine	Hydralazine	Lidocaine
Methoserpidine	Methyldopa	Oxprenolol
Prazosin	Procainamide	Propranolol
Reserpine	Veratrum	

Antipsychotic agents		
Butyrophenones	Phenothiazines	

Sedatives and hypnotics		
Barbiturates	Benzodiazepines	Chloral hydrate
Chlorazepate	Chlormethiazole	Ethanol

Steroids and hormones		
Corticosteroids	Danazol	Oral contraceptives
Prednisone	Norethisterone	Triamcinolone

Stimulants and appetite suppressants		
Amphetamine	Cocaine	Diethylpropion
Fenfluramine	Phenmetrazine	Caffeine

Neurological agents		
Amantadine	Baclofen	Bromocriptine
Carbamazepine	Levodopa	Methsuximide
Tetrabenazine	Phenytoin	

Other miscellaneous agents		
Acetazolamide	Choline	Cyproheptadine
Disulfiram	Interferon	Methysergide
Meclizine	Pizotifen	

Course and prognosis

Points to note
- Average age of onset late 20s, although depression may occur at any age.
- Later-onset depression may be milder, more chronic, more likely to be associated with life events, more likely to have a subclinical prodrome.
- Untreated depressive episodes typically last 6–13 months.
- Most treated depressive episodes last <3 months.
- Episodes of recurrent depression tend to be shorter (4–16wks).
- Number of prior episodes predicts risk of subsequent episodes: one episode, 60% → second episode; two episodes, 70% → third episode; three episodes, 90% → fourth episode.
- One of the most important predictors is the course and duration of previous episodes, as longitudinal studies suggest successive episodes can be remarkably similar.
- Risk of recurrence is greater when there are residual symptoms after remission (about a third of cases) such as low mood, anxiety, sleep disturbance, reduced libido, and physical symptoms (headache, fatigue, gastrointestinal upset).
- There is good evidence that modern antidepressant treatments (the SSRIs) impact significantly upon all these quoted figures, reducing the length of depressive episodes.
- If treatment is given long term, incidence of residual symptoms is lower, there are fewer recurrent episodes, and chronicity may be as low as 4%.

Mortality
- Suicide rates for severe depressive episodes vary between reports but may be up to 15% (i.e., up to 20 times more likely than in the general population), with a slightly higher rate for those who have required hospital admission (15–19%). For less severe episodes the rates are much lower.
- Overall death rate for patients with depression is higher than the general population (SMR 1.37–2.49) with the cause of death usually due to suicide, drug and alcohol problems, accidents, cardiovascular disease, respiratory infections, and thyroid disorders.

Prognostic factors
Better outcome
Advanced age of onset, acute onset, mild episodes, no psychotic symptoms, brief hospital stay, no co-morbid Axis I or Axis II psychiatric disorders, a history of solid friendships during adolescence, a history of good social functioning for the previous five years, current stable family functioning.

Poorer outcome

Insidious onset, "neurotic" depression, severe episodes, residual symptoms, low self-confidence, any co-morbidity (but especially anxiety disorders, alcohol or drug problems, personality disorders, or debilitating physical illness), lack of social supports, multiple prior episodes, more than one prior hospital admission; males are more likely to have a chronically impaired course.

Management principles

Initial assessment

Complete history

Key areas of inquiry include:

- Any clear psychosocial precipitants.
- Current social situation.
- Current mood symptoms.
- Degree of functional impairment.
- Any co-morbid psychiatric disorder (esp. dysthymia).
- Any co-morbid substance use/abuse/dependence.
- Any previous mood symptoms or episodes (including "subclinical" periods of low or elevated mood), their course and duration.
- Any previous effective and/or ineffective treatments.
- General medical history.
- Family history of mood disorder.
- Review of all current medications.

Mental status examination (see 📖 p. 48)

Focused inquiry about subjective mood symptoms, somatic symptoms, psychotic symptoms, anxiety symptoms. Objective assessment of psychomotor retardation/agitation, cognitive functioning (MMSE, if indicated). Also consider depression severity rating scales.

Lethality risk assessment

Careful and crucial evaluation of the following:

- Any suicidal or homicidal ideation, intent, or plans.
- Access to means for suicide/homicide, potential lethality of such means.
- History of previous attempts, potential lethality of such attempts.
- Family history of suicide, recent exposure to suicide.
- Clinical factors that increase risk: psychotic symptoms (especially command hallucinations), severe anxiety, panic attacks, alcohol/substance use.
- Assessment of patient's strengths and motivation to seek help or follow safety plan.

Establish therapeutic alliance

Especially critical in a patient population whose symptoms can include poor motivation, poor self-care, decreased attention and/or memory, the potential for self-harm, and a general pessimism or even hopelessness regarding the effectiveness of treatment.

Determination of treatment setting

After careful consideration of all the aforementioned factors, the site of treatment is chosen (ideally by joint agreement of both clinician and patient) that provides the greatest opportunity for safe and effective care. Possible settings range from ambulatory clinics, to intensive day programs, to hospitalization, which is usually reserved for patients with serious potential lethality or inability to care for self and can be involuntarily mandated if admission criteria of the local jurisdiction are met.

Physical examination

Focused on possible differential diagnoses (see 📖 p. 294).

Initial labwork and studies

Focused on the exclusion of potentially treatable causes (see 📖 *p. 294*) or secondary problems (e.g., appetite loss, alcohol abuse, etc).

- Standard tests: CBC with differential, electrolytes, LFTs, TFTs, B_{12}, folate.
- Additional tests: (if indicated by history or physical signs) Urine toxicology, thyroid antibodies, antinuclear antibodies, syphilis serology, CT/MRI, EEG, LP, HIV and hepatitis testing, dexamethasone suppression test (Cushing's disease), cosyntropin stimulation test (Addison's disease).

Hospital admission for depression

Major depressive episodes can be severe enough to require hospital admission, at times through involuntary commitment. All psychiatrists should be well versed in the criteria for and due process of such commitments in their local jurisdiction and should (along with their clinical support staff) always be prepared for this possibility. As for all psychiatric disorders, issues of safety and the provision of effective treatment will govern the decisions about whether a patient can remain in the ambulatory setting.

Common reasons for hospital admission

- Serious risk of suicide (see 📖 pp. 60, 756—for assessment of suicide risk).
- Serious risk of harm to others.
- Significant self-neglect.
- Severe depressive symptoms.
- Severe psychotic symptoms.
- Lack or breakdown of social supports.
- Initiation of ECT.
- Treatment-resistant depression (where inpatient monitoring is needed).
- Urgent need to address co-morbid conditions (e.g., poorly managed or complex medical conditions, other psychiatric conditions).
- Need for inpatient detoxification.

Points to note

- Often due to symptoms of low self-esteem or guilt, some depressed patients may decline hospital admission because they feel "unworthy" of such an intense level of clinical care and attention and would therefore "take up a valuable bed." Sympathetic reassurance that this is not the case and that the clinician believes the patient's symptoms are severe enough to deserve the benefits of hospital admission may avoid unnecessary involuntary commitment procedures.
- Some patients (or their relatives) may demand admission to hospital. Although sometimes due to personality factors, this may also be due to erroneous ideas of what can be reasonably achieved in the hospital setting (e.g., intensive psychotherapy for a specific issue, comprehensive diagnostic testing), or reflect undisclosed factors that have created a social crisis. A nonconfrontational approach in eliciting the reasons behind such demands may reveal other important issues that may help the disposition process, including those that may be more effectively addressed by other services (e.g., emergency shelters, respite housing, etc.).
- With significant risk of harm to self or others, admission should be to a ward where close observation and monitoring of the patient are possible.

- The inpatient milieu is often not the quiet sanctuary patients might have imagined, prompting some to demand prompt discharge from the hospital. This situation may lead to difficult decisions, balancing the risk of self-harm against the use of involuntary commitment. Careful assessment of a patient's insight into his or her illness, capacity to seek additional support when symptoms are worse, and issues of substance abuse and other psychiatric co-morbidity are critical in this decision process and can allow for more flexible disposition planning, such as initiating an intensive day program and/or temporary residence with family members or friends.

Treatment of the depressive disorders

Acute phase treatment

Once a positive diagnosis has been made, possible treatments should be discussed with the patient. The range of initial treatment modalities includes psychotherapy, pharmacotherapy, or a combination of the two. If clinically indicated, ECT should also be considered. Initial treatment selection should be based on the severity of symptoms and the patient's preference.

The goal of treatment in the acute phase is nothing less than remission of depressive symptoms and return of the patient to his or her former level of social and occupational functioning. Toward this end, regular and frequent follow-up is needed to carefully assess the extent of response (possibly with the aid of depression symptom severity rating scales). Should a moderate response not be observed after the first four to eight weeks, the treatment regimen should be reappraised and strategically adjusted. Regular and frequent monitoring of response along with further periodic treatment reappraisals and revisions every four to eight weeks in the case of poor or partial response; therefore, monitoring needs to be performed throughout the entire acute phase of treatment, until the patient has a full response to treatment and symptom remission is achieved.

Choosing psychotherapy as initial treatment

- Usually for patients with mild to moderate depressive symptoms.
- Patient preference should guide specific psychotherapy choice.
- Psychosocial stressors, personal history, relationship difficulties, degree of psychological mindedness can also suggest specific modalities.
- CBT and IPT repeatedly shown to be effective in treating depression.
- If poor or partial response, consider addition of antidepressant trial.

Choosing an antidepressant as initial treatment

The following are guidelines. Be certain to discuss risks, benefits, and alternatives, and refer to literature for updates.

- All available antidepressants (see 📖 p. 314) have generally comparable efficacy both within a given class and across classes.
- Selection of a specific antidepressant agent typically depends upon:
  - Patient factors such as age, sex, co-morbid physical illness(es), especially cardiac, renal, liver, or neurological, previous responses to antidepressants.
  - Tolerability issues.
  - Presenting symptoms, such as insomnia (more sedative agent), anergia/hypersomnia (more activating agent), anxious or obsessive (possibly SSRI), suicidal (avoid TCAs), etc.
  - Physician familiarity, which allows for better patient education in anticipation of possible adverse effects, enhancing adherence.
- Patients should be specifically informed that the onset of an antidepressant's beneficial effects can take up to several weeks, during which depressive symptoms may continue to worsen. Knowing this in advance can prevent demoralization and enhance adherence in many patients.

- Starting doses are typically low to enhance tolerability.
- If poor or partial response, consider increase in dose if tolerated.
- If poor or partial response, consider addition of psychotherapy.
- If persisting poor or partial response, increase dose further, up to maximum recommended or tolerated dose. An adequate clinical trial of an antidepressant is considered at least six weeks at this dose.
- If persisting poor or partial response, consider switching to a different antidepressant (non-MAOI), either from same class or from another class and perform an adequate clinical trial.
- If, despite these trials, response continues to be poor or partial, additional non-MAOI trials can be made. Alternatively, addition of another non-MAOI antidepressant can be made to the current antidepressant, being cautious of any expected drug-drug interactions.
- If these efforts fail, trial of a MAOI may be warranted (see 📖 *p. 314* for cautions and recommended timeframes to "washout" prior antidepressant).
- Alternatively, various augmentation strategies can be attempted (📖 *p. 312*).
- If these efforts fail, ECT should be strongly considered.

Choosing to combine psychotherapy and antidepressant treatment

- Anecdotal evidence and indirect data have long suggested that "combination" treatment is the optimal way to treat recurrent depression.
- Recent studies specifically designed to investigate and compare treatments for depression strongly support this perception, finding higher rates of remission and lower rates of recurrence in depressed patients treated with the combination of an antidepressant and psychotherapy (CBT or IPT in most studies) versus either treatment alone.[1]
- As further evidence emerges that supports the superiority of combining psychotherapy and antidepressant therapy in the treatment of depression, "combination" treatment should become standard practice, and clinicians may one day have to justify their reasons for not choosing to combine these treatment modalities.

Choosing ECT as initial treatment

- ECT should be considered as a first-line therapy for severe major depressive disorder when there are debilitating neurovegetative symptoms (e.g., significant weight loss and nutritional compromise from reduced appetite, profound psychomotor retardation, catatonic stupor, etc).
- Also should be considered when the patient has high potential lethality issues (e.g., intense suicidality, clear evidence of repeated suicide attempts, significantly aggressive behavior) or prominent psychotic features.

1 Three key studies in this regard are the Pittsburgh Maintenance Therapies in Recurrent Depression study (see Frank E. *et al.*, Three-year outcomes for maintenance therapies in recurrent depression, *Arch Gen Psych* **47**, 1093–1099, 1990), the Geriatric Depression Study (see Reynolds C.F. III *et al.*, Nortriptyline and interpersonal psychotherapy as maintenance therapies for recurrent major depression: a randomized controlled trial in patients older than 59 years, *JAMA* **281**, 39–45, 1999), and the Treatment of Chronic Depression study (see Keller M.B. *et al.*, A comparison of nefazodone, the cognitive behavioural-analysis system of psychotherapy, and their combination for the treatment of chronic depression, *NEJM* **342**, 1462–1470, 2000).

- In these above circumstances, problematic issues of consent to treatment must be considered and resolved (see Chapters 17 and 18 on forensic psychiatry).
- ECT should also be considered a treatment choice for severely depressed patients who are pregnant, who have responded well to prior ECT course(s), who have responded poorly to adequate trials of antidepressants, or in situations where a particularly rapid response is needed.

Continuation phase treatment

Upon full response to treatment and remission of depressive symptoms, care for the depressed patient enters the continuation phase, roughly defined as the 16–20 weeks following remission.

The goal of treatment in the continuation phase focuses on the prevention of relapse during the vulnerable period following symptomatic recovery. Evidence suggests that as many as 25% of patients effectively treated with an antidepressant medication to the point of recovery will relapse within two months if that medication is discontinued soon after recovery. For this reason, it is strongly recommended that all patients who are successfully treated for a depressive episode with an antidepressant medication continue that medication at its therapeutic dose for at least 16–20 weeks following full remission. Studies have also suggested that psychotherapies thought to be "time-limited" (CBT, IPT) are effective at preventing relapse either when continued beyond the acute phase or when added to antidepressant treatment following recovery.

During the continuation phase, assessment visits may be scheduled less frequently (every 6 to 8 weeks), if appropriate. Regardless of modality, key components of follow-up during the continuation phase should include:

- Maintaining the therapeutic alliance.
- Screening for the return of any depressive symptoms.
- Providing further education about depression and its treatment.
- Enhancing treatment adherence.
- Screening for and addressing any side-effects of medication.
- Encouraging regular patterns of activity (e.g., through aerobic exercise) and rest (e.g., through improved sleep hygiene).
- Identifying any unmet needs for specific practical support, counseling (e.g., marital, grief, stress management) or psychotherapy.
- Identifying and addressing any significant co-morbidity.
- Promoting understanding of and adaptation to the psychosocial effects of symptoms and their sequelae.

Maintenance phase treatment and future risk

Despite having recovered from a depressive episode and having sustained that recovery for several months without relapse of symptoms, most patients potentially remain at risk for another depressive episode at some point in their life. This risk is substantially increased by the following recognized factors:

- Number of prior depressive episodes.
- Psychotic features when depressed.
- Residual symptoms or dysthymia.
- Co-morbid medical or psychiatric conditions.
- Significant family history of major depressive disorder.

For patients with increased risk of recurrence or for those with significant lethality issues or functional impairments when depressed, treatment(s) effective in the acute and continuation phases should be maintained beyond the timeframe of the typical continuation phase and possibly indefinitely.

The goal of treatment in the maintenance phase is prevention of recurrence of further depressive episodes. Antidepressant(s) successfully used in prior phases are typically maintained at the same doses, and reassurance should be given to patients that there is no evidence of any specific long-term problems with such a course of action. In the maintenance of the "time limited" psychotherapies, sessions are scheduled less frequently (i.e., monthly as opposed to weekly), although psychodynamic therapies may be maintained at the original frequency to further explore predisposing psychological factors.

As in the continuation phase, assessment visits may be scheduled less frequently, possibly every two to four months for stable patients if appropriate, and the same key components of follow-up as described earlier continue to apply.

Deciding to discontinue active treatment

Whether and when active treatment should be discontinued depends again on the risk factors identified above in the discussion of maintenance treatment. Other relative factors include the overall balance between the patient's perceived benefits of treatment and variable tolerability of any adverse effects. Ideally, the decision to discontinue active treatment should be a collaborative decision between the psychiatrist (and/or psychotherapist) and the patient.

Maintenance antidepressant treatment is best discontinued through a gradual taper over a period of at least several weeks (or even several months in the case of agents with a short half-life). This is not only to avoid the discontinuation symptoms that can be associated with such medications (see 📖 p. 327), but also to allow for the early detection of any depressive symptoms that may warrant return to maintenance level doses.

Maintenance psychotherapy should also be discontinued in a manner appropriate to the specific type of psychotherapeutic modality, while also being sensitive to the individual needs of the patient.

Regardless of treatment type(s), discontinuation of active treatment must incorporate psycho-education about depressive disorders and the risk for further episodes. The specific signs and symptoms that were (in retrospect) "distant early warnings" for the previous depressive episode(s) should be carefully reviewed with the patient, as well as any psychosocial stressors or behavioral habits which may have played a key role in producing depression. Lastly, a reasonable plan to again access help and treatment should be clearly established in the event that symptoms recur. One option in this regard is regularly scheduled check-up visits for several months following the actual termination of active treatment, to allow for periodic reassessment of any symptoms and overall functional status.

Treatment considerations for specific clinical features (1)

Depression with psychotic features

- Increased risk for suicide and recurrence than in nonpsychotic depression.
- ECT should be considered first-line therapy, as evidence supports the superior efficacy of ECT to pharmacotherapy in this patient group, with significant benefit in 80–90% of cases. Issues of consent, however, can preclude the immediate use of ECT, and its role is often that of a second-line treatment after partial response or failure of combination pharmacotherapy.
- Combination treatment of an antidepressant plus an antipsychotic is generally recommended, although this is based on earlier studies which showed efficacy (almost comparable to ECT) of combinations of high-dosed TCA + first generation antipsychotic. Concerns for the side-effects and toxicities of such agents are significant, however, and available evidence for combination treatment with newer, better tolerated, agents (SSRI + atypical antipsychotic) is lacking. Hopefully, studies currently underway can help define a clear strategy for combination pharmacotherapy with these newer agents.
- It can be helpful to start an antipsychotic agent (as for an acute psychotic episode see 📖 Chapter 6) a few days before starting an antidepressant. This can allow a period of assessment (to exclude a primary psychotic disorder), may improve compliance (when psychotic symptoms are seen to improve with medication), avoids potential worsening of psychotic symptoms with an antidepressant (in some predisposed individuals), and may help identify those patients who may respond to an antipsychotic alone.
- Antipsychotic side-effects may mask improvement in depressive symptoms, and combinations of antidepressant + antipsychotic may worsen side-effects common to both (e.g., sedation, anticholinergic effects). *Lowest effective dose* of antipsychotic is advocated (e.g., around 2–4mg haloperidol or equivalent), and careful dose titration is warranted.
- Once acute psychotic symptoms have resolved, a lower dose (and possible discontinuation) of antipsychotic may be indicated, particularly if patients begin to manifest side-effects not seen in the acute phase, with careful monitoring for recurrence of psychotic symptoms.
- When combination treatment has been successful, maintenance involves a clinically effective antidepressant coupled with the lowest effective antipsychotic dose. In view of the severity of the disorder, treatment is often maintained indefinitely, although long-term studies are lacking.

Depression with melancholic features (see 📖 p. 284)

- Because of its putative endogenous etiology, historically thought to respond better to the somatic therapies than to psychotherapy.

- TCAs were long thought to be the agents of choice, although SSRIs have been shown to have comparable efficacy and improved tolerability.
- The widely held perception that this presentation responds poorly to MAOIs is based on a limited number of studies.

Depression with atypical features

- As atypical features (increased sleep and fatigue, increased appetite and weight, marked mood reactivity and sensitivity to emotional rejection) are common in bipolar depression, the clinician should thoroughly screen for bipolar disorder and review possible indicators before treatment.
- Best evidence is for the use of phenelzine or another MAOI (see 📖 *p. 322* for guidance on prescribing/dietary advice). However, SSRIs or bupropion are better tolerated, safer to use, and thought to have comparable efficacy.
- TCAs have traditionally been regarded as less effective. However, some individuals may respond well, and the best evidence is for the use of imipramine.

Depression with catatonic features

- Need to rule out general medical conditions that can present with the symptoms of catatonia (encephalitis, hypercalcemia, hepatic encephalopathy, homocysteinuria, DKA, neoplasms, head trauma, cerebrovascular disease).
- If the patient is taking antipsychotics, consider possibility of acute dystonic reaction or NMS, see 📖 *pp. 1064, 1066.*
- May be life threatening in severity, as it can lead to malnutrition, exhaustion, hyperpyrexia, and significant self-harm or harm to others (through automatisms and excitement). Close and careful supervision is needed.
- Benzodiazepines (typically lorazepam, administered IM or IV if needed) often can provide immediate relief.
- ECT has been shown to be effective even after a few treatments and may be administered daily.
- Upon resolution, consider antidepressant maintenance, possibly combined with an antipsychotic agent or lithium.

Treatment considerations for specific clinical features (2)

Depression with co-morbid anxiety

- Co-morbid anxiety disorders and symptoms are frequently seen with depressive disorders, impairing functioning still further. Fortunately, most first-line antidepressants are also effective at treating anxiety disorders.
- As SSRIs, SNRIs, and TCAs may initially increase anxiety symptoms, low-dose initiation and slow up titration should be considered, if possible.
- With co-morbid OCD symptoms, consider SSRI or clomipramine.
- MAOI can be considered if several trials of first-line agents are ineffective.
- Bupropion has potential anxiogenic side-effects and should generally be avoided.

Depression with seasonal pattern

- In the Northern Hemisphere, typical recurrence of depressive episodes in January/ February (winter depression), remitting in spring. Younger patients at higher risk, with greater prevalence at higher latitudes.
- Symptoms are generally mild to moderate with prominent anergia, low self-esteem, hypersomnia, increased appetite (including carbohydrate craving) and weight gain. It is unclear whether this constitutes a separate subtype of depressive disorder (the controversial "seasonal affective disorder"), or whether it is simply a manifestation of atypical depression.
- Light therapy can be tried for mild to moderate episodes as a primary form of treatment in the outpatient setting (see 💭 p. 338). For more severe episodes, however, it should be used as an adjunct to antidepressant therapy.
- Of the antidepressants, fluoxetine and bupropion (generally considered to be more activating) have been shown to be effective treatments.

Dysthymia and double depression

There are special considerations for dysthymic disorder (💭 p. 286) and double depression (meeting criteria for both dysthymia and MDD, 💭 p. 284):

- Historically, perceived as primarily a psychologically-determined disorder that warranted long-term, insight oriented psychotherapy.
- Recent studies, however, support the efficacy of "time-limited" psychotherapies (such as CBT and IPT) as well as antidepressant therapy, and especially their combination, in treating dysthymia.
- Best evidence exists for the use of phenelzine, but response rates vary (30–70%). Reasonable first-line agents include the SSRIs and bupropion.
- Given available data that only 10–15% of dysthymic patients are in remission one year after initial diagnosis and that ~25% of dysthymic patients never attain a complete recovery, it can be conceived as a kind of treatment-resistant depression warranting long-term maintenance treatment.

Premenstrual dysphoric disorder

- Proposed as a category for further study in DSM-IV-TR, the essential features encompass debilitating depressive mood symptoms (sad or irritable mood, tearful lability, anxious tension, social withdrawal), neurovegetative symptoms (anergy, hyperphagia, sleep dysregulation), and physical symptoms (breast tenderness, bloating, muscle/joint pain).
- Typical pattern with onset during the week prior to menses (last week of the luteal phase) and remission by midmenses (follicular phase).
- Important to rule out the following general medical conditions that can produce dysphoria and fatigue exacerbated during the premenstrual period: anemia, systemic lupus erythematosus, endometriosis, migraine, polycystic ovarian disease, hypoglycemia, Cushing's disease, thyroid disorders, cancers, and other endocrine disorders.
- Onset typically in 30s, and if untreated, symptoms tend to worsen over time, increasing in duration, possibly becoming a major mood disorder.
- Conservative treatment involves lifestyle changes: regular exercise and dietary adjustment (avoid caffeine and simple sugars, smoking cessation).
- Oral contraceptive agents can be recommended through referral to PCP or OB/GYN, with follow-up for any further mood symptoms.
- SSRIs have been shown to be effective treatments, either as maintenance monotherapy or administered in luteal-phase dosing (two-week intervals).

Treatment-resistant depression

Variously defined as the failure to respond to adequate trials of two to four (or more) different antidepressants (plus or minus ECT), one thing is agreed upon: treatment-resistant depression is unfortunately common and associated with significant personal and societal burdens. The consequences of resistant depression include profoundly reduced quality of life, excessive strain on relationships (which may lead to break-up of families), significant personal financial strain and economic impact on annualized health care costs, increased physical co-morbidity, increased risk of suicide, therapeutic alienation (making further interventions difficult due to difficulties forming a therapeutic alliance), and high use of psychiatric services (often without clear benefit).

Management of treatment resistance

- Review diagnostic formulation. Is the diagnosis correct?
- Review prior treatment adequacy. Appropriate doses and durations?
- Check patient understanding and adherence. Serum levels may help.
- Review biopsychosocial case formulation. Are there any maintaining factors (e.g., social, physical, psychological) that are not being addressed? Psychological and social interventions, particularly when psychosocial factors appear paramount, may be important (and often overlooked or undisclosed) aspects of management.
- Rescreen for co-morbid medical or psychiatric disorders including substance abuse issues, sleep patterns, etc.

Treatment options

Continue monotherapy at maximum tolerable dose

This may mean exceeding usual maximum dose (especially in patients with partial response).

Add psychotherapy

Add psychotherapy to treatment plan, if not already incorporated.

Change antidepressant

Trial of different antidepressant (see previous sections), followed (after appropriate washout) by trial of MAOI if no effective response.

Lithium augmentation

Usual dose 600–900mg/day, response generally observed within two to three weeks.

Atypical antipsychotic augmentation

Usually at relatively low daily dose, response generally observed within two to three weeks.

Other augmentative agents

These include the following:
- Liothyronine (T3): Usual dose 5–25 micrograms/day to start (max 75 micrograms), response generally observed within three weeks.
- Pindolol (a beta-blocker with $5HT_{1A}$ autoreceptor effects): Usual dose 5–10mg/day, possible response within one to two weeks.

- Lamotrigine: Usual dose 20–100mg/day, response generally observed within 6 weeks.
- Stimulants (methylphenidate, dextroamphetamine): Usually at half normal doses, response generally observed within one to two weeks.

Combining antidepressants from different classes

Caution is advised, due to possible serious adverse reactions (e.g., serotonin syndrome 📖 *p. 1070*).

ECT

An effective option that should always be considered.

New physical treatments

Such as vagus nerve stimulation, transcranial magnetic stimulation, repetitive transcranial magnetic stimulation have mixed study results and further studies of long-term outcomes are needed.

Antidepressants

Assumed mode of action

All currently available antidepressants appear to exert their antidepressant action by increasing the availability of monoamines (5HT, NA and DA) via one or more of the following:

- Presynaptic inhibition of reuptake of 5HT, NA, or DA.
- Antagonist activity at presynaptic autoreceptor/inhibitory 5HT or NA receptor sites, which enhances neurotransmitter release.
- Inhibition of monoamine oxidase, reducing neurotransmitter breakdown.
- Increasing the availability of neurotransmitter precursors.

Although this net increase occurs almost immediately following administration, initial resolution of depressive symptoms generally takes 10–20 days, implying therapeutic effect involves mechanisms possibly related to receptor regulation over time and changes in intracellular signaling.

Selectivity v. specificity

Although the newer antidepressants are more selective than the TCAs and MAOIs in their pharmacological effects, this should not be confused with them being more specific for any particular type of depressive symptoms. All antidepressants have potential unwanted side-effects. The clinical challenge is finding the balance between efficacy in treating psychiatric symptoms and minimizing iatrogenic problems.

For example, patients may not be able to tolerate therapeutic levels of TCAs due to anticholinergic side-effects. Similarly, GI upset or sexual dysfunction may limit the usefulness of SSRIs in some individuals. Ideally, a practitioner may be able to leverage medication side-effects for therapeutic effect (e.g., histaminergic sedation of citalopram or mirtazapine). Also, clinicians may choose to use combinations of antidepressants to enhance antidepressant effects or even offset side-effects (e.g., trazodone added to an SSRI in a patient with insomnia).

Cautionary notes

Particular caution is necessary in prescribing for certain patient groups such as those with renal or hepatic impairment; cardiac problems; epilepsy; pregnant or breastfeeding women; the elderly; children; and those on other medications that may interact with antidepressants. There are also well-recognized problems such as weight gain (📖 *p. 1048*), hyponatremia (📖 *p. 1076*), sexual dysfunction (📖 *p. 1052*), and withdrawal syndromes (📖 *p. 1074*).

Combining/switching antidepressants

An adequate washout period is required when switching to or from the MAOIs, whereas it is usual to cross-taper between other antidepressants (i.e., gradually reducing the dose of one, while slowly increasing the dose of the other). During this process, or when combining antidepressants, side-effects may be enhanced (due to pharmacokinetic effects) and it is possible to induce the serotonin syndrome (see 📖 *p. 1070*).

Washout times between antidepressant trials with MAOIs

Initial medication	Switching to	Minimum Washout
Antidepressant with long half-life metabolites (e.g., fluoxetine)	MAOI	5 weeks
Antidepressant without long half-life metabolites (e.g., TCAs, SNRIs, paroxetine, fluvoxamine, citalopram, escitalopram, etc.)	MAOI	2 weeks
MAOI	MAOI	2 weeks
MAOI	Non-MAOI	2 weeks

The following pages outline the main groups of antidepressants. This information should be used as a guide and the clinician is always advised to consult manufacturers' data sheets, or more detailed formularies, for less common problems or specific details of administration. Risks, benefits, and alternatives should be routinely discussed and documented. For information regarding depression and youth, please refer to Chapter 16.

2004 FDA BLACK BOX WARNING

In clinical studies, antidepressants increased the risk of suicidal thinking and behavior in children and adolescents with depression and other psychiatric disorders. A combined analysis of studies involving nine antidepressants showed that in people under 18 this risk was 4% for those taking antidepressants compared to 2% for those taking a sugar pill. Anyone considering the use of any antidepressant in a child or adolescent must balance this risk with the clinical need. Patients who are starting therapy should be observed closely. Families and caregivers should discuss with the doctor any observations of worsening depression symptoms, suicidal thinking and behavior, or unusual changes in behavior.

**In 2006, the FDA's Psychopharmacologic Drugs Advisory Committee (PDAC) voted in favor of expanding drug label warnings to include young adults up to age 25. The new data on adults came from a meta-analysis involving 372 drug-company studies and nearly 100,000 patients. The panel also advised the FDA to require that the drug labels carry information regarding the risks (including suicide) associated with not treating depression.

Selective serotonin reuptake inhibitors

Common mode of action and effects/side-effects

- Reuptake inhibition leads to increased neurotransmitter (primarily 5HT) in the synaptic cleft and expression via various receptor types:
  - **$5HT_{1A}$** Antidepressant, anxiolytic, anti-obsessive, antibulimic effects.
  - **$5HT_2$** Agitation, akathisia, anxiety/panic, insomnia, sexual dysfunction.
  - **$5HT_3$** Nausea, GI upset, diarrhea, headache.

Advantages

Ease of dosing; well tolerated when compared to TCAs; less cardiotoxic; fewer anticholinergic side-effects; low toxicity in overdose.

Disadvantages

Can cause nausea, gastrointestinal upset, headache, restlessness, insomnia, sexual dysfunction, and weight gain. Potential for discontinuation syndrome (see 🕮 p. 327).

Contraindications

Manic episode, concomitant use of MAOIs.

Cautions

Variable inhibitory effects on hepatic P450 (particularly CYP2D6) enzymes. Consideration should be made when prescribed with other drugs that undergo extensive liver metabolism. Increased risk of gastrointestinal bleed in the elderly and in those with a history of this condition.

Fluoxetine (Prozac®, Sarafem®)

Half-life
84hrs (active metabolite, norfluoxetine 4–16 days).

Formulations
Tablets 10mg; capsules 10/20/40mg. Also available in elixir (20mg/5mL), weekly capsule (90mg), and single-pill combination with olanzapine (Symbyax 6/25, 12/25, 6/50, 12/50mg).

Starting dose
20mg (consider 5–10mg in the elderly, children, medically compromised, or if significant anxiety).

Dose range
20–80mg (usually qam dosing).

P450 considerations
Inhibits 2D6 (strong), 1A2 (moderate), 2C19 (moderate). Substrate of 2C8/9 (major), 2D6 (major).

Warning
Due to long half-life, wait five weeks after discontinuation of fluoxetine before initiating an MAOI, thioridazine, or mesoridazine.

Pearls

Fluoxetine has the longest half-life, withdrawal syndrome less likely, increased energy or activation early in dosing, occasional weight loss, weekly dosing may enhance compliance.

Paroxetine (Paxil®, Paxil CR®, Pexeva®)

Half-life

21hrs (up to 65hrs with CR).

Formulations

Tablets 10/20/30/40mg (tablets 12.5/25/37.5mg CR). Elixir 10mg/5mL.

Starting dose

20mg or 25mg CR (consider 10mg in the elderly, children, medically compromised, or if significant anxiety).

Dose range

20–60mg or 25–75mg CR (usually qhs dosing).

P450 considerations

Substrate of 2D6 (major). Inhibits 2D6 (strong) and 2B6 (moderate).

Warning

Only SSRI that is Category D in pregnancy due to increased risk for teratogenesis, particularly cardiac malformations.

Pearls

Beware of significant p450 interactions. Anticholinergic properties may contribute to constipation, dry mouth, sedation, and confusion. Weight gain common. Short half-life contributes to withdrawal syndrome. Main advantage of CR is reduction of side-effects (especially nausea).

Sertraline (Zoloft®)

Half-life

26hrs (active metabolite, N-desmethylsertraline 62–104hrs).

Formulations

Tablets 25, 50, 100mg. Elixir 20mg/mL.

Starting dose

50mg (consider 25mg in the elderly, children, medically compromised, or if significant anxiety).

Dose range

50–200mg (usually qam dosing).

P450 considerations

Substrate of 2C19 (major) and 2D6 (major). Inhibits 2B6 (moderate), 2C19 (moderate), 2D6 (moderate), 3A4 (moderate).

Pearls

Moderately alerting. Most dopaminergic activity of all the SSRIs, which may contribute to its therapeutic actions.

Fluvoxamine (Luvox®)

Half-life
15–20hrs.

Formulations
Tablets 25/50/100mg.

Starting dose
50mg (consider 25mg in the elderly, children, medically compromised, or if significant anxiety).

Usual dose range
50–300mg (bid dosing if >150mg).

P450 considerations
Substrate of 1A2 (major) and 2D6 (major). Inhibits 1A2 (strong) and 2C19 (strong).

Warning
Contraindicated concurrent use of pimozide, thioridazine, mesoridazine, or cisapride. Do not use MAOI within 14 days.

Pearls
Moderately sedating. Only SSRI with bid dosing (with doses >150mg). Primary FDA approval for OCD.

Citalopram (Celexa®)

Half-life
24–48hrs.

Formulations
Tablets 10/20/40mg. Elixir 10mg/5mL.

Starting dose
20mg (consider 10mg in the elderly, children, medically compromised, or if significant anxiety).

Dose range
20–60mg (either qam or qhs dosing).
P450 considerations.
Substrate of 2C19 (major) and 3A4 (major).

Pearls
Tends to be slightly sedating/anxiolytic (as a result of histaminergic activity from the R-enantiomer of the molecule).

Escitalopram (Lexapro®)

Half-life
27–32hrs (Active metabolite, S-desmethylcitalopram 59hrs).

Formulations
Tablets 5/10/20mg. Elixir 1mg/mL.

Starting dose
10mg (consider 5mg in the elderly, children, medically compromised, or if significant anxiety).

Dose range
10–20mg (usually qam dosing).

P450 considerations
Substrate of 2C19 and 3A4.

Pearls
Tends to be slightly activating (likely due to the absence of the histaminergic R-enantiomer). Generally well tolerated with few drug-drug interactions.

Tricyclic antidepressants (TCAs)

Common mode of action and effects/side-effects

- Reuptake inhibition leads to increased neurotransmitter (primarily 5HT and NE) in the synaptic cleft and expression via various receptor types:
  - 5HT/NE (and DA).
  - Antidepressant and anxiolytic effects.
  - M1 (cholinergic) antagonism.
  - Dry mouth, blurred vision, constipation, urinary retention, drowsiness, confusion, memory problems, palpitations, tachycardia.
  - NE (noradrenergic) antagonism.
  - Drowsiness, postural hypotension, tachycardia, sexual dysfunction
  - 5HT$_2$ antagonism.
  - Anxiolytic, reduced sexual dysfunction, sedation.
  - H$_1$ (histaminergic) antagonism.
  - Drowsiness, weight gain.

Advantages

Well-established efficacy and evidence base. Usually single daily dose. Generic forms available, which tends to reduce cost.

Disadvantages

Toxicity in overdose; may be less well tolerated than SSRIs; slows cardiac conduction (due to quinidine-like properties); lowers seizure threshold. Potential for postural hypotension and anticholinergic side-effects.

Contraindications

Acute MI, heart block, arrhythmias, ischemic heart disease, severe liver disease, narrow-angle glaucoma, pregnancy, and lactation.

Cautions

Cardiovascular disorders, hepatic/renal dysfunction; endocrine disorders (hyperthyroidism, adrenal tumors, diabetes); urinary retention; prostatic hypertrophy; constipation; glaucoma; seizure disorders; psychotic disorders; patients with suicidal ideation; elderly (use lower doses).

Monitoring

It is good practice to monitor cardiac (BP, pulse, EKG), hepatic/renal function, electrolytes, CBC, and weight during long-term therapy.

Tricyclic antidepressants (TCAs)

Drug	Half life (hrs)	Formulations	Usual starting dose	Usual maintenance dose	Maximum daily dose	Therapeutic blood level (ng/mL)	Notes
Amitriptyline*** (Elavil)	9–27 18–44 (metab)	T 10/25/50/75/ 100/125/150mg Inj 10mg/mL	25–75mg (qhs or bid-tid)	50–150mg	300mg	100–250 (with metab) Toxic >500(utility controversial)	Sedating. Metabolized to nortriptyline. Also useful in nocturnal enuresis, chronic pain, migraines, insomnia
Clomipramine*** (Anafranil)	32 69 (metab)	C 25/50/75mg	25mg/qhs	50–150mg/d (divided or qhs)	250mg		Most SSRI-like. Can be given IV/IM. Approved for OCD
Doxepin*** (Sinequan)	6–8 28–52 (metab)	C 10/25/50/75/ 100/150mg S 10mg/mL	25–75mg qhs	150–300mg (divided if >150mg/d)	300mg	110–250 (with metab) Toxic >500 (utility controversial)	Sedating. Also comes in topical form for pruritis associated with some dermatitis.
Imipramine*** (Tofranil)	4–18	T 10/25/50/50mg C 75/100/125/ 150mg	25–75mg (qhs or bid-tid)	150–300mg (divided or qhs)	300mg	150–250 (with metab) Toxic >500	Metabolized to desipramine; useful for nocturnal enuresis; blood levels relevant; orthostatic hypotension common
Trimipramine*** (Surmontil)	16–40	C 25/50/100mg	25–75mg/qhs	50–150mg/d (divided or qhs)	200mg (outpt) 300mg (inpt)		Sedating.
Amoxapine** (Asendin)	8–16 30 (metab)	T 25/50/100/150mg	50mg/d (divide bid-tid)	200–300mg/d (divided if >300mg/d)	400mg (outpt) 600mg (inpt)	>200 (with metab) (utility controversial)	Metabolite has significant dopamine blocking activity; may cause EPS
Desipramine**	7–60	T 10/25/50/75/100/ 150mg	25–75mg/qhs	100–200mg/d	300mg	50–300	Less anticholinergic; blood levels
Maprotiline** (Ludiomil)	43 60–90 (metab)	T 25/50/75mg	25–75mg/d (divide bid - tid)	75–150mg/d (divide bid-tid)	150mg (outpt) 225mg (inpt)		Sometimes categorized as a tetracyclic. May have increased risk of seizures.
Nortriptyline** (Aventyl, Pamelor)	18–44	C 10/25/50/75mg S 10mg/5mL	25–50mg qhs	75–150mg (qhs or divided)	150mg	50–150 Toxic >500	Blood levels relevant. Fewer anticholinergic side-effects.
Protriptyline** (Vivactil)	54–92	T 5/10mg	5–10mg tid	5–10mg tid-qid	60mg	70–250 (utility controversial)	Potentially activating (useful if anergic). May exacerbate anxiety/agitation.

Key: T = tablets; C = capsules; S = oral suspension/solution; SR = modified release capsules; Inj = injectable form; *** tertiary amines; ** secondary amines

Monoamine oxidase inhibitors (MAOIs)

Common mode of action

- Irreversible inhibition of MAO-A (acts on NA, DA, 5HT, and tyramine) and MAO-B (acts on DA, tyramine, phenylethylamine, benzylamine), leading to accumulation of monoamines in synaptic cleft.

Side-effects

Risk of hypertensive crisis

The exact mechanism unknown, but it is proposed that tyramine causes an excessive release of norepinephrine/catecholemines in the peripheral nervous system. Therefore, foods high in tyramine and certain medications should be avoided.

- Sources of dietary **tyramine** (avoid these): Food that has been aged, fermented, pickled, cured or smoked; cheese (except cottage and cream cheese); beer (especially from tap); wine (especially red); concentrated yeast extract; liver; dried meats (sausage, salami, pepperoni); nonfresh fish (pickled or smoked herring); broad beans (fava beans); yogurt; certain fruits/vegetables (avocado, sauerkraut, banana peels, figs, raisins, over-ripened fruit); fermented soy products (soy sauce, miso).
- **Medications**: Antidepressants (e.g., SSRI/SNRIs, TCAs, mirtazapine, buproprion, St. Johns Wort); analgesics (e.g., tramadol, methadone, propoxyphene, meperidine, cyclobenzaprine); antitussives or decongestants (e.g., dextromethorphan, pseudoephedrine, phenylephrine); diet pills; stimulants (e.g., methylphenidate); or other sympathomimetics (e.g., amphetamines, dopamine, epinephrine, isoproterenol, methyldopa, dextroamphetamine, ephedrine, etc.).

Other side-effects

Anticholinergic side-effects, hepatotoxicity, insomnia, anxiety, appetite suppression, weight gain, postural hypotension, ankle edema, sexual dysfunction, possible dependency.

Indications

Usually used as second-line therapy for treatment-resistant depression (particularly atypical symptoms)/anxiety disorders.

Cautions

Avoid in cardiovascular disease, hepatic failure, poorly controlled hypertension, hyperthyroidism, porphyria, pheochromocytoma.

Advantages

Well-established efficacy in a broad range of affective and anxiety disorders.

Disadvantages

Dietary restrictions and drug interactions.

Other significant drug interactions

Note: variable—always check data sheets.

Antidiabetics, antiepileptics, antihypertensives, antipsychotics, barbiturates, benzodiazepines, beta-blockers, buspirone, cimetidine, dopaminergics, morphine, $5HT_1$ agonists (rizatriptan, sumatriptan).

MAOIs

Drug	Class	Half Life (hrs)	Formulations	Usual starting dose	Usual maintenance dose	Max. daily dose	Notes
Isocarboxazid (Marplan)	MAOI	36	T 10mg	10mg bid	10–40mg/d (divided bid-qid)	60mg	Hydrazine derivative – less stimulating. Effective for co-morbid anxiety.
Phenelizine (Nardil)	MAOI	12	T 15mg	15mg tid	15mg qod-tid	90mg	Hydrazine derivative – less stimulating. Effective for co-morbid anxiety.
Tranylcypromine (Parnate)	MAOI	2.5	T 10mg	10mg bid	10mg tid	60mg	Most stimulating (amphetamine-related), and therefore useful in atypical depression. Do not give after 3 p.m. More rapid onset of therapeutic effect, however, increased risk of severe hypertensive reactions.
Selegiline (Emsam)	MAOI	25	Transdermal 6/9/12mg	6mg/24hr patch	6–9mg/24hr	12mg/24hr	MAOI diet required for >6mg only.

Key: T = tablets, Transdermal = patch. Note: It is estimated that 20mg of tranylcypromine = 40mg of isocarboxazid = 45mg phenelzine.

Other antidepressants

Serotonin/noradrenaline reuptake inhibitors (SNRIs)

Mode of action
- At low doses—acts as a reuptake inhibitor on 5HT (like an SSRI).
- At moderate doses—acts as a reuptake inhibitor on 5HT and NE.
- At high doses— acts as a reuptake inhibitor on 5HT, NE, and DA.

Common adverse effects
Nausea, GI upset, constipation, loss of appetite, dry mouth, dizziness, agitation, insomnia, sexual dysfunction, headache, nervousness, sweating, weakness.

Venlafaxine (Effexor®, Effexor XR®)
Half-life
5hr (11hr for metabolite).

Formulations
25/37.7/50/75/100mg (37.5/75/150mg XR).

Starting dose
37.5mg bid (or 75mg qam for XL formulation).

Dose range
75–375mg divided bid-tid (or 75–225mg XR qam).

P450 considerations
Substrate 2D6 and 3A4.

Warning
Monitor blood pressure (risk increases for diastolic hypertension in doses >200mg/d). Caution in glaucoma secondary to mydriasis. Risk of fatal overdoses may be higher than SSRIs (but lower than TCAs).

Pearls
May be more effective in treatment-resistant depression; potential for significant withdrawal syndrome; once-daily dosing of XL formulation improves compliance; useful when treating co-morbid pain syndromes.

Duloxetine (Cymbalta®)
Half-life
12hr.

Formulations
20/30/60mg.

Starting dose
30mg qam.

Dose range
40–120mg/d either once daily or bid.

P450 considerations
Substrate 2D6 and 1A2; inhibits 2D6 (moderate).

Warning
Potential hepatotoxicity (i.e., cases of severe elevations of liver enzymes or liver injury with a hepatocellular, cholestatic or mixed pattern have been reported). Caution in glaucoma secondary to mydriasis.

Pearls
No evidence that doses greater than 60mg/day confer any additional benefit. Monitor blood pressure for dose-dependent elevations. Useful when treating co-morbid pain syndrome or urinary incontinence.

Serotonin antagonist/reuptake inhibitors (SARIs)
Mode of action
- $5HT_{1A/1C/2A}$ antagonism—more sedating/anxiolytic, less sexual dyfunction.
- 5HT agonism through the active metabolite.
  (*m*chlorophenylpiperazine)—antidepressant effect.
- alpha$_1$ antagonism—orthostatic hypotension.
- H$_1$ antagonism—sedation and weight gain.

Common adverse effects
Priapism (see 🕮 *p. 1054*); sedation; orthostatic hypotension; otherwise similar to TCAs (but less anticholinergic and cardiotoxic).

Trazodone (Desyrel®)
Half-life
5–9hrs.

Formulations
50/100/150/300mg.

Starting dose
50mg qhs-tid.

Dose range
150–300mg/d (qhs-tid); Max dose 600mg (inpatient).

P450 considerations
Substate 3A4; inhibits 2D6 (moderate).

Warning
Warn male patients of risk of priapism (1:6000).

Pearls
Often not tolerated as monotherapy for depression since many patients cannot tolerate sedation. Commonly used in lower doses off label for insomnia.

Noradrenergic and specific serotonergic antidepressant (NaSSA)
Mode of action
- Alpha$_2$ antagonism—increases 5HT and NE release (antidepressant).
- Alpha$_1$ antagonism—orthostatic hypotension.
- M$_1$ antagonism—anticholinergic side-effects.
- $5HT_{2A/C}$ antagonism—more sedating/anxiolytic, less sexual dysfunction.
- 5HT$_3$ antagonism—reduced nausea/GI upset.
- H$_1$ antagonism—sedation and weight gain.

Common adverse effects
Sedation, increased appetite, weight gain. Less common: transaminase elevation, jaundice, edema, orthostatic hypotension, tremor, myoclonus, blood dyscrasias.

Mirtazapine (Remeron®)
Half-life
20–40hr.

Formulations
Tablets (or Sol-Tab) 15/30/45mg.

Starting dose
7.5–15mg qhs.

Dose range
15–45mg qhs.

P450 considerations
Substrate 1A2, 2D6, 3A4.

Warning
Rare agranulocytosis. If a patient develops a sore throat, fever, stomatitis or signs of infection accompanied by neutropenia, Remeron should be discontinued and the patient should be closely monitored.

Pearls
Weight gain, sedation may be greater at lower doses. Low toxicity in overdose, less sexual dysfunction and GI upset. Useful for patients with co-morbid insomnia, weight loss, or agitation. Sometimes used as an adjunct to improve SSRI-related side-effects (e.g., sexual dysfunction, insomnia, GI upset).

Noradrenergic and dopaminergic reuptake inhibitor (NDRI)
Mode of Action
• NE/DA reuptake inhibition—antidepressant effects.

Common adverse effects
Agitation/insomnia, dry mouth, GI upset (nausea, vomiting, abdominal pain, constipation), hypertension (esp. if concomitant use of nicotine patches), risk of seizures (0.4%), disturbance of taste.

Buproprion (Wellbutrin®, Wellbutrin SR®, Wellbutrin XL®, Zyban®)
Half-life
10–14hr (20–27hr metabolite).

Formulations
75/100mg; SR 100/150/200mg; XL 150/300mg.

Starting dose
Wellbutrin SR 100mg bid (or XL 150mg qam).

Dose range
150–450mg/d.

P450 considerations
Substrate 2B6.

Warning
Increased risk of seizures in Immediate-Release Wellbutrin at a total daily dosage >450mg, individual doses >150mg, or by sudden large increments in dose. Seizure incidence is 0.4% at 300–450mg (tenfold increased risk at 450–600mg). Wellbutrin SR and XL formulations may have equal only slightly higher seizure risk when compared to other antidepressants. Risk of seizures is increased in patients with epilepsy, eating disorders, CNS tumor, head trauma, severe hepatic cirrhosis, abrupt discontinuation of alcohol/benzodiazepines, use with medications which lower seizure threshold, stimulants, or hypoglycemics.

Pearls
May be activating (useful in patients with psychomotor retardation or hypersomnia); may be useful in impulse disorders and addiction cravings; treatment of nicotine dependence (and possibly withdrawal from other stimulants); may be useful in ADHD; sexual dysfunction is lower than SSRIs; may worsen psychosis in some patients.

<u>FINISH</u> Mnemonic for recognition of antidepressant discontinuation syndrome

Flu-like symptoms
  fatigue, lethargy, malaise, muscle aches, headaches, diarrhea
Insomnia
Nausea
Imbalance
  gait instability, dizziness/lightheadedness, vertigo
Sensory disturbances
  paresthesia, "electric shock" sensations, visual disturbance
Hyperarousal
  anxiety/agitation

Berber, M.J. (1998). FINISH: remembering the discontinuation syndrome. Flu-like symptoms, Insomnia, Nausea, Imbalance, Sensory disturbances, and Hyperarousal (anxiety/agitation). *J Clin Psychiatry* **59**, 255.

ECT (1)—background and indications

Electroconvulsive therapy (ECT)

ECT is a highly effective treatment for depression (particularly with psychotic or catatonic features), which may act more rapidly than antidepressant medication. Advances in brief anesthesia and neuromuscular paralysis have led to improved safety and tolerability. Decline in the use of ECT reflects the influence of nonevidence based factors on the choice of treatment modalities rather than being an indicator of its efficacy. A classic systematic review of 153 studies (~6000 patients)[1] found the treatment response of ECT to be superior to other modes of treatment: ECT (72%), TCAs (65%), MAOIs (50%), placebo (23%).

Mode of action

Specific mode of action is unknown. ECT does cause a wide range of effects on neurotransmitters with net functional increases in monoamine systems (NA, 5HT, DA), GABA, ACh, endogenous opioids (increase/altered binding of met-enkephalin and beta-endorphin), and adenosine (A1 purinoceptors). Also profound effects on the neuroendocrine system, with release of hypothalamic, pituitary, and adrenal hormones.

Indications

- Depressive episode: severe episodes, need for rapid definitive antidepressant response (e.g., due to failure to eat or drink in depressive stupor; high suicide risk), failure of drug treatments, patient inability to tolerate side-effects of drug treatment (e.g., during pregnancy), previous history of poor response to pharmacotherapy or good response to ECT, patient preference.
- Other indications: mania, including mixed episodes (50–60% effective), schizophrenia and schizoaffective disorder, catatonia, neuroleptic malignant syndrome, neurological crises (e.g., extreme Parkinsonian symptoms: on-off phenomena), intractable seizure disorders (as ECT acts to raise seizure threshold).

Contraindications

There are no absolute contraindications. Certain medical conditions, however, may increase the risk of serious complications by variously compromising the functional status of organ systems transiently affected by ECT. These conditions include: recent MI, cardiac arrythmias, other unstable cardiac conditions, severe pulmonary disease, recent cerebral infarction (especially hemorrhagic), any illness that already increases intracranial pressure, acute/impending retinal detachment, any unstable vascular aneurysm or malformation, pheochromocytoma, osteoporosis, recent fractures, and temporomandibular joint problems.

---

1 Wechsler, H., Grosser, G.H., Greenblatt, M. (1965). Research evaluating antidepressant medications on hospitalized mental patients: a survey of published reports during a five-year period. *Journal of Nervous and Mental Disease* **141**, 231–239.

ECT—an historical perspective

The use of convulsive treatments for psychiatric disorders has at its origin the clinical observation of apparent antagonism between schizophrenia (then dementia praecox) and epilepsy. It appeared that patients who had a seizure were relieved of their psychotic symptoms and Meduna noted increased glial cells in the brains of patients with epilepsy compared to reduced number in those with schizophrenia. In 1934 he induced a seizure with an injection of camphor-in-oil in a patient with catatonic schizophrenia, and continued this treatment every 3 days. After the fifth seizure the patient was able to talk spontaneously and began to eat and care for himself for the first time in 4 years, making a full recovery with 3 further treatments. Chemically induced convulsive treatments using camphor or metrazol (pentylenetetrazol) became accepted for the treatment of schizophrenia, but were not without problems. Cerletti and Bini introduced the use of "electric shock" to induce seizures in 1938, and soon this method became the standard. Initially ECT was unmodified (i.e., without anesthetic or muscle relaxant), but because of frequent injury, and advances in brief anesthesia, the current procedure is the more humane modified ECT. Indications have also changed, with the majority of patients receiving ECT due to severe depressive illness, although it is also effective in other conditions (see opposite).

ECT (2)—problems and treatment course

Limitations
Time-limited action (tends to dissipate after a couple of weeks, hence need for follow-up medication, or maintenance treatment), issues of consent to treatment (see Chapters 17 and 18).

Side-effects
- Early: Some transient loss of short-term memory/retrograde amnesia usually resolves completely (64%), headache (48%, if recurrent, use simple analgesics), temporary confusion (27%), nausea/vomiting (9%), clumsiness (5%), muscular aches.
- Late: Loss of long-term memory (rare, see opposite).
- Mortality: No greater than for general anesthesia in minor surgery (1:10,000) and is usually due to cardiac complications in patients with known cardiac disease (hence need for close monitoring).

ECT as acute phase treatment
- Rarely will a single treatment be effective to relieve the underlying disorder (but this does occasionally occur).
- ECT is usually given three times a week, reduced to twice a week or once a week once symptoms begin to respond. This limits cognitive problems, and there is no evidence that treatments of greater frequency enhance treatment response.
- Treatment of depression usually consists of 6–12 treatments.
- Treatment-resistant psychosis and mania may require up to 20 (or more) treatments.
- Catatonia usually resolves in 3–5 treatments.

Continuation and maintenance ECT
- Although evidence is limited, many psychiatrists recommend maintenance ECT (e.g., once a week, or every 2 weeks, for 4 months or more) when a patient has responded well to ECT, and when drug treatments have been ineffective prior to ECT.
- Usually patients are aware of how effective ECT has been for them and a collaborative approach can be established (balancing frequency of ECT against return of symptoms and side-effects, especially memory problems).

Does ECT cause brain damage?

ECT is not the devastating purveyor of wholesale brain damage that some of its detractors claim. For the typical individual receiving ECT, no detectable correlates of irreversible brain damage appear to occur. Still, there remains the possibility that either subtle, objectively undetectable persistent defects, particularly in the area of autobiographical memory function, occur, or that a rarely occurring syndrome of more pervasive persistent deficits related to ECT use may be present.

From Devanand, D.P., Dwork, A.J., Hutchinson, E.R., *et al.* (1994). Does ECT alter brain structure? *AJP* **151**, 957–970.

ECT (3)—pretreatment evaluation

Psychiatric component

Establish relative indications for ECT

Through careful diagnosis on basis of thorough review of systems and history of present illness, current symptoms and clinical features, assessment of current functional impairment and/or lethality risk, review of previous pharmacological treatments (number, types, adequacy of trials, degrees of response), any past treatment course of ECT (technique, frequency, number, tolerance, efficacy).

Assessment of target symptoms

Often through established symptom severity rating scales (e.g., Hamilton Rating Scale for Depression [HAM-D]) to track response during the treatment course and help determine when to conclude acute phase treatment.

Baseline cognitive evaluation

Of the faculties most likely to be affected by ECT (typically through scoring MMSE before and throughout ECT course).

Review of psychiatric medications

And recommended adjustments to this regimen in light of possible effects upon and safety during ECT (see 📖 p. 336).

Medical component

Focused medical history

To screen for any known medical conditions (or current physical symptoms suggestive of conditions) that may put the patient at potential increased risk of adverse outcome. As in prescreening for outpatient surgical procedures, this largely is focused on cardiac, pulmonary, and neurologic conditions and symptoms, but also includes inquiry into skeletal integrity, retinal conditions, and TMJ/jaw/dental conditions.

Focused surgical/anesthetic history

To assess patient's capacity to safely tolerate anesthesia, any past complications. Personal and family history of malignant hyperthermia also reviewed.

Complete physical examination

That also includes brief dental examination for loose, damaged, or missing teeth, presence of bridges or dentures.

Standard initial studies

Include CBC with differential, electrolytes, EKG.

Additional studies

If warranted include the following:
- Serum pregnancy test, TFTs, complete metabolic panel, lipid panel.
- Spinal films depending on patient's age or skeletal history.
- Chest films in patients with known or suspected pulmonary disease.
- Brain imaging if suggested by neurological exam or history.
- Cardiac tress testing (exercise treadmill, persantine thallium, etc.).

Consultation with cardiology service
To evaluate and manage known cardiovascular disease before and during course of ECT.

Informed consent

Discussion of the procedure
Including general description, expected benefits, potential risks (including cognitive and other adverse effects, including death), alternative treatment options (including no treatment), specific individual indications and rationale for suggesting ECT.

Written informed consent is standard
It should be clear to patient that he or she can withdraw consent at any time prior to or during acute treatment. Separate written informed consent required for maintenance ECT.

When capacity to consent is in question
Independent consultation is helpful. Involuntary treatment (with surrogate consent and due legal/judicial review) may need to be pursued in some cases.

ECT (4)—notes on treatment

ECT Electrode placement

Bilateral or bitemporal placement

Electrodes
positioned on the
same point on both sides

4cm

Midpoint

Unilateral placement

Nondominant
hemisphere

Notes: The choice of bilateral or unilateral electrode placement remains controversial, although the balance of the evidence points to bilateral electrode placement being preferable in terms of speed of action and effectiveness. There is no doubt that unilateral ECT is associated with substantially less memory impairment, however modern brief pulse, low energy stimuli have reduced the memory impairment commonly associated with the old sine wave stimulation. There may well be regional differences in ECT policy, but the usual reasons for using unilateral/bilateral electrode placement are summarized below:

Electrode placement	Bilateral	Unilateral (nondominant hemisphere)
When to use:	Speed of response a priority.	Speed of response less important.
	Failure of unilateral ECT.	Previous good response to unilateral ECT.
	Previous good response to bilateral ECT without significant memory problems.	Where minimizing memory impairment is critical (e.g., evidence of cognitive impairment, outpatient treatment).
	Where determination of cerebral dominance is difficult.	

Energy dosing

Because the higher the stimulus used, the greater the likelihood of transient cognitive disturbance, and because once the current is above seizure threshold, further increases only contribute to post-ECT confusion, there are a number of dosing strategies used. Local policy and the type of ECT machine used will dictate which method is preferred. For example:

- Dose titration–This is the most accurate method, delivering the minimum stimulus necessary to produce an adequate seizure, and is therefore to be preferred. Treatment begins with a low stimulus, with the dose increased gradually until an adequate seizure is induced. Once the approximate seizure threshold is known, the next treatment dose is increased to abut 50–100% (for bilateral) or 100–200% (for unilateral) above the threshold. The dose is only increased further if later treatments are sub-therapeutic.
- Age dosing—Selection of a predetermined dose calculated on the basis of the patient's age (and the ECT machine used). The main advantage is that this is a less complex regime. However, there is the possibility of overdosing (i.e., inducing excessive cognitive side-effects) because seizure threshold is not determined.

As ECT itself raises the seizure threshold, the dose is likely to rise by an average of 80% over the length of a treatment course. Higher (or lower) doses will also be needed when the patient is taking drugs that raise (or lower) the seizure threshold (see 📖 p. 336).

Effective treatment

It was once thought that any seizure length was therapeutic; however, this is no longer considered to be the case and specific measurement of duration in monitored and recorded.

EEG monitoring

This is the gold standard with a typical ictal EEG having four phases: build-up of energies; "spike and wave" activity (mixed high voltage spike activity with high voltage 3–6Hz slow waves); trains of lower voltage slow waves; and an abrupt end to activity followed by electrical "silence." This will usually last 35–130s, with motor seizure ~720% shorter in duration.

Timing of convulsion

Where EEG monitoring is not used, the less reliable measure of length of observable motor seizure is used, with an effective treatment defined as a motor seizure lasting at least 20 seconds (from end of ECT dose to end of observable motor activity).

Cuff technique

Often underused technique involving isolation of a forearm or leg from the effects of muscle relaxant, by inflation of a blood pressure cuff to above systolic pressure. As the isolated limb does not become paralyzed, the seizure can be more easily observed.

When a subtherapeutic treatment is judged to have occurred, the treatment is repeated at different energy settings (see Energy dosing above).

Psychiatric drugs and ECT

Note: Ensure anesthetist is fully informed of all medication the patient is currently taking.

Drugs that raise seizure threshold
- **Benzodiazepines/barbiturates**
  Best avoided during ECT, or reduced to the lowest dose possible.
- **Anticonvulsants**
  Continue during ECT, but higher ECT stimulus will usually be needed.
  Drugs that lower seizure threshold.
- **Antipsychotics**
  Continue if clinically indicated.
  Increased risk of hypotension and post-ECT confusion.
  Clozapine should be suspended 24hrs before ECT.
- **Antidepressants**
  TCAs, SSRIs, MAOIs—continue if clinically indicated.
  Increased risk of hypotension and post-ECT confusion (especially TCAs).
  Moclobemide should be suspended 24hrs before ECT.
- **Lithium**
  Best avoided as may increase cognitive side-effects and increase likelihood of neurotoxic effects of lithium.

Other physical treatments

Light therapy (phototherapy)

First introduced in 1984 for the treatment of "seasonal affective disorder" (SAD) by Rosenthal,[1] on the basis that bright light therapy might ameliorate symptoms of winter depression, due to effects on circadian and seasonal rhythms mediated by melatonin. Recent research has suggested that the effects of phototherapy may be independent of melatonin and produce a "phase advance" in circadian rhythms (hence treatment may be best given first thing in the morning). It is usually administered by use of a light box (alternatives include light visors), Optimal intensity of light appears to be 10,000 lux. Ideal treatment duration is for 30 minutes (at 10,000 lux) a day. Although treatment response is generally noticeable within five days, ideal length of treatment course is still under investigation. For patients with seasonal depressive symptoms, maintenance therapy is recommended throughout the winter months with possible discontinuation in the spring. Patients receiving light therapy should be sure to avoid exposure to bright light during nighttime.

Adverse effects

Headache and visual problems (e.g., eye strain, blurred vision), particularly at 10,000 lux, can occur but usually resolve during first week; if persistent, reduce duration or intensity of exposure. Rarely, increased irritability, induction of hypomania or mania, increased thoughts of suicide (possibly due to alerting effect and increased energy).

Indications

Major depressive disorder with seasonal pattern (see 📖 p. 310), circadian rhythm disorders (see 📖 p. 490), possibly other depressive disorders.

Contraindications

Marked agitation, insomnia, history of hypomania/mania.

Vagus nerve stimulation (VNS) therapy

Approved by the FDA for severe, recurrent unipolar and bipolar depression in July 2005. Left cervical vagus nerve stimulation is accomplished through leads attached to a pulse generator implanted in the left chest area. The electrical impulses generated are mild (usually 0.5 ms pulse-width, at 20–30Hz, with 30s stimulation periods alternating with 5min breaks) and automatic. Response rates of 40–46% have been shown for treatment-resistant depressive disorder after 10 weeks to 9 months, with a remission rate of 29% at one year, suggesting that the effectiveness of VNS may have a slow trajectory.[2] VNS may be combined with essentially all existing treatments for depressive disorders. It has been safely used with antidepressants (including MAOIs) and can be temporarily shut off to allow for ECT and restarted immediately post-ECT.

1 Rosenthal, N.E., Sack, D.A., Gillin, J.C., et al. (1984). Seasonal affective disorder. A description of the syndrome and preliminary findings with light therapy. *Archives of General Psychiatry* **41**, 72–80.
2 George, M.S., et al. (2000). Vagus nerve stimulation: a new tool for brain research and therapy. *Biol Psychiatry* **47**, 287–295. Marangell, L.B., et al. (2002). Vagus nerve stimulation (VNS) for major depressive episodes: one year outcomes. *Biol Psychiatry* **51**, 280–287.

Adverse effects

Surgical complications (wound infection, transient left vocal cord paresis), asystole (rare; 1:1000 implants during initial lead testing). Side-effects related to stimulation may include voice alteration (e.g., mild hoarseness is common), pain, cough, and dysphagia. Rare hypomanic or manic symptoms, usually responsive to temporary reduction in VNS intensity.

Indications

As long-term adjunctive treatment for treatment-resistant unipolar and bipolar depression (as defined by at least four treatment failures over the lifetime course of depressive illness). Also for pharmacoresistant epilepsy.

Contraindications

Not approved for psychotic depression or schizoaffective disorder. (Paranoid ideation militates against the implantation of a device).

Relative contraindications

Unstable Axis II disorders, given need for adherence to a surgical intervention with a slow trajectory of response.

Postimplant precautions

MRI of spine or joints prohibited given nature of implant; MRI of brain may be possible with special send-receive coils. In the event of prolonged nonresponse, the device can be turned off and left in place. Should the patient elect, the pulse generator can be explanted; however, the stimulus electrode is left in place, as attempted removal risks injury to the left vagus nerve. Consequently, MRI precautions remain indefinitely.

Repetitive transcranial magnetic stimulation (rTMS)

Continues to be researched and is under review by the FDA. However, the difference in stimulation parameters used across reported studies make comparisons difficult.[3] The rationale for treatment is either to increase activity in the left dorsolateral prefrontal cortex (using high-frequency stimulation, e.g., 20Hz) or to reduce activity in the right dorsolateral prefrontal cortex (using low-frequency stimulation, e.g., 1Hz). Initial results in treatment-resistant depression ought to be viewed with caution, although this mode of therapy presents an attractive alternative to ECT, without the accompanying risks and adverse effects.

Adverse effects

Minimal, but patients often report headache. Risk of motor convulsions. Inconvenience of daily therapy for four to six weeks.

Indications

Experimental treatment for treatment-resistant depression; possible use in treatment of treatment-resistant auditory hallucinations and the negative symptoms of schizophrenia.

Contraindications

Epilepsy.

3 Holtzheimer, P.E., III, Russo J., Avery, D.H. (2002). A meta-analysis of repetitive transcranial magnetic stimulation of the treatment of depression. *Psychopharmacology Bulletin* **35**, 149–169.

Recommended further reading

1 Cain, R.A. (2007). Navigating the Sequenced Treatment Alternatives to Relieve Depression (STAR*D) study: practical outcomes and implications for depression treatment in primary care, *Prim Care* **34**(3): 505–19, iv.
2 Kennedy, S.H., Giacobbe, P. (2007). Treatment resistant depression—advances in somatic therapies, *Ann Clin Psychiatry* **19**(4): 279–87.

Bipolar disorders

Introduction

Bipolar affective disorder (once commonly known as manic depression or manic depressive illness) is one of the most common, severe, and persistent psychiatric illnesses. In the public mind, it is associated with notions of "creative madness," and indeed it has affected many creative people—both past and present. Appealing as such notions are, most people who battle with the effects of the disorder would rather live a "normal" life, free from the unpredictability of mood swings.

Dr. Jekyll and Mr. Hyde-like in its presentation, the symptoms vary considerably from one person to the next, but are relatively consistent from one manic or depressive episode to the next within the same patient. The variety of presentations makes bipolar disorder one of the most difficult conditions to diagnose. More than in any other psychiatric disorder, the clinician needs to pay attention to the patient's life history, including functional status during periods of well-being. Moreover, because of a patient's tendency to confuse more functional, high-energy periods of hypomania with one's best self, clinicians need to obtain third-party information from family and friends whenever possible.

In the classical "couple" presentation, relatively longer periods of depression alternate with shorter-lived periods of mania. The symptoms of mania characteristically include excessively elevated and/or irritable mood, a decreased need for sleep, pressured speech, increased libido, reckless behavior without regard for consequences, and grandiosity (see Mania/manic episode 📖 p. 347). More severe manic episodes are typically characterized by thought disturbances and psychotic symptoms. On the basis of a single episode, it may be difficult to distinguish a manic episode with psychotic symptoms from schizoaffective disorder (📖 p. 256). The vast majority of people who experience mania also suffer from recurrent episodes of depression. Between these highs and lows, patients usually experience periods of full remission, which at times may extend for years or even decades.

The diagnosis of bipolar I disorder is used when an individual has experienced at least one clear-cut manic episode. The classic presentation of bipolar I disorder appears, however, to be but one pole of a broader spectrum of mood disorders (see Bipolar spectrum disorder 📖 p. 358). Some individuals experience only milder—hypomanic—episodes (see Hypomania/hypomanic episode 📖 p. 350). The diagnosis bipolar II disorder is used when there is a history of hypomania and major depressive episodes; the diagnosis of cyclothymia (see Cyclothymic disorder 📖 p. 356) is used when there are oscillations between hypomania and briefer, subclinical depressive episodes.

Full assessment should take account of issues including the number of previous episodes, the average length of episodes, the average time between episodes, the level of psychosocial and vocational functioning between episodes, previous responses to treatment (especially treatment of early depressive episodes), family history of psychiatric problems, and current (and past) use of alcohol and drugs.

Although at the present time there is no cure for bipolar disorder, for most cases effective treatment is possible and can substantially decrease the associated morbidity and mortality, both from suicide and other causes such as heart disease. Over time, a significant minority of people with bipolar disorder develop severe and persistent functional impairments and warrant specific rehabilitative services. In general, however, the specific aims of treatment are to treat acute episodes as vigorously as needed to achieve remission and then to institute a preventive therapy plan to decrease the frequency, severity, and psychosocial consequences of mood episodes and to improve psychosocial functioning between such episodes.

Famous people who have publicly stated they have bipolar disorder

Buzz Aldrin, astronaut; **Tim Burton**, artist, movie director; **Francis Ford Coppola**, director; **Patricia Cornwell**, writer; **Ray Davies**, musician; **Robert Downey, Jr.,** actor; **Carrie Fisher**, writer, actor; **Larry Flynt**, magazine publisher; **Connie Francis**, actor, musician; **Stephen Fry**, actor, author, comedian; **Stuart Goddard (Adam Ant)**, musician; **Linda Hamilton**, actor; **Kay Redfield Jamison**, psychologist, writer; **Ilie Nastase**, athlete (tennis), politician; **Axl Rose**, musician; **Ben Stiller**, actor, comedian; **Gordon Sumner** (Sting), musician, composer; **Jean-Claude Van Damme**, athlete (martial arts), actor; **Tom Waits**, musician, composer; **Brian Wilson**, musician, composer, arranger.

Famous people (deceased) who had a confirmed diagnosis of bipolar disorder

Louis Althusser, 1918–1990, philosopher, writer; **Clifford Beers**, 1876–1943, humanitarian; **Neal Cassady**, 1926–1968, writer; **Graham Greene**, 1904–1991, writer; **Frances Lear**, 1923–1996, writer, editor, women's rights activist; **Vivien Leigh**, 1913–1967, actor; **Robert Lowell**, 1917–1977, poet; **Burgess Meredith**, 1908–1997, actor, director; **Spike Milligan**, 1919–2002, comic actor, writer; **Theodore Roethke**, 1908–1963, writer; **Don Simpson**, 1944–1996, movie producer; **David Strickland**, 1970–1999, actor; **Joseph Vasquez**, 1963–1996, writer, movie director; **Mary Jane Ward**, 1905–1981, writer; **Virginia Woolf**, 1882–1941, writer.

Other famous people who are thought to have had bipolar disorder

William Blake, Napoleon Bonaparte, Agatha Christie, Winston Churchill, T.S. Eliot, F. Scott Fitzgerald, Cary Grant, Victor Hugo, Robert E. Lee, Abraham Lincoln, Samuel Johnson, Marilyn Monroe, Wolfgang Amadeus Mozart, Isaac Newton, Plato (according to Aristotle), Edgar Allen Poe, St. Francis, St. John, St. Theresa, Rod Steiger, Robert Louis Stevenson, Mark Twain, Alfred, Lord Tennyson, Vincent van Gogh, Walt Whitman, Tennessee Williams.

Historical perspective

The condition now referred to as bipolar affective disorder has been described since ancient times. Hippocrates described such people as "amic" and "melancholic." Proposed connections between melancholia and mania are described in the writings of Aretaius of Cappadocia (c.150 B.C.) and Paul of Aegina (625–690). Theories of psychopathology at that time were based in the "humors," with melancholia caused by excess of "black bile" and mania by excess of "yellow bile."

18th–19th century

Despite the view of some clinicians in the 18th century that melancholia and mania were interconnected (e.g., Robert James, 1705–1776), it was not until the middle of the 19th century before this connection was more widely accepted. In 1854 Jules Baillarger (1809–1890) published a paper in the *Bulletin of the Imperial Academy of Medicine* describing "la folie à double forme," closely followed two weeks later by a paper in the same journal by Jean-Pierre Falret (1794–1870), who claimed that he had been teaching students at the Salpetrière about "la folie circulaire" for 10 years. Although the two men were to continue arguing about who originated the idea, they at least agreed that the illness was characterized by alternating periods of melancholia and mania, often separated by periods of normal mood. In 1899, Emil Kraepelin comprehensively described "manic-depressive insanity" in the sixth edition of his textbook *Psychiatrie: Ein Lehrbuch für Studirende und Ärzte*. In the fifth edition he had already divided severe mental illnesses into those with a "deteriorating" course (e.g., schizophrenia and related psychoses) and those with a "periodic" course (e.g., the mood disorders). It was his view that the mood disorders "represented manifestations of a single morbid process."

20th century

At the turn of the 20th century, hopes were high that understanding of the pathophysiology of mental illness might be within reach. In 1906, the German microbiologist August Wassermann discovered a method of detecting syphilitic infection in the CNS, and in the same year an effective treatment was developed by Paul Ehrlich using arsenic compounds. Syphilis was, at that time, one of the most common causes of severe (often mania-like) psychiatric symptoms ("general paralysis of the insane"). Reliably diagnosing and treating such a condition was a huge step forward. In cases of manic-depressive illness, however, neuropathologists failed to find any structural brain abnormalities. Although some still maintained it was a physical illness, caused by disruptions in biological functioning, the pervasive "new" psychodynamic theories regarded functional illnesses (e.g., schizophrenia and manic-depressive illness) as illnesses of the mind, not the brain. The idea that they could be understood and treated only if the traumatic childhood events, repressed sexual feelings, or interpersonal conflicts were uncovered, influenced psychiatric thinking for over half a century.

Drug treatments for bipolar disorder

It was not until specific drug treatments for these "functional illnesses" were found that psychiatry came full circle again, and new life was breathed into the old search for biological mechanisms. In 1949 John Cade published a report on the use of lithium salts in manic patients (curiously, based on an incorrect animal model), but it took nearly three decades, and the work of many psychiatrists, including Mogens Schou in Denmark and Ronald Fieve in the United States, before lithium would become the mainstay of treatment for manic-depressive illness. Indeed, the FDA's approval of lithium salts in 1970 led to a dramatic increase in the diagnosis of bipolar disorder in the United States. Equally significant was the observation by Ronald Kuhn that when patients with "manic-depressive psychosis" were treated with imipramine they could switch from depression to mania. That this did not occur in most patients with depression suggested that there was a different biological mechanism underlying depressive illness compared to manic-depressive illness. With different pharmacological agents treating different psychiatric disorders, the stage was set for classifying psychiatric disorders in line with their presumed differing etiologies. The quest had begun to understand the biological mechanisms and, in doing so, to develop better treatments.

Bipolar disorders in the DSM-IV-TR

DSM-IV-TR provides a categorical classification of the bipolar affective disorders by dividing them into types based on criteria sets with defining features. Basic to this classification scheme are the concepts of the manic episode (see p. 347), the hypomanic episode (see p. 350), the mixed episode (see p. 348), and the major depressive episode (see p. 282), each uniquely defined by a specified criteria set of symptoms. Although all bipolar affective disorders are defined by the occurrence of at least some manic or hypomanic symptoms, they are divided into the following types by the number, duration, and etiology (if known) of the manic, hypomanic, mixed, and/or depressive symptoms present.

Bipolar I disorder

Occurrence of at least one manic or mixed episode, although may also have hypomanic or major depressive episodes.

Bipolar II disorder

Occurrence of one or more major depressive episodes and at least one hypomanic episode.

Cyclothymia (p. 356)

Occurrence of numerous periods of hypomanic symptoms and numerous periods of depressive symptoms, but no manic or major depressive episodes.

Substance-induced mood disorder with manic or mixed features

Prominent manic or mixed symptoms arising during or within one month of substance intoxication or withdrawal or otherwise etiologically related to medication use.

Mood disorder due to a general medical condition with manic or mixed features

Prominent manic or mixed symptoms arising as a direct physiological consequence of a medical condition as evident from labwork, physical exam, or history.

Bipolar disorder not otherwise specified

Prominent bipolar symptoms that do not clearly meet the criteria for any of the aforementioned bipolar disorders or that have an indeterminable etiology. DSM-IV-TR also includes very rapid mood cycling (not meeting minimal episode duration criteria) and manic or mixed episodes superimposed on primary psychotic disorders within this category.

Mania/manic episode

DSM-IV-TR lists the specific diagnostic criteria set for a manic episode and includes additional criteria/descriptors to allow the clinician to further qualify the current or most recent episode (📖 see p. 351).

DSM-IV-TR criteria for manic episode

- A distinct period of abnormally and persistently elevated, expansive, or irritable mood, lasting at least one week (or any duration if hospitalization is necessary).
- During the period of mood disturbance, three (or more) of the following symptoms have persisted (four if the mood is only irritable) and have been present to a significant degree:
  - Inflated self-esteem or grandiosity.
  - Decreased need for sleep (e.g., feels rested after only three hours of sleep).
  - More talkative than usual or pressure to keep talking.
  - Flight of ideas or subjective experience that thoughts are racing.
  - Distractibility (e.g., attention too easily drawn to unimportant or irrelevant external stimuli).
  - Increase in goal-directed activity (either socially, at work or school, or sexually) or psychomotor agitation.
  - Excessive involvement in pleasurable activities that have a high potential for painful consequences (e.g., engaging in unrestrained buying sprees, sexual indiscretions, or foolish business investments).
- The symptoms do not meet criteria for a mixed episode.
- The mood disturbance is sufficiently severe to cause marked impairment in occupational functioning or in usual social activities or relationships with others, or to necessitate hospitalization to prevent harm to self or others, or there are psychotic features.
- The symptoms are not due to the direct physiological effects of a substance (e.g., a drug of abuse, a medication, or other treatment) or a general medical condition (e.g., hyperthyroidism).

Note: Manic-like episodes that are clearly caused by somatic antidepressant treatment (e.g., medication, electroconvulsive therapy, light therapy) should not count toward a diagnosis of bipolar I disorder.

Psychotic symptoms

In its more severe form, mania may be associated with psychotic symptoms (usually mood-congruent, but may also be incongruent):

- Grandiose ideas may be delusional, related to identity or role (with "special powers" or religious content).
- Suspiciousness may develop into well-formed persecutory delusions.
- Pressured speech may become so great that clear associations are lost and speech becomes incomprehensible.
- Irritability and aggression may lead to violent behavior.
- Preoccupation with thoughts and schemes may lead to self-neglect, to the point of not eating or drinking, and inability to maintain adequate living condtions.
- Catatonic behavior—also termed "manic stupor."
- Total loss of insight.

Mixed episode

DSM-IV-TR characterizes a mixed episode as the co-occurrence of the specific criteria sets for a manic episode and a major depressive episode (see 📖 p. 282). Also included are additional criteria/descriptors to allow the clinician to further qualify the current or most recent episode (see 📖 p. 351).

DSM-IV-TR criteria for mixed episode

- The criteria are met both for a manic episode and for a major depressive episode (except for duration) nearly every day during at least a one-week period.
- The mood disturbance is sufficiently severe to cause marked impairment in occupational functioning or in usual social activities or relationships with others, or to necessitate hospitalization to prevent harm to self or others, or there are psychotic features.
- The symptoms are not due to the direct physiological effects of a substance (e.g., a drug of abuse, a medication, or other treatment) or a general medical condition (e.g., hyperthyroidism).

Note: Mixed-like episodes that are clearly caused by somatic antidepressant treatment (e.g., medication, electroconvulsive therapy, light therapy) should not count toward a diagnosis of bipolar I disorder.

Typical presentations of a mixed episode can include:
- Depression plus over-activity/pressure of speech.
- Mania plus agitation and reduced energy/libido.
- Dysphoria plus manic symptoms (with exception of elevated mood).
- Rapid cycling (fluctuating between mania and depression—four or more episodes/yr) Note: "Ultra-rapid" cycling refers to the situation when fluctuations are over days or even hours.

Hypomania/hypomanic episode

Finally, DSM-IV-TR lists the specific diagnostic criteria set for a hypomanic episode and includes additional criteria/descriptors to allow the clinician to further qualify the current or most recent episode (see 📖 p. 351).

DSM-IV-TR criteria for hypomanic episode

- A distinct period of persistently elevated, expansive, or irritable mood, lasting throughout at least four days, that is clearly different from the usual nondepressed mood.
- During the period of mood disturbance, three (or more) of the following symptoms have persisted (four if the mood is only irritable) and have been present to a significant degree:
  - Inflated self-esteem or grandiosity.
  - Decreased need for sleep (e.g., feels rested after only three hours of sleep).
  - More talkative than usual or pressure to keep talking.
  - Flight of ideas or subjective experience that thoughts are racing.
  - Distractibility (e.g., attention too easily drawn to unimportant or irrelevant external stimuli).
  - Increase in goal-directed activity (either socially, at work or school, or sexually) or psychomotor agitation.
  - Excessive involvement in pleasurable activities that have a high potential for painful consequences (e.g., the person engages in unrestrained buying sprees, sexual indiscretions, or foolish business investments).
- The episode is associated with an unequivocal change in functioning that is uncharacteristic of the person when not symptomatic.
- The disturbance in mood and the change in functioning are observable by others.
- The episode is not severe enough to cause marked impairment in social or occupational functioning, or to necessitate hospitalization, and there are no psychotic features.
- The symptoms are not due to the direct physiological effects of a substance (e.g., a drug of abuse, a medication, or other treatment) or a general medical condition (e.g., hyperthyroidism).

Note: Hypomanic-like episodes that are clearly caused by somatic anti-depressant treatment (e.g., medication, electroconvulsive therapy, light therapy) should not count toward a diagnosis of bipolar II disorder.

The clinical reality of manic-depressive illness is that it is far more disabling and infinitely more complex than the current psychiatric nomenclature would suggest. Cycles of fluctuating moods and energy levels serve as a background to constantly changing thoughts, behaviors, and feelings. The illness encompasses the extremes of human experience. Thinking can range from florid psychosis, or "madness," to patterns of unusually clear, fast, and creative associations, to retardation so profound that no meaningful mental activity can occur. Behavior can be frenzied, expansive, bizarre, and seductive, or it can be seclusive, sluggish, and dangerously suicidal. Moods may swing erratically between euphoria and despair or irritability and desperation. The rapid oscillations and combinations of such extremes result in an intricately textured clinical picture. Manic patients, for example, are depressed and irritable as often as they are euphoric; the highs associated with mania are generally only pleasant and productive during the earlier, milder stages.

Dr Kay Redfield Jamison (1993) *Touched With Fire: Manic-Depressive Illness and the Artistic Temperament*. New York: The Free Press, Macmillan, pp 47–48.

DSM-IV-TR bipolar disorders classifications

Bipolar I disorder
Single manic episode
Most recent episode, hypomanic
Most recent episode, manic
Most recent episode, mixed
Most recent episode, depressed
Most recent episode, unspecified

Bipolar II disorder
Most recent episode, hypomanic
Most recent episode, depressed

Cyclothymic disorder
Bipolar disorder not otherwise specified

Bipolar disorder

Etiology

Factors identified as important include:

- Genetic—First-degree relatives are seven times more likely to develop the condition than the general population (i.e., 10–15% risk). Children of a parent with bipolar disorder have a 50% chance of developing a psychiatric disorder (genetic liability appears shared for schizophrenia, schizoaffective, and bipolar affective disorder). Siblings have comparable risks. MZ twins: 33–90% concordance; DZ twins: ~23%.
- Neurotransmitters—NA, DA, 5HT, and glutamine have all been implicated. Brain-derived neurotrophic factor (BDNF) may contribute to lessening the potential for longer-term neuronal consequences.
- HPA axis—Given the effects of environmental stressors, and of exogenous steroids, a role has also been suggested for glucocorticoids and other stress-related hormonal responses.

Etiological theories

Abnormal "programmed cell death"

Animal studies have recently shown that antidepressants, lithium, and valproate indirectly regulate a number of factors involved in cell survival pathways (e.g., CREB, BDNF, Bcl-2, and MAP kinases) perhaps explaining their delayed long-term beneficial effects (via underappreciated neurotrophic effects, especially in the frontal cortex and the hippocampus[1]). Neuroimaging studies also indicate cell loss in these same brain regions. This suggests that bipolar affective disorder may be the result of abnormal programmed cell death (apoptosis) in critical neural networks involved in the regulation of emotion, which in turn may be accelerated by the stress of prolonged episodes of illness. Mood stabilizers and antidepressants may act to stimulate cell survival pathways and increase levels of neurotrophic factors that improve cellular resilience.

"Kindling"

An older hypothesis,[2] also drawing on animal models, suggests a role for neuronal injury, through mechanisms identified in studies of electrophysiological kindling and behavioral sensitization. A genetically predisposed individual experiences an increasing number of minor neurological insults (e.g., due to drugs of abuse, excessive glucocorticoid stimulation, to acute or chronic stress, or other factors), which eventually result in mania. After the first episode, sufficient neuronal damage may persist, allowing for recurrence with or without minor environmental or behavioral stressors (much like epilepsy), which may in turn result in further injury. This view provides an explanation for later episodes becoming more frequent and more likely to occur independent of life stress, why anticonvulsants may be useful in preventing recurrent episodes, and suggests that treatment should be as early as possible and long term.

---

1 Manji, H.K. and Duman, R.S. (2001). Impairments of neuroplasticity and cellular resilience in severe mood disorders: implications for the development of novel therapeutics. *Psychopharmacology Bulletin* **35**, 5–49.

2 Post, R.M. and Weiss, S.R. (1989). Sensitization, kindling, and anticonvulsants in mania. *J Clin Psychiatry* **50**, Suppl: 23–30.

Epidemiology

Lifetime prevalence 0.3–1.5% (0.8% bipolar I; 0.5% bipolar II); males:females (bipolar II and rapid cycling more common in females; first episodes: males tend to be manic, females depressive); no significant racial differences; age range 15–50 + yrs (peaks at 15–19 yrs and 20–24 yrs; mean 21 yrs).

Prodrome

When attempting to differentiate from depressive disorders, the following features (especially in combination) are **suggestive of potential bipolar disorder**:

- Early age of depression onset.
- Psychotic depressive episode before age 25.
- Postpartum depression.
- Rapid cycling or >5 depressive episodes.
- Atypical features.
- Seasonal pattern.
- Antidepressant-induced hypomania.
- Refractory to >3 antidepressant trials after initial positive response.
- Treatment-resistant depression.
- Family history of bipolar disorder.
- Periodic impulsivity or irritability.

Course

Extremely variable. The first episode of bipolar I disorder is about equally likely to be manic/mixed or depressive in nature. (In bipolar II disorder, the first recognized episode is almost always a depression.) This may be followed by many years (5 or more) without a further episode, but the length of time between subsequent episodes typically begins to narrow.

Survey data uniformly document that there is usually a 5–10yr interval between age at onset of illness and age at first treatment or first admission to hospital. Generally, for people with a history of recurrent depression the risk of "converting" to a bipolar diagnosis is greatest before age 30. Nevertheless, even when there is a history of five or more depressive episodes, there is at least a 5% chance of still experiencing a hypomania or mania. It is known that untreated patients may have more than 10 episodes in a lifetime, and that the duration and period of time between episodes stabilizes after the fourth or fifth episode. Although the prognosis is better for treated patients, there still remains a high degree of unpredictability.

Morbidity/mortality
Morbidity and mortality rates are high, in terms of lost work, lost productivity, effects on marriage (increased divorce rates) and the family, with attempted suicide in 25–50%, and completed suicide in ~10% (males > females usually during a depressive or mixed episode). Often significant co-morbidity—especially drug/alcohol misuse and anxiety disorders, both of which significantly increase risk of suicide.

Investigations
As for depression; full physical and routine blood tests to exclude any treatable cause, including CBC, glucose, electrolytes, Ca^{2+}, TFTs, LFTs, and drug screen. Less routine tests: urinary copper (to exclude Wilson's disease [rare]), ANA (SLE), infection screen (RPR, HIV test). CT/MRI brain (to exclude tumors, infarction, hemorrhage, MS)—may show hyperintense subcortical structures (especially temporal lobes), ventricular enlargement and sulcal prominence; EEG (baseline and to rule out epilepsy). Other baseline tests prior to treatment should include EKG and creatinine clearance.

Management
See specific sections (📖 *pp. 363–375*) for management principles, other issues, and treatment of acute manic episodes, depressive episodes, prophylaxis, and psychotherapeutic interventions.

Prognosis
Within the first two years of first episode, 40–50% of patients experience another manic episode. 50–60% of patients on lithium gain control of their symptoms (7% no recurrence; 45% some future episodes; 40% with little effect on risk of recurrence). Often, the cycling between depression and mania accelerates with age.
- *Poor prognostic factors*: poor employment history; alcohol abuse; psychotic features; depressive features between periods of mania and depression; evidence of depression; male sex, treatment noncompliance.
- *Good prognostic factors*: manic episodes of short duration; later age of onset; few thoughts of suicide; few psychotic symptoms; few co-morbid physical problems, good treatment response and compliance.

Cyclothymic disorder

Previously regarded as a disorder of personality ("cyclothymic temperament"—see opposite) mainly because of its early age of onset and relative stability throughout adult life, cyclothymia is now considered to be a mood disorder. The diagnosis is difficult to establish without a prolonged period of observation or an unusually good account of the individual's past behavior.

DSM-IV-TR criteria for cyclothymic disorder

- For at least two years, the presence of numerous periods with hypomanic symptoms (see 📖 p. 350) and numerous periods with depressive symptoms that do not meet criteria for a major depressive episode. Note: In children and adolescents, the duration must be at least one year.
- During the aforementioned two-year period (one year in children and adolescents), the person has not been without the symptoms for more than two months at a time.
- No major depressive episode, manic episode, or mixed episode has been present during the first two years of the disturbance.
  Note: After the initial two years (one year in children and adolescents) of cyclothymic disorder, there may be superimposed manic or mixed episodes (in which case both bipolar I disorder and cyclothymic disorder may be diagnosed) or major depressive episodes (in which case both bipolar II disorder and cyclothymic disorder may be diagnosed).
- The symptoms are not better accounted for by schizoaffective disorder and are not superimposed on schizophrenia, schizophreniform disorder, delusional disorder, or psychotic disorder not otherwise specified.
- The symptoms are not due to the direct physiological effects of a substance (e.g., a drug of abuse, a medication) or a general medical condition (e.g., hyperthyroidism).
- The symptoms cause clinically significant distress or impairment in social, occupational, or other important areas of functioning.

Clinical features

- Persistent instability of mood, with numerous periods of mild depression and mild elation, not sufficiently severe or prolonged to fulfill the criteria for bipolar affective disorder or recurrent depressive disorder.
- The mood swings are usually perceived by the individual as being unrelated to life events.

Epidemiology

Prevalence 3–6% of general population. Age of onset: usually early adulthood (i.e., teens or 20s), but sometimes may present later in life. More common in the relatives of patients with bipolar affective disorder.

Course

Onset is often gradual, making it difficult to pinpoint exactly when symptoms began. The alternating ups and downs may fluctuate in hours, weeks, or months. Because the mood swings are relatively mild and the periods of mood elevation may be enjoyable (with increased activity and productivity, self-confidence, and sociability), cyclothymia frequently fails to come to medical attention. Often the person may present either because of the impact of the depressive episodes on their social and work situations, or because of problems related to co-morbid drug or alcohol misuse. Usually runs a chronic course, persisting throughout adult life. In some cases symptoms may cease temporarily or permanently, or develop into more severe mood swings meeting the criteria for bipolar affective disorder or recurrent depressive disorder.

Management

- If pharmacological treatment is contemplated, this usually consists of a trial of a mood stabilizer (e.g., lithium), either singly or in combination with antipsychotic medication or potent benzodiazepines. When antipsychotic medications are used, concerns about tardive dyskinesia have led to preferential use of the atypical antipsychotics—which all have been shown to be effective antimanic agents—instead of the older antipsychotic compounds.
- Recently there has been a tendency to use anticonvulsants such as valproate, carbamazepine, or lamotrigine, as these may be better tolerated. Not all anticonvulsants are effective, however, and gabapentin was singularly ineffective as an antimanic. As yet there is no clear evidence to suggest any of these approaches is superior to lithium unless there is a clear history of lithium resistance.
- Psycho-education and several focused forms of psychotherapy have been shown to reduce recurrence risk. More traditional forms of insight-orientated psychotherapy also may help patients to understand the condition, and allow them to develop better ways of coping.
- There is often a reluctance to continue to take medication because this not only treats the depressive episodes, but also may be perceived as "blunting" creativity, productivity, or intellectual capacity.

Kraepelin's "cyclothymic temperament"

These are the people who constantly oscillate hither and thither between the two opposite poles of mood, sometimes "rejoicing to the skies," sometimes "sad as death." Today lively, sparkling, beaming, full of the joy of life, the pleasure of enterprise, and the pressure of activity, after some time they meet us depressed, enervated, ill-humored, in need of rest, and again a few months later they display the old freshness and elasticity.

Emil Kraepelin (1896). Manic-Depressive Insanity and Paranoia. (Extract from translation of the 8th edition of Kraepelin's textbook *Psychiatrie*).

"Bipolar spectrum disorder"

One view of the affective disorders is that they consist of a continuum (see below). Such definitions provide alternative views and are currently under research.

Proposed clinical features

"Bipolar spectrum disorder" is characterized by:[1]
• At least one major depressive episode.
• No spontaneous hypomanic or manic episodes.

And a history including some of the following

• A family history of bipolar disorder in a first-degree relative.
• Antidepressant-induced mania or hypomania.
• Hyperthymic personality[2] (at baseline, nondepressed state).
• Recurrent major depressive episodes (>3).
• Brief major depressive episodes (on average, <3 months).
• Atypical depressive symptoms (DSM-IV criteria).
• Psychotic major depressive episodes.
• Early age of onset of major depressive episode (< age 25).
• Postpartum depression.
• Antidepressant "wear-off" (acute but not prophylactic response).
• Lack of response to up to three antidepressant treatment trials.

Management

Patients with features of bipolar spectrum disorder may represent a subset of patients who do not respond well to antidepressants (often precipitating a switch to a hypomanic or manic episode) and for whom an anticonvulsant may be the drug of choice (e.g., valproate—see 📖 p. 384).

The "affective continuum"

Dysthymia
Unipolar depression
Atypical depression
Psychotic depression   } Unipolar spectrum disorder
Recurrent depression
Bipolar spectrum disorder
Bipolar II
Bipolar I

Recommended further reading

1 Ghaemi, S.N., Ko, J.Y., Goodwin, F.K. (2002). "Cade's disease" and beyond: misdiagnosis, antide-pressant use, and a proposed definition for bipolar spectrum disorder. *Can J Psychiatry* **47**, 125–34.
2 Characterized by cheerful, optimistic personality style, tendency to become easily irritated, extroverted and sociable, and requiring little sleep (less than 6 hours/night).

Differential diagnosis of bipolar disorders

Other psychiatric disorders

There are many other psychiatric disorders and conditions that share some of the manic or hypomanic affective and/or neurovegetative features of bipolar disorders:

- ADHD.
- Anxiety disorders.
- Conduct disorder.
- Dementias.
- Dissociative disorders (dissociative fugue, dissociative identity disorder).
- Eating disorders.
- Impulse control disorders.
- Personality disorders (paranoid, schizotypal, antisocial, borderline, histrionic, narcissistic).
- Schizoaffective disorders.
- Schizophrenia and other psychotic disorders.
- Sleep disorders.
- Sexual disorders (paraphilias, exhibitionism, frotteurism, voyeurism).
- Substance-use disorders.

General medical conditions

Some patients who have manic or hypomanic symptoms can also have one or more general medical conditions, and it can at times be difficult to discern how much to attribute these symptoms (especially neurovegetative) to a primary bipolar disorder or to the medical condition. A temporal association (onset, exacerbation, remission) between the condition and the manic symptoms can help guide the clinician, especially if the condition is known to have a direct association with the development of such symptoms (see Table 8.1).

Pharmacological causes of manic/hypomanic symptoms

Finally, many substances (prescribed for a medical condition, used recreationally, or through environmental exposure) can induce manic or hypomanic symptoms. A listing of such pharmacological agents is given in Table 8.2.

Table 8.1 General medical conditions with manic/hypomanic features

Endocrine	
Acromegaly	Hyperthyroidism
Cushing's disease	Addison's disease
Hyperparathyroidism	Hypoparathyroidism
Hyperglycemia	Carcinoid
Pheochromocytoma	Menopausal symptoms
Perimenstrual syndromes	Hypercalcemia
Prolactinoma	
Infectious/Inflammatory	
Influenza	Tertiary syphilis
Mononucleosis	Hepatic encephalopathy
HIV/AIDS	Rheumatoid arthritis
Encephalitis	Toxoplasmosis
Systemic lupus erythematosus	HSV encephalopathy
Neurological	
Multiple sclerosis	Stroke (esp. right sided)
Head trauma	Brain tumors
Wilson's disease	Huntington's disease
Epilepsy (esp. complex partial)	Delirium
Nutritional deficiencies/Metabolic deficiencies	
Folate deficiency	B_{12} deficiency
Other	
Porphyrias	

Table 8.2 Pharmacological causes of manic or hypomanic symptoms

Analgesics and anti-inflammatory agents		
Tramadol	Indomethacin	Phenylbutazone
Opiates		

Antibiotic/antiviral agents		
Isoniazid	Chloroquine	Clarithromycin
	Dapsone	

Anticholinesterases		
Cimetidine	Diphenoxylate	Lysergide
Mebeverine		Salbutamol

Antidepressant agents		

Gastrointestinal agents		
Cimetidine	Metoclopramide	Ranitidine

Cardiac and antihypertensive agents		
Captopril	Clonidine	Digitalis
Diltiazem	Hydralazine	Lidocaine
Reserpine	Methyldopa withdrawal	Propranolol
Procainamide		

Sedatives *in withdrawal*		
Barbiturates	Benzodiazepines	Ethanol

Steroids and hormones		
Corticosteroids	Danazol	Oral contraceptives
Prednisone	Norethisterone	Dexamethasone
Testosterone		

Stimulants and appetite suppressants		
Amphetamine	Cocaine	Diethylpropion
Fenfluramine	Caffeine	Methylphenidate

Neurological agents		
Amantadine	Baclofen	Bromocriptine
Carbamazepine	Levodopa	Phenytoin

Respiratory agents		
Aminophylline	Ephedrine	Pseudoephedrine

Other miscellaneous agents		
Cyclosporine	Cyclizine	Cyproheptadine
Disulfiram	Interferon	Methysergide

Management principles

Acute episodes

Management of acute episodes depends upon the nature of the presentation (See Treatment of acute manic episodes 📖 *p. 368*, Hypomania/hypomanic episode 📖 *p. 350*, and Treatment of depressive episodes 📖 *p. 370*). Often the manic episodes are of a nature and degree that hospital admission will be necessary (for criteria and considerations see Hospital admission 📖 *p. 366*).

Special consideration should also be given to certain specific issues related to the clinical presentation, the presence of concurrent medical problems, and particular patient groups, both in terms of setting and choice of treatment (see Other issues affecting management decisions 📖 *p. 364*). Issues of maintenance (see Maintenance 📖 *p. 372*) should be considered, and this may sometimes involve not only pharmacological, but also psychotherapeutic interventions (see Psychotherapeutic interventions 📖 *p. 374*).

Outpatient follow-up

Once the diagnosis has been clearly established, possible physical causes excluded, and the presenting episode effectively treated, follow-up has a number of key aims:

- Establishing and maintaining a therapeutic alliance.
- Monitoring the patient's psychiatric status.
- Providing education regarding bipolar disorder.
- Enhancing treatment compliance.
- Monitoring side-effects of medication and ensuring therapeutic levels of any mood stabilizer.
- Identifying and addressing any significant co-morbid conditions.
- Promoting regular patterns of activity and wakefulness.
- Promoting understanding of and adaptation to the psychosocial effects of bipolar disorder.
- Identifying new episodes early.
- Reducing the morbidity and sequelae of bipolar disorder.

Relapse prevention

A key part of psychiatric management is helping patients to identify precipitants or early manifestations of illness, so that treatment can be initiated early. This may be done as part of the usual psychiatric follow-up, or form part of a specific psychotherapeutic intervention (see Psychotherapeutic interventions 📖 *p. 374*) (e.g., insomnia may often be either a precipitant, or an early indicator, of mania or depression—education about the importance of regular sleep habits and occasional use of an hypnotic (see Chapter 11) to promote normal sleep patterns may be useful in preventing the development of a manic episode). Other early or subtle signs of mania may be treated with the short-term use of benzodiazepines or antipsychotics. A good therapeutic alliance is critical, and the patient, who often has good insight, ought to feel that they can contact their clinician as soon as they are aware of these early warning signs.

Other issues affecting management decisions

Specific clinical features

Certain clinical features will strongly influence the choice of treatment. For issues of substance misuse or other psychiatric morbidity these should be addressed directly (see specific sections).

Psychotic symptoms

It is not uncommon for patients to experience delusions and/or hallucinations during episodes of mania and a significant minority of depressive episodes also are psychotic. Management: Mood stabilizer with/without an antipsychotic, consider ECT, if severe consider admission to hospital.

Catatonic symptoms

Management: During a manic episode ("manic stupor"), admit to hospital, exclude medical problem, clarify psychiatric diagnosis, if diagnosis clear treat with ECT and/or benzodiazepine.

Rapid cycling

Defined as four or more discreet mood episodes per year. Occurs in 10–20% of patients with bipolar disorder. Women>>Men. Worse long term prognosis. Initial rule out of medical conditions should be completed (e.g., hypothyroidism, multiple sclerosis, etc.). Other factors may contribute (e.g., SSRI treatment or substance abuse). Valproate and lamotrigine have been found to be more effective than other mood stabilizers.

Risk of suicide

Assess nature of risk (see 📖 p. 60), note association with rapid cycling mood. If significant risk, or unacceptable uncertainty, admit to hospital (or if in hospital, increase level of observation), consider ECT.

Risk of violence

Assess nature of risk (see 📖 p. 866). Note increased risk with rapid mood cycling, paranoid delusions, agitation, and dysphoria. Admit to hospital, consider need for secure setting.

Substance-related disorders

Co-morbidity is high, often confusing the clinical picture. Substance misuse may lead to relapse both directly and indirectly (by reducing compliance). Equally, alcohol consumption may increase when on lithium.
Management: Address issues of misuse; if detoxification considered, admit to hospital as risk of suicide may be increased.

Other co-morbidities

Personality disorders, anxiety disorder, ADHD, conduct disorder.

Concurrent medical problems

The presence of other medical problems may affect the management either by exacerbating the course or severity of the disorder or by complicating pharmacological treatment (e.g., issues of tolerability and drug interactions).

Cardiovascular/renal/hepatic disorders
May restrict the choice of drug therapy or increase the need for closer monitoring.

Endocrine disorders
For example, hypo/hyperthyoidism.

Infectious diseases
For example, HIV-infected patients may be more sensitive to CNS side-effects of mood stabilizers.

Use of steroids
For inflammatory conditions (e.g., asthma, inflammatory bowel disease) may exacerbate mood symptoms.

Special patient groups

Children and adolescents (see 📖 p. 756)
Although not extensively studied in these age groups, clinical experience indicates that lithium and other antimanic therapies are effective. The long-term effects of these treatments on development have not been fully studied. Lithium may be excreted more quickly, allowing more rapid dose adjustments, but therapeutic levels are the same as for adults. Youth may be at particular risk for weight gain, particularly when treated with atypical antipsychotics. Risks associated with other adjunctive agents (e.g., antipsychotics, antidepressants, benzodiazepines) should be considered separately. ECT is rarely used, but may be effective. Education, support, and other specific psychosocial interventions should be considered (usually involving family, teachers, etc.)

The elderly (see 📖 p. 586)
When a first manic episode occurs in a patient after age 60, there is often evidence of previous depressive episodes in their 40s and 50s. Full physical examination is necessary to exclude medical causes (especially CNS disorders). Older patients may be more sensitive to the side-effects of lithium (particularly neurological) and may require lower therapeutic levels (i.e., below 0.7mmol/L). Atypical antipsychotics have received a "black box" warning that cautions about the risk of increased mortality (~2%) in controlled studies of elders with dementia.

Pregnancy and lactation (see 📖 p. 504)
Consider ECT as first line for treatment of significant manic, depressed, or psychotically depressed episodes. Teratogenic risks of lithium probably have been exaggerated. Atypical antipsychotics and lamotrigine may have the safest profiles, but further research is needed.

Hospital admission

Frequently, acute manic episodes require hospital admission (often on a compulsory basis because of loss of insight and inability to make informed choices about the need for treatment). Issues of safety and the provision of effective treatment will govern the decisions about whether a patient can remain in the community.

Points to note

- Patients with symptoms of mania/hypomania or depression often have impaired judgment (sometimes related to psychotic symptoms), which may interfere with their ability to make reasoned decisions about the need for treatment.
- Risk assessment includes not only behaviors that may cause direct harm (e.g., suicide attempts or homicidal behavior), but also those that may be indirectly harmful (e.g., overspending, sexual promiscuity, excessive use of drugs/alcohol, driving while unwell).
- The relapsing/remitting nature of the disorder makes it possible to work with the patient (when well) and their family to anticipate future acute episodes and agree to a treatment plan, should they occur.

Clinical features and situations where admission may be necessary

- High risk of suicide or homicide.
- Illness-related behavior that endangers relationships, reputation, or assets.
- Lack of capacity to cooperate with treatment (e.g., directly due to illness, or secondary to availability of social supports/outpatient resources).
- Lack (or loss) of psychosocial supports.
- Severe psychotic symptoms.
- Severe depressive symptoms.
- Severe mixed states or rapid cycling (days/hours).
- Catatonic symptoms.
- Failure of outpatient treatment.
- A need to address co-morbid conditions (e.g., physical problems, other psychiatric conditions, inpatient detoxification).

Suitable environment?

During an acute manic episode, a routine, calm environment is desirable (but not always possible). A balance should be struck between avoidance of overstimulation (e.g., from outside events, TV, radio, lively conversations) and provision of sufficient space to walk or exercise in order to use up excess energy. Where possible, access to alcohol and drugs should be restricted. Patients may find regular observations by staff overly intrusive, feel uncomfortable in a busy ward, and make requests of staff that may well be reasonable but not practical. The psychiatrist needs to adopt a pragmatic approach, listening to concerns, and balancing risks. Sometimes this may result in a difficult decision about whether to detain a patient to a hospital environment, which, although far from ideal, is the "least worst" option. Because manic individuals can be uncannily aware of less-than-honest responses, yet uncompromising in negotiations, it is often best to tell unpleasant truths (i.e., "You must stay here in the hospital for at least five days") in a calm manner and not to engage in long debates aimed at reaching consensus.

Treatment of acute manic episodes

First-line treatment

Lithium (see 📖 p. 376)

Lithium remains the first-line treatment for acute mania, with a response rate of at least 50% across all patients, and up to 80% among more treatment-responsive subsets (e.g., nonpsychotic first- or second-episode patients without a history of cycling and minimal depressive features.) Note: At least two weeks of treatment is necessary to reach maximal effectiveness for manic patients. Due to this delayed effect, especially for severe mania or psychotic symptoms, with associated acute behavioral disturbance, addition of an antipsychotic or a benzodiazepine is usually required.

Predictors of good response: Previous response to lithium, compliance with medication, family history of mood disorder, euphoria (not dysphoria), lack of psychotic symptoms or suicidal behavior.

Antipsychotics

As in acute behavioral disturbance (see 📖 p. 1110), antipsychotics are useful in the rapid control of severely agitated or psychotic patients with bipolar disorder.[1] As noted previously, the high frequency of EPS and risk of TD has driven the field's preference for atypical antipsychotics over older agents such as haloperidol or chlorpromazine. Atypical antipsychotics—unlike the older drugs—also have been shown to reduce the risk of relapse following successful acute phase therapy. When the more commonly used atypical antipsychotics are ineffective, the antimanic efficacy of clozapine should not be overlooked. Documentation of weight, waist size, and pretreatment blood sugar and lipid profiles are recommended to facilitate monitoring if longer-term therapy with atypical antipsychotics is subsequently indicated.

Benzodiazepines

Another approach to reduce the need for antipsychotics is the adjunctive use of benzodiazepines. Clonazepam and lorazepam are the most widely studied compounds, either alone or in combination with lithium, and are effective, in place of, or in conjunction with, an antipsychotic, to sedate the acutely agitated manic patient while waiting for the effects of other primary mood-stabilizing agents. The fact that lorazepam is well absorbed after intramuscular injection (unlike other benzodiazepines) has made it particularly useful for some very agitated patients.

---

1 Gelenberg, A.J. and Hopkins, H.S. (1996). Antipsychotics in bipolar disorder. *Journal of Clinical Psychiatry* **57**(Suppl.), 49–52.

ECT

ECT has been shown to be the most rapidly effective treatment option for patients with severe mania.[2] Current practice reserves ECT for clinical situations in which pharmacological treatments may not be possible, such as pregnancy or severe cardiac disease, or when the patient's illness is refractory to drug treatments.

Use of anticonvulsants

Valproate (see 📖 p. 384)

Valproate became the most commonly used mood stabilizer by psychiatrists in the United States in the late 1990s, although its longer-term efficacy still is not convincingly established. Valproate is about as effective as lithium in head-to-head studies of acute phase therapy and certainly should be considered the treatment of choice for patients who are intolerant of or not responsive to lithium. Valproate is generally well tolerated, although some caution is needed in treatment of patients with alcoholism and liver disease. Valproate also is well suited for combined treatment regimes, keeping in mind the caveat that it essentially doubles plasma levels of lamotrigine.

Predictors of good response: May be more effective in particular patients, e.g., those with "rapid cycling"—where some consider it "first line"—dysphoric mania, mixed episodes, stable or decreasing frequency of manic episodes, or less severe forms of bipolar spectrum disorders.

Carbamazepine (see 📖 p. 386)

Carbamazepine or its derivative, oxcarbazepine, may be effective, either alone or in combination with lithium or antipsychotics.[3] It may be better tolerated in patients with co-morbid drug or alcohol problems or obesity.

Predictors of good response: Previous response to carbamazepine, poor compliance (due to wide therapeutic window), absence of psychotic symptoms, secondary mania (e.g., drug-induced, neurological disorder, brain injury), dysphoria, "mixed" episode, rapid cycling, episode part of schizoaffective disorder.

Other

There is no current evidence to recommend use of gabapentin in bipolar disorder (mania or hypomania). Lamotrigine is approved for preventive therapy of bipolar I disorder (prevention greater for depressive than manic relapses). Controlled studies suggest acute antidepressant effects as well, but the level of empirical support is not sufficient to justify formal FDA indication. The jury is still out on topiramate, which has shown some promise in both depressed and manic bipolar patients, but has failed to garner sufficient evidence of efficacy in larger-scale controlled trials. Topiramate is best known for its effect in promoting weight loss.

---

2 Mukherjee, S., Sackeim, H.A., Schnur, D.B. (1994). Electroconvulsive therapy of acute manic episodes: a review of 50 years' experience. *AJP* **151**, 169–176.

3 McElroy, S.L. and Keck, P.E. Jr. (2000). Pharmacologic agents for the treatment of acute bipolar mania. *Biol Psychiatry* **48**, 539–557.

Treatment of depressive episodes

The pharmacological treatment of depressive episodes in bipolar disorder represents a particular challenge.[1] Although the antidepressants that are used to treat major depressive episodes are widely thought to be effective in the treatment of bipolar depression, there is surprisingly little prospective research, and some of the studies have yielded contradictory findings. In fact, only one antidepressant—fluoxetine—is specifically approved for treatment of bipolar depression and that indication is limited to the use of fluoxetine in combination with olanzapine.

In general, antidepressants are recommended for use only in combination with mood stabilizers to lessen the risk of treatment-emergent affective switches (TEAS). Naturalistic studies suggest that response rates tend to be lower (than observed in major depressive disorder), perhaps partly because of the risk of precipitating a manic episode or inducing/accelerating rapid cycling. When symptoms are milder, it may be worth considering focused psychological interventions instead of pharmacotherapy (as in unipolar depression, 🕮 p. 304).

Alternatively, lamotrigine and several of the atypical antipsychotics are currently being used as monotherapies for patients with bipolar depression. Although the antidepressant effects of lamotrigine have been inconsistent in larger scale controlled studies, both olanzapine and quetiapine have shown definite efficacy in placebo-controlled studies (the former drug was not given an FDA indication because of the superior performance of the fluoxetine-olanzapine combination; the latter was approved for therapy of both bipolar I and bipolar II depressions in late 2005).[2,3]

Initial management

- If severely depressed, suicidal, or when urgent treatment necessary, consider ECT.
- If patient is currently "drug-free," consider initiation of either a mood stabilizer (e.g., lithium or valproate).
- If patient already on prophylaxis, optimize (ensure compliance), check serum levels, exclude/treat associated problems (e.g., hypothyroidism).
- If depressive symptoms persist, then consider addition of an antidepressant or an additional mood stabilizer.

Choice of antidepressant

Although evidence is scarce, most clinicians favor either the SSRIs or bupropion because of superior tolerability, greater safety in overdose,

1 Thase, M.E. Pharmacotherapy of bipolar depression: an update. Curr. Psychiatry Rep. **8**(6), 478–488, 2006.

2 Calabrese J.R., Keck, P.E., MacFadden, W., Minkwitz, M., Ketter, T.A., Weisler, R.H., Cutler, A.J., Mccoy, R., Wilson, E., Mullen, J. (2005). A randomized, double-blind, placebo-controlled trial of quetiapine in the treatment of bipolar I or II depression. Am J Psychiatry. **162**, 1351–1360.

3 Thase, M.E., MacFadden, W., Weisler, R.H., Chang, W., Paulsson, B., Khan, A., Calabrese, J.R., for the Bolder II Study Group. (2006). Efficacy of quetiapine monotherapy in bipolar I and II depression: A confirmatory double-blind, placebo-controlled study (the Bolder II study). J. Clin. Psychopharm. **26**(6), 600–609.

and—in all likelihood—less tendency to cause TEAS than the TCAs[3]. Recent data suggest that venlafaxine—perhaps because of its noradrenergic effects—may be more likely to cause TEAS than the other newer antidepressants.[4] In general, choice will depend on issues of previous response, side-effects (both desired and undesired), and tolerability issues. When newer antidepressants are ineffective and ECT is not a therapeutic option, clinicians should not forget the therapeutic potential of the MAOIs for patients with more difficult-to-treat episodes of bipolar depression.

Additional mood stabilizer

Although only a handful of controlled clinical trials comparing standard treatments for depression in patients with bipolar disorder are lacking, it is a widely accepted practice to add a second mood stabilizer (e.g., lamotrigine, valproate, or carbamazepine) to the treatment regimens of patients with bipolar disorder. Recent evidence suggests monotherapy with lamotrigine may have utility in the treatment of refractory bipolar depression.[5]

Note: Be alert for evidence of lithium toxicity, even at "normal" serum levels (see 📖 p. 380).

ECT

- Perhaps the best-established treatment for more refractory cases of bipolar depression, ECT also should not be overlooked (especially in severe cases). Because relapse almost invariably follows successful treatment within six to nine months, it is important to ensure that preventive therapy is initiated.
- ECT has been reported to cause memory impairment, acute confusion, and other neurological problems in patients on lithium; hence lithium should be withdrawn prior to treatment.
- Anticonvulsants oppose the desired convulsant effects of ECT and should also be withdrawn prior to treatment.

Alternative strategies/treatment resistance

Other suggested strategies include: the use of adjunctive triiodothyronine (T3)—even if there is no evidence of (sub)clinical hypothyroidism.[6] For treatment-resistant depressive episodes, principles of management are as for unipolar depression (see 📖 p. 312).

3 C.B., Evans, D.L., Gyulai, L., *et al.* (2001). Double-blind, placebo-controlled comparison of imipramine and paroxetine in the treatment of bipolar depression. *AJP* **158**, 906–912.
4 Post, R.M., Altshuler, L.L., Leverich, G.S., Frye, M.A., Nolen, W.A., Kupka, R.W., Suppes, T., McElroy, S., Keck, P.E., Denicoff, K.D., Grunze, H., Kitchen, C.M.R., Mintz, J. (2006). Mood switch in bipolar depression: comparison of adjunctive venlafaxine, bupropion and sertraline. *Br J Psychiatry.* **189**, 124–131.
5 Calabrese, J.R., Vieta, E., Shelton, M.D. (2003). Latest maintenance data on lamotrigine in bipolar disorder. *Eur Neuropsychopharmacol.* **13** Suppl 2, S57–S66.
6 Bauer, M., Berghofer, A., Bschor, T., *et al.* (2002). Supraphysiological doses of L-thyroxine in the maintenance treatment of prophylaxis-resistant affective disorders. *Neuropsychopharmacology* **27**, 620–628.

Maintenance treatment of bipolar disorder

Primary aim

Prevention of recurrent episodes (either mania or depression).

Indications

Following effective remission of a manic episode. Also strongly recommended for patients with bipolar II disorder. (APA Guidelines 2004[1]).

First-line treatment

Lithium (see 📖 p. 376)

To date, lithium remains the first-line choice for maintenance treatment in patients with a "classical" course of illness. Some subtypes of what has become known as the "bipolar spectrum" may not respond as well to lithium. These include patients with "mixed mania" (i.e., depressive symptoms during manic episodes) and patients with "rapid cycling" mania. Emerging evidence would seem to suggest a role for anticonvulsants in these patients.

Second-line treatments

Valproate

Has demonstrated efficacy in rapid cycling bipolar disorder and the added confidence of being the most widely prescribed therapy for bipolar depression, although unequivocal evidence of successful prophylaxis has not yet emerged.

Carbamazepine

Appears to be effective in the long-term treatment of bipolar disorder, with an overall response rate of 63%.[2] Although it does not have world-wide approval as yet, carbamazepine may be more effective in the treatment of bipolar spectrum than classical bipolar disorder.

Lamotrigine

Efficacy established in a pair of controlled studies for prevention of depressive and, to a lesser extent, mania following discontinuation of other psychotropic medications.[3]

Other anticonvulsants

There have been promising reports on the efficacy of oxcarbazepine. At this time, there remains no convincing evidence for efficacy with topiramate, gabapentin, tiagabine, or pregabalin in the treatment of bipolar disorder.

---

1 American Psychiatric Association: Practice Guidelines for the Treatment of Psychiatric Disorders, American Psychiatric Association. 2004.
2 Dunn, R.T., Frye, M.S., Kimbrell, T.A., *et al.* (1998). The efficacy and use of anticonvulsants in mood disorders. *Clinical Neuropharmacology* 21, 215–235.
3 Goodwin, G.M., Bowden, C.L., Calabrese, J.R., Grunze, H., Kasper, S., White, R., Greene, P., Leadbetter, R. (2004). A pooled analysis of 2 placebo-controlled 18-month trials of lamotrigine and lithium maintenance in bipolar I disorder. *J Clin Psychiatry* 65, 432–441.

Atypical antipsychotics

Over the past several years several of the atypical antipsychotics have been approved for longer term use after successful acute phase therapy.

Alternative/augmentative agents

Alternative treatment strategies, or potential augmentative agents, include a number of other compounds, which may have some clinical utility, but for which the evidence remains weak. These include: calcium channel antagonists such as verapamil, nifedipine, and nimodipine; thyroid hormones.

Risks of discontinuation

With long-term treatment it is essential that patients are well informed about the risks and implications of stopping medication. Substantial evidence exists that abrupt discontinuation of lithium is associated with an increased risk of relapse. The risk, particularly of mania, may be minimized by gradually reducing the lithium dose. Although comparable studies are not available for the anticonvulsants, a similarly cautious approach would seem advisable.

Suicide prevention

Because patients with bipolar disorder represent a group at high risk of suicide, it is reasonable to ask whether the above treatment strategies reduce the occurrence of suicidal acts. Retrospective and prospective studies do suggest that long-term lithium therapy reduces the risk of suicide, and may even reduce the known associated risk of cardiovascular disease. At present there is still little data available on the antisuicidal effects of the anticonvulsants in bipolar disorder. Prospective studies looking at the issue of outcome in bipolar disorder suggest that lithium may be significantly superior to carbamazepine in this regard.

Psychotherapeutic interventions

Most patients will struggle with some of the following issues

- Emotional consequences of significant periods of illness and receiving the diagnosis of a chronic psychiatric disorder.
- Developmental deviations and delays caused by past episodes.
- Problems associated with stigmatization.
- Problems related to self-esteem.
- Fear of recurrence and the consequent inhibition of normal psychosocial functioning.
- Interpersonal difficulties.
- Issues related to marriage, family, childbearing, and parenting.
- Academic and occupational problems.
- Other legal, social, and emotional problems that arise from illness-related behaviors.

For some patients, a specific psychotherapeutic intervention (in addition to usual psychiatric management and social support) will be needed to address these issues. Approaches include: psychodynamic, interpersonal, and cognitive behavioral therapies. In addition, couple therapy, family therapy, and group therapy may be indicated for some patients. The selection of appropriate interventions is influenced by the local availability of such treatments, as well as the patient's needs and preferences.

Key elements of selected interventions
CBT
Time limited, with specific aims: educate the patient about bipolar disorder and its treatment, teach cognitive behavioral skills for coping with psychosocial stressors and associated problems, facilitate compliance with treatment, and monitor the occurrence and severity of symptoms.

Interpersonal and social rhythm therapy
To reduce lability of mood by maintaining a regular pattern of daily activities (e.g., sleeping, eating, physical activity, and emotional stimulation). Recent evidence suggests these psychotherapeutic interventions provide improved long-term outcomes.[1]

Family therapies
Usually brief, include psycho-education (of patient and family members) with specific aims: accepting the reality of the illness, identifying precipitating stresses and likely future stresses inside and outside the family, elucidating family interactions that produce stress on the patient, planning strategies for managing and/or minimizing future stresses, and bringing about the patient's family's acceptance of the need for continued treatment.

---

1 Frank, E., Kupfer, D.J., Thase, M.E., Mallinger, A.G., Swartz, H.A., Fagiolini, A.M., Grochocinski, V., Houck, P., Scott, J., Thompson, W., Monk T. (Sept. 2005). Two-year outcomes for interpersonal and social rhythm therapy in individuals with bipolar I disorder. *Archives of General Psychiatry* **62**(9), 996–1004.

Support groups

These may provide useful information about bipolar disorder and its treatment. Patients may benefit from hearing the experiences of others, struggling with similar issues. This may help them to see their problems as not being unique, understand the need for medication, and access advice and assistance with other practical issues. In the United States, groups such as NAMI (www.nami.org), Depression and Bipolar Support Alliance (www.dbsalliance.org), and the Child and Adolescent Bipolar Foundation (www.bpkids.org) provide both support and educational material to patients and their families. For therapeutic considerations in youth, please refer to Chapter 16, Child and adolscent psychiatry.

Lithium

Despite problems with tolerability, lithium[1] still remains the gold standard in the treatment of bipolar affective disorder against which other treatments are measured. The effectiveness of long-term treatment with lithium is supported by at least nine controlled, double-blind studies.[2,3] This evidence far exceeds the available support for other possible alternatives to lithium treatment, although the last decade has seen an emerging body of research supporting the use of anticonvulsant, antipsychotic, or sedative agents.

Mode of action

Uncertain; numerous effects on biological systems (particularly at high concentrations). Lithium can substitute for Na^+, K^+, Ca^{2+}, Mg^{2+} and may have effects on cell membrane electrophysiology. Within cells, lithium interacts with systems involving other cations, including the release of neurotransmitters and second messenger systems (e.g., adenylate cyclase, inositol 1,4,5,-triphosphate, arachidonate, protein kinase C, G proteins and calcium), effectively blocking the actions of transmitters and hormones. There is also a reduction in receptor up-regulation, perhaps explaining lithium's value as an adjunctive treatment.

Pharmacokinetics

Half-life: 18–24 hours (can increase to >36hrs in elderly or in renal impairment). Not protein bound. Bioavailability not affected by food. Elimination: 90–98% of drug is excreted unchanged in the urine.

Drug interactions

Increased plasma concentration (risk of toxicity even at therapeutic serum levels)

ACE inhibitors/angiotensin II antagonists, analgesics (especially NSAIDs and COX-2 inhibitors), antidepressants (especially SSRIs), antiepileptics, antihypertensives (e.g., methyldopa), antipsychotics (especially haloperidol), calcium-channel blockers, diuretics (especially thiazides), metronidazole, methyldopa, antibiotics (especially tetracyclines).

Decreased plasma concentration (risk of decreased efficacy)

Antacids, theophylline, caffeine, chlorpromazine, bicarbonate, sodium-containing products.

---

1 The use of lithium salts in the treatment of "psychotic excitement" is usually credited to John Cade in 1949 (*Medical Journal of Australia* **2**, 349–352). However, this was a rediscovery of the application of lithium to the treatment of "insanity" first described by W.A. Hammond in 1871 ("The treatment of insanity" in *A Treatise on Diseases of the Nervous System*, New York: Appleton, 325–384). The use of a specific agent for a specific disorder heralded the start of the modern era of psychopharmacology. First approved by the FDA in 1970 for treatment in "manic depresssion."
2 Price, L.H. and Heninger, G.R. (1994). Lithium in the treatment of mood disorders *NEJM* **331**, 591–598.
3 Burgess, S,. Geddes, J,. Hawton, K., *et al.* (2002). *Lithium for Maintenance Treatment of Mood Disorders.* The Cochrane Library, 1 Oxford: Update Software.

Other interactions

Anti-arrhythmics (e.g., amiodarone: increased risk of hypothyroidism), antidiabetics (may sometimes impair glucose tolerance), antipsychotics (increased risk of EPS), parasympathomimetics (antagonizes neostigmine and pyridostigmine), MAOI (malignant hyperthermia), iodine salts (increase risk of hypothyroidism), neuromuscular-blocking agents (prolong blockade), sibutramine (risk of serotonin syndrome), others.

Initiating and monitoring lithium therapy

Prior to commencing lithium therapy

Renal function (BUN/Cr), thyroid function (TSH), pregnancy test (in women of child-bearing age), and EKG (for patients >50 yr). Also consider CBC with differential, electrolytes, urinalysis and 24-hour creatinine clearance (CrCl).

Starting dose

Usually start 300mg bid. Titrate dosage upwards (e.g., increase weekly in increments of 300mg/d) as indicated by plasma lithium level, clinical response, and side-effects.

Lithium levels

Check lithium level approximately 5 days after starting the medication and 5 days after each dosage adjustment. Blood samples should be trough levels 12 hours following the last dose. In acute stabilization, usual effective dose is approximately 1800mg/d in divided doses (target lithium level ~0.8–1.4 mmol/L). In maintenance phase, usual dosing range is 900–1200mg/d (target lithium level ~0.6–1.2 mmol/L). Of note, the optimal therapeutic lithium level may vary from patient to patient, however, a higher rate of relapse has been shown in healthy adults maintained at levels of <0.4mmol/L. Target lithium levels for the elderly and for patients with special medical considerations are generally lower. Actual dose also depends on preparation used (as molar availability varies even when milligram amounts are the same)—see opposite.

Maintenance monitoring

Once a therapeutic serum level (0.6–1.2mmol/L) has been established, ongoing lithium levels, renal function, and thyroid function must be followed.

During the first 6 months: check renal function and lithium level every 2–3 months, and thyroid function once or twice.

After the first 6 months: check renal function, thyroid function, and lithium level every 6–12 months or whenever clinically indicated.

Information for the patient

Starting lithium should be fully discussed with the patient, highlighting the relevant issues discussed in the pages following on adverse effects. Emphasis should be on a number of issues:
- How and when to take their dose,
- What to do if a dose is missed,
- Common side-effects and signs of toxicity,
- Potential long-term complications and thus the need for regular monitoring of blood levels, kidney, and thyroid functioning,
- What medications/illnesses may change blood levels,
- Effects of dehydration and dietary considerations,
- Appropriate contraceptive measures and dialogue about pregnancy risks,
- A reminder of these issues is usually given in the form of a pamphlet or information handout.

Lithium preparations

Preparation	Formulation	Available dosages
Eskalith	Capsule	300mg
Eskalith CR	Tablet (controlled release)	450mg (scored)
Lithobid	Tablet (slow release)	300mg
Lithium carbonate	Capsule	150/300/600mg
Lithium citrate	Syrup (contains alcohol)	300mg/5mL

Other dosing considerations
- Immediate-release formulations are usually initiated in divided doses (bid-tid), however, may be switched to qhs if tolerated.
- Controlled-release formulations may be given once daily at bedtime or divided bid.
- Sustained release formulations may reduce side-effects (especially GI distress) by lowering peak levels.
- When switching a patient from immediate-release capsules to controlled-release formulation, give the same total daily dose when possible.
- Rapid discontinuation of lithium increases relapse.
- May be most useful in patients with euphoric mania (versus those with mixed state or rapid cycling).
- Due to the delayed onset of action, often given in conjunction with benzodiazepines, antipsychotics, or valproic acid for the treatment of acute mania.
- Low-dose lithium may be an effective augmenting agent in the treatment of depression.

Lithium—adverse effects

Lithium has a narrow therapeutic window and has the potential of being highly toxic at supratherapeutic drug levels. Therefore, safe and effective therapy requires regular monitoring of serum levels. Up to 75% of patients treated with lithium will experience some side-effects.[1]

Dose-related side-effects

Polyuria/polydypsia (reduced ability to concentrate urine due to antidiuretic hormone [ADH] antagonism), weight gain (effects on carbohydrate metabolism and/or edema), cognitive problems (e.g., dulling, impaired memory, poor concentration, confusion, mental slowness), tremor, sedation/lethargy, impaired coordination, gastrointestinal distress (e.g., nausea, vomiting, dyspepsia, diarrhea), hair loss, benign leukocytosis, hypercalcemia, acne, and edema.

Management

Usually managed by lowering the dose, or altering the dose schedule or formulation. If side-effects persist, additional medications may be necessary: propranolol (tremor), thiazide diuretic or amiloride (nephrogenic diabetes insipidus), topical antibiotics or retinoic acid (acne). GI problems can be managed by administering lithium with meals or switching formulations (sustained release or lithium citrate). Patients with tremor at therapeutic lithium levels should avoid caffeine.

Cardiac conduction problems

Usually benign EKG changes (e.g., nonspecific T-wave changes, widening of QRS). Rarely, exacerbation of existing arrhythmias or induction of new arrhythmias due to conduction deficits at the SA or AV nodes. Lithium is contraindicated in heart failure, sick sinus syndrome, and severe cardiovascular disease.

Long-term effects

Renal function

Approximately 10–20% of patients on long-term therapy demonstrate morphological kidney changes (interstitial fibrosis, tubular atrophy, and sometimes glomerular sclerosis.), however, rarely clinically significant. There are case reports in which patients have developed irreversible renal failure after 10 years or more of treatment.

Subclinical/clinical hypothyroidism

5–35% of patients on lithium develop hypothyroidism. Thyroid dysfunction tends to appear 6–18 months after initiation of lithium. More frequent in women and patients >50 years old. Even though lithium-induced hypothyroidism is generally reversible upon discontinuation, it does not constitute an absolute contraindication for continuing lithium treatment as the associated hypothyroidism is readily treated with thyroxine.[2] It is worth noting that, in addition to the classic signs and symptoms of hypothyroidism,

---

1 Goodwin, F.K. and Jamison, K.R. *Manic-Depressive Illness*. London: Oxford University Press, 1990.
2 Jefferson, J.W. (ed.) *Lithium Encyclopedia for Clinical Practice*, 2nd ed. Washington, American Psychiatric Press, 1987.

patients with bipolar disorder are also at risk of developing depression and/or rapid cycling as a consequence of suboptimal thyroid functioning.[3]

Toxicity

The usual upper therapeutic limit for 12-hour postdose serum lithium level is 1.2mmol/l. With levels >1.5mmol/l most patients will experience some symptoms of toxicity; >2.0mmol/l definite, often life-threatening, toxic effects occur. There is often a narrow therapeutic window where the beneficial effects outweigh the toxic effects.

Early signs and symptoms

(Approx 1.5–2.0mmol/L) tremulousness, anorexia, nausea/vomiting, diarrhea (sometimes hematemesis) with associated dehydration and lethargy.

As lithium levels rise (>2.0mmol/L)

Severe neurological complications—restlessness, muscle fasciculation/myoclonic jerks, choreoathetoid movements, marked hypertonicity. This may progress to ataxia, dysarthria, increased lethargy, drowsiness, and confusion/delirium. Hypotension and cardiac arrhythmias generally precede circulatory collapse. As levels climb above 2.5mmol/L, there is serious risk of seizures, coma, permanent neurological impairment or even death.

Management

• Prevention by patient psycho-education; e.g., maintaining hydration and salt intake, avoiding certain medications (see 📖 p. 376) and being watchful for early signs and symptoms of toxicity.

• Careful adjustment of lithium dosage may be all that is required in mild toxicity.

• In moderate to severe toxicity (e.g., following overdose), rapid steps to reduce serum lithium level are urgently necessary. This may involve forced diuresis with intravenous isotonic saline and electrolyte repletion. There is no antidote, however; **hemodialysis** is the treatment of choice in cases where toxicity is severe or accompanied by significant renal failure.

Teratogenicity

The much-quoted 400-fold increased risk of **Ebstein's anomaly** (a congenital malformation of the tricuspid valve) due to first trimester lithium exposure,[4] now appears to be substantially less than first reported—at most an eightfold relative risk[5]. Other reported second and third trimester problems include polyhydramnios, premature delivery, thyroid abnormalities, nephrogenic diabetes insipidus, and floppy baby syndrome. The estimated risk of major congenital anomalies for lithium-exposed babies is 4–12% compared with 2–4% in control groups. Even so, lithium today is considered a first-line treatment of bipolar disorder during pregnancy.

3 Bocchetta, A., Bernardi, F., Pedditzi, M., et al. (1991). Thyroid abnormalities during lithium treatment. Acta Psychiatr Scand. **83**, 193–198.
4 Weinstein, M.R. (1980). In: Johnson FN (ed.) Handbook of Lithium Therapy. MTP Press, 421–429.

Management

A careful balance needs to be struck between the risks of teratogenicity and the risks of relapse following discontinuation. Cohen et al. (1994)[5] suggested guidelines:

- mild, stable forms of bipolar disorder—lithium may be tapered down and stopped prepregnancy,
- moderate risk of relapse—lithium should be tapered and discontinued during the first trimester (4–12 weeks after last menstrual period),
- severe forms of bipolar disorder, who are at high risk of relapse— lithium should be maintained during pregnancy (with informed consent, appropriate counseling, prenatal diagnosis and detailed ultrasound and echocardiography at 16–18 weeks gestation). During pregnancy, lithium levels should be monitored every 2–4 weeks; weekly in the last month; and every few days before and after delivery.[6]

5 Cohen, L.S., Friedman, J.M., Jefferson, J.W., et al. (1994). A reevaluation of risk of in utero exposure to lithium. *JAMA* **271**, 146–150.
6 Yonkers, et al., (2004). Management of bipolar disorder during pregnancy and the postpartum period. *Am J Psychiatry* **161**, 608–620.

Valproate/valproic acid

Valproic acid was the first FDA-approved antiepileptic drug (AED) for the treatment of acute mania. To this day, it remains a first-line agent in the treatment of bipolar disorder. Furthermore, there is data to suggest that it may be more effective than other mood stabilizing agents in mixed episodes and rapid cycling. Beyond mood stabilization, it is also indicated in various seizure disorders and migraine headaches.

Mode of action

Uncertain. Modulates voltage-sensitive sodium channels, acts on second-messenger systems, and increases bioavailability of GABA (or mimics action at postsynaptic receptor sites) in the central nervous system.

Pharmacokinetics

Rapidly absorbed when taken orally (peak serum level 1–5hr) with a plasma half-life of 6–16 hrs. Time to steady-state 2–3 days. Highly protein bound (80–90%) and has non-linear, saturation-dependent kinetics. Extensively metabolized by the liver.

Interactions

- Decreased serum levels with carbamazepine, cholestyramine, phenytoin, rifampin, primidone, topiramate.
- Raised serum levels with felbamate, clarithromycin, chlorpromazine, antidepressants (especially TCAs, fluoxetine).
- Toxicity may be precipitated by other highly protein-bound drugs (e.g., aspirin), which can displace valproate from its protein-binding sites.

Side-effects and toxicity

Dose-related side-effects

GI upset (anorexia, nausea, dyspepsia, vomiting, diarrhea), elevated LFTs, tremor, dizziness, ataxia, asthenia, headache, and sedation—if persistent, may require dose reduction, change in preparation, or treatment of specific symptoms (e.g., beta-blocker for tremor; H_2-blocker for dyspepsia).

Unpredictable side-effects

Mild leukopenia and thrombocytopenia (reversible upon drug reduction/discontinuation), hair loss (usually transient; consider treatment with multivitamin with Zinc/Selenium), increased appetite, and weight gain.

Rare, idiosyncratic side-effects

Irreversible hepatic failure, pancreatitis, agranulocytosis, polycystic ovarian syndrome/hyperandrogenism, and teratogenicity.

Teratogenicity see 📖 p. 392

Toxicity/overdose

Wide therapeutic window, hence unintentional overdose is uncommon. Hemodialysis may be needed as toxicity can proceed to heartblock, coma, and even death.

Treatment guidelines

- Before starting: CBC with platelets, LFTs, and pregnancy test (in women of child-bearing age). Also consider baseline EKG and coagulation labwork (if history of bleeding).
- Acute Mania: Load 15–20mg/kg/day (or approximately 750–1000mg) divided in bid dosing (or qhs with extended-release). May load 30mg/kg/d in the inpatient setting.
- Nonacute: Initiate 250–500mg/day divided in bid dosing (or qhs with extended-release), then titrate upwards.
- Although there is no well-established correlation between serum concentrations and mood-stabilizing effects, clinicians will generally target 50–120mcg/mL.
- Extended release formulations (e.g., Depakote ER) should be administered once daily using a dose 8–20% higher than the total daily dose of the immediate-release formulation.
- If GI upset is a problem, consider changing to enteric-coated or slow-release formulation.

Monitoring

- VPA level: Measure five days after start of medication, five days after change in dose, or whenever addition/discontinuation of other interacting drugs.
- CBC: baseline, at two months, and then two to three times/year.
- LFTs: baseline, at two months, and then two to three times/year.
- Other: Follow weight, fasting glucose, and fasting lipids annually. Consider testosterone in women with symptoms of hyperandrogenism or menstrual irregularities. Consider ammonia level if mental status changes. Check platelet counts and coagulation labwork prior to planned surgeries or as clinically indicated. Consider amylase in patient with GI discomfort.

Valproate/valproic acid preparations

Preparation	Active agent	Available dosages
Depakote	Divalproex sodium	Caps 125/250/500mg
Depakote Sprinkles	Divalproex sodium	Caps 125mg
Depakote ER	Divalproex sodium	Tabs 250/500mg
Depakene	Valproic acid	Caps 250mg
Depakene Elixir	Valproic acid	Liq 250mg/5mL
Depacon	Sodium valproate	IV 100mg/mL

Carbamazepine

Although psychiatrists have been using carbamazepine as a second or third line mood stabilizer for years, only recently did Equetro™ earn FDA approval for the treatment of acute manic and mixed episodes associated with bipolar I disorder. Carbamazepine is also approved for use in various seizure disorders and trigeminal neuralgia.

Pharmacokinetics

Peak plasma concentrations usually 4–12 hrs (depending on formulation), may be as late as 26 hrs. Plasma half-life 18–55hrs. With long-term use, carbamazepine **induces its own metabolism**, decreasing the half-life 5–26 hrs. The pharmacokinetics of extended-release carbamazepine is linear over the single dose range of 200–800mg. 76% protein-bound. Metabolized by the liver; cytochrome P450 3A4 is the major isoform.

Mode of action

Uncertain. Modulates sodium and calcium ion channels, receptor-mediation of GABA and glutamine, and various intracellular signaling pathways.

Interactions

- Carbamazepine decreases the plasma levels of many drugs metabolized by the liver, e.g., antipsychotics, BZDs (except clonazepam), TCAs, other anticonvulsants, hormonal contraceptives, thyroid hormones.
- Carbamazepine serum concentrations can be increased by certain drugs e.g., erythromycin, calcium channel blockers (diltiazem and verapamil, but not nifedipine or nimodipine), SSRIs.
- Contraindicated in use with MAOI, nefazodone, protease inhibitors, azole antifungals.

Side-effects and toxicity

Unpredictable side-effects

Antidiuretic effects leading to hyponatremia (6–31%), probably more common in the elderly, sometimes developing many months after starting treatment; decrease in total and free thyroxin levels; increase in free cortisol levels (rarely clinically significant).

Idiosyncratic side-effects

Agranulocytosis, aplastic anemia, hepatic failure, exfoliative dermatitis (e.g., Stevens-Johnson syndrome), and pancreatitis (these side-effects usually occur within the first three to six months of treatment, rarely after longer periods). Routine blood monitoring does not reliably predict blood dyscrasias, hepatic failure, or exfoliative dermatitis—patient education about early symptoms and signs essential.

Other rare side-effects

Systemic hypersensitivity reactions, cardiac conduction problems, psychiatric symptoms, extremely rare renal problems (failure, oliguria, hematuria, and proteinuria).

Teratogenic effects (see 📖 p.392)
Toxicity/overdose

Early signs: dizziness, ataxia, sedation, and diplopia. Acute intoxication may present as marked irritability, stupor, or even coma. May be fatal in overdose (if >6g ingested). Symptoms of overdose: nystagmus, ophthal-moplegia, cerebellar/extrapyramidal signs, impairment of consciousness, convulsions, respiratory depression, cardiac problems (tachycardia, hypotension, arrhythmias/conduction disturbances), GI upset, and other anticholinergic symptoms. Significant overdose requires emergency medical management (i.e., close monitoring, symptomatic treatment, gastric lavage, and possible hemodialysis.)

Treatment guidelines for carbamazepine

- Prior to starting: CBC, liver/kidney/thyroid functions, pregnancy test, baseline Na. Consider EKG.
- Initiate with a dose of 200mg bid, then increase 200mg/day at weekly interval. Divide dosing bid (extended release formulation) or tid-qid (immediate release formulation). Usual total daily dosage range is 800–1,200mg. Maximum daily dose is 2,000mg/day, however doses higher than 1,600mg/day are generally not recommended.
- Although there is no well-established correlation between serum concentrations and mood-stabilizing effects, clinicians will generally target a trough level of 4–15 mcg/mL.

Monitoring

- Carbamazepine level: Measure five days after start of medication, five days after change in dose, or whenever addition/discontinuation of other interacting drugs.
- CBC with platelets: baseline, then every two weeks for two months, then every three months.
- LFTs: baseline, then every two weeks for two months, then every three to six months.
- BMP: baseline, then every six months.
- TFTs: baseline, then every six months.
- Other: Consider obtaining baseline and regular iron levels. Obtain EKG as clinically indicated (e.g., >45 years of age, cardiac history, etc.). Baseline and periodic eye exams recommended.

Carbamazepine preparations

Preparation	Formulation	Available dosages
Tegretol	Tablet (also in chewable form)	100/200mg
Tegretol Elixir	Suspension	100mg/5mL
Tegretol XL	Extended release tablet	100/200/400mg ER
Carbatrol	Extended release capsule	100/200/300mg ER
Equetro	Extended release capsule	100/200/300mg ER
Carbamazepine	Tablet (also in chewable form)	100/200mg
Carbamazepine	Suspension	100mg/5mL

Oxcarbazepine

Oxcarbazepine has the identical chemical structure of carbamazepine, and differs only in that it contains a keto-group substitution in the 10–11 position. Because it tends to be better tolerated and does not appear to confer the same adverse risk profile, this newer antiepileptic drug has been used increasingly as an alternative agent in the treatment of Bipolar disorder. Unfortunately, it is not as well studied, but early evidence suggests that it has similar mechanism to carbamazepine.

Mode of action

Unknown. In vitro studies suggest that the active metabolite blocks voltage-sensitive sodium channels.

Pharmacokinetics

Time to peak serum level 3–13 hours. The half-life is 2–9 hours. Steady state plasma concentrations are reached within 2–3 days when given bid. Approximately 40% protein bound. Oxcarbazepine is rapidly metabolized in the liver to its active metabolite (10-monohydroxy-oxcarbazepine) which is primarily responsible for the medication's pharmacological effect.

Interactions

- Oxcarbazepine may reduce serum levels of calcium channel blockers, clarithromycin, protease inhibitors, and oral contraceptives.
- Contraindicated in use with MAOI.

Side-effects and toxicity

Most common side-effects

Dizziness, somnolence, diplopia, fatigue, nasea, vomiting, ataxia, abnormal vision, abdominal pain, tremor, dyspepsia, and abnormal gait. These were typically mild-moderate in severity.

Idiosyncratic side-effects

Association with cognitive adverse events including psychomotor slowing, difficulty concentrating, speech/language difficulties, somnolence/fatigue, coordination abnormalities (e.g., ataxia and gait disturbances).

Serious side-effects

Clinically significant hyponatremia (sodium <125 mEq/L) has been observed in 2.5% of patients in controlled trials (generally during the first 3 months of treatment). Of those patients who are allergic to carbamazepine, 35–30% will have a reaction to oxcarbazepine.

Other rare side-effects

Serious dermatological reactions (including Stevens-Johnson syndrome and toxic epidermal necrolysis) have been reported.

Teratogenic effects see 📖 p. 392

Treatment guidelines for oxcarbazepine
- Prior to starting: pregnancy test (in women of child-bearing age) and serum electrolytes with sodium level.
- Initiate with a dose of 300mg bid, then increase 300–600mg/day at weekly intervals. Usual total daily dosage is 1,200mg/day divided bid. Doses >2,400mg/d are generally not advised.

Monitoring
- Electrolytes: baseline, at one month, and then every three months (or as clinically indicated for signs/symptoms of hyponatremia; e.g., nausea, malaise, headache, lethargy, obtundation). Of note, however, most patients who develop hyponatremia are initially asymptomatic.

Oxcarbazepine preparations

Preparation	Formulation	Available dosages
Trileptal	Tablet (scored)	150/300/600mg
Trileptal Elixir	Liquid	300mg/5mL

Lamotrigine

Indicated for the maintenance treatment of bipolar disorder to delay the time to occurrence of mood episodes (depression, mania, hypomania, mixed episodes). There is some evidence that lamotrigine may be more effective than other mood stabilizers in preventing depressive episodes in bipolar disorder. Evidence is supported by two multicenter, double-blind, placebo-controlled studies in adult patients who met DSM-IV criteria for bipolar I disorder. The effectiveness in the acute treatment of mood episodes has not been established.

Mode of action

Unknown. Inhibits voltage-gated sodium channels and glutamate release. Also has weak inhibitory effect at 5-HT$_3$ receptors.

Pharmacokinetics

Rapidly and completely absorbed after oral administration with negligible first-pass metabolism (absolute bioavailability is 98%). The bioavailability is not affected by food drug administration. Peak plasma concentrations occur anywhere from 1–5 hours following. Half-life 24 hours, and time to steady state is 5–8 days. Drug is 55% protein bound.

Interactions

- Certain medications have been shown to increase clearance of lamotrigine (meaning level of lamotrigine is reduced): carbamazepine (40%), oxcarbazepine (30%), phenobarbital (40%), phenytoin (50%), ritonavir, methsuximide, rifampin, primidone, and certain estrogen-containing oral contraceptives.
- **Valproate decreases the clearance of lamotrigine** (more than doubles the elimination half-life of lamotrigine). Accordingly, if administered to a patient receiving valproate, lamotrigine must be given at a reduced dosage, of no more than half the dose used in patients not receiving valproate, even in the presence of drugs that increase the apparent clearance of lamotrigine.

Side-effects and toxicity

Most common side-effects

Dizziness, headache, blurred or double vision, lack of coordination, sleepiness, nausea, vomiting, insomnia, and rash.

Rare side-effects

Rare incidence of multiorgan failure and various degrees of hepatic failure. Some cases has been fatal or irreversible, however, the majority of these deaths occurred in association with other serious medical events, making it difficult to identify the initial cause.

Risk of rash

Approximately 10–14% of patients receiving lamotrigine will develop a rash. Although the majority of rashes are benign, some individuals may develop a serious skin reaction that requires hospitalization. Among these rashes include Stevens-Johnson syndrome, toxic epidermal necrolysis, angioedema, and a rash associated with a variable number of the following systemic manifestations (e.g., fever, lymphadenopathy, facial swelling, hematologic, and hepatologic abnormalities). Rarely, deaths have been reported.

These serious skin reactions are most likely to occur within the first 2–8 weeks of treatment. It has been suggested that the risk of rash increases with coadministration with valproate, exceeding the recommended initial dose, or exceeding the recommended dose escalation. Although most rashes resolve even with continuation of treatment, it is not possible to predict reliably which rashes will prove to be serious or life threatening. Accordingly, **lamotrigine should ordinarily be discontinued at first sign** of rash, unless the rash is clearly not drug related. Discontinuation of treatment may not prevent a rash from becoming life threatening or permanently disabling/disfiguring. It is recommended that lamotrigine not be restarted in patients who discontinued due to rash associated with prior treatment with lamotrigine, unless the potential benefits clearly outweigh the risks.

Other rare side-effects
Serious hypersensitivity reactions, blood dyscrasias (neutropenia, leukopenia, anemia, thrombocytopenia, pancytopenia, and, rarely, aplastic anemia and pure red cell aplasia), withdrawal seizures.

Teratogenic effects see 📖 p. 392

Treatment guidelines for lamotrigine
- Prior to starting: pregnancy test (in women of child-bearing age).
- *As monotherapy*: Start 25mg/day for weeks 1 and 2. Increase to 50mg/day for weeks 3 and 4. Increase to 100mg/day for week 5. Increase to 200mg for week 6 and onward. Target dose: 200mg.
- *With valproate*: Start 25mg every other day for weeks 1 and 2. Increase to 25mg/day for weeks 3 and 4. Increase to 50mg/day for Week 5. Increase to 100mg/day for week 6 and onward. Target dose: 100mg.
- *With carbamazepine* (and/or phenytoin, phenobarbital, primidone, rifampin) and NOT taking Valproate: Start 50mg/day for weeks 1 and 2. Increase to 100mg/day for week 3 and 4. Increase to 200mg/day for Week 5. Increase to 300mg for week 6. Increase to 400mg for week 7 and onward. Target dose: 400mg/day (usually given in bid divided dose).
- If a patient has discontinued lamotrigine for a period of more than five half-lives, it is recommended that initial dosing recommendations and guidelines be followed.
- Although there is no well-established correlation between serum concentrations and mood-stabilizing effects, antiepileptic therapeutic serum levels are 8–10mcg/mL.

Monitoring

- Drug levels: The value of monitoring plasma concentrations has not been established. Because of the possible pharmacokinetic interactions, however, monitoring of the plasma levels of concomitant drugs may be indicated, particularly during dosage adjustments.
- Prior to initiation of treatment, the patient should be instructed that a rash or other signs or symptoms of hypersensitivity (e.g., fever, lymphadenopathy, hives, painful sores in the mouth or around the eyes, or swelling of lips or tongue) may herald a serious medical event and that the patient should be seen by a physician immediately to determine if lamotrigine should be discontinued.

Lamotrigine preparations

Preparation	Formulation	Available dosages
Lamictal	Tablet (chewable available)	25/100/150/200mg; 2/5/25mg (CH)
Lamotrigine	Tablet (chewable available)	2/25mg

Teratogenicity of antiepileptics

Unfortunately, there are no large-scale, clinically controlled studies comparing the relative risks of each antiepileptic drug (AED) during pregnancy.

The European and International Registry of Antiepileptic Drugs in Pregnancy surveillance system suggests that the risk for major congenital malformations is higher with valproic acid (6.1%) when compared to carbamazepine (2.3%) or lamotrigine (2.9%).[1] Most notably, there is an estimated 1–2% estimated risk for neural tube defect among infants born to mothers receiving valproate during the first trimester of pregnancy (as compared with 0.14–0.2% in the general population). Frequently, patients are not even aware they are pregnant at the time of fetal neural tube closure (i.e., 17–30 days postconception). This highlights the importance of discussing potential teratogenic effects with all women of child-bearing age and monitoring contraceptive status, even if they do not intend to become pregnant.

1 Morrow, J. (2004). Getting it right for children born to mothers with epilepsy: morphology. Epilepsia **45**(Suppl3), 206.

There is less solid evidence that carbamazepine also may carry a 0.5% elevated risk of spina bifida. The Center for Disease Control strongly recommends at least 0.4mg of folic acid daily to be given to all women of childbearing age, as this has shown to reduce the risk of spina bifida. Certain AEDs (phenobarbital, phenytoin, primidone, and carbamazepine) are competitive inhibitors of prothrombin precursors, which pose a risk of neonatal hemorrhage. Therefore, most experts recommend administering Vitamin K 20mg daily to pregnant patients taking these medications (and 1mg IM to the newborn). Though lamotrigine and oxcarbazepine have been used in Europe for at least a decade, there is little information available on their safety in pregnancy. Other AED-related complications include neonatal irritability, jitteriness, feeding difficulties, hypotonia, hepatic toxicity, hypoglycemia, limb malformations, craniofacial abnormalities, and growth and development difficulties.

Atypical antipsychotics

All atypical antipsychotics are FDA approved for use in the treatment of schizophrenia, however, some now carry FDA approved indications for acute mania, bipolar mania, bipolar depression, and bipolar maintenance. Atypical antipsychotic medications include:

- Clozapine (Clozaril®).
- Olanzapine (Zyprexa®).
- Risperidone (Risperdal®).
- Quetiapine (Seroquel®).
- Ziprasidone (Geodon®).
- Aripiprazole (Abilify®).
- Paliperidone (Invega®).

Refer to Chapter 6, Schizophrenia and related psychoses for detailed pharmacologic parameters and side-effect profiles of these medications.

Anxiety and stress-related disorders

Introduction

Anxiety disorders are highly prevalent and disabling psychiatric conditions. The lifetime prevalence and 12-month prevalence of any anxiety disorder is approximately 25% and 18%, respectively, resulting in substantial morbidity, functional impairments, and utilization of health care services. Fortunately, treatments for many anxiety disorders are some of the most effective in psychiatry.

Although anxiety disorders frequently share common features (physiological/autonomic reactivity, avoidance behaviors, apprehension), the DSM-IV has divided them into the following categories based upon the differential involvement of feared objects or situations and distinct constellations of symptoms:

- Phobias—characterized by excessive fear related to specific objects or situations.
- Panic disorder—involves recurrent episodes of spontaneous sudden increase in fear associated with autonomic symptoms.
- Generalized anxiety disorder (GAD)—a pattern of pervasive worry.
- Obsessive-compulsive disorder (OCD)—anxiety-producing intrusive thoughts or images (obsessions) and anxiety-neutralizing repetitive behaviors (compulsions).
- Post-traumatic stress disorder (PTSD)—involves the threat of death, injury, severe harm and a resultant fear, helplessness, or horror.

We can all be empathic toward those with anxiety disorders in that we have all experienced symptoms of anxiety. Anxiety is a highly adaptive phenomenon, similar to physical pain, capable of protecting us from harm and motivating us to achieve our goals. The many individuals who suffer from anxiety disorders, however, experience excessive and inappropriate anxiety, causing marked distress and/or substantial interference in their day-to-day lives.

Points to note

- "Symptoms" are common in the general population.
- Co-morbidity is frequent (other anxiety disorders, mood disorders, substance use, personality disorders).
- May often present with physical symptoms.
- Must be recognized if they are to be treated appropriately.
- Management will usually involve a combined approach (pharmacological and psychological).

Table 9.1 Twelve-month prevalence and severity of *DSM-IV* and WMH-CIDI disorders in 9282 respondents (Kessler *et al.* 2005[1]). WMH-CIDI (World Health Organization Composite International Diagnostic Interview). Values are expressed as percentage (standard error). Percentages in the three severity columns are repeated as proportions of all cases and sum to 100% across each row.

| | Total | Severity | | |
		Serious	Moderate	Mild
Anxiety disorders				
Panic disorder	2.7(0.2)	44.8(3.2)	29.5(2.7)	25.7(2.5)
Agraphobia without panic	0.8(0.1)	40.6(7.2)	30.7(6.4)	28.7(8.4)
Specific phobia	8.7(0.4)	21.9(2.0)	30.0(2.0)	48.1(2.1)
Social phobia	6.8(0.3)	29.9(2.0)	38.8(2.5)	31.3(2.4)
Generalized anxiety disorder	3.1(0.2)	32.3(2.9)	44.6(4.0)	23.1(2.9)
Post-traumatic stress disorder	3.5(0.3)	36.6(3.5)	33.1(2.2)	30.2(3.4)
Obsessive-complusive disorder	1.0(0.3)	50.6(12.4)	34.8(14.1)	14.6(5.7)
Seperation anxiety disorder	0.9(0.2)	43.3(9.2)	24.8(7.5)	31.9(12.2)
Any anxiety disorder ||	18.1(0.7)	22.8(1.5)	33.7(1.4)	43.5(2.1)

1 Kessler R.C., *et al.* (2005). Lifetime prevalence and age-of-onset distributions of DSM-IV disorders in the National Co-morbidify Survey Replication. *Arch Gen Psychiatry* **62**, 593–602.

Historical perspective

The history of anxiety disorders is embedded in the history of the "neuroses," which were first described in 1777 by William Cullen to mean any disease of the nervous system without a known organic basis. The history of the neuroses is tightly bound to the (re)discovery of hypnosis (formerly thought of as "faith healing"). The work of Franz-Anton Mesmer [1734–1815] ("mesmerism") and James Braid [1795–1860] ("braidism") was brought to France by Azam in 1859, coming to the attention of Charcot, whose experiments with "hysterics" would have a profound influence on one particular assistant—Sigmund Freud. Freud's first paper, published in 1886, shortly after his return to Vienna, was of a case of "traumatic hysteria" in a male patient. It was his *Studies on Hysteria*, written with Josef Breuer and published in 1895, which provided the starting point of all his subsequent major concepts of psychoanalytical theory—including repression, psychic reality, and the subconscious.

Sigmund Freud

Freud used the term "neuroses" to describe conditions that reflected anxiety and its various defenses, including conversion, repression, and displacement. The use of the term "neurosis" in American psychiatry was gradually deemphasized as the Diagnostic and Statistical Manual (DSM) evolved. In the original DSM in 1952, anxiety disorders were described in the "psychoneurotic disorders" category. Anxiety was defined as a "danger signal felt and perceived by the conscious portion of the personality." The various ways in which the patient expressed their anxiety, were listed as "reactions," including anxiety, dissociative, conversion, phobic, and obsessive-compulsive reactions. The association between anxiety disorders and neuroses endured until DSM-IV, when the "neuroses" terminology was dropped and anxiety disorders emerged as their own separate entity.

The origins of anxiety

Throughout the 20th century, analysts and behaviorists debated over the origins of anxiety. While psychoanalytic/psychodynamic formulations described anxiety as a threat to the ego and the manifestation of unconscious conflict, behaviorists argued that anxiety disorders were expressions of conditioned fear and were reinforced and triggered throughout life. John Watson, the father of behaviorism, explained anxiety via his classical conditioning study of Little Albert, an 11-month-old boy, which involved the pairing of a furry rat to an unconditioned loud noise. The conditioned fear generalized to other furry animals. Watson argued that he had produced an animal phobia in Little Albert, as manifested by the child's later fear of rabbits and other furry animals (representing the generalization of a conditioned fear.) Watson proposed that anxiety arose out of traumatic learning situations and then persisted to influence behavior throughout life.

A combination of bench research as well as pharmacological trials gradually led to a broader understanding of the role of several brain "systems" in the pathophysiology of anxiety disorders, including the norepinephric, limbic, and serotonergic systems. A growing literature that included neurophysiology and lesion studies revealed the importance of the central norepinephric system in anxiety disorders. Stimulation and blockage of the locus ceruleus led to the onset and decrease of panic attacks, respectively. The arrival of the benzodiazepines in the 1950s and their widespread use and efficacy illuminated the role of GABA in anxiety. The role of serotonin in anxiety was later highlighted following the efficacy of clomipramine in the treatment of OCD. The fact that clomipramine was the most serotonergic of the TCAs, paved the way for the second-generation antidepressants (the SSRIs) to be used to treat anxiety disorders (previously thought only to be amenable to psychological approaches).

1980s

In the 1980s, neuroimaging studies demonstrated underlying functional changes in OCD patients (in the frontal cortex [left orbital gyrus] and bilateral caudate nuclei), which "normalized" after successful treatment with medication (and interestingly with CBT techniques—although this took longer). For many patients with panic attacks, structural and functional changes were found in the temporal lobes. These findings resonated with the long-held observation that symptoms of anxiety disorders (e.g., anxiety, panic, somatic symptoms, depersonalization/derealization) were often reported in other "organic" conditions (e.g., temporal lobe epilepsy). A greater understanding of the significant role of the amygdala and other limbic structures in both normal emotion regulation as well as in disorders of emotion continues to evolve. Furthermore, a growing understanding of the neural mechanisms involved in fear suggests that anxiety disorders may result from a loss of cortical control over a primitive fear system. Animal conditioning and human neuroimaging studies suggest the presence of prewired survival responses and signals stored in the amygdala, as well as stress-induced abnormalities in the hippocampus that, taken together, contribute to the expression of anxiety disorder symptoms.

The present day

The current view of anxiety disorders encompasses a biopsychosocial model of illness. Not only are anxiety disorders heritable, but early environmental influences (including "social" factors like maternal deprivation) can alter the sensitivity of physiological stress responses in adulthood. Hence, the experience of stressors (psychological or physical) may lead (e.g., through the effects of "stress hormones" such as cortisol, and other neurophysiological mechanisms) to alterations in the structure and/or function of the brain, which in turn manifest as clinical symptoms (i.e., behavioral and/or emotional change).

Panic disorder (1)[1–7]

Description

Panic disorder is a chronic and distressing psychiatric condition characterized by panic attacks that are followed by at least one month of concern about future panic attacks or the implications and consequences of these attacks. Panic attacks may result in significant behavioral changes, such as avoidance of specific situations for fear of having a panic attack. Panic attacks are associated with physiological (i.e., heart palpitations) and somatic symptoms (i.e., cardiac) as well as anticipatory anxiety and frequently, agoraphobia (situations from which escape may be difficult or where a panic attack may occur are either avoided or endured with significant distress). Symptoms of panic disorder cause significant impairment in social and occupational functioning.

Clinical features

Clinical presentation

Panic attacks are accompanied by physical symptoms, including the following: heart palpitations and elevated heart rate; sweating; trembling or shaking; feeling of shortness of breath or smothering; feeling of choking; chest pain or discomfort; nausea or abdominal distress; feeling dizzy, unsteady or faint; derealization; depersonalization; fear of loss of control or going crazy; fear of dying; paresthesias (numbness or tingling sensation); chills or hot flashes. Limited symptom panic attacks include a subset (less than 4) of the 13 symptoms. Panic attacks may have a sudden onset and can occur during sleep. Concerns about future attacks may result in agoraphobia. Agoraphobia most often develops within 1 year of onset of panic attacks. Symptoms of panic disorder often wax and wane, though the course may be chronic for some individuals.

DSM-IV-TR criteria for panic attack

Note: A panic attack is not a codable disorder. Code the specific diagnosis in which the panic attack occurs A discrete period of intense fear or discomfort, in which four (or more) of the following symptoms developed abruptly and reached a peak within 10 minutes:

(1) palpitations, pounding heart, or accelerated heart rate
(2) sweating
(3) trembling or shaking
(4) sensations of shortness of breath or smothering
(5) feeling of choking
(6) chest pain or discomfort
(7) nausea or abdominal distress
(8) feeling dizzy, unsteady, lightheaded, or faint
(9) derealization (feelings of unreality) or depersonalization (being detached from oneself)
(10) fear of losing control or going crazy
(11) fear of dying

---

(12) paresthesias (numbness or tingling sensations)
(13) chills or hot flushes

DSM-IV-TR criteria for panic disorder

A. Both (1) and (2):

(1) recurrent unexpected panic attacks

(2) at least one of the attacks has been followed by 1 month (or more) of one (or more) of the following:

  (a) persistent concern about having additional attacks

  (b) worry about the implications of the attack or its consequences (e.g., losing control, having a heart attack, "going crazy")

  (c) a significant change in behavior related to the attacks

    —the attacks cannot be due to a substance, a general medical condition, or be better explained by another Axis 1 disorder.

    —the disorder can occur with or without agoraphobia (anxiety about being in places or situations from which escape might be difficult (or embarrassing) or in which help may not be available in the event of having an unexpected or situationally predisposed panic attack or panic-like symptoms).

Diagnosis

A clinical diagnosis should include the following: psychiatric interview, review of symptoms, physical exam and history.

Differential diagnosis

Anxiety due to a general medical condition; substance-induced anxiety disorder; other anxiety disorders; psychotic disorders; social phobia; specific phobia; generalized anxiety disorder; obsessive-compulsive disorder; post-traumatic stress disorder; separation anxiety disorder; delusional disorder. Medical conditions that may lead to panic attack-like symptoms (hyperthyroidism, congestive heart failure [CHF], chronic obstructive pulmonary disease [COPD], myocardial infarction [MI]).

Co-morbidity

10–65% have at least one co-morbid psychiatric disorder. Common co-morbid conditions include the following: major depression (10–65%); bipolar disorder; substance-related disorder; social phobia and generalized anxiety disorder (15–30%); specific phobia (2–20%); obsessive-compulsive disorder (0–10%); post-traumatic stress disorder (2–10%). Co-morbid medical conditions may include irritable bowel syndrome; COPD; hyperthyroidism; cardiac arrhythmias; dizziness. A later onset of the disorder is associated with a greater frequency of co-morbid conditions.

Panic disorder (2)

Epidemiology

In the general population the prevalence of panic disorder is approximately 1 to 4%. Prevalence in a primary care or medical setting is higher (up to 60% in cardiac clinics). In the general population agoraphobia is present in 50% of those with panic disorder. In clinical samples, a higher rate of agoraphobia is present. Studies suggest a bimodal distribution of incidence, with one peak in late adolescence and another smaller peak in adulthood (mid 30s). The prevalence is greatest in those 25–44 years of age. Male/female ratio is at least 2:1. Recurrent mild subclinical symptoms of panic disorder are found in approximately 3.6% of the population.

Etiology

Causes

The causes of panic disorder remain to be fully elucidated; however there are several hypotheses regarding its etiology and pathogenesis. Panic disorder is associated with sensitivity to inhaled CO_2, which may lead to hyperventilation. This exaggerated response has been linked to abnormalities in cholinergic receptors, which regulate physiological responses to CO_2 intake. The subjective experience of hyperventilation may precipitate panic disorder symptoms. Prefrontal and sub-cortical alterations in blood flow may be affected by hypercapnia.

Genetics

Panic disorder is highly familial. Panic disorder is 8 times more likely in first-degree relatives of those with the diagnosis. Panic disorder is 20 times more likely in first degree relatives if illness onset was prior to age 20. Studies suggest genetic and non-genetic factors are important in risk for developing panic disorder.

Treatment

Psychotherapy

Cognitive behavior therapy (CBT) is a preferred and effective treatment for panic disorder. Behavior therapy (BT) and CBT are equally effective in reducing anxiety in panic disorder. However, CBT, in comparison to BT, is associated with lower drop out rates and is superior in reducing depressive symptoms.

Pharmacotherapy

Pharmacotherapy is an effective treatment for panic disorder. There are no differences in efficacy or in compliance rates between the use of Benzodiazapines (BDZs), TCAs, and SSRIs. Long-term treatment with BDZs should be used with caution due to the increasing risks of physical dependence and withdrawal, as well as memory impairment. SSRIs are preferred to BDZs and TCAs for long-term use due to a more favorable side-effect profile. Maintenance treatment is recommended for approximately 12–24 months and, in some cases, indefinitely. The doses used are similar to those used to treat major depression.

Combination therapy
The combination of CBT and pharmacotherapy is slightly more effective than CBT alone for all symptom categories but not for quality of life in the short term. Long-term follow up studies examining the efficacy of CBT, pharmacotherapy, and their combination are limited.

Prognosis

Studies suggest poor outcome and that full remission occurs in 10–35% of patients. Early onset is associated with a longer duration of illness compared to late onset.

Panic disorder—management guidelines

Combination of pharmacological and psychological treatments may be superior to single approach.

Pharmacological[1,2]

- SSRIs (e.g., sertraline, fluoxetine, fluvoxamine, citalopram) are recommended as the drugs of choice. In view of the possibility of initially increasing panic symptoms, start with low dose and gradually increase. Beneficial effect may take 3–8 weeks.
- Alternative antidepressants TCAs (e.g., imipramine or clomipramine) have been shown to be 70–80% effective (possible alternatives include: desipramine, doxepin, nortryptiline, or amitriptyline). MAOIs (e.g., phenelzine) may be superior to TCAs (for severe, chronic symptoms).
- BDZs (e.g., alprazolam or clonazepam) should be used with caution (due to potential for abuse/dependence/cognitive impairment) but may be effective for severe, frequent, incapacitating symptoms. Use for one to two weeks in combination with an antidepressant may "cover" and provide symptomatic relief until the antidepressant becomes effective. Note: "Antipanic" effects do not show tolerance, although sedative effects do. Clonazepam and Diazepam, due to longer half-lives, can "self-taper" and therefore are less likely to cause adverse withdrawal effects during cessation of medication trial.
- If initial management is ineffective consider change to a different class agent (i.e., TCA, SSRI, MAOI) or combination (e.g., TCA+lithium, SSRI+TCA, watching carefully for "serotonin syndrome"). If treatment-resistant, consider alternative agent (e.g., carbamazepine, valproate, gabapentin, low-potency BDZ [diazepam—may need high dose], venlafaxine, inositol, verapamil).
- If successful continue treatment for ~1yr before trial discontinuation (gradual tapering of dose). Do not confuse "withdrawal" effects (10–20% of patients) with re-emergence of symptoms (50–70% of patients). If symptoms recur, continue for ~1yr before considering second trial discontinuation. (Note: Patient may wish to continue treatment, rather than risk return of symptoms).

Psychological[2,3,4]

- Behavioral methods: to treat phobic avoidance by exposure, use of relaxation, and control of hyperventilation (have been shown to be 58–83% effective[5]).
- Cognitive methods: teaching about bodily responses associated with anxiety/education about panic attacks, modification of thinking errors.
- Psychodynamic methods: there is some evidence for brief dynamic psychotherapy, particularly "emotion-focused" treatment (e.g., "panic-focused psychodynamic psychotherapy"), where typical fears of being abandoned or trapped are explored.

Issues of co-morbidity

- In view of high levels of co-morbidity, treatment of these conditions should not be neglected.
- For the other anxiety disorders and depression, this issue is somewhat simplified by the fact that SSRIs and other antidepressants have been shown to be effective for these conditions too. However, behavioral interventions (e.g., for OCD, social phobia) should also be considered.
- Alcohol/substance abuse may need to be addressed first, but specific treatment for persistent symptoms of panic should not be neglected.

Emergency treatment of an acute panic attack

- Maintain a reassuring and calm attitude (most panic attacks spontaneously resolve within 30 minutes).
- If symptoms are severe and distressing consider prompt use of BDZs (immediate relief of anxiety may help reassure the patient, provide confidence that treatment is possible, and reduce subsequent "emergency" presentations).
- If "first presentation," excludes medical causes (may require admission to hospital for specific tests).
- If panic attacks are recurrent, consider differential diagnosis for panic disorder and address underlying disorder (may require psychiatric referral).

Recommended further reading

1 Pollack, M.H., Allgulander, C., Bandelow, B., et al. (2003). WCA recommendations for the long-term treatment of panic disorder. *CNS Spectr.* **8**, 17–30.

2 Ballenger, J.C. *et al.* Panic disorder and agoraphobia. In *Treatments of Psychiatric Disorders* (2nd ed.) Vol.2. Washington DC: American Psychiatric Press, 1997. pp 1421–1452.

3 Mitte, K. (2005). A meta-analysis of the efficacy of psycho-and pharmacotherapy in panic disorder with and without agoraphobia. *Journal of Affective Disorders* **88**, 27–45.

4 Barlow, D.H. and Craske, M.G. *Mastery of Your Anxiety and Panic.* Center for Stress and Anxiety Disorders, State University for New York at Albany, 1988.

5 American Psychiatric Association. Diagnostic and statistical manual of mental disorders. 4th ed., text revision (DSM-IV-TR). Washington DC: American Psychiatric Association, 1994.

6 Battaglia, M., Ogilari, A. (2005). Anxiety and panic: from human studies to animal research and back. *Neuroscience and Biobehavioral Reviews* **29**, 169–179.

7 Hettema, J.M., Neale, M.C., Kendler, K.S. (2001). A Review and Meta-Analysis of the Genetic Epidemiology of Anxiety Disorders. *Am J Psychiatry* **158**, 1568–1578.

Agoraphobia[1–6]

Description

Agoraphobia is characterized by anxiety about being unable to escape from situations or places or get help in the event of a panic attack. This anxiety may result in avoidance of the situation or place, or may be endured with great difficulty. Agoraphobia may occur within the context of panic attacks or may occur without a history of panic attacks.

Clinical features

Avoidance of situations or places that cause significant impairment in social or occupational functioning. Agoraphobia is most often diagnosed in females compared to males.

Diagnosis

A clinical diagnosis should include the following: psychiatric interview, review of symptoms, physical exam and history. Special attention should be paid to agoraphobia in the absence of panic.

Differential Diagnosis

Social phobia, specific phobia, obsessive-compulsive disorder, generalized anxiety disorder, delusional disorder, separation anxiety disorder, major depressive disorder.

Co-morbidity

Agoraphobia is most often present in individuals with panic disorder and may be a risk factor for panic disorder.

Epidemiology

According the 2006 National Epidemiological Survey on Alcohol and Related Conditions 12-month prevalence of agoraphobia without panic disoder was 0.05%. Lifetime prevalence was 0.17%.

Etiology

Genetics

Agoraphobia, panic disorder and generalized anxiety disorder may have common genetic correlates.

Treatment

Psychotherapy

In vivo exposure and cognitive behavior therapy is recommended for agoraphobia.

Pharmacotherapy

SSRIs are a first line agent. Higher dosages of SSRIs may be effective in reducing phobic avoidance, compared to dosages used to treat mood disorders. Benzodiazepines in non-sedative doses may also be used.

Prognosis

Individuals with agoraphobia may show earlier onset of panic disorder, have a worse course of illness and poor treatment outcomes.

Recommended further reading

1 American Psychiatric Association. Diagnostic and statistical manual of mental disorders. 4th ed, text revision (DSM-IV-TR). Washington DC: American Psychiatric Association, 1994.

2 Bienvenu, J.O., Onyike, C.U., Stein, M.B., Chen, L-S., Samuels, J., Nestadt, G., Eaton, W.W. (2006). Agoraphobia in adults: incidence and longitudinal relationship with panic. *British Journal of Psychiatry* **188**, 432–438.

3 Grant, B.F., Hasin, D. S., Stinson, F.S., Dawson, D.A., Goldstein, R. B., Smith, S., Huang, B., Saha, T.D. (2006). The epidemiology of DSM-IV Panic Disorder and Agoraphobia in the United States: Results from the National Epidemiological Survey on Alcohol and Related Conditions. Journal of Clinical Psychiatry, **67**, 363–374.

4 Hettema, J.M., Prescott, C.A., Myers, J.M., Neale, M.C., Kendlar, K.S. (2005). The structure of genetic and environmental risk factors for anxiety disorders in men and women. Archives of General Psychiatry, **62**, 182–189.

5 Mitte K. A meta-analysis of the efficacy of psycho-and pharmacotherapy in panic disorder with and witout agoraphobia. (2005). *Journal of Affective Disorders*, **88**, 27–45.

6 Schmidt, N.B. & Cromer, K.R. (in press). Assessing the clinical utility of agoraphobia in the context of panic disorder. Depression and Anxiety.

Specific phobia[1-4]

Description

Specific phobia is a condition characterized by fear of well-defined, specific objects or situations. Exposure to the phobic stimulus provokes anxiety and may lead to a panic attack. Children may not recognize that this anxiety reaction is excessive. The aversive stimulus is often avoided or, if tolerated, may be experienced as frightening. These symptoms cause significant impairment in psychosocial functioning and in children under age 18, must persist for at least 6 months. There are five subtypes of specific phobia: animal type (i.e., spiders), natural environment type (i.e., weather), blood-injection type, situational type (i.e., trains, flying, bridges) and other type (i.e., vomiting).

Clinical features

Clinical presentation

Individuals with specific phobias often avoid the feared object or situation, thus interfering with social and occupational functioning. Children with specific phobia may exhibit anxiety as crying, freezing or clinging behaviors in response to the feared object or situation. A history of fainting response has been found in 75% of individuals with blood-injury phobias. This response manifests itself as heart rate acceleration and increased blood pressure followed by heart rate deceleration and decrease in blood pressure.

Diagnosis

A clinical diagnosis should include the following: psychiatric interview, review of symptoms, physical exam and history.

Differential diagnosis

Panic disorder with agoraphobia, separation anxiety disorder, social phobia, post-traumatic stress disorder, obsessive-compulsive disorder, hypochondriasis, anorexia nervosa, bulimia nervosa, schizophrenia, other psychotic disorders.

Co-morbidity

Specific phobias are frequently co-morbid with other disorders, especially anxiety, mood, and substance-related disorders. Frequently, the specific phobia leads to less distress and discomfort compared to the other disorders. Most specific phobias involve multiple fears and there is growing evidence that an increasing number of fears are associated with higher co-morbidity. Recent studies also suggest that there are differences in co-morbidity among young female individuals depending upon the type of phobia, with animal phobias most often co-morbid with other anxiety disorders (25%; n = 2064) and affective disorders (22%; n = 2064).

DSM-IV-TR criteria for specific phobia

A. Marked and persistent fear that is excessive or unreasonable, cued by the presence or anticipation of a specific object or situation (e.g., flying, heights, animals, receiving an injection, seeing blood).

B. Exposure to the phobic stimulus almost invariably provokes an immediate anxiety response, which may take the form of a situationally bound or situationally predisposed panic attack.

Note: In children, the anxiety may be expressed by crying, tantrums, freezing, or clinging.

C. The person recognizes that the fear is excessive or unreasonable.

Note: In children, this feature may be absent.

D. The phobic situation(s) is avoided or else is endured with intense anxiety or distress.

E. The avoidance, anxious anticipation, or distress in the feared situation(s) interferes significantly with the person's normal routine, occupational (or academic) functioning, or social activities or relationships, or there is marked distress about having the phobia.

F. In individuals under age 18 years, the duration is at least 6 months. and cannot be better accounted for by another Axis 1 diagnosis.

Specify type: Animal Type, Natural Environment Type (e.g., heights, storms, water), Blood-Injection-Injury Type, Situational Type (e.g., airplanes, elevators, enclosed places), Other Type (e.g., phobic avoidance of situations that may lead to choking, vomiting, or contracting an illness; in children, avoidance of loud sounds or costumed characters). See *p. 411*

Epidemiology

Lifetime prevalence in the general population is from 7.2% to 12.5% (DSM-IV[2]). Specific phobia often begins in childhood or adolescence and may vary based on subtype. Age of onset peaks in childhood and in the mid-20s. Prevalence is usually higher in women versus men (2:1). Prevalence rates differ for specific phobia subtypes; for example, approximately 75–90% of individuals with Animal and Natural Environment Type and Situational Type are female and approximately 55–70% of individuals with the Blood Injection-Injury Type are female.

Etiology

Causes

The causes of specific phobia remain to be fully elucidated; however, there are several hypotheses regarding its etiology and pathogenesis. Experiencing a traumatic event, observing others, reactions to a feared situation or object, or being informed or warned about the dangers of a feared situation or object may predispose individuals to specific phobia. Specific phobias may be maintained because of avoidance of the feared object or situation. Dysregulation in the neural processes that affect fear circuitry, including the amygdala, may also contribute to specific phobia symptoms. Neurotransmitters associated with amygdala function (monamine receptors, amino acid receptors) may also affect the etiology of specific phobia. Genetic factors include allelic variation in monamine receptors.

Evolutionary preparedness and emotional learning may play in important role in the etiology of specific phobia subtypes.

Genetics

Specific phobia is familial. A two- to three-fold increased risk for specific phobia has been found in relatives of specific phobia probands compared to relatives of control probands. Offspring of anxious parents may also have increased rates of specific phobia. The generalized subtype of specific phobia may be more familial. Studies suggest that both genetic and nongenetic factors contribute to risk for developing specific phobia.

Treatment

Psychotherapy

Recent studies of evidence-based treatments for specific phobia suggest that in vivo exposure therapy is most effective. A new exposure technique that may be as effective as in vivo exposure is virtual reality exposure. Behavior therapies are also effective, though findings at long-term follow-up (greater than one year) have been mixed. Effective treatment for claustrophobia includes interceptive exposure and adjunct cognitive behavior therapy. Muscle tension may be helpful for blood phobias. Systematic desensitization may improve subjective anxiety in phobic individuals.

Pharmacotherapy

Medication has limited efficacy for phobias. There is some evidence that Benzodiazepines reduce anxiety when confronting a feared stimulus or situation (i.e., flying). However, research has found that subsequent encounters with the feared stimulus or situation are not improved. More recently, trials of D-cycloserine have shown promise in accelerating fear extinction during exposure.

Combination therapy

There is limited evidence for the efficacy of combined psychotherapy and pharmacotherapy in the treatment of specific phobia.

Prognosis

Relapse over time is expected. High drop-out rates and problems with treatment adherence may account for a poor prognosis. Recent evidence suggests that increasing numbers of fears, regardless of content, are associated with greater disability and impairment.

Recommended further reading

1 American Psychiatric Association. Diagnostic and statistical manual of mental disorders. 4th ed, text revision (DSM-IV-TR). Washington DC: American Psychiatric Association, 1994.

2 Stinson, F.S., Dawson, D.A., Patricia, Chou S., et al. (2007). The epidemiology of DSM-IV specific phobia in the U.S.A.: Results from the National Epidemiologic Survey on Alcohol and Related Conditions. *Psychology Med* **37**(7): 1047–49.

3 Choy, Y., Fyer, A.J., Lipsitz, J.D. (2007). Treatment of specific phobia in adults. *Clinical Psychology Review* **27**, 266–286.

4 Barlow, D.H. *Clinical Handbook of Psychological Disorders*. New York: Guilford, 1993.

Specific phobias—selected glossary

Accidents	Dystychiphobia
Animals	Zoophobia
Ants	Myrmecophobia
Automobiles	Amaxophobia, motorphobia
Bees	Apiphobia, melissophobia
Birds	Ornithophobia
Blood	Hemophobia
Bridges	Gephyrophobia
Cats	Felinophobia
Choking/being smothered	Anginaphobia, pnigophobia, pnigerophobia
Contamination, dirt, or infection	Molysomophobia, mysophobia
Creepy, crawly things	Herpetophobia
Crossing streets	Agyrophobia
Darkness	Nyctophobia, scotophobia
Dentists	Dentophobia, Odontophobia
Depth	Bathophobia
Doctors	Iatrophobia
Dogs or rabies	Cynophobia
Everything	Panophobia, panphobia, pamphobia
Feathers	Pteronophobia
Flying	Aviophobia
Forests, at night	Nyctohylophobia
Frogs	Batrachophobia
Hair, fur, or animal skins	Chaetophobia, Trichophobia, doraphobia
Horses	Equinophobia, hippophobia
Hospitals	Nosocomephobia
Injections	Trypanophobia
Jumping	Catapedaphobia
Lightning and thunder	Brontophobia, karaunophobia
Moths	Mottephobia
Needles	Aichmophobia, belonephobia
Open high places	Aeroacrophobia
Operations: surgical	Tomophobia
Place: enclosed	Claustrophobia
Railways/trains	Siderodromophobia
Rain	Ombrophobia, Pluviophobia
Rats	Zemmiphobia
Reptiles	Herpetophobia
Snakes	Ophidiophobia
Spiders	Arachnophobia
Vomiting	Emetophobia
X-rays	Radiophobia

Social phobia (social anxiety disorder)[1–4]

Description

Social phobia (SP) is a chronic disabling psychiatric condition characterized by avoidance of social situations and evaluation by others driven by a fear of humiliation or embarrassment. These symptoms cause significant impairment in psychosocial functioning and, in individuals under the age of 18, the symptoms persist for at least 6 months.

Clinical features

Clinical presentation

Patients with SP may seem self-focused upon physical examination and may be reluctant to reveal symptoms of SP because they consider them embarrassing. Individuals may believe that their symptoms of anxiety (e.g., sweating) are conspicuous to others. Individuals with generalized SP fear most social situations. Non-generalized SP is restricted to one or several social situations.

DSM-IV-TR criteria for social phobia

A. A marked and persistent fear of one or more social or performance situations in which the person is exposed to unfamiliar people or to possible scrutiny by others. The individual fears that he or she will act in a way (or show anxiety symptoms) that will be humiliating or embarrassing.

Note: In children, there must be evidence of the capacity for age-appropriate social relationships with familiar people and the anxiety must occur in peer settings, not just in interactions with adults.

B. Exposure to the feared social situation almost invariably provokes anxiety, which may take the form of a situationally bound or situationally predisposed panic attack. Note: In children, the anxiety may be expressed by crying, tantrums, freezing, or shrinking from social situations with unfamiliar people.

C. The person recognizes that the fear is excessive or unreasonable.

Note: In children, this feature may be absent.

D. The feared social or performance situations are avoided or else are endured with intense anxiety or distress.

E. The avoidance, anxious anticipation, or distress in the feared social or performance situation(s) interferes significantly with the person's normal routine, occupational (academic) functioning, or social activities or relationships, or there is marked distress about having the phobia.

F. In individuals under age 18 years, the duration is at least 6 months. and cannot be due to substance use, a general medical condition, or be better explained by another Axis 1 disorder.

If a general medical condition or another mental disorder is present, the fear in Criterion A is unrelated to it, e.g., the fear is not of stuttering, trembling in Parkinson's disease, or exhibiting abnormal eating behavior in anorexia nervosa or bulimia nervosa.

Diagnosis

A clinical diagnosis should include the following: psychiatric interview, review of symptoms, physical exam and history.

Differential diagnosis

Panic disorder with agoraphobia, agoraphobia without a history of panic disorder, separation anxiety disorder, generalized anxiety disorder, specific phobia, pervasive developmental disorder, schizoid personality disorder, avoidant personality disorder, anxiety disorder not otherwise specified, performance anxiety, stage fright, shyness.

Co-morbidity

81% of individuals with SP have an additional psychiatric diagnosis. More than 50% with SP have a lifetime history of phobias. 15–20% with SP have a lifetime history of major depressive disorder or alcohol abuse. Common co-morbid conditions may include the following: major depression, dysthymia, mania, agoraphobia, simple phobia, panic disorder, eating disorders, alcohol abuse, and drug abuse.

Epidemiology

Lifetime prevalence in the general population is from 3% to 13%. The incidence is approximately 7.8% each year. SP often begins in adolescence. Early onset may be associated with more severe and generalized SP. Females are just as likely or more likely to have SP than males. Quality of life is poorer relative to other phobic disorders.

Etiology

Causes

The causes of SP remain to be fully elucidated; however there are several hypotheses regarding its etiology and pathogenesis. Temperaments such as shyness and behaviors such as increased inhibition, may be factors affecting the development of social anxiety. Individuals with SP may have limited social skills that contribute to a limited capacity to identify emotional expressions and engage in appropriate social behavior. SP may be maintained because of negative thoughts that impair social performance and bias perception of social interactions and situations. Dysregulation in the neural processes that affect fear circuitry, including the amygdala, may also contribute to SP symptoms. Altered neurotransmitter function (serotonin and dopamine) may also affect the expression of personality traits that contribute to symptoms of SP. Neuroimaging studies suggest structural and functional alterations in emotional processing and affective regulatory brain regions.

Genetics

SP is familial. A two- to three-fold increased risk for SP has been found in relatives of SP probands compared to relatives of control probands. Offspring of anxious parents may also have increased rates of SP. The generalized subtype of SP may be more familial. Studies suggest that both genetic and non-genetic factors contribute to risk for developing SP.

Treatment

Psychotherapy

CBT involving cognitive restructuring, exposure to feared objects or situations, and relaxation are recommended as a first-line intervention.

Pharmacotherapy

First line treatment is SSRIs. Clinical trials have demonstrated efficacy of sertraline, paroxetine and fluvoxamine. If acute treatment is effective it is recommended that treatment is continued for at least 12 months. Longer-term treatment is recommended if symptoms persist or accompanied by co-morbid psychiatric conditions. Early onset of SP may also require long-term treatment with SSRIs.

For acute treatment, MAOIs have been efficacious but have been associated with adverse events and are generally intended for refractory patients. Few studies have assessed the efficacy of BDZs. Current literature suggests BDZs may be useful for treatment refractory SP and may be helpful as augmenting agents. Further research and larger sample sizes are necessary in order to determine which agents, other than SSRIs, are most efficacious and tolerable for long-term treatment.

Prognosis

The course of SP is frequently continuous and tends to follow a pattern of exacerbations associated with life stressors and demands. Although SP can lead to substantial impairments with employment and relationships, there are equivocal findings regarding the long-term outcome of SP with treatment.

Recommended further reading

1 American Psychiatric Association. Diagnostic and statistical manual of mental disorders. 4th ed, text revision (DSM-IV-TR). Washington (DC): American Psychiatric Association (1994).
2 Van Ameringen, M., Allgulander, C., Bandelow, B., *et al.* (2003). WCA recommendations for the long-term treatment of social phobia. *CNS Spectrums* **8** (Suppl 1), 40–52.
3 Brunello, N., den Boer, J.A., Judd, L.L., *et al.* (2000). Social phobia: diagnosis and epidemiology, neurobiology and pharmacology, co-morbidity and treatment. *Journal of Affective Disorders* **60**, 61–74.
4 Barlow, D.H., *Clinical Handbook of Psychological Disorders.* New York: Guilford, 1993.

Generalized anxiety disorder[1–3]

Description

GAD is a chronic disabling psychiatric condition characterized by excessive anxiety and worry that is difficult to control. The worry is generally related to a number of events or activities and is associated with at least three of the following symptoms: restlessness, fatigue, decreased concentration, irritability, muscle tensions, or sleep disturbance. These symptoms persist for at least 6 months and cause significant impairment in psychosocial functioning.

Clinical features

Clinical presentation

Patients with GAD often present with physical symptoms (e.g., muscle tension) and sleep disturbance.

DSM-IV-TR Diagnosis for GAD

A. Excessive anxiety and worry (apprehensive expectation), occurring more days than not, for at least six months, about a number of events or activities (such as work or school performance).

B. The person finds it difficult to control the worry.

C. The anxiety and worry are associated with three (or more) of the following six symptoms (with at le`ast some symptoms present for more days than not for the past six months). Note: Only one item is required in children.

   1. Restlessness or feeling keyed up or on edge.
   2. Being easily fatigued.
   3. Difficulty concentrating or mind going blank.
   4. Irritability.
   5. Muscle tension.
   6. Sleep disturbance (difficulty falling or staying asleep, or restless unsatisfying sleep).

- The symptoms must cause impairment. The worry cannot be due to another Axis I disorder or worrying about other Axis I disorders (e.g., worrying about having a panic attack with panic disorder).
- The disturbance is not due to the direct physiological effects of a substance (e.g., a drug of abuse, a medication) or a general medical condition (e.g., hyperthyroidism) and does not occur exclusively during a mood disorder, a psychotic disorder, or a pervasive developmental disorder.

Diagnosis

A clinical diagnosis should include the following: psychiatric interview, review of symptoms, and medical history.

Differential diagnosis

Panic disorder, social phobia, obsessive-compulsive disorder, anorexia nervosa, hypochondriasis, somatization disorder, separation anxiety disorder, post-traumatic stress disorder, adjustment disorder, mood disorder, psychotic disorder, general medical condition, substance-induced anxiety disorder.

Co-morbidity

90% with lifetime GAD have a lifetime history of least one co-morbid psychiatric disorder. 66.3% with current GAD have a current diagnosis of at least one co-morbid psychiatric disorder. Common co-morbid conditions include the following: major depression, agoraphobia, simple phobia, social anxiety disorder, panic disorder, dysthymia, mania, alcohol abuse, and drug abuse. Nonpsychiatric co-morbidities may include headache, backache, gastrointestinal distress (e.g., irritable bowel syndrome), joint pain, migraine, or sleep disturbance.

Epidemiology

Lifetime prevalence in the general population is approximately 5 to 6 %. The incidence is approximately 3% each year. GAD frequently occurs before age 25 and the incidence increases at 35–45 years of age. GAD is the most common anxiety disorder diagnosed in the elderly. The male to female ratio is approximately 3:4.

Etiology

Causes

The causes of GAD remain to be fully elucidated; however, there are several hypotheses regarding its etiology and pathogenesis. Animal and human studies suggest that GABA, glutamate, monoamine and/or neuropeptide dysregulation may be involved in GAD. Abnormalities of neural processes involved in fear circuitry, such as the amygdala, may also contribute to GAD symptoms. Altered neurotransmitter function may also affect the expression of personality traits that contribute to symptoms of GAD. Neuroimaging studies suggest altered structure and function in regions implicated in emotion processing (e.g., limbic regions) and affective regulation (e.g., prefrontal cortex). Other neurobiological factors include loss of regulatory control of cortisol (HPA axis) in approximately 1/3 of GAD patients (DMST—reduced cortisol suppression). Possible sustained activation of stria terminalis (increased startle) following prolonged CRF stimulation (chronic stress). Abnormalities in the "behavioral inhibition system" (septohippocampal-Papez circuit-amygdala). Neurotransmitter abnormalities (e.g., GABA activity, dysregulation of 5-HT systems, CCK). Psychological factors include the experience of unexpected negative events (e.g., early death of parent, rape, war) or chronic stressors (dysfunctional family/marriage). Overprotective or parenting lacking warmth and responsiveness (theoretically leading to low perceived control over events).

Genetics

GAD is a highly familial disorder. GAD is present in approximately 19.5% of first-degree relatives. Relative risk in family members of affected children is approximately 5.6%, which is considered large relative to other anxiety disorders. Studies suggest that both genetic and nongenetic factors contribute to risk for developing GAD.

Treatment

Psychotherapy

Cognitive behavior therapy (CBT), involving cognitive restructuring, exposure to worry thoughts, and relaxation are recommended as a first-line intervention.

Pharmacotherapy

Recent meta-analyses have demonstrated that antidepressants, including paroxetine, venlafaxine, and imiprimine, are more efficacious than placebo in the treatment of GAD. SSRIs currently stand as first line agents in the treatment of GAD in similar does to those used to treat major depression. Traditionally, benzodiazepines and azathirones, such as buspirone, were considered first-line agents for the treatment of GAD. Benzodiazepines, however, are not recommended for long term use because of side-effects that may include tolerance, physical dependence, memory impairment and withdrawal. Azathirones have been found to be helpful in the treatment of GAD but less so than benzodiazepines. Continued research comparing various treatments is ongoing.

Combination therapy

There is limited evidence for the efficacy of combined psychotherapy and pharmacotherapy in the treatment of GAD.

Prognosis

Co-morbid medical and psychiatric conditions are poor prognostic factors.

Recommended further reading

1 American Psychiatric Association. Diagnostic and statistical manual of mental disorders. 4th ed, text revision (DSM-IV-TR). Washington DC: American Psychiatric Association, 1994.

2 Karczinski, F., Lima, M.S., Souza, J.S., Cunha, A., Schmitt, R.. Antidepressants for generalized anxiety disorder. Cochrane Database of Systematic Reviews 2003, Issue 2, Art. No.: CD003592. DOI: 10.1002/14651858.CD003592.

3 Barlow, D.H. Clinical Handbook of Psychological Disorders. New York: Guilford, 1993.

Obsessive-compulsive disorder (1)[1-4]

Description
OCD is a disabling psychiatric condition characterized by obsessions (recurrent intrusive thoughts, ideas or images) and compulsions (repetitive ritualistic behaviors). These symptoms cause significant impairment in terms of time (>1 hr/day), distress, and interference in functioning.

Clinical features
Clinical presentation
OCD is a clinically heterogenous disorder, characterized by at least four temporally stable symptom dimensions, including: contamination/washing (fears about dirt, germs, or illness and excessive cleaning rituals), aggressive/sexual obsessions and related compulsions (excessive worries about danger, catastrophic events, such as death or illness happening to self or loved ones; intrusive and disturbing sexual thoughts or images), hoarding and collecting (concerns about discarding objects or personal items), and symmetry/ordering (worries that things are not symmetrical or "just right"). These symptoms may overlap and most patients with OCD will report ego-dystonic symptoms (they recognize that the obsessions and compulsions are excessive and unreasonable). It is traditionally understood that patients with OCD are attempting to neutralize the anxiety caused by their obsessions by carrying out their compulsions.

DSM-IV-TR diagnosis of OCD

A. Either obsessions or compulsions:
Obsessions as defined by (1), (2), (3), and (4):
(1) recurrent and persistent thoughts, impulses, or images that are experienced, at some time during the disturbance, as intrusive and inappropriate and that cause marked anxiety or distress.
(2) the thoughts, impulses, or images are not simply excessive worries about real-life problems.
(3) the person attempts to ignore or suppress such thoughts, impulses, or images, or to neutralize them with some other thought or action.
(4) the person recognizes that the obsessional thoughts, impulses, or images are a product of his or her own mind (not imposed from without as in thought insertion).
Compulsions as defined by (1) and (2):
(1) repetitive behaviors (e.g., hand washing, ordering, checking) or mental acts (e.g., praying, counting, repeating words silently) that the person feels driven to perform in response to an obsession, or according to rules that must be applied rigidly.
(2) the behaviors or mental acts are aimed at preventing or reducing distress or preventing some dreaded event or situation; however, these behaviors or mental acts either are not connected in a realistic way with what they are designed to neutralize or prevent or are clearly excessive.

B. At some point during the course of the disorder, the person has recognized that the obsessions or compulsions are excessive or unreasonable. Note: This does not apply to children.

C. The obsessions or compulsions cause marked distress, are time consuming (take more than 1 hour a day), or significantly interfere with the person's normal routine, occupational (or academic) functioning, or usual social activities or relationships.

D. If another Axis I disorder is present, the content of the obsessions or compulsions is not restricted to it (e.g., preoccupation with food in the presence of an eating disorder; hair pulling in the presence of trichotillomania; concern with appearance in the presence of body dysmorphic disorder; preoccupation with drugs in the presence of a substance use disorder; preoccupation with having a serious illness in the presence of hypochondriasis; preoccupation with sexual urges or fantasies in the presence of a paraphilia; or guilty ruminations in the presence of major depressive disorder). Cannot be due to effect or substances or a general medical condition.

Diagnosis

A clinical diagnosis should include the following: psychiatric interview with patient; interview with family members, if possible; symptom rating and monitoring of severity over time using the Yale-Brown Obsessive-Compulsive Scale (Y-BOCS) or the Dimensional Yale Brown Obsessive-Compulsive Scale (DY-BOCS); review of systems, with special attention to neurological and infectious disease signs, symptoms, and history.

Differential diagnosis

Tourette's/tic disorders; obsessive-compulsive personality disorder (OCPD) (ego-syntonic); OCD spectrum disorders (including trichotillomania, onychiophagia [nail biting], chronic skin picking, other impulse control disorders, body dysmorphic disorder); eating disorders; psychotic disorders; depressive and anxiety disorders; pervasive developmental disorders; rarely, basal ganglia disease.

Co-morbidity

Common co-morbid conditions include the following: OCPD and other personality disorders; major depression and other mood disorders; other anxiety disorders; OCD spectrum disorders; tic disorders; eating disorders.

Obsessive-compulsive disorder (2)

Epidemiology

Prevalence rate is approximately 2% worldwide. Most cases of OCD begin prior to adulthood and approximately one third to one half of adult OCD cases have a childhood onset, with approximately 20% of cases starting by age 10. The age of onset is bimodal: between ages 6 and 15 for males and between ages 20 and 29 for females.

Etiology

Causes

There are several hypotheses regarding the etiology and pathophysiology of OCD.

A serotonergic hypothesis, due to the effectiveness of serotonin reuptake inhibitors in treating OCD, suggests that dysregulation of the 5HT system and/or 5HT/DA systems are potentially involved in the development and expression of the disorder.

Recent genetic studies implicate glutamate receptor abnormalities. Abnormalities in cortical-striatal-thalamo-cortical (CSTC) circuitry have been consistently implicated in the pathophysiology of OCD. Specifically, it is postulated that there is an imbalance in the basal ganglia pathways, with increased "tone" in the direct basal ganglia pathway and a decreased "tone" in the indirect pathway. Both structural and functional neuroimaging studies have consistently implicated the following components of CSTC circuitry: basal ganglia, thalamus, orbital frontal cortex, and anterior cingulate.

Basal ganglia abnormalities, have been supported by underlying functional changes in OCD patients (in the frontal cortex [left orbital gyrus] and bilateral caudate nuclei), which normalized after successful treatment with medication (and interestingly with CBT techniques—although this took longer). Further support of a basal ganglia role in OCD is its frequent association with several basal ganglia illnesses, including tic disorders, Huntington's chorea, and Sydenham's chorea. Anterior cingulate hyperactivity has been reported at rest and during symptom provocation; it is postulated that this aberrant anterior cingulate activity reflects dysfunctional action monitoring and both conflict and error related activity.

More recent evidence points to the dysregulation of limbic circuitry associated with washing and hoarding symptoms and more frontal-striatal abnormalities associated with checking and symmetry symptoms.

Genetics

OCD is highly familial and is considered a complex genetic disorder. Twin studies indicate that monozygotic twins have a higher concordance rate than dizygotic twins (80–87% versus 47%–50%, respectively). Family studies of both adult and pediatric probands suggest that the lifetime prevalence in case relatives versus control relatives is substantially greater (five- to seven-fold more frequent).

Treatment

Psychotherapy

CBT involving graded exposure to anxiety-provoking stimuli and ritualizing prevention (ERP) is recommended as a first-line intervention. Meta-analyses have found that ERP showed an equal or greater impact on OCD symptoms and impairment, compared to medication. The effects of psychotherapy have been shown to endure after the cessation of treatment, whereas there is a high rate of relapse once medication is discontinued.

Pharmacotherapy

First-line agents include SSRIs: fluoxetine, sertraline, fluvoxamine, paroxetine, citalopram, and escitalopram and the TCA, clomipramine. Maintenance therapy for at least 1–2 years. Relapses common and long-term treatment advised after two relapses. There is anecdotal evidence for improved efficacy with higher dosages of SSRIs compared to dosages used to treat mood disorders. Augmentation of SSRIs with atypical antipsychotics have also proven efficacious in some treatment refractory cases.

Combination therapy

Expert consensus guidelines recommend starting treatment with either CBT or with the combination of CBT and pharmacotherapy; this decision depends upon the severity of the OCD and any co-morbid conditions that may benefit from pharmacotherapy.

Prognosis

Many patients have a chronic waxing and waning course. Approximately one-third to one-half of patients with a pediatric onset will have symptoms that continue into adulthood. Approximately 15% of patients have progressive deterioration in occupational and social functioning. Approximately 5% of patients have an episodic course with minimal or no symptoms between episodes.

Recommended further reading

1 Kessler, R.C., Berglund, P., Demier, O., Jin, R., Merikangas, K.R., Walters, E.E. (2005). Lifetime prevalence and age-of-onset distributions of DSM-IV disorders in the National Co-morbidity Survey Replication. *Arch Gen Psychiatry* **62**, 593–602.

2 Mataix-Cols, D., Roario-Campos, M.C., Leckman, J.F. (2005). A Multidimensional Model of Obsessive-Compulsive Disorder. *Am J Psychiatry* **162**, 228–238.

3 American Psychiatric Association. Diagnostic and statistical manual of mental disorders. 4th edition, text revision (DSM-IV-TR). Washington DC: American Psychiatric Association, 1994.

4 Bartz, J.A., Hollander, E. Is obsessive-compulsive disorder an anxiety disorder? (2006). *Progress in Neuro-Psychopharmacology and Biological Psychiatry* **30**, 338–352.

"Stressor" and "trauma" related disorders

Introduction

Adaptation to life's challenges is at the core of psychiatry. Failure to adapt causes or worsens the symptoms of most psychiatric disorders. The challenges can be categorized as either stressors or traumas.

Stressors

Stressors are universal life events that strain a person's biopsychosocial well-being. Examples include having a chronic disease, losing a loved one, the birth of a child, or changing a job. As a result of the stressor, the person must cope with the change and adapt to the new situation. Most times, the person fairs well and moves on with their lives. However, sometimes the stressor overwhelms the person, leading to psychiatric symptoms. This result is more likely when the stressor is chronic or when there are multiple stressors occurring simultaneously.

Traumas

Traumas are more intense than stressors. Traumas are defined in the DSM-IV by a strict, two part criteria.

- First, there must be an event(s) that involves actual or threatened death or serious injury, or a threat to the physical integrity of self or others.
- Second, the person's response to the traumatic event must involve intense fear, helplessness, or horror.

Examples of traumas include natural disasters, abuse, or terrorist attacks. Traumas are more common than expected. Even using the strict DSM-IV criteria, 50–80% of the population experiences a trauma during their lives.

Traumas are usually described as either single episode or chronic because of the difference in effect.

- Single episode traumas are often sudden and severe in nature, but they are also rarer and time limited. They are unexpected and produce an intense, overwhelming terror but resolve and are not likely to recur. These types of traumas are more likely to cause post-traumatic stress reactions. Examples of single episode traumas include being robbed at gunpoint or being in an earthquake.
- Chronic traumas are repeated, often expected, traumas of an interpersonal nature. They produce a persistent terror that often causes different psychiatric symptoms, like personality changes, somatic complaints, and dissociation. Examples of chronic traumas include child abuse, combat, and domestic abuse.

Traumas, whether single episode or chronic, can result in a large variety of psychiatric problems and diagnoses. Those with histories of trauma can have problems with substance use, depression/dysthymia, anxiety disorders, eating disorders (especially anorexia), somatoform disorders, borderline personality disorder, antisocial personality disorder, sexual disorders, and dissociative disorders. In addition, traumas are associated with increased medical problems and increased morbidity/mortality. Therefore, it is extremely important to screen for traumas and their sequelae and to treat them aggressively.

Adjustment disorders

Key features

Adjustment disorders are impairments caused by difficulty adjusting to a stressor or stressors that are beyond "normal" but not severe enough to warrant another diagnosis. The person's symptoms are in-between those seen in a normal reaction and those seen a more "primary" psychiatric diagnosis, such as a mood or an anxiety disorder. As a result, the diagnosis is subject to interpretation. It can be either under or over-diagnosed depending on one's views of what is a "normal" reaction and what constitutes impairment.

The symptoms of an adjustment disorder must appear within 3 months of the onset of the stressor. They typically resolve within 6 months, although they can linger if the stressor is chronic or results in long lasting consequences. The causes of adjustment disorders are very person specific. A stressor causing impairment in one person might not in another. Treatment is important to prevent chronic problems or the development of a more debilitating, "primary" psychiatric diagnosis.

Prevalence

- 2–8% of general population.
- In adults, women: men = 2:1; 1:1 in children and adolescents.
- 10–30% of psychiatric outpatients.
- 5% of medical population.
- In twin studies, some evidence for environmental and genetic factors.

Differential diagnosis

- Event must be a stressor.
- Substance-related disorder.
- Major depressive disorder.
- Conduct disorder.
- Brief psychotic disorder.
- Academic problem.
- Generalized anxiety disorder.
- Identity problem.
- Panic disorder.
- Somatization disorder.
- Acute stress disorder/PTSD.
- General medical condition.

Treatment

Psychotherapy

This is often the mainstay of treatment. There is a focus on supportive psychotherapy and finding supportive measures (e.g., making use of community and financial resources). Group therapy can be useful in preventing isolation. Interpersonal psychotherapy is used for working on interactions with others and cognitive behavior therapy for correcting cognitive distortions.

Pharmacological

Medications (e.g., antidepressants or anxiolytics) are used to treat specific symptoms if they are persistent or distressing. They are generally used for a short duration.

Prognosis

The majority recover within three months. Five-year follow-up studies indicate recovery in 70% of adults and 40% of adolescents. Unfortunately, 20% of adults and 45% of adolescents develop primary psychiatric diagnoses (i.e., mood disorders, anxiety disorders, and alcoholism).

DSM-IV-TR diagnosis of adjustment disorder

A. The development of emotional or behavioral symptoms in response to an identifiable stressor(s) occurring within three months of the onset of the stressor(s).

B. These symptoms or behaviors are clinically significant as evidenced by either of the following:
   (1) After exposure to the event(s)/stressor(s), the behavioral or emotional symptoms seem in excess of what would be normally expected.
   (2) Significant social, functioning, or occupational impairment.

C. The disturbance does not meet the criteria for another specific Axis I disorder or is not part of a preexisting Axis I or Axis II disorder.

D. The behavioral or emotional symptoms do not represent bereavement.

E. Once the event(s)/stressor(s) has terminated, the symptoms do not last more than an additional 6 months.

Specify if:

Acute: Lasts less than 6 months.

Chronic: Lasts for 6 months or longer. By definition the disturbance can not last longer then 6 months. Only use the chronic specifier if the disturbance is in response to a chronic event(s)/stressor(s).

• With anxiety.
• With depressed mood.
• With disturbance of conduct.
• With mixed anxiety and depressed mood.
• With mixed disturbance of emotions and conduct.
• Unspecified.

"Normal" and "complicated" grief

Introduction

According to the DSM-IV-TR, bereavement disqualifies one from having an adjustment disorder. This is because the grief of losing a loved one is expected to cause some psychological problems and impairment in functioning. Grief causes many symptoms including: mood lability (e.g., crying, irritability), depressive symptoms (e.g., dysphoria, poor appetite, poor concentration, hopelessness, guilt), sleep difficulties (e.g., insomnia, sleep continuity disturbances), dissociative symptoms (e.g., shock, numbing), psychotic symptoms (e.g., hearing or seeing the loved one), and somatic symptoms (e.g., weakness, pain). These symptoms tend to peak within the first few months of grieving and improve over time. "Normal" grief lasts an average of 6 months but can last upwards of 12 months. Grief reactions are common, seen in 60% of people who experience the sudden, unexpected death of a close relative or friend (Breslau, *Arch Gen Psych*, 1998).

Given that these are the symptoms of "normal" grief, it is difficult to say when the person's grief is severe enough to warrant a psychiatric diagnosis, known as complicated grief. A general guideline is that the symptoms of complicated grief are more intense, prolonged, and/or beyond what is seen in "normal" grief. A useful set of criteria for diagnosing complicated grief has been proposed by Holly Prigerson (*JAMA*, 2001). While her criteria are not universally held and are not in the DSM-IV, they are helpful diagnostically.

Risk Factors

- Prior history of a psychiatric diagnosis.
- Intense symptoms early in the grieving process.
- Limited social supports.
- Unfamiliarity with death.
- A sudden or unexpected death.

Treatment

Psychotherapy

For "normal grief" usually family and community supports are typically sufficient. Some may make use of bereavement groups.

For "complicated grief," often supportive or grief therapy is used, either individual or group based. CBT, interpersonal psychotherapy, and psychodynamic psychotherapy can also be used.

Pharmacological

- "Normal grief": symptom specific and short-term use.
- "Complicated grief": treat as one would major depressive disorder.

**Proposed DSM-IV-TR diagnostic criteria
for complicated grief**

A. Person has experienced the death of a significant other and response
   involves 3 of the 4 following symptoms experienced at least daily or
   to a marked degree:
   1. intrusive thoughts about deceased,
   2. yearning for deceased,
   3. searching for deceased,
   4. excessive loneliness since the death.
B. In response to the death, 6 of the following 11 symptoms experienced at least daily or to a marked degree:
   1. purposelessness, feelings of futility about future,
   2. subjective sense of numbness, detachment, or absence of
      emotional responsiveness,
   3. difficulty acknowledging the death (disbelief),
   4. feeling life is empty or meaningless,
   5. feeling that part of oneself has died,
   6. shattered worldview (lost sense of security, trust, control),
   7. assumes symptoms or harmful behaviors of, or related to,
      the deceased,
   8. excessive irritability, bitterness, or anger related to the death,
   9. avoidance of reminders of the loss,
   10. stunned, shocked, dazed by the loss,
   11. life is not fulfilling without the deceased.
C. Duration of disturbance (symptoms listed) is at least six months.
D. The disturbance causes clinically significant impairment in social,
   occupational, or other important areas of functioning.

Trauma disorders

Historical perspective

There are written accounts of PTSD symptoms from ancient times, and there is clear documentation of a PTSD-like disorder known as "Da Costa's syndrome" from the Civil War era. However, trauma disorders were not widely studied until the late 19th century. In 1859, Paul Briquet first linked "hysteria" to histories of trauma. Then, in 1887 Jean-Martin Charcot described how traumas could result in a "hypnoid state" (today known as dissociation) that was central in hysterical reactions. Pierre Janet, who is known as the "father" of trauma disorders, expanded on these ideas. He described how extreme emotional arousal results in a failure to integrate traumatic memories into declarative memory. He also discussed how traumatic memories remain in the unconscious, intruding on the person's life and interfering with their functioning, until they are integrated into declarative memory.

After the initial focus in the late 19th century, trauma disorders essentially disappeared from study until the World Wars provided a fresh impetus to study the effects of trauma. In 1941 Abram Kardiner published *The Traumatic Neuroses of War*, which defined PTSD for the 20th century. Later, in the wake of the Vietnam War, the diagnostic category of PTSD was added to the DSM-III (APA, 1980). It incorporated insights from a number of trauma areas, including the "rape trauma syndrome," the "battered woman syndrome," the "Vietnam veterans' syndrome" and the "abused child syndrome." Also, the category of dissociative disorders was created at the time of the DSM-III, though the importance of trauma in their etiology was not initially emphasized. Acute stress disorder was added later to the DSM-IV.

Prevalence

Traumas are not as ubiquitous as stressors, but are still very common. Between 50 and 90% of the population is exposed to a trauma and many are traumatized multiple times. 10% of men and 6% of women have experienced four or more types of trauma. Traumas are more likely to happen to teens and young adults, as well as to males. Men are more likely to experience combat or assaults, women are more likely to be raped.

Initial traumatic assessment

Key features

One can see a variety of symptoms in the initial hours to days after a trauma. People commonly present with intense physical symptoms (e.g., pain, GI problems, insomnia, and autonomic instability) and emotional symptoms (e.g., agitation, poor concentration, mood lability, depression, and dissociation).

Risk factors for development of trauma disorders

Pretrauma risk factors

Include younger age, lower educational or socioeconomic level, trauma or abuse history, and psychiatric history.

- For men their race, family psychiatric history, and lower IQ (especially in combat populations) are also risk factors.
- For women, the only additional risk factor is being female.

Peritrauma risk factors
The proximity/interpersonal nature of threat, severity (especially in combat situations), chronicity, dissociation at time of trauma (biggest predictor of future problems), perceived helplessness, and risk of death.

Initial treatment
Goal
Treat initial symptoms and prevent future psychiatric issues.

Initial assessment
You need to determine what the experience was, how the person is handling the trauma, determine the risk factors, and determine lethality.

Psychotherapy
- Supportive psychotherapy, psycho-education, assisting in obtaining resources reduces symptoms and engages the person in care.
- Encouraging people to rely on their own strengths, existing supports, and own judgment may also aid in recovery.
- Critical Incident Stress Debriefing (CISD) is often a standardized intervention after a trauma. Of note, the debriefing aspect has been studied, and it was found that discussing the event may worsen symptoms.
- Cognitive behavior therapy: can be preventative if done within 2–3 weeks of the trauma.

Pharmacological
- Should be limited to symptom management.
- Propranolol may prevent PTSD, Benzodiazepines may decrease symptoms.

Prognosis
- Recovery is the rule, but it takes time.
- Symptoms decrease most rapidly in the first 12 months.
- Median time for remission: men = 12 months, women = 48 months.
- 7.8% of trauma victims go on to develop PTSD.

Acute stress disorder

Key features

Acute stress disorder (ASD) serves to identify those who are having substantial difficulties soon after a trauma. The diagnostic criteria include the three core problems also seen in PTSD, namely intrusive recollections (e.g., nightmares, flashbacks), avoidance of reminders of the trauma, and hyperarousal (e.g., hypervigilance, exaggerated startle response). However, ASD differs from PTSD in two ways.

- In ASD the symptoms are present for less than a month, in comparison to >1 month for PTSD.
- Secondly, the criteria for ASD emphasize dissociative symptoms, like depersonalization and dissociative amnesia, more than PTSD does.

Prevalence

Roughly between 7 and 33% of trauma sufferers develop ASD and 75–85% of people with ASD go on to develop PTSD. A decent predictor of PTSD. Of note, people can develop PTSD without having ASD.

Differential diagnosis

- PTSD.
- Personality disorders.
- Major depressive disorder (MDD).
- Malingering/factitious disorder.
- Complicated grief.
- Substance use.
- Adjustment disorder.
- Dissociative disorders.
- Brief psychotic episode.

Diagnostic tools

- Acute Stress Disorder Interview (ASDI)—structured interview.
- Acute Stress Disorder Scale (ASDS)—self-report measure.

Treatment

Psychotherapy

There is good evidence that CBT limits the development of PTSD. There is some evidence in favor of exposure-based therapies. There are some case report and small trials in favor of EMDR (eye-movement desensitization and reprocessing)

Pharmacological

Although research is limited, there is some support for the use of SSRIs, and benzodiazepines can be used symptomatically for anxiety and insomnia.

DSM-IV-TR criteria for acute stress disorder

A. The person has been exposed to a traumatic event in which both of the following were present:
   (1) the person experienced, witnessed, or was confronted with an event or events that involved actual or threatened death or serious injury, or a threat to the physical integrity of self or others.
   (2) the person's response involved intense fear, helplessness, or horror.

B. Either while experiencing or after experiencing the distressing event, the individual has three (or more) of the following dissociative symptoms:
   (1) a subjective sense of numbing, detachment, or absence of emotional responsiveness.
   (2) a reduction in awareness of his or her surroundings e.g., "being in a daze").
   (3) derealization.
   (4) depersonalization.
   (5) dissociative amnesia (i.e., inability to recall an important aspect of the trauma).

C. The traumatic event is persistently re-experienced in at least one of the following ways: recurrent images, thoughts, dreams, illusions, flashback episodes, or a sense of reliving the experience; or distress on exposure to reminders of the traumatic event.

D. Marked avoidance of stimuli that arouse recollections of the trauma (e.g., thoughts, feelings, conversations, activities, places, people).

E. Marked symptoms of anxiety or increased arousal (e.g., difficulty sleeping, irritability, poor concentration, hypervigilance, exaggerated startle response, motor restlessness).

F. The disturbance causes clinically significant distress or impairment in social, occupational, or other important areas of functioning or impairs the individual's ability to pursue some necessary task, such as obtaining necessary assistance or mobilizing personal resources by telling family members about the traumatic experience.

G. The disturbance lasts for a minimum of 2 days and a maximum of 4 weeks and occurs within 4 weeks of the traumatic event.

H. The disturbance is not due to the direct physiological effects of a substance (e.g., a drug of abuse, a medication) or a general medical condition, is not better accounted for by brief psychotic disorder, and is not merely an exacerbation of a preexisting Axis I or Axis II disorder.

Post-traumatic stress disorder

Key features

Post-traumatic stress disorder (PTSD) is a devastating psychiatric illness that causes marked impairment. It develops in the aftermath of a trauma, which according to the DSM-IV requires an actual or threatened death or serious injury as well as a severe emotional response. However, this definition can be limiting. For example, those who have watched a disaster or have recently lost a loved one can also develop PTSD. PTSD incorporates the same clusters of symptoms seen in acute stress disorder, namely intrusive recollections, avoidance (which includes emotional numbing and dissociative symptoms), and hyperarousal. Unlike ASD, these symptoms must be present for greater than a month and dissociation plays less of a role in the diagnosis.

Neurobiological and physiological changes

- Altered brainwave activity (EEG).
- Decreased volume of the hippocampus (5–10%).
- Increased activation of the right amygdala and occipital area.
- Decreased activation of left Broca's area.
- Changes in stress hormones that are opposite to depression.
  - Thyroid and opioid function enhanced.
  - Higher levels of epinephrine and norepinephrine.
  - Lower levels of cortisol.
  - Increased suppression on dexamethasone suppression test.

Prevalence

PTSD is present in about 7.8% of the population (National Co-morbidity Survey). The rates depend on the type of trauma. (Refer to peri-traumatic risk factors). PTSD affects Women > Men = 2:1 (females: 10.4% and males: 5%). Higher rates due to greater exposure to violence are seen in African Americans, Native Americans, and Alaska natives. PTSD sufferers are more likely to have a lower socioeconomic status, live in an inner-city, or be combat veterans. About 5–15% more experience sub-clinical PTSD. There is evidence of family risk (if parent has, child more likely to develop) and twin studies support a genetic contribution.

Co-morbidity

Rare to find in isolation. 84% have another lifetime diagnosis. Most common are MDD, alcohol abuse/dependence, social phobia, and agoraphobia.

Diagnosis

- PTSD checklist – self report scale.
- Impact of Events Scale (IES) – self report scale.
- Davidson Trauma Scale – self report scale.
- Clinician-Administered PTSD Scale (CAPS) – structured interview.
- Structured Interview for PTSD – structured diagnostic interview.

Differential diagnosis
- ASD.
- Personality disorders.
- MDD and dysthymia.
- Malingering/factitious disorder.
- Complicated grief.
- Substance use.
- Adjustment disorder.
- Dissociative disorders.
- Schizophrenia.
- Bipolar disorder.
- Other anxiety disorders.

Treatment
Psychotherapy
- CBT is considered the mainstay of treatment. It involves confronting and modifying the distorted threat appraisal process and irrational beliefs about guilt.
- Exposure therapies are effective in 60–70% of patients, although may increase symptoms in some people.
- Eye movement desensitization and reprocessing (EMDR) has been shown in meta-analyses to have efficacy similar to CBT.
- Psychodynamic psychotherapy may be used to explore the connection between the trauma and its effects, unfortunately randomized, controlled research is limited.
- Hypnotherapy: one meta-analysis demonstrated efficacy.

Pharmacotherapy
- SSRIs are the mainstay of treatment, helping between 40–85% of the people. They help with each of the three symptom clusters of PTSD, though least helpful with avoidance.
- TCAs and MAOIs may also be useful, but there is less evidence and have greater side-effects.
- BDZs are logical choices for anxiety and insomnia. However, they run risks of causing dependence, increasing the risk of PTSD with early treatment, and causing the worsening of symptoms when withdrawing.
- Atypical antipsychotics, anticonvulsants, α2-adrenergic agonists and β–blockers may help with specific symptoms.

Prognosis
58% recover within nine months, but 15–25% have a chronic course.
Outcome depends on initial symptom severity. Recovery is helped by:
- Good social support.
- Absence of "maladaptive" coping mechanisms (e.g., avoidance, denial, not talking about problems, thought suppression or rumination).
- No further traumas (including secondary problems like physical health, disability, disfigurement, disrupted relationships, economic problems, litigation).

PTSD is a relapsing illness, with an average of 3.3 episodes over 20 years.
Sufferers are six times more likely to attempt suicide compared to controls and PTSD results in more suicide attempts than other anxiety disorder.

DSM-IV criteria for post-traumatic stress disorder

The person has been exposed to a traumatic event in which both of the following have been present:
- the person experienced, witnessed, or was confronted with an event or events that involved actual or threatened death or serious injury, or a threat to the physical integrity of self or others,
- the person's response involved intense fear, helplessness, or horror. Note: In children, this may be expressed instead by disorganized or agitated behavior.

The traumatic event is persistently re-experienced in one (or more) of the following ways:
- recurrent and intrusive distressing recollections of the event, including images, thoughts, or perceptions. Note: In young children, repetitive play may occur in which themes or aspects of the trauma are expressed,
- recurrent distressing dreams of the event. Note: In children, there may be frightening dreams without recognizable content,
- acting or feeling as if the traumatic event were recurring (includes a sense of reliving the experience, illusions, hallucinations, and dissociative flashback episodes, including those that occur upon awakening or when intoxicated). Note: In young children, trauma-specific reenactment may occur,
- intense psychological distress at exposure to internal or external cues that symbolize or resemble an aspect of the traumatic event, physiological reactivity on exposure to internal or external cues that symbolize or resemble an aspect of the traumatic event.
C. Persistent avoidance of stimuli associated with the trauma and numbing of general responsiveness (not present before the trauma), as indicated by three (or more) of the following:
    (1) efforts to avoid thoughts, feelings, or conversations associated with the trauma,
    (2) efforts to avoid activities, places, or people that arouse recollections of the trauma,
    (3) inability to recall an important aspect of the trauma,
    (4) markedly diminished interest or participation in significant activities,
    (5) feeling of detachment or estrangement from others,
    (6) restricted range of affect (e.g., unable to have loving feelings),
    (7) sense of a foreshortened future (e.g., does not expect to have a career, marriage, children, or a normal life span).
D. Persistent symptoms of increased arousal (not present before the trauma), as indicated by two (or more) of the following:
    (1) difficulty falling or staying asleep,
    (2) irritability or outbursts of anger,
    (3) difficulty concentrating,
    (4) hypervigilance,
    (5) exaggerated startle response.

E. Duration of the disturbance (symptoms in Criteria B, C, and D) is more than one month.

F. The disturbance causes clinically significant distress or impairment in social, occupational, or other important areas of functioning.

Specify if:

Acute: if duration of symptoms is less than 3 months.

Chronic: if duration of symptoms is 3 months or more.

Specify if:

With delayed onset: if onset of symptoms is at least 6 months after the stressor.

Disorders of extreme stress not otherwise specified (DESNOS), aka complex PTSD

Introduction

Prior to the DSM-III, hysteria was used as the category for those with complex biological and psychological reactions to trauma. In the DSM-III, this concept was abandoned. Instead, those with complicated trauma reactions were given multiple diagnoses, including PTSD, somatoform disorders, dissociative disorders, and personality disorders. As a result, 84% of those with PTSD carry another psychiatric diagnosis, and 44% meet criteria for at least three other diagnoses. This has resulted in both diagnostic and treatment problems for many trauma victims.

As a result, the concept of a complex PTSD response was developed. The symptoms often include depression, shame, mood lability, aggression, dissociation, problems with intimacy, somatic complaints, and an inability to experience pleasure. Research has validated this concept, and the category of disorders of extreme stress not otherwise specified (DESNOS) is included under the "associated features and disorders" section of the DSM-IV.

DESNOS is useful as a "meta-diagnosis." It (re)consolidates a number of related symptoms into one category. Also, it is helpful in treatment because DESNOS patients often have a worse prognosis and require more intensive care. More research needs to be done into this disorder, but it may be a useful diagnostic construct for these complex patients.

Prevalence

70+% of those with PTSD will experience DESNOS symptoms.

Diagnosis

- Scheduled Interview of Disorders of Extreme Stress (SIDES)
- Self-Report Inventory for Disorders of Extreme Stress (SIDES-SR)

Phase oriented treatment

- Stabilization and symptom management:
    - medications, dialectical behavior therapy (DBT),
    - mindfulness training, stress inoculation training.
- Using language to create narratives of life's events.
- Recognize repetitive patterns in one's life.
- Make connections between internal states and actions:
    - e.g., aggression, sex, eating, gambling, cutting.
- Identify traumatic memory nodes and treat via:
    - exposure therapy, EMDR, body oriented work.
- Learn to how to create interpersonal connections.

Disorders of extreme stress not otherwise specified proposed criteria

A. Alterations in regulating affective arousal:
    (1) chronic affect dysregulation
    (2) difficulty modulating anger
    (3) self-destructive and suicidal behavior
    (4) difficulty modulating sexual involvement
    (5) impulsive and risk-taking behaviors
B. Alterations in attention and consciousness:
    (1) amnesia
    (2) dissociation
C. Somatization
D. Chronic characterological changes:
    (1) alterations in self-perception: chronic guilt and shame; feelings of self-blame, of ineffectiveness, and of being permanently damaged
    (2) alterations in perception of perpetrator: adopting distorted beliefs and idealizing the perpetrator
    (3) alterations in relations with others:
        (a) an inability to trust or maintain relationships with others
        (b) a tendency to be revictimized
        (c) a tendency to victimize others
E. Alterations in systems:
    (1) despair and hopelessness
    (2) of previously sustaining beliefs

Dissociative disorders

Introduction

Dissociation is an area that started to be studied in the late 19th century, especially in relation to hysteria and hypnosis. The term *dissociation* is usually attributed to Pierre Janet, who hypothesized that there are "idea complexes existing outside of consciousness." Today, dissociation is defined as "a disruption in the usually integrated functions of consciousness, memory, identity, or perception." It is an unconscious defense mechanism that occurs when people are put in stressful or traumatic situations. The internal conflict caused by the situation forces the person's mind to separate incompatible or unacceptable knowledge, information, or feelings into the unconscious. The memories can become buried in the unconscious, only to resurface later.

Dissociation occurs along a spectrum of utility. It can be part of the range of normal experience and a useful coping mechanism, such as depersonalization at the time of an accident. Or dissociation can be overapplied and interfere with normal functioning. Chronic dissociators frequently have a history of abuse and/or neglect, often as young children. It is hypothesized that the child learns to use dissociation as a means to deal with the traumas. Afterwards, dissociation becomes a "normal" defense mechanism. It is then used even when situations are not traumatic and results in a substantial degree of impairment.

Types of dissociation

Multiple types, which overlap but are distinct entities.

Depersonalization

Persistent or recurrent experiences of feeling detached from, and as if one is an outside observer of, one's mental processes or body.

Derealization

Alteration in perception or experience of the world so that it seems unreal.

Dissociative amnesia

One or more episodes of inability to recall important personal information, usually of a traumatic or stressful nature, too excessive to be explained by ordinary forgetfulness.

Somatic dissociation

Altered perceptions of parts of the body. They present as physical deficits that defy physiologic explanation by examination, laboratory tests, and imaging studies. Today classified as somatic disorders.

Emotional dissociation

Blunting of intense emotional states. Can result in alexithymia, which is the inability to recognize/describe one's own emotions.

Identity dissociation

Existence of two or more distinct identities or personalities that have control over the person.

Diagnosis

Clinician-administered interviews

- Structured Clinical Interview for DSM-IV Dissociative Disorders-Revised (SCID-D-R).
- Dissociative Disorder Interview Schedule (DDIS).

Clinician-administered measures

- Clinician Administered Dissociative States Scale (CADSS).

Self-report instruments

- Dissociative Experiences Scale (DES) – most commonly used and studied scale.

Dissociative amnesia

Key features

Formerly known as "psychogenic amnesia," the hallmark of dissociative amnesia is a disruption in the continuity of memories. Patients have recurrent episodes of forgetting important personal information or events when they are under extreme stress. They will often report gaps in their personal history. Dissociative amnesia can be difficult to differentiate from medical causes of amnesia, but it has a couple of unique features. The patient's memory loss is almost always anterograde (i.e., limited to the period following the trauma) in dissociative amnesia. Also, patients with dissociative amnesia do not have problems learning new information.

Prevalence

The exact prevalence is unknown but 4–40% of general population experience amnesia after a trauma. It appears to be most common among young adults.

Co-morbid problems
- Confusion.
- Emotional distress.
- Depression.
- Disturbed relationships.
- Sexual dysfunction.
- Employment problems.
- Aggression.
- Self-injurious behaviors and suicide attempts.

Risk factors
- Chronic, interpersonal abuse as a child.
- Susceptibility to hypnosis.
- No specific genes have been associated with vulnerability.

Evaluation
- Often a diagnosis of exclusion.
- History and physical.
- Blood and urine tests for dementia/delirium.
- EEG for seizure disorder.
- Head CT or MRI for brain injury or malignancy.
- Use of a dissociative scale (e.g., DES).

Differential diagnosis
- Dementia/delirium.
- Cerebral infections/neoplasms.
- Epilepsy.
- Postconcussive amnesia.
- Anoxic injury.
- Metabolic disorders.
- Substance induced.
- Sleep-related amnesia.

- Other dissociative disorders.
- ASD or PTSD.
- Somatoform disorders.
- Malingering/factitious disorder.

Treatment

Psychotherapy

Initially use supportive therapy remembering that many spontaneously recover. If this does not work, some use hypnosis or sodium amytal, to "abreact" the patient. Once memory is restored, work begins on integrating dissociated memories.

Pharmacological

There are no medications that prevent or cure the amnesia and treatment is often symptom related.

Prognosis

The majority will recover their memories through spontaneous recovery or through therapy. A minority develop chronic dissociative amnesia and this depends on present life circumstances, presence of other psychiatric disorders, and the severity of stresses associated with the amnesia.

DSM-IV-TR diagnostic criteria

The predominant disturbance is one or more episodes of inability to recall important personal information, usually of a traumatic or stressful nature, that is too excessive to be explained by ordinary forgetfulness.

The disturbance does not occur exclusively during the course of dissociative identity disorder, dissociative fugue, post-traumatic stress disorder, acute stress disorder, or somatization disorder and is not due to the direct physiological effects of a substance (e.g., a drug of abuse, a medication) or a neurological or other general medical condition (e.g., amnestic disorder due to head trauma).

The symptoms cause clinically significant distress or impairment in social, occupational, or other important areas of functioning.

Subtypes

Localized: Cannot recall events that took place within a limited period of time (several hours or 1–2 days) following a traumatic event.
Selective: The patient can remember some, but not all of the events that took place during a limited period of time.
Generalized: The person cannot recall anything in his/her entire life.
Continuous: The amnesia covers the entire period without interruption from a traumatic event in the past to the present.
Systematized: The amnesia covers only certain categories of information, such as all memories related to a certain location or to a particular person.

Depersonalization disorder

Introduction

During depersonalization there is a profound unreality or foreignness of one's body. Patients feel as if they are watching a movie of themselves and/or their consciousness is outside of themselves (a.k.a. doubling). It often coexists with derealization. It is related to a history of early trauma, although there is debate as to the strength of the correlation. Depersonalization is seen in other psychiatric diagnoses, including panic disorder, borderline personality disorder, PTSD, ASD, and other dissociative disorders. It can also occur in normal individuals during sleep deprivation, during the use of certain anesthetics, in experimental laboratory conditions, and during emotionally stressful situations. Thus, depersonalization is a common experience. It warrants diagnosis only when it causes distress or interferes with functioning.

Prevalence

Half of American adults have experienced depersonalization but only 2.4% meet criteria for the disorder. Females are diagnosed twice as often as males.

Evaluation and differential diagnosis

Same as for dissociative amnesia.

Diagnosis

Depersonalization Severity Scale (DSS)—discriminates between depersonalization disorder and other trauma disorders.

Treatment

Psychotherapy

There is typically spontaneous resolution. Insight-oriented psychodynamic psychotherapy, cognitive behavior therapy, and hypnosis can be used and relaxation techniques may also be helpful.

Pharmacotherapy

Symptom based treatment.

Prognosis

Most recover completely; some develop a chronic form.

Dissociative identity disorder

(Formerly known as multiple personality disorder)

Dissociative identity disorder (DID) is the most controversial of the dissociative disorders, if not psychiatric disorders in general. This is true for a number of reasons. Its presentation can be both dramatic and bizarre, making the concept of separate personalities difficult to believe. Since 1980s there has been a large increase in the number of people diagnosed with DID, making the diagnostic accuracy questionable. Then, there is the question of whether alters, the term used to describe the "separate" personalities, are merely a therapeutic construct used to help integrate different aspects of a person. As a result, there is a fair amount of disbelief and mistrust in the diagnosis even amongst psychiatrists.

Etiology

DID is most commonly caused by severe and prolonged abuse, neglect, or a combination of both during early childhood. The theory is that a child learns to dissociate their identity during these traumas in order to cope. As a result, a separate part of the child experiences the trauma while the primary identity escapes. Over time, the traumatized part organizes into a separate personality capable of autonomous action. Many different identities can form in this manner.

Presentation

DID does not have to be dramatic. The symptoms are often subtle, and the patient may try to minimize or conceal them. DID patients typically present with a wide range of symptoms from PTSD and dissociation to dysthymia, panic attacks, hallucinations, mood lability, somatoform symptoms, and eating disorder symptoms. As a result, the DID patient often carries a number of different diagnoses and has had a variety of treatments before DID is recognized.

The other identities or alters typically emerge in the face of a stressor or trauma. The "switch" is often sudden, and the alters can be very different from the primary identity. They can be of different genders, sexual orientations, ages, and ethnicities. They often have different temperaments, use of language, and even physical characteristics (e.g., posture and handedness). The primary personality may not be aware of the alters and may experience "lost time" when they are in control.

Prevalence

May be as high as 1–3% of the general population and 1–20% of inpatient population. In adults, there is an 8–9:1 female to male sex ratio, but is 1:1 in children.

There is a suggestion that many patients may spend 5–12 years in treatment before being diagnosed.

Evaluation and differential diagnosis

Similar to that of other dissociative disorders.

Treatment

According to the International Society for the Study of Trauma and Dissociation, the overall goal of treatment is "better integrated functioning." The ultimate goal is referred to as "final fusion," which is marked by the shift from multiple identities to a unified sense of self. This work is most often long-term, occurring over years.

Three stages of DID treatment
• Safety, stabilization, and symptom reduction.
• Working directly and in depth with traumatic memories.
• Identity integration and rehabilitation.

Psychotherapy
The most commonly used is psychodynamic psychotherapy although CBT, DBT, systemic desensitization, imagery, and hypnotherapy can be added to the treatment.

Pharmacotherapy
Medications are used as "shock absorbers" to treat symptoms and only partial response to medications is the rule. Many of these patients receive polypharmacy.

Prognosis

There are no long-term outcome studies. However, there are suggestions that the earlier the diagnosis and treatment, the better the prognosis, and that symptoms often lessen by middle age.

DSM-IV-TR criteria

A. The presence of two or more distinct identities or personality states (each with its own relatively enduring pattern or perceiving, relating to, and thinking about the environment and self).
B. At least two of these identities or personality states recurrently take control of the person's behavior.
C. Inability to recall important personal information that is too extensive to be explained by ordinary forgetfulness.
D. The disturbance is not due to the direct physiological effects of a substance (e.g., blackouts or chaotic behavior during alcohol intoxication) or general medical condition (e.g., complex partial seizures). Note: in children, the symptoms are not attributable to imaginary playmates or other fantasy play.

False memory syndrome

Introduction

A topic related to the treatment of trauma disorders is the false-memory-syndrome debate. The question is whether memories "recovered" during treatment are accurate. This question dates back to the late 19th century when the sexual abuse of children came into public discussion. Even at that point, there was much debate, and Alfred Fournier described "pseudologica phantastica" in children who were thought to have falsely accused their parents of incest.

According to proponents of the false memory syndrome, people who have no actual history of abuse can come to adamantly believe that they do. This problem arises when therapists suggest the possibility of abuse to a vulnerable patient. The patient then seizes onto this notion, and the idea becomes fact. Proponents of the false memory syndrome, most notably the False Memory Syndrome Foundation, cite a handful of experimental studies showing the inexactitude of memory, and its ability to be implanted. Also, they point out that 25% of DID patients recall abuse before the age of 3, and 25% recall ritual satanic abuse. Both very early memories and ritual abuse are extremely rare and nearly impossible in 25% of the DID population.

The research

The literature supports a middle ground in this debate. Traumatic memories are not exact replicas of what happened. They are fragmentary and not as well encoded as regular memories. Thus, when these memory fragments are recalled, they are subject to interpretation. For example, while the person may accurately remember the occurrence of abuse, the details are inexact. As a result, the person may reach inaccurate conclusions in an attempt to process their partially recovered memories. This can lead to improper accusations and hurt families.

Treatment implications

The concept of memory interpretation is important to remember when treating a patient with repressed memories. Although it is important to treat the trauma, it is just as important not to overextend what is known. Therapists must inform patients that these memories might not be accurate and be very careful not to make suggestions of abuse.

Eating and impulse control disorders

Anorexia nervosa (1)—overview

Key features

Anorexia nervosa (AN) is a condition, usually in young women, characterized by inability to sustain a minimally adequate body weight, marked distortion of body image or overvaluation of thinness, and engaging in weight loss behaviors.

Mortality in patient groups is significantly higher than in matched population groups. AN may be associated with concurrent substance use disorders, depression, and personality disorders.

Epidemiology

M:F = 1:10; typical age of onset: 15–19 years (rarely > 30 years > 30 years < 12 years).

Prevalence ~0.3% of adolescent and young women in U.S. and Western Europe.

Diagnostic criteria

- Low body weight—at least 15% less than that expected by population norms for age and sex or growth charts; body mass index (BMI) of 17.5 or less (see opposite for calculation).
- Intense fear of becoming fat or gaining weight—fear persists despite being underweight.
- Disturbance in the way shape and weight are experienced, undue influence of weight on self-evaluation, denial of seriousness of problem.
- Amenorrhea in females, reduced sexual interest or impotence, or delay of onset of puberty in prepubertal children.
- Two subtypes—restricting type in which individual maintains low body weight by food restriction or excessive exercise; binge-eating/purging type in which the individual regularly engages in binge eating and/or purging behavior (self-induced vomiting or the misuse of laxatives, diuretics or enemas).

Etiology

Psychological factors

- Individual factors—anxiety, difficulties in emotion regulation, disturbed body image, eating problems in early life, negative self evaluation, general psychiatric morbidity, adverse life events (however, there is no excess of childhood physical or sexual abuse in anorexic patients when compared to psychiatric controls).
- Temperamental factors—perfectionism, obsessionality, harm avoidance and reward dependence behaviors.
- Family factors—enmeshment, rigidity, overemphasis on weight, shape and eating, lack of conflict resolution, weak generational boundaries.
- Sociocultural factors—emphasis on slimness and physical appearance as promoting, precipitating, and/or maintaining factors in the disorder.

Biological factors

- Genetic factors—AN is familial with aggregation attributable largely to genetic factors, and linkage analyses pointing to specific genes. Concordance rates for MZ and DZ twins are 65% and 32%, respectively; and range from 6–10% in female siblings.
- Disturbances in serotonergic function, which may persist even after recovery; dopaminergic factors also are implicated.

Differential diagnosis

- GI disorders (e.g., inflammatory bowel disease, malabsorption syndromes, superior mesenteric artery syndrome, etc.).
- Endocrine disorders (e.g., diabetes mellitus, hyperthyroidism, Addison's disease, etc.).
- Occult malignancies.
- Chronic infections.
- Substance-related disorders.
- Other psychiatric disorders (e.g., depression, schizophrenia, bulimia nervosa).

BMI[*]

BMI is a number calculated from a person's weight and height. BMI provides an indicator of body fatness and is used to screen for weight categories that may lead to health problems. To calculate BMI the following formulas are used:

$$\text{BMI} = \frac{\text{Weight (in kilograms)}}{\text{Height (in meters)}^2}$$

or

$$\text{BMI} = \frac{\text{Weight (in pounds)} \times 703}{\text{Height (in inches)}^2}$$

BMI	Weight Category
Less than 18.5	Underweight
18.5–24.9	Normal Weight
25–29.9	Overweight
30–40	Obese
>40	Morbidly Obese

* BMI is calculated the same way for children and adults, but for children and teens BMI age- and sex-specific percentiles are used: http://www.cdc.gov/growthcharts.

Anorexia nervosa (2)—physical consequences

Common problems

Mainly due to the effects of starvation:

- Cardiovascular—Bradycardia, orthostatic hypotension, EKG changes (sinus bradycardia, arrhythmias, QTc prolongation), Echocardiogram findings (mitral valve prolapse, pericardial effusion).
- Gastrointestinal—Constipation, abdominal bloating, delayed gastric emptying.
- Endocrine and metabolic—Hypothermia, dependent edema, altered thyroid function, hypercortisolemia, amenorrhea, delay in puberty, arrested growth, electrolyte disturbance (hypokalemia, hypophosphatemia, hypomagnesemia), osteopenia, osteoporosis (current recommended treatment is weight restoration and calcium with vitamin D supplementation)
- Renal—↑ or ↓ urinary volume, renal failure (rare), higher risk of renal calculi.
- Reproductive—Amenorrhea (due to hypothalamic dysfunction with low levels of FSH, LH, and estrogen); low testosterone in males, delayed puberty, infertility, higher rates of pregnancy and neonatal complications.
- Neurological—Peripheral neuropathy, structural brain changes (enlarged ventricles, decreased gray and white matter (mostly reversible with weight gain)), nonspecific EEG changes, seizures (rare).
- Hematologic—Anemia, leukopenia, thrombocytopenia.

Mainly due to the effects of vomiting:

- Cardiovascular—Arrhythmias; EKG changes (hypokalemia induced QT interval and T wave changes, supraventricular and ventricular ectopic rhythms, torsades de pointes), cardiomyopathy (ipecac users).
- Gastrointestinal—Enlarged salivary glands, reflux, bloating, esophagitis, gastritis, blood streaked vomitus, bowel irregularities, acute gastric or esophageal rupture.
- Endocrine and metabolic—Hypokalemia, hypochloremic alkalosis, hypomagnesemia, hypophosphatemia (mainly due to stimulant laxative abuse).

Physical signs of vomiting

- Eroded dental enamel/periodontal disease.
- Calluses on dorsum of hand (Russell's sign).
- Salivary gland enlargement.
- Seripheral edema.
- Abdominal bloating.

Physical signs of starvation

- Emaciation.
- Dry skin.
- Acrocyanosis.
- Brittle hair and nails.
- Hair loss on scalp.
- Hypercarotinemia (yellow skin).
- Lanugo (fine, downy body hair).
- Hypothermia.
- Hypotension.
- Bradycardia.
- Peripheral neuropathy.
- ± hyperactivity.

Anorexia nervosa (3)—assessment

Full psychiatric history

- Confirm the diagnosis of an eating disorder and establish circumstances around weight loss.
- Assess dietary habits; weight history; episodes of restricting food; binge eating; purging; use of laxatives, diet pills, diuretics, and ipecac; exercise regimen.
- Pertinent history includes assessment of risk of self-harm/suicide, history of abuse, history of drug and alcohol abuse, family history of eating disorders.

Commonly reported psychiatric symptoms

- Depressive and anxious symptoms.
- Concentration and memory difficulties.
- Irritability.
- Low self-esteem.
- Reduced energy.
- Insomnia.
- Social withdrawal.
- Obsessiveness regarding food and eating.

Full medical history

- Focus on the medical complications of malnutrition (□ p. 450).
- Specifically inquire about menstrual history, dizziness, GI symptoms, syncope, electrolyte abnormalities, and ER visits.

Common symptoms elicited on review of systems

- Amenorrhea.
- Cold hands and feet.
- Weight loss.
- Gastric distress.
- Constipation, bloating.
- Dry skin.
- Hair loss.
- Headaches.
- Fainting or dizziness.
- Fatigue.

Physical examination

- Determine weight and height (calculate BMI—see □ p. 449).
- Assess vital signs and physical signs of starvation and vomiting (□ p. 451).
- Routine and focused laboratory assessment (see opposite).

Routine laboratory assessments

CBC with diff and platelets: Hgb/hct may be ↑ in dehydration although it can be ↓ reflecting anemia. Leukopenia (due to bone marrow suppression) with relative lymphocytosis; thrombocytopenia.

Glucose: Hypoglycemia (if prolonged starvation and low glycogen stores).

LFTs: Possible elevation (nutritional hepatitis).

Serum electrolytes: ↑BUN (dehydration), hyponatremia (excess water intake or SIADH that reverses with refeeding), ↓Cr (low lean body mass), hypokalemic hypochloremic metabolic alkalosis (vomiting), metabolic acidosis (laxative abuse).

TFTs: Most common pattern is normal (nl) TSH, nl/↓T4, ↓T3, ↑rT3. (usually corrects upon refeeding so hormone replacement generally not indicated).

Calcium, magnesium, phosphorus: May be ↓ especially upon refeeding.

EKG: Bradycardia, QT_c prolongation.

Additional studies as indicated: (e.g., urinalysis, SED rate).

Albumin/total protein: Usually normal.

Cholesterol: May be elevated—secondary to ↓T3 levels, low cholesterol binding globulin, and leakage of intrahepatic cholesterol.

Drug screening: To consider substance co-morbidity.

Iron studies: If significant anemia.

DEXA scan: If longstanding amenorrhea.

Anorexia nervosa (4)—management

General principles

- Weight restoration is the cornerstone of treatment for low weight patients.
- Most patients are treated as outpatients at varying levels of intensity (e.g., partial hospital, intensive outpatient, individual treatment).
- Consider specialized eating disorder hospitalization in patients with markedly low weight or with medical or psychiatric instability (see criteria below).
- A multidisciplinary team approach is the standard of care and includes a psychiatrist, psychotherapist, dietitian, and primary care physician.
- Psychotherapy—There is no strong evidence for any psychotherapeutic approach. Family therapy is recommended for children and adolescents. CBT may be helpful for adults.
- Pharmacology—No evidence of efficacy for any medication to ameliorate core symptoms of AN. SSRIs may be useful for managing co-morbid anxiety and/or depression in weight-restored patients only, but the evidence is weak. Some evidence that second-generation antipsychotics may decrease obsessional thinking and anxiety in low-weight patients.

Criteria for admission to hospital

- Extremely low body weight: less than 85% of ideal body weight or a BMI < 17.5.
- Acute medical instability.
  - Rapid, excessive weight loss (~10% weight loss within 3 months).
  - Psychosis or significant risk of suicide.
  - Other serious psychiatric co-morbidities.
  - Failure of outpatient treatment.
  - Involuntary admission is considered when compulsory refeeding is needed to medically stabilize patient and/or decision making capacity is impaired.

Refeeding syndrome

A potentially lethal consequence of refeeding characterized by cardiovascular decompensation (myocardium weakened in starvation) and serious electrolyte disturbances (including hypophosphatemia, which produces abnormalities in cardiac contractility) that can lead to heart failure, severe fluid retention, and multiorgan system collapse. Risk is highest in early refeeding and when using TPN.

General inpatient refeeding guidelines

- Controlled weight gain of 1–1.5kg/week in hospitalized patients and 0.25–0.5kg/week in outpatients.
- Intake levels begin around 35kcal/kg/day and increase by 200–300kcal every 3–5 days (working with a nutritionist).
- Medical monitoring with daily attention to vital signs, cardiovascular status (including edema), and gastrointestional symptoms.
- Electrolyte and mineral level monitoring frequently during early re-feeding.

Prognosis

- Approximately 45–60% recover over 5–10 years, 20–30% continue to have residual moderate symptoms and 10–20% remain chronically ill.
- Anorexia nervosa has one of the highest mortality rates (~5.6% per decade of illness) of any psychiatric disorder. Women with anorexia nervosa are 12 times more likely to die and have a suicide rate 57 times higher than women of a similar age group in the general population.
- Poor prognostic factors include:
  - Late age of onset.
  - Chronicity of illness.
  - Lower initial minimum weights.
  - Bulimic features (vomiting, purgative abuse).
  - Obsessive-compulsive personality features.

Bulimia nervosa

Key features

Characterized by recurrent episodes of binge eating, with compensatory behaviors and overvalued ideas about ideal body shape and weight. Often there is a past history of anorexia nervosa (30–50%), but body weight usually is normal.

Epidemiology

Prevalence 1–1.5% of women, 0.1% of men; onset in adolescence or early adulthood.

Etiology

Similar to anorexia nervosa, but also evidence for associated personal or family history of obesity, and family history of affective disorder or substance abuse. Possible "dysregulation of eating," related to serotonergic and dopaminergic mechanisms.

Diagnostic criteria

- Binge eating (ingestion, in a discrete period of time, a large amount of food given the circumstances paired with a sense of loss of control over eating during the episode).
- Persistent and frequent inappropriate compensatory behaviors to undo the effects of binge eating.
- Binge eating and inappropriate compensatory behaviors are both frequent (at least twice a week) and persistent (duration of at least three months).
- Self-evaluation is unduly affected by body shape and weight.
- The disturbance does not occur exclusively during episodes of anorexia nervosa.
- Two subtypes:
  - Purging type; in which the individual regularly engages in binge eating or purging behavior (self-induced vomiting or the misuse of laxatives, diuretics, or enemas).
  - Nonpurging type; in which the individual engages in fasting or excessive exercise to compensate for binge eating.

Physical signs

- Similar to physical consequences and signs of vomiting in anorexia nervosa (📖 p. 453).
- Investigations—as for AN (📖 p. 455).

Differential diagnosis

- GI disorders (e.g., inflammatory bowel disease, peptic ulcers, etc.).
- Occult malignancies (e.g., brain tumors).
- Intestinal infection.
- Connective tissue disorders (e.g., scleroderma, etc.).
- Substance-related disorders.
- Other psychiatric disorders (e.g., depression, anorexia nervosa, impulse control disorders, etc.).

Co-morbidity
- Anxiety disorders (especially social phobia).
- Depressive disorders.
- Substance abuse disorders.
- Personality disorders (especially borderline personality disorder).

Treatment
General principles
- Assessment: Full psychiatric and medical evaluation (as for anorexia nervosa, 📖 p. 454).
- Management: Outpatient management is typical. Hospital admission may be indicated for acute medical instability, extremely refractory symptoms, suicidality, or severe co-morbid psychiatric illness.
- Nutrition counseling: Includes the development of a structured, balanced meal plan to reduce dietary restriction and urges to binge and purge.
- Psychotherapy (the cornerstone of treatment):
  - CBT has a strong evidence base and is effective in addressing the core symptoms of bulimia nervosa.
  - Interpersonal Therapy (IPT) appears to be effective long-term, but acts less quickly (see Chapter 21 on psychotherapy, 📖 p. 1020).
  - "Guided self-help" may be a useful first step (e.g., bibliotherapy, on-line programs) in the absence of available CBT.

Pharmacotherapy
Antidepressants are effective in reducing binge eating and purging behaviors, with SSRIs considered to be the safest. Fluoxetine (at doses of 60mg) is the best studied and currently is the only FDA approved medication for bulimia nervosa. There is some initial evidence supporting topiramate.[1]

Prognosis
Short term reduction of binge eating and purging behaviors for patients treated with psychosocial or pharmacological interventions is approximately 50–70%. There are high rates of relapse (30–85%), reflecting a frequently waxing and waning course of the illness.

Long-term prognostic data are limited, but in clinical studies more than 50% of patients do not meet criteria for bulimia nervosa at the end of study. Onset of illness in adolescence is associated with a better outcome, while co-morbid depression is associated with a poorer outcome. Bulimia nervosa does not appear to be associated with increased relative mortality.

The SCOFF[2] questions

These questions are useful as a screening tool for eating disorders (highly sensitive for both anorexia nervosa and bulimia nervosa) in primary care. A score of 2+ "yes" answers indicates that a more detailed history is indicated (before considering treatment or referral).
- Do you make yourself sick (vomit) because you feel uncomfortably full?
- Do you worry you have lost control over how much you eat?
- Have you recently lost more than 14 pounds in a 3-month period?
- Do you believe yourself to be fat when others say you are too thin?
- Would you say that food dominates your life?

Recommended further reading

1 Tata, A.L., Kockler, D.R. (2006). *Ann Pharmacother*. Nov; **40**(11), 1993–1997.
2 Morgan, J.F., Reid, F., Lacey, J.H. (1999). The SCOFF questionnaire: assessment of a new screening tool for eating disorders. *BMJ* **319**, 1467–1468.

Impulse control disorders (1)[1]

Impulse control disorders (ICDs) are disorders in which a person acts on a certain impulse that is potentially harmful but that he or she cannot resist. They are a pattern of repetitive behaviors and impaired inhibition of these behaviors.

General criteria for ICDs include[1]

- The failure to resist an impulse to perform some act that is harmful to the individual or others;
- An increasing sense of arousal or tension prior to committing or engaging in the act;
- An experience of pleasure, gratification, or release of tension at the time of committing the act.

DSM-IV-TR includes intermittent explosive disorder, kleptomania, pyromania, pathological gambling, and trichotillomania under the ICD category.

Intermittent explosive disorder (IED)[1]

IED represents individuals who have extreme explosive anger out of proportion to the actual event. For example, a person who feels insulted by a co-worker may go into the lunch area and rip down the cabinets and throw the chairs, only to later feel very guilty and embarrassed. IED may have a lifetime prevalence up to 2–11%, and occurs most often in young men. Episodes are typically infrequent in occurrence, and last 20 minutes or less. Other symptoms may include tingling, tremor, palpitations, chest tightness, head pressure, hearing an echo.

Diagnostic criteria

- Several discrete episodes of failure to resist aggressive impulses that result in serious assaultive acts or destruction of property.
- The degree of aggressiveness expressed during the episodes is grossly out of proportion to any precipitating psychosocial stressors.
- Not due to another disorder or substance use.

Differential diagnosis

ADHD, bipolar disorder, conduct disorder, personality disorder

Treatment

Evaluate and treat co-morbid disorders. IED is challenging to treat, and most efforts are focused on minimizing aggression. There is some evidence for the use of mood stabilizers (lithium, divalproex, maybe carbamazepine), phenytoin, SSRIs, β-blockers (if brain damage is present), α_2-agonists (clonidine), and antipsychotics.

Kleptomania[1,2]

Failure to resist impulses to steal items that are not needed for their personal use or monetary value. Usually women, mean age 36, mean duration of illness 16 years (often childhood onset). Accounts for about 5% of stealing in United States.

Diagnostic criteria

- Recurrent failure to resist impulses to steal objects that are not needed for personal use or for their monetary value.
- Increasing sense of tension immediately before committing the theft.
- Pleasure, gratification, or relief at the time of committing the theft.
- The stealing is not committed to express anger or vengeance and is not in response to a delusion or a hallucination.
- The stealing is not better accounted for by conduct disorder, a manic episode, or antisocial personality disorder.

Differential diagnosis

Shoplifting (actions are usually well planned and motivated by need or monetary gain), antisocial personality disorder, OCD, depression.

Co-morbidity

Eating disorders, substance abuse, depression. May be precipitated by major stressors (e.g., loss events).

Treatment

SSRIs (e.g., fluoxetine); psychotherapy (e.g., CBT, family therapy).

Pyromania[1,3]

The presence of multiple episodes of deliberate and purposeful fire-setting, leading to property damage, legal consequences, and injury or loss of life. It is rare in children; more common in male adolescents, particularly those with poor social skills, learning difficulties, and parental psychopathology. Prevalence in this age group is 2.4–3.5%. Peak age range is 12–14 years old. Adolescents are reported to set about 60% of fires in major U.S. cities.

Diagnostic criteria

- Deliberate and purposeful fire setting on more than one occasion.
- Tension or affective arousal before the act.
- Fascination with, interest in, or attraction to fire and its situational contexts.
- Pleasure, gratification, or relief when setting fires, or when witnessing or participating in the aftermath.
- Fires are not set for financial gain, to express socio-political ideology, to conceal criminal activity, as an expression of anger or vengeance, to improve one's living circumstances, and are not due to delusions or hallucinations, or as a result of impaired judgment.
- Fire setting is not better accounted for by conduct disorder, a manic episode, or antisocial personality disorder.

Differential diagnosis
Conduct disorder, ADHD, adjustment disorder, other major affective or psychotic disorder.

Co-morbidity
Substance abuse or dependence, past history of sexual or physical abuse, antisocial personality disorder.

Treatment
Should address any underlying or co-morbid psychiatric disorder. Psychotherapeutic intervention may be helpful (e.g., CBT).

Recommended further reading

1 Dell'Osso, B. et al. (2006). Epidemiologic and clinical updates on impulse control disorders: a critical review. Eur Arch Psychiatry Clin Neurosci **256**, 464–475.
2 McElroy, S.L., Pope, H.G. Jr, Hudson, J.I., et al. (1991). Kleptomania: a report of 20 cases. AJP **148**, 652–657.
3 Puri, B.K., Baxter, R., Cordess, C.C. (1995). Characteristics of fire setters. A study and proposed multi-axial psychiatric classification. Brit Jour of Psychiatry **166**: 393–6.

Impulse control disorders (2)

Pathological gambling disorder[1]

Persistent and recurrent maladaptive patterns of gambling behavior that may lead to significant personal, family, and occupational difficulties. The disorder is thought to begin in adolescence, where the prevalence is 4–7%. Prevalence in adults is reported around 1–3%, whereas about 86% of the U.S. population consider themselves recreational gamblers.

Highly co-morbid with multiple psychiatric disorders (e.g., depression, substance use, bipolar disorder).

Diagnostic criteria

- Preoccupation with gambling (thinking of past gambling experiences, planning the next experience, or thinking of ways to get money to gamble).
- Needing to gamble with larger amounts of money to get the same feeling of excitement.
- Unsuccessful attempts to stop gambling or to cut down.
- Restlessness or irritability when trying to cut down or stop gambling.
- Gambling to escape from problems or to relieve feelings of anxiety, depression, or guilt.
- Chasing losses (return after losing to get even).
- Lying to family or friends about gambling.
- Committing illegal acts to finance gambling.
- Has lost or jeopardized a significant relationship, job, or career or educational opportunities because of gambling.
- Relies on family or friends for money to relieve financial problems caused by gambling.
- The gambling behavior is not better accounted for by a manic episode.

Co-morbidity

Mood disorders, ADHD, substance abuse or dependence, other impulse control disorders, cluster B personality disorders.

Treatment

Exclusion and treatment of any co-morbid psychiatric disorder. Proposed specific treatments to control addictive behavior include SSRIs (e.g., fluoxetine, fluvoxamine, paroxetine, citalopram), lithium, clomipramine, and naltrexone. CBT also may help reduce preoccupation with gambling.

Trichotillomania[2]

Recurrent pulling of one's own hair, exacerbated by stress or relaxation (e.g., reading, watching TV). Feelings of tension are relieved by pulling hair. Usually involves the scalp, but may include eyelashes, eyebrows, axillae, pubic, and any other body regions. In children, F = M, often with a limited course. In adults, F(3.4%) > M (1.5%), with a chronic or episodic course. Lifetime prevalence rate of 1–2%.

Diagnostic criteria
- Recurrent pulling out of one's hair resulting in noticeable hair loss.
- An increasing sense of tension immediately before pulling out the hair or when attempting to resist the behavior.
- Pleasure, gratification, or relief when pulling out the hair.
- The disturbance is not better accounted for by another mental disorder and is not due to a general medical condition (e.g., a dermatological condition).
- The behavior causes clinically significant distress or impairment in social or occupational functioning.

Associated features
Examining hair root, pulling strands between teeth, trichophagia (eating hairs), nail biting, scratching, gnawing, excoriation.

Differential diagnosis
OCD, Tourette's syndrome, pervasive developmental disorder (e.g., autism), stereotyped behavior, factitious disorder.

Co-morbidity
Depressive disorder, generalized anxiety disorder, OCD, personality disorder.

Treatment
Address any co-morbid disorder. CBT/ behavioral modification (substitution, positive/negative reinforcement) is key to treatment. There is some evidence for use of SSRIs, clomipramine, pimozide, risperidone, and lithium.

Recommended further reading

1 Grant, Jon E. and Potenza, Marc N. Impulse control disorders: Clinical characteristics and pharmacological management. *Annals of Clinical Psychiatry.* **16**(1), Jan-Mar 2004, 27–34.
2 Walsh, K.H. and McDougle, C.J. (2001). Trichotillomania. Presentation, etiology, diagnosis and therapy. *Am J Clin Dermatol* **2**, 327–333.

Sleep disorders

Introduction

Functions of sleep

Sleep and sleep-wake rhythms are found in all higher animals. Among these organisms, some functions of sleep are held in common:

- Use of a sleeping period as a way to help match animals to their environment.
  - For example, humans are awake during the day when they can rely on their vision whereas rodents are awake at night when they can rely on smell and touch.
- Use of sleep and quiet wakefulness as a way to physically restore the body.
  - For example, sleep deprivation is associated with impaired glucose metabolism and altered immune function.
- Use of sleep to optimize waking function and cognition.
  - For instance, sleep deprivation may lead to decreased alertness and decision making capacity.

Clinical assessment of sleep

Sleep history

An accurate clinical history is the foundation of the proper diagnosis and treatment of a sleep disorder.

- Current symptoms: nature, severity, duration, frequency, time course, exacerbating and reliving factors, effect on daily life and/or impairments.
- 24-hour history: the circumstances of sleep and wakefulness. Sleep-related questions may include activities prior to bedtime that may prove incompatible with restful sleep, sleep latency (or, the time it takes to fall asleep), number/duration/timing of nighttime awakenings, snoring, limb movements, and other behaviors during sleep.
- Daytime-related questions may include naps, difficulty staying awake, inadvertent sleep episodes, use of alarms clocks, periods of confusion, and amount of time needed to fully awaken.
- Regularity and timing of sleep-wake behaviors over time.
- Bed partner history: the reporting of breathing problems (choking, snoring, gasping), limb or muscle movement during sleep as well as complex behaviors such as sleep walking/talking, changes in mood, substance use.
- Family history of sleep disorders.
- Medication use, including timing and recent changes.
- Substance use, including the timing and use of caffeine, nicotine, alcohol, and illicit substances.
- Previous treatments and their effects on sleep disorders.

Actigraphy

- Method to measure motor activity, usually through an activity meter worn on the wrist. Data collected by this device may reveal general patterns of sleep and wakefulness.

Sleep diary

- Record created by the patient detailing his/her sleep-wake pattern over a period of weeks. Information included in the diary: daily activities, sleep/wake times, naps, exercise, mealtimes, and use of caffeine/nicotine/alcohol/other substances.

Polysomnography (PSG)

- A polysomnogram includes at least one channel of electroencephalography (EEG) to measure brain activity, electrooculography (EOG) to measure eye movements, and electromyography (EMG) to measure muscle tone, usually in the submentalis muscles.
- Additional channels of PSG may measure nasal-oral airflow or nasal pressure, chest and abdominal movement to measure breathing, oximetry to measure oxygen desaturation, and additional EMG channels of the anterior tibilias muscles to evaluate for movements before or during sleep.
- Polysomnography is indicated for the evaluation of patients with suspected sleep apnea and in some cases of parasomnia. It is not routinely indicated for restless legs syndrome, circadian rhythm sleep disorders, and insomnia; in these disorders the diagnosis relies on the clinical history.

Multiple Sleep Latency Test (MSLT)

- MSLT is a variant of polysomnography used to evaluate daytime sleepiness. EEG, EOG, and EMG data is recorded while the patient is allowed to nap four to five times at two-hour intervals throughout the day. The sleep latency and presence or absence of rapid eye movement sleep for each nap is noted.
- Mean sleep latency values >10 minutes are considered normal, while values <8 minutes suggest clinically significant sleepiness. The presence of REM sleep in at least two naps may indicate the presence of narcolepsy.

Stages of normal sleep

- Sleep normally cycles through a pattern of stages. The different stages of sleep may be seen in polysomnography, as revealed by EEG.
- Sleep is divided in Rapid Eye Movement (REM) sleep and nonrapid eye movement (NREM) sleep. REM and NREM sleep alternate every 90–100 minutes throughout the night.
- NREM sleep is further subdivided into 4 stages of decreasing arousability:
  - Stage 1 is viewed as a transitional sleep stage.
  - Stage 2 occupies the majority of NREM sleep.
  - Stages 3 and 4 are "deep" sleep.
- Normal sleep stages, as characterized on PSG:
  - Wakefulness: low-voltage, fast frequency EEG pattern (alpha pattern), voluntary eye movements, tonic muscle tone.
  - Stage 1 NREM sleep: small increase in EEG amplitude with slowing of EEG frequency, slow rolling eye movements in EOG channels.
  - Stage 2 NREM sleep: increase in amplitude and further slowing of EEG frequencies, presence of "K complexes" (isolated large-amplitude slow waves) and "sleep spindles" (episodic bursts of fast EEG activity), reduction in muscle tone.
  - Stage 3 NREM sleep: large amplitude, slow EEG activity also known as "delta" or "slow-wave sleep" that comprises 20–50% of a 30-second epoch, low muscle tone, EOG pattern mirrors EEG activity.
  - Stage 4 NREM sleep: same as stage 3 sleep, except delta activity constitutes >50% of an epoch.
  - REM sleep: return of fast-frequency, mixed voltage EEG activity similar to Stage 1 NREM sleep. Phasic rapid eye movements are characteristically seen. Muscle tone is essentially absent aside from muscle twitches.

Insomnia

Note: The International Classification of Sleep Disorders Second Edition (ICSD-2) is commonly used by sleep medicine practitioners as a diagnostic manual. As the sleep medicine field encompasses practitioners from various fields, including psychiatry, pulmnology, and neurology, this manual allows medical personnel to use a standardized manual from which to draw information. However, in deference to the use of the DSM IV-TR by psychiatrists, reference has been made to both ICSD and DSM definitions when applicable. Although the information contained in these two manuals is generally consistent, some differences in sleep disorder classification are present.

Thus, naming by classifications will be denoted as follows: International Classification of Sleep Disorders Second Edition (ICSD-2) first followed by [DSM IV-TR] in brackets.

Insomnia [primary insomnia]

DSM IV-TR contains two diagnoses that fall under this category: Primary Insomnia and Insomnia Related to Axis I or II. DSM critieria state that the predominant complaint of difficulty initiating/maintaining sleep, or nonrestorative sleep, must be present for at least 1 month and be associated with impairment of functioning.

Under the ICSD, insomnia is defined as:
- Insomnia symptoms may consist of difficulty falling asleep, nighttime awakenings, inadequate sleep quality or sleep duration.
- Insomnia causes significant distress or impairment in functioning.
- Adequate opportunity for sleep exists.

Epidemiology

Prevalence of insomnia symptoms is 30–40% in the general population. Prevalence of insomnia disorder is 5–10%.

Risk factors

Risk factors include female sex, advanced age, unemployment, co-morbid illnesses, genetics, psychosocial stressors, and counterproductive sleep habits.

Pathophysiology

- Physiological model proposes that insomnia is a disorder of increased arousal.
- Cognitive-behavioral model propose that insomnia arises from the interaction of predisposing factors, external precipitating factors, and cognitive-behavioral perpetuating factors.

Consequences

Insomnia is a risk factor for developing depressive, anxiety, and substance abuse disorders. Insomnia is associated with motor vehicle accidents, work absenteeism, and reduced quality of life.

Clinical assessment and diagnosis

The clinical assessment relies on careful history taking. Review of the insomnia history, including a 24-hour perspective. Symptoms, chronology, alleviating and exacerbating factors, and previous treatments should be assessed. In addition, sleep/wake times, regularity of these hours, and daytime activities should also be questioned.

- Evaluation of underlying psychiatric, medical, co-morbid sleep disorders should be performed.
- Medication and substance use history must also be ascertained.
- Sleep-wake diaries, actigraphy, and polysomnography may also play a role in making the diagnosis.

Differential diagnosis

The differential diagnosis list is broad.

- Primary insomnia refers to a disorder in which the chief complaint is insomnia in the absence of another disorder as a possible cause.
- Secondary insomnia arises from other causes, including many psychiatric illnesses. Medical diseases such as congestive heart failure, COPD, stroke, Parkinson's disease, chronic renal failure, diabetes, hyperthyroidism, arthritis, and fibromylagia may cause insomnia.
- Substance use including alcohol, caffeine, nicotine, and stimulants must be considered.
- Medications such as antidepressants, decongestants, corticosteroids, and statins may also cause insomnia.

Treatment of insomnia

- Pharmacological management should focus on short-term use (2–4 weeks), followed by a gradual taper and discontinuation of medication.
- For primary insomnia, the first-line choice is a short-acting benzodiazepine receptor agonist, such as zoplidem, eszopiclone, or zaleplon. A sedating antidepressant such as doxepin or amitriptyline may be used adjunctively. A third-line choice is gabapentin or tiagabine.
- Psychological and behavioral treatments may be used alongside medications.
- Sleep restriction therapy maximizes sleep efficiency by restricting time spent in bed with strict bedtime and waking hours.
- Stimulus control therapy reinforces connections between sleep and the sleep environment; the patient is told to use the bed/bedroom for sleep and sex only and to enter the bedroom only when sleepy. If still awake after 20 minutes, the patient must leave the bedroom until sleepy once more.
- Cognitive therapy uses psychological methods to both challenge and change misconceptions about sleep and insomnia. A combination of behavioral and cognitive techniques may also be utilized.

Hypersomnias of central origin (1)—narcolepsy

ICSD-2 names three types of hypersomnia of central origin: Narcolepsy, Idiopathic Hypersomnia, and Recurrent Hypersomnia.
- In ICSD-2 narcolepsy is further defined as occurring with cataplexy, without cataplexy, due to a medical condition, or unspecified; these distinctions are not made in the DSM IV-TR, which simply lists the diagnosis as narcolepsy.

DSM IV-TR contains three diagnoses that fall under this category: Narcolepsy, Primary Hypersomnia, and Hypersomnia Related to an Axis I or II disorder.

Narcolepsy

Definition

The DSM criteria for narcolepsy include: irresistible attacks of refreshing sleep that occur daily over at least three months; and the presence of cataplexy and/or recurrent rapid eye movement intrusions in the transition between sleep and wakefulness, as manifested by sleep paralysis and hypnopompic or hypnagogic hallucinations.

In ICSD, narcolepsy is defined as a complaint of irresistible attacks of refreshing sleep occurring on a daily basis for at least three months in addition to the following based on laboratory findings:
- On the multiple sleep latency test (MSLT), mean sleep latency is ≤8 minutes, and two or more sleep-onset rapid-eye-movement periods are found in patients who have had at least 6 hours of sleep the night before the test. CSF hypocretin-1 levels ≤110 pg/mL or one-third of mean control values are also considered to be diagnostic.
- Cataplexy, which is defined as a transient loss of muscle tone that occurs suddenly in response to strong emotion.

Epidemiology
- Narcolepsy with cataplexy occurs in 0.02% to 0.18% of the U.S. population. Males and females are equally affected.
- Prevalence of narcolepsy without cataplexy, narcolepsy due to a medical condition, and unspecified narcolepsy are unknown.

Risk factors
Narcolepsy with cataplexy is associated with human leukocyte antigen (HLA) subtypes DR2/DRB1*1501 and DQB1*0602. First-degree relatives of patients with these subtypes have a 10- to 40-fold increased risk for narcolepsy with cataplexy.

Pathophysiology
Narcolepsy with cataplexy is linked to a loss of hypothalamic neurons that contain hypocretin. An underlying autoimmune process may lead to elimination of the hypocretin cells.

Consequences
Significant impact on psychosocial functioning with negative effects on social interactions and work.

Clinical assessment and diagnosis

- Patients commonly present with excessive daytime sleepiness. This symptom may manifest as nodding off or falling asleep in low-stimulation environments. Urges to sleep, known as sleep attacks, irritability, poor concentration or memory, and automatic behavior, characterized by nonsensical behavior performed while sleepy, may also characterize the disorder.
- Cataplexy may range from total body collapse to more localized muscular involvement such as ptosis or slurred speech. While any strong emotional stimuli can trigger an event, laughter is a common trigger. Note: These are manifestations of REM elements intruding on the transition from sleep to wakefulness or vice versa.
- Hypnagogic (occur as patient transitions from wakefulness to sleep) or hypnopompic (occur as patient transitions from sleep to wakefulness) hallucinations, especially of a visual nature, may occur. Auditory and tactile hallucinations may also occur. Note: These are manifestations of REM elements intruding on the transition from sleep to wakefulness or vice versa.
- Sleep paralysis, or the inability to move, during the the transition from sleep to wakefulness may occur. Note: These are manifestations of REM elements intruding on the transition from sleep to wakefulness or vice versa.
- Polysomnography is performed to rule out other sleep disorders such as sleep apnea, periodic limb movement disorder, and REM sleep disorder.
- MSLT, in which a patient is presented with four or five 20-minute nap opportunities every two hours in the morning and afternoon, will show a sleep latency of eight minutes or less.

Differential diagnosis

- For excessive daytime sleepiness: sleep apnea, idiopathic hypersomnia, periodic limb movement disorder, insufficient sleep, depression, neurodegenerative disorder.
- For cataplexy: transient ischemic attack, seizure, vestibular disorder.

Treatment

Pharmacologic treatment for daytime sleepiness includes: modafinil (Provigil®), sodium oxybate/GHB (Xyrem®), and traditional stimulants including methylphenidate, dextroamphetamine, and methamphetamine. Note: use of traditional stimulants may be accompanied by side-effects such as rebound hypersomnia and tachyphylaxis. Sodium oxybate, TCAs, SSRIs may be used in the treatment of cataplexy.

Behavioral treatments include: regular sleep schedule, scheduled daytime naps, and elimination of shift work.

Hypersomnias of central origin (2)

Idiopathic hypersomnia

Definition
Idiopathic hypersomnia is defined by the following: excessive daytime sleepiness occurring for at least three months on an almost daily basis; Multiple Sleep Latency Test showing mean sleep latency <8 minutes and <2 sleep onset REM periods; polysomnography results exclude other causes of sleepiness.

Epidemiology
Prevalence is unknown.

Risk factors
A possible familial link may exist.

Pathophysiology
Etiology is unknown, but daytime sleepiness may be preceded in some patients by a viral illness such as Guillain-Barre syndrome or mononucleosis.

Consequences
Significant impact on psychosocial functioning with negative effects on social interactions and work.

Clinical assessment and diagnosis
As in narcolepsy, the main complaint of this disorder is excessive daytime sleepiness. Unlike patients with narcolepsy, idiopathic hypersomnia patients do not present with cataplexy, reduced CSF hypocretin levels, or nocturnal sleep disruption. Furthermore, if these patients take naps, they are characterized as unrefreshing.
- Polysomnography reveals normal to increased total sleep time without the sleep fragmentation commonly seen in patients with narcolepsy. The MLST shows a short sleep latency but no evidence of sleep onset REM periods.

Differential diagnosis
Narcolepsy, sleep-related breathing disorders, insufficient sleep, periodic limb movement disorder, depression.

Treatment
Treatment of excessive daytime sleepiness in idiopathic hypersomnia follows that of narcolepsy.

Recurrent hypersomnia
This category includes both Kleine-Levin syndrome and menstrual-related hypersomnia.
- Kleine-Levin syndrome is an idiopathic disorder primarily seen in adolescent males. Patients present with periods of daytime sleepiness in conjunction with hyperphagia, hypersexuality, and aggression. While not sleeping patients may also manifest confusion, stupor, and irritability. They then have periods in which they are asymptomatic. Polysomnography shows long total sleep time, high sleep efficiency, and decreased slow-wave sleep. The disorder is usually self-limited.

- Menstrual-related hypersomnia is characterized by daytime sleepiness in the days preceding menstruation. Etiology and prevalence are not known. Treatment with medication that blocks ovulation, such as oral contraceptives, may be beneficial.

Sleep-related breathing disorder (breathing-related sleep disorder)

Definition

DSM IV-TR defines the sleep disorders that fall under this category as sleep-related breathing conditions that lead to disruption in sleep, as manifested by excessive sleepiness or insomnia. Specific examples include obstructive and central sleep apneas as well as central alveolar hypoventilation syndrome. This diagnosis should be coded on both Axis I and Axis III.

Obstructive sleep apnea (OSA)

Definition

OSA is defined as repetitive episodes of obstruction in the upper airway that occur during sleep, resulting in snoring, apneic periods, gasping, and choking, and ultimately sleep disruption. The disruption in sleep results in daytime symptoms including sleepiness and fatigue.

- An obstructive apnea is defined as a significantly decreased or lack of airflow (less than 25% of a normal breath) for at least 10 seconds at the nose and mouth, despite efforts to breathe. An obstructive hypopnea is defined as a decrease in airflow, usually at least 30% of baseline. Both apneas and hypopneas are associated with a 4% or greater decrease in blood oxygen saturation.
- The Apnea Hypopnea Index (AHI) is a measure of syndrome severity and is defined as the total number of apneas and hypopneas per hour of sleep. An AHI with fewer than 5 events per hour of sleep is normal. An AHI of 5–15 events per hour of sleep is defined as mild OSA, 16–30 events per hour as moderate OSA, and greater than 30 events per hour as severe OSA.

Epidemiology

Estimates of prevalence vary based on the criteria used to define the disorder. In one study in which the disorder was defined as having an AHI >5 in addition to excessive daytime sleepiness, prevalence was estimated at 24% of men and 9% of women.

- The ratio of men to women with OSA is 2:1.

Risk factors

The major risk factor is obesity. Other risk factors include head and neck structural abnormalities, such as enlarged tonsils or adenoids, increased neck circumference, menopause, hypothyroidism, smoking (causes inflammation, swelling, and narrowing of the upper airway), sedative or alcohol use (causes relaxation of the musculature of the upper airway), Marfan syndrome, and Down syndrome.

Pathophysiology

Upper airway narrowing during sleep causes OSA. In turn, this narrowing may be secondary to a variety of factors such as bulky soft tissue in the oropharynx, craniofacial abnormalities, and decreased pharyngeal muscle tone.

Consequences

- Increased risk of hypertension secondary to repeated triggering of the sympathetic nervous system.
- Increased risk of motor vehicle accidents.
- Decreased neurocognitive function with negative effects on vigilance, coordination, and executive functioning.
- A possible relationship between OSA and depression may exist. Up to 20% of patients presenting with depressive symptoms may have OSA and vice versa.

Clinical assessment and diagnosis

- Patients may complain of snoring, choking, snorting, or breathing cessation at night (noted by their bed partner) as well as sleepiness, fatigue, and insomnia.
- Physically patients may present with obesity, retro/micrognathia, enlarged tonsils, elongated soft palate, or right heart failure.
- On polysomnography breathing disordered events are usually marked by an arousal on EEG and by a drop in oxyhemoglobin saturation. Paradoxical movement of the chest and abdomen and bradytachycardia may also be seen.

Differential diagnosis

Depression, chronic sleep deprivation, narcolepsy, insomnia.

Treatment

- Lifestyle interventions such as weight loss, avoidance of sleep deprivation, supine sleeping position, alcohol, or sedatives, as well as smoking cessation.
- Pharmacologic interventions include treating any medical conditions that may be contributing to OSA, such as hypothyroidism and allergic rhinitis.
- Positive pressure delivered through a nasal or nasal-oral mask pneumatically splints open the airway during sleep. Options include Continuous Positive Airway Pressure (CPAP) and Bilevel Positive Airway Pressure (BiPAP). CPAP and BiPAP are considered first-line therapy.
- Second-line therapies, include oral appliances to change the position of the tongue and mandible in order to maximize the airway opening and surgery, such as uvulopalatopharyngoplasty.

Sleep-related movement disorder

(Dyssomnia not otherwise specified)

DSM-IV-TR includes both restless legs syndrome and periodic limb movements in this category. They fall under an NOS label because they do not fit under defined categories of dyssomnias, such as insomnia, hypersomnia, narcolepsy, and circadian rhythm disorders.

Restless legs syndrome (RLS)

Definition

Four criteria are required for diagnosis:

- an urge to move the legs commonly accompanied with unpleasant sensation in the legs.
- exacerbation of sensations during rest or inactivity.
- relief of sensations with movement.
- increased sensations in the evening or night.

Epidemiology

- Three to five percent of adults of Northern European descent.
- Female to male ratio 1.5–2:1.

Risk factors

- Secondary RLS may be associated with iron deficiency anemia, rheumatoid arthritis, end-stage renal disease, or pregnancy.
- Medication use including sedating antihistamines, dopamine-receptor antagonists, and antidepressants (especially serotonergic).

Pathophysiology

Possible mechanisms include: impaired transport and intracellular use of iron in the central nervous system; an autosomal dominant inheritance pattern; hypodopaminergic state.

Consequences

- Increased risk of insomnia and daytime sleepiness.
- Increased risk of depression (13 times higher in men with RLS versus men without RLS).
- Eighty percent of RLS patients also have periodic limb movement disorder.

Clinical assessment and diagnosis

- RLS is a clinical diagnosis. Common descriptions of sensory symptoms include achy, itchy, or "creepy-crawly" sensations in the legs. Symptoms tend to worsen in the evening, particularly when patient is trying to go to sleep. Complaints of sleep disturbance, especially sleep onset insomnia, are therefore common. Relief may occur with movement and stimulation of the legs by rubbing or hot baths.
- Suggested Immobilization Test (SIT) may be helpful in assessing the severity of RLS. The patient lies supine for one hour and does not move legs unless necessary. Meanwhile, he/she rates sensory complaints every five minutes while an EMG of anterior tibialis is taken.

Differential diagnosis
- To consider with motor restlessness: akathisia, anxiety disorder, attention deficit hyperactivity disorder, periodic limb movement disorder.
- To consider with sensory symptoms: peripheral neuropathy, opiate withdrawal.

Treatment
- Treat reversible causes of RLS such as iron deficiency, medication-related symptoms, and opiate withdrawal.
- Lifestyle modifications include limited caffeine and alcohol intake 12 hours prior to bedtime and preventing sleep deprivation.
- First-line therapy for RLS includes long-acting dopaminergic agonists such as pramipexole, ropinirole, and pergolide. Of note, these medications must be used with caution in psychotic patients because they may exacerbate psychosis.
- Adjunctive medications include gabapentin, opiates, and benzodiazepines.

Periodic limb movement disorder (PLMD)
Definition
PLMD is defined by sleep disturbance or daytime fatigue in the setting of polysomnographic findings of stereotyped, repetitive limb movements. Limb movements must be 0.5–5 seconds in duration, occur in a sequence of at least 4 movements, and be separated by intervals of 5 to 90 seconds. A periodic limb movement arousal index of greater than 15 events per hour is also required.

Epidemiology
Prevalence is not known, although up to 34% of people over the age of 60 may be affected.

Risk factors
- Increased risk with advancing age.
- Increased risk of periodic limb movements during sleep with restless legs syndrome (80–90% of patients), REM sleep behavior disorder (70%), and narcolepsy (45–65%).
- Medication use, including selective serotonin reuptake inhibitors, lithium, TCAs, and dopamine-receptor antagonists, may lead to or aggravate periodic limb movements.
- Low level of iron in the central nervous system may exacerbate periodic limb movements.

Pathophysiology
Etiology is not known, although a connection with dopaminergic impairment has been hypothesized.

Consequences
- Insomnia or hypersomnia secondary to nonrestful sleep.
- Disturbance of bed partner's sleep.
- Increased risk of depression, memory and attention deficits.

Clinical assessment and diagnosis
- Periodic limb movements usually occur in the lower extremities, commonly involving extension of the big toe with partial flexion of ankle, knee, or hip. Movements can also occur in the upper extremities. The patient is usually unaware of movement.
- Patients may complain of difficulty with sleep onset or sleep maintenance. Fatigue and excessive daytime sleepiness may also accompany the condition.
- In addition to the clinical presentation, polysomnographic evidence of limb movements as set by the definition of the disorder is necessary for diagnosis.

Differential diagnosis
Sleep starts, fragmentary myoclonus, seizure disorder.

Treatment
- Medication options include benzodiazepines, dopaminergic agents, and gabapentin.

Parasomnias (1)

Classification of Parasomnias:
- DSM-IV-TR divides parasomnias into the four categories: nightmare disorder, sleep terror disorder, sleepwalking disorder and parasomnias not otherwise specified.
- Another approach to understanding parasomnias, as used in the ICSD-2, is to distinguish between parasomnias associated with NREM sleep versus REM sleep. Disorders that arise in NREM sleep include confusional arousals, sleepwalking, and sleep terrors. Disorders that arise in REM sleep include nightmare disorder, recurrent isolated sleep paralysis, and REM sleep behavior disorder. The latter two disorders are classified in DSM-IV-TR as parasomnia not otherwise specified.

Confusional arousals

Definition
Mental confusion occurring upon arousal or awakening from sleep.

Epidemiology
Prevalence is 17% in children up to 13 years of age and ranges from 2.9–4.2% in those over 15 years of age.

Risk factors
Genetic factors, shift work, insomnia, hypersomnia, circadian rhythm disorder, mood disorder, substance abuse, sleep deprivation.

Pathophysiology
Etiology is unknown, although a familial component may exist.

Consequences
- Children with this disorder may develop sleepwalking as adolescents.
- Significant social, school, and work impairment may result.

Clinical assessment and diagnosis
- Confusional arousals commonly arise in the earlier part of the sleep cycle. On EEG, arousal episodes may correlate with delta waves, theta or alpha activity.
- Three variants found in adults include excessive sleep inertia, abnormal sleep-related sexual behavior, and sleep-related violence.

Differential diagnosis
Seizure disorder, sleepwalking, sleep terrors.

Treatment
- The decision to treat is based on impairment or distress as well as the degree of danger to individual or others.
- A regular sleep schedule, avoidance of sleep deprivation, safe sleep and home environment (e.g., locking of windows, sleeping on the ground floor) may be beneficial.

Sleepwalking

Definition
Ambulation that occurs during sleep and is associated with at least one of the following: difficulty arousing the individual, mental confusion upon awakening, amnesia of the episode, routine behaviors occurring at inappropriate times, inappropriate or dangerous behaviors.

Epidemiology
Prevalence peaks between 5–10 years of age. 10–20% of children and 1–4% of adults are affected.

Risk factors
A significant genetic component exists.

Precipitating factors
Include sleep deprivation, central nervous system insult such as stroke or trauma, hyperthyroidism, migraines, stress, irregular sleep schedules, and the use of lithium, anticholinergics, and phenothiazines.

Pathophysiology
Etiology is unknown.

Consequences
Possible injury to the individual or co-habitors, disruption of bed partner's sleep.

Clinical assessment and diagnosis
- Sleepwalking usually arises during slow-wave sleep and thus commonly starts in the first few hours of sleep.
- Goal-directed activity such as attempts to use bathroom may occur. The individual's eyes may be open.
- On EEG, arousal from slow-wave sleep followed by an increase in autonomic activity may be seen. Polysomnography can help to determine if precipitants such as seizure disorder, periodic limb movements, or a breathing disorder may be triggering arousal.

Differential diagnosis
Sleep terrors, REM sleep behavior disorder, sleep related epilepsy, malingering.

Treatment
- The decision to treat is based on impairment or distress as well as the degree of danger to the individual or others.
- A regular sleep schedule, avoidance of sleep deprivation, safe sleep and home environment (e.g., locking of windows, sleeping on the ground floor) may be beneficial.
- Clonazepam and other benzodiazepine receptor agonists can be used without tolerance developing in the individual.

Parasomnias (2)

Sleep terrors

Definition
An episode of terror commonly associated with a loud cry that occurs with autonomic or behavioral arousal. In addition, at least one of the following must also be present: difficulty arousing individual, mental confusion upon awakening, amnesia of episode, or dangerous behaviors.

Epidemiology
Prevalence is 5% of children and 1–2% of adults.

Risk factors
A genetic component exists.

Precipitants
May include a breathing disorder such as OSA.

Pathophysiology
Etiology is unknown.

Consequences
Social impairment, possible injury to individual or co-habitors.

Clinical assessment and diagnosis
- Sleep terrors usually arise during slow-wave sleep and thus commonly start in the first few hours of sleep.
- Episodes usually start with arousal followed by a loud cry or scream. Increased autonomic activity, such as elevated heart or respiratory rate, diaphoresis, and increased muscle tone may follow. Confusion during the event and amnesia of the event are common.
- On EEG, arousal from slow-wave sleep followed by an increase in autonomic activity may be seen. Polysomnography can help to determine if precipitants such as periodic limb movements or a breathing disorder may be triggering arousal. It may also help to exclude REM sleep behavior disorder.

Differential diagnosis
Sleepwalking, confusional arousals, REM sleep, behavior disorder, seizure disorder, nocturnal panic attack, malingering.

Treatment
- The decision to treat is based on impairment or distress as well as the degree of danger to the individual or others.
- A regular sleep schedule, avoidance of sleep deprivation, safe sleep and home environment (e.g., locking of windows, sleeping on the ground floor) may be beneficial.
- Clonazepam and other benzodiazepine receptor agonists can be used without tolerance developing in the individual.

Nightmare disorder

Definition
- Recurrent awakenings with recollection of disturbing dreams.
- No confusion or disorientation upon awakening and clear recollection of dream content are present.
- Disorder is also marked by either delayed return to sleep following episode or occurrence of episode in latter half of sleep.

Epidemiology
- Prevalence is 5% in adults and is higher in women.
- Seventy-five percent of children report having at least one nightmare during childhood. Generally, nightmares decrease in frequency and intensity with age.
- Of note, nightmares are seen in at least 50% of individuals with PTSD.

Risk factors
PTSD or acute stress disorder, female sex, low socioeconomic status, antidepressants, dopamine-receptor agonists.

Pathophysiology
Etiology is unknown.

Consequences
Sleep avoidance, insomnia, depression, daytime sleepiness.

Clinical assessment and diagnosis
Clinical history, including evaluation for a traumatic event.

Differential diagnosis
Sleep terrors, sleep paralysis, REM sleep behavior disorder.

Treatment
- Medication: prazosin.
- Imagery rehearsal, in which new versions of a nightmare are re-scripted during the day.

Circadian rhythm sleep disorders

Classification

DSM-IV-TR divides circadian rhythm sleep disorders into four subtypes: delayed sleep phase, jet lag, shift work, and unspecified types. ICSD-2 makes similar divisions, but also includes other subdivisions, including advanced sleep phase.

Background

- Circadian, or 24-hour, rhythms underlie physiology. The sleep-wake cycle is one example of a circadian rhythm. In mammals the suprachiasmatic nucleus (SCN) acts as a pacemaker to maintain a self-sustaining rhythm.
- The SCN also synchronizes the endogenous rhythm to the 24-hour day. Light, the strongest synchronizing agent, can delay circadian rhythms if exposure occurs in the first half of the night. Similarly, light exposure in the second half of the night may advance the rhythm. In addition, melatonin exposure in the early evening can phase advance, while exposure in the early morning can phase delay.

Delayed sleep phase type

Definition

Habitual sleep-wake times are delayed, usually by more than two hours, relative to socially accepted times. Typically the patient may have difficulty falling asleep and prefer later wake-up times; however, once asleep sleep is normal. When allowed to choose a preferred schedule, the patient will demonstrate a delayed but stable circadian phase.

Epidemiology

More common in adolescents and young adults, with a prevalence of 7–16%. Mean age of onset is 20 years. Prevalence in the general population is <1%.

Risk factors

Genetic factors, bright light exposure in the evening, minimal light exposure in the morning, caffeine or stimulant use, shift work, travel across time zones.

Pathophysiology

Etiology is unknown.

Consequences

Difficulty conforming to required school and work schedules.

Clinical assessment and diagnosis

- A stable delay of the sleep period coupled with an inability to fall asleep and awaken at socially accepted times forms the diagnosis. Patients may fit the description of extreme "night owls."
- Sleep log or actigraphy for at least seven days will show a stable delay in the sleep period.

Differential diagnosis

Normal sleep, insomnia, depression.

Treatment
- Chronotherapy: bedtime is delayed by three hours every two days until the desired sleep time is achieved.
- Exposure to bright light in the early morning and dark in the evening.
- Melatonin administered in the evening can phase advance sleep-wake times.

Advanced sleep phase type

Definition
Advance in the sleep period relative to desired sleep/wake times, resulting in early morning awakenings and the inability to stay awake until a desired bedtime. When allowed to choose a schedule, patients will demonstrate advanced, but stable, sleep-wake patterns.

Epidemiology
Prevalence increases with age. Prevalence in the general population is unknown.

Risk factors
Genetic factors, environmental factors.

Pathophysiology
Etiology is unknown.

Consequences
Difficulty conforming to conventionally accepted times for social interaction.

Clinical assessment and diagnosis
- A stable advancement of the sleep period coupled with an inability to fall asleep and awaken at socially accepted times forms the diagnosis. Patients may fit the description of extreme "morning larks."
- Sleep log or actigraphy for at least seven days will show a stable advance in the sleep period.

Differential diagnosis
Normal sleep, insomnia, depression.

Treatment
- Chronotherapy: bedtime is advanced by two hours every two days until the desired sleep time is achieved.
- Exposure to bright light in the early evening.

Reproductive psychiatry and sexuality

Introduction

Reproductive psychiatry and sexuality is a developing area of psychiatry. This field is at the intersection of gynecology, urology, obstetrics, and family practice. Therefore, criteria and definitions from the professional societies in these fields are also referred to throughout this chapter. This is an area of a great deal of recent research, and its clinical importance is only now being recognized. Much of this chapter focuses on female reproductive psychiatry. However, that does not mean that there are not significant reproductive and sexual aspects to psychiatric disorders in men. The disorders that we identify are limited by those that we look for. A bias that male psychiatry would not be affected by reproduction and hormones has been present for over a century in the West. Clinical observations made in the absence of this preconception, and studies designed to test this are necessary. Until these are done, the minimal inclusion of male reproductive psychiatry in this chapter signifies only a lack of knowledge, not a lack of effect.

Disorders related to menstruation

Premenstrual symptoms

The physical signs and symptoms that affect up to three-quarters of women with regular menstrual cycles. The most common presentations are abdominal bloating (present in 90% of women with any symptoms), breast tenderness and headaches. These mild symptoms do not usually interfere with a woman's ability to function.

Management

Premenstrual symptoms that do not meet premenstrual syndrome (PMS) or premenstrual dysphoric disorder (PMDD) criteria (see below) are initially conservatively managed unless there is significant psychiatric co-morbidity. This management involves a diet low in salt, fat, caffeine, and sugar; restriction of alcohol and tobacco; exercise; and measures to reduce stress.

If there is failure to adequately respond to conservative management after two to three months, consider medicating with SSRIs.

Menstrual-related disorders

Premenstrual syndrome (PMS) and premenstrual dysphoric disorder (PMDD)

To diagnose a menstrual-related disorder, one must:
• Establish that signs and symptoms are those characteristic of these disorders.
• Prospectively document that the signs and symptoms occur only in the luteal phase and the first few days of menses.
• To be a disorder, the symptoms must impair some aspect of the women's life.
• Exclude hormone or drug ingestion.
• Exclude other possible diagnoses.

Premenstrual syndrome (PMS)

Clinically significant PMS occurs in 20–30% of women. PMS is characterized by the presence of both physical and behavioral symptoms that recur in the second half of the menstrual cycle, and often the first few days of menses. Most common behavioral symptoms are fatigue, labile mood, irritability, tension, depressed mood, increased appetite, forgetfulness, and difficulty concentrating (see table). These symptoms must be severe enough to impair the patient's social and occupational functioning. Most common criteria used: UCSD criteria for PMS.[1]

Women with PMS have a higher incidence of affective and anxiety disorders and are at greater risk to have them in the future. The reason for this correlation is not yet known.

Frequency of premenstrual symptoms*

SYMPTOM	FREQUENCY, % of Cycles
Fatigue	92
Irritability	91
Bloating	90
Anxiety and/or tension	89
Breast tenderness	85
Mood lability	81
Depression	80
Food cravings	78
Acne	71
Increased appetite	70
Oversensitivity	69
Swelling	67
Expressed anger	67
Crying easily	65
Feeling of isolation	65
Headache	60
Forgetfulness	56
Gastrointestinal symptoms	48
Poor concentration	47
Hot flashes	18
Heart palpitations	14
Dizziness	14

* Mortola, J.F. et al (1990). Diagnosis of premenstrual syndrome by a simple prospective reliable instrument. *Obstet Gynecol* **72**, 302.

Recommended further reading

1 Mishell, D.R. (2005). Epidemiology, and etiology of premenstrual disorders. *Managing the Spectrum of Premenstrual Symptoms, A Clinician's Guide*, 📖 pp. 4–9, San Antonio: Dannemiller Foundation/MedPro Communications.

Premenstrual dysphoric disorder (PMDD)

PMDD (called late luteal phase dysphoric disorder in the DSM III) is distinguished from PMS by the prominent presence of one or more marked affective symptoms: notably depressed mood, anxiety, affective lability, and/or irritability or anger. PMDD occurs in between 2–8% of women with regular menstrual cycles. There is no evidence for cultural, ethnic, or socioeconomic differences in prevalence.

Note: the criteria require behavioral symptoms only; the presence of physical symptoms is not required. PMDD may occur in the presence of other psychiatric disorders if it is not an exacerbation of these disorders. It is a research diagnosis in the DSM-IV, and can be coded as depressive disorder, not otherwise specified.

PMDD, DSM-IV-TR

This syndrome of physical symptoms associated with depressed or irritable mood, labile affect, loss of interest, impaired concentration and other symptoms occurs regularly prior to menses, remits shortly before menses, and is absent during the week after menses. It is often considered a severe form of normal PMS in women

---

Etiology

A genetic vulnerability conferring increased sensitivity to normal changes in hormone levels throughout the menstrual cycle. This causes alterations in the normal cyclic ovarian steroid interactions with central neurotransmitters and neurohormones. Cyclic changes in ovarian steroids alone do not lead to PMS/PMDD. Most evidence supports involvement of the serotinergic system, endorphins and GABA and the renin-angiotensin-aldosterone system. The autonomic and peripheral nervous systems may be involved in certain symptoms.

Minimal or no evidence for the following etiologies: Trace vitamin and element deficiencies, personality factors, and stress. Stress also has little effect on PMS severity, and PMS is more likely to cause stress than vice versa.

Morbidity

These disorders can extend over a women's entire reproductive cycle, from approximately age 14 to 50. Symptoms are relatively constant between cycles, and can cause an aggregate total of years of disability over a lifetime. This negatively affects quality of life and can have both direct and indirect economic consequences.

Psychiatric consultation

Consultation for already diagnosed premenstrual symptoms is rare unless emotional symptoms are marked and/or there are vegetative symptoms, suicidal ideation, or a frequent inability to function.

Differential diagnosis

Up to 40% of women presenting to a physician with presumed PMS have another mood disorder; many meet the criteria for a depressive or anxiety disorder.[1]

PMDD can be a premenstrual exacerbation of an underlying psychiatric disorder or of a medical condition. Medical disorders such as migraine, chronic fatigue syndrome, and irritable bowel syndrome can have exacerbations prior to or during menses. Rule out perimenopause, gynecological disorders (dysmenorrhea, postpartum status, polycystic ovary disease, and endometriosis) and hypothyroidism and nutrient deficiencies (e.g., manganese, magnesium, B vitamins, vitamin E, and linoleic acid).

Investigations

There are no specific tests diagnostic of premenstrual disorders. Prospective charting of daily symptoms for at least two menstrual cycles is essential to confirm the cyclical pattern. If menses are not regular and/or if they have length <25 days or >36 days, referral should be made for a reproductive endocrine evaluation.

Laboratory tests

For concomitant medical conditions (chemistry profile, cbc, and TFTs) may be warranted. Consultation with a gynecologist or primary care provider for a physical exam and exclusion of medical disorders is appropriate.

Assessment tools

Prospective Record of the Impact and Severity of Menstruation (PRISM), the Calendar of Premenstrual Experiences (COPE), and the Daily Record of Severity of Problems (DRSP). The DRSP is available on line at http://www.pmdd.factsforhealth.org/have/dailyrecord.asp

Recommended further reading

1 Keenan, P.A., Stern, R.A., Janowsky, D.S., Pedersen, C.A. (1992). Psychological aspects of premenstrual syndrome. I: Cognition and memory. *Psychoneuroendocrinology* **17**, 179–187.

Treatment of PMS and PMDD

First-line therapy

- SSRIs are effective for PMDD, with fluoxetine the most studied. At a dose of 20mg/d the overall response is 60–75%. Fluoxetine is approved by the FDA for PMDD. Other SSRIs and venlaxafine (an SNRI) have been shown to be effective in placebo controlled trials.
- Luteal phase therapy: therapy in the luteal phase alone, starting 14 days prior to the expected next menses, and terminating with the onset of menses.

If ineffective:

- Try a second SSRI.
- If treating daily, try intermittent treatment; if treating intermittently, try daily treatment.

Second-line therapy

- Alprazolam (0.25mg tid or qid) for luteal phase depression.
- For severe PMDD, refractory to other treatment, refer to a specialist. Potential treatments include: "Medical oophoriectomy" with a GnRH agonist (e.g., leuprolide, danazol). There are significant side-effects related to hypoestrogenism (e.g., hot flashes, long-term effects of estrogen deficiency—osteoporosis, etc.). For patients who respond well, treatment can continue over the long term (>6 months) with continuous add-back of estrogen (+ progesterone when indicated) to decrease and/or prevent these side-effects. For rare, refractory cases with severe disabling symptoms, surgical bilateral oophoriectomy may be considered.

Other promising possible treatments or adjuncts:

RCTs initially failed to demonstrate the effectiveness of OCP in treating PMS or PMDD. Newer placebo-controlled trials are showing that a 24-day (rather than 21-day) hormonal formulation is efficacious for PMDD.[1]

- Diuretics for severe edema—e.g., fursemide, spironolactone; danazol for mastalgia.
- There is some evidence for the efficacy of vitamin B_6 (no more than 100mg/d), vitamin E, calcium, vitamin D, and magnesium.
- No evidence for multiple other treatment options including progesterone treatment, ginko biloba, evening primrose oil, essential free fatty acids.

Recommended further reading

1 Yonkers, K.A., Brown, C., *et al.* (2005). Efficacy of a New Low-Dose Oral Contraceptive With Drospirenone in Premenstrual Dysphoric Disorder. *Obstet Gynecol* **106**(3), 492–501.

Psychiatry and pregnancy

Overview

Pregnancy is a significant life event, yet psychiatric admissions and completed suicide are less common in pregnancy than at other times. There may be subclinical mild anxiety or mood disturbance, worse in the third and first trimesters. There is a 10% risk of clinically significant depression in the first trimester associated with past history of depression, previous abortion, previous intra-uterine loss, or unwanted pregnancy. Third trimester depression may persist as postpartum depression.

Normal pregnancy

Although there is usually an increase in symptoms of anxiety and depression during pregnancy, these are quite normal. They are usually related to "adjustment" in the first trimester and "fears" in the third trimester. Unless there is a past history of psychiatric illness, there is no reported increase in the incidence of psychiatric disorders.[1] Risk factors in addition to personal history of psychiatric disorders include family history of depression; ambivalence about the pregnancy; lack of marital, family, or social supports. Treatment for adjustment-related anxiety and depression will usually focus on psychosocial interventions. Specific psychiatric disorders should be identified and treated appropriately (see Prescribing in pregnancy 📖 pp. 508–9).

Pseudocyesis[2]

A condition in which a woman firmly believes herself to be pregnant and develops objective pregnancy signs (abdominal enlargement, menstrual disturbance, apparent fetal movements, nausea, breast changes, labor pains, uterine enlargement, cervical softening, urinary frequency, positive pregnancy test) in the absence of pregnancy.

Differential diagnosis

This diagnosis cannot be made without the collaboration of an obstetrician to rule out other disorders that include ectopic pregnancy, corpus luteal cyst, placenta previa, pituitary tumor, pelvic tumor.

Etiology

Regarded as a somatoform disorder or variant of depression, it may present as a complication of postpartum depression or as psychosis with amenorrhoea. It may be related to Couvade's syndrome in expectant fathers (see 📖 p. 104). However, there is no delusional aspect to Couvade's syndrome; the expectant father knows that he is not pregnant.

Treatment

This tends to include supportive or insight-orientated psychotherapy and a trial of an antidepressant.

---

1 Klein, M.H. and Essex, M.J. (1995). Pregnant or depressed? The effect of overlap between symptoms of depression and somatic complaints of pregnancy on rates of depression in the second trimester. *Depression* **2**, 308–314.
2 Small, G.W. (1986). Pseudocyesis: an overview. *Can J Psych* **31**, 452–457.

"Postpartum blues"

This is not a clinical psychiatric disorder. In fact, it can be considered "normal" for the postpartum period since 50–80% of new mothers experience this syndrome. It is a transient period, starting within a few days of birth, usually peaking at 4–5 days after delivery and lasting up to 14 days postpartum, of mild depressive symptoms, irritability, anxiety, mood lability, increased sensitivity, fatigue and crying spells (often for no apparent reason).

It can be differentiated from depression by its transience and low-level symptoms. Be more suspicious that this may herald the onset of postpartum depression (PPD) if the woman has a history of depression. There is a correlation between severe baby blues and later PPD. A heightened, euphoric mood in the first days postpartum is also correlated with later PPD. The "postpartum blues" require only reassurance and encouragement to rest adequately. If symptoms do not resolve within two weeks, or become worse, then the woman should be evaluated for postpartum depression. There is weak evidence that "postpartum blues" may be related to rapid postpartum reductions in levels of estrogen, progesterone, and prolactin. Some women may be more sensitive to these changes than others.

Effects of postpartum psychiatric disorders

Anxiety, depression, and psychosis are all potential postpartum psychiatric disorders, and are discussed in the following pages. In addition to the usual negative effects of psychiatric disorders (diminished quality of life, decreased productivity, etc,), there are impaired mother-infant interactions in 10–25% of women with postpartum psychiatric disorders. Specifically, maternal rejection of the baby, insecure attachment, and cognitive or behavioral problems in children may result.

Postpartum anxiety disorders

Panic disorder and obsessive-compulsive disorder can arise or recur in the postpartum period. These disorders are frequently co-morbid with PPD and may worsen the prognosis.

Postpartum depression (PPD)

Introduction

Postpartum depression is common, and occurs following more than 1 in 8 pregnancies with a peak at 3–4 weeks postpartum.

The DSM-IV classifies it as a subset of MDD with the modifier "with postpartum onset." This is specified as the onset of MDD (see Chapter 7 on depression, 📖 p. 271) within four weeks after birth. Other classifications have used postnatal time periods of up to two years.

Diagnosis

Sleep disturbance, weight loss, and loss of energy may be difficult to differentiate from normal sequela of pregnancy and having a neonate. Evaluate insomnia by asking if a woman is able to sleep when her baby sleeps. Loss of weight associated with PPD is often accompanied by having to force oneself to eat or not enjoying the taste of food. Energy level can decrease to the degree that a woman does not get out of bed for hours.

The clinical features are those of other depressive episodes, although thought content may include worries about the baby's health or her ability to cope adequately with the baby or thoughts of harming the baby. These thoughts are not usually revealed unless questioned about directly. They are not usually predictive of suicide or infanticide; however, a woman with these thoughts should be evaluated for postpartum psychosis. There may be a significant anxiety component. As with all MDD, prior/current diagnosis of anemia and thyroid dysfunction must be ruled out. This is particularly important during the postpartum period as loss of blood accompanies delivery, and there is a doubling of incidence of thyroid disorders over the general population presenting following pregnancy. 90% of cases last less than one month; 4% last greater than one year.

Risk factors

A major risk factor is a personal history of MDD. Multiple lesser risk factors include: conflict in relationship with partner, stressful life events in the previous 12 months, lack of perceived support from friends and family for the pregnancy, unsupportive partner emotionally and/or financially, not living with a partner, ambivalence toward or unwanted pregnancy, poor relationship with one's own mother, congenitally malformed infant, high number of visits to the prenatal clinic, severe "baby blues," previous postpartum psychosis. No evidence for association with obstetric complications or with any mode of delivery.

Women may be hesitant to mention how badly they are feeling to health care providers out of fear that they will lose custody of the child, though this almost never happens.

Pathogenesis

Interaction of genetic susceptibility, life events, and hormonal changes. No hormone has been consistently identified as the cause of PPD (some evidence that unusual sensitivity to withdrawal of gonadal steroids is the precipitant).

Prevention

For women with one or more previous episodes of PPD the recurrence risk is 25–50%. Treat at-risk women with an SSRI immediately after birth, and/or initiate psychotherapy toward the end of pregnancy. Review risks and benefits of treatment and potential side-effects to mother and baby. Postnatal counseling by individuals with specific training in postnatal disorders may be preventative. Education about PPD does not reduce the risk.

Note: Always ask about thoughts of self-harm or harming the baby.

Management

Early identification and close monitoring of those "at risk" is key (use of Edinburgh Postnatal Depression Scale in primary care setting—see 📖 p. 506).

Psychotherapy: Interpersonal therapy (IPT): a 12-week course with particular focus on role transition.[1] Marital therapy may be indicated, and education of the partner about PPD is felt to always be useful. Group therapy and support groups may also be helpful, but this has not been studied. Family and marital therapy may also be useful. There are associations between paternal postpartum depression and maternal PPD, and vice versa.

Pharmacotherapy v. psychotherapy

One RCT[2] showed 6 CBT sessions were equal in efficacy to 20mg/d of fluoxetine.

If a woman has been treated successfully for MDD with a particular drug in the past, then it should be restarted unless a woman prefers one with more evidence about effects during lactation. As with all patients, women should be closely monitored during the first weeks of starting an antidepressant due to the risk of suicide. A clinical response should occur from 2–6 weeks after initiation of therapy. ECT in postpartum women is effective with few adverse effects for mother or infant. ECT is particularly recommended when rapid treatment is necessary, for psychotic symptoms or acute mania, and in mothers at risk of suicide or infanticide. There are no effects of ECT on breast milk. Alternative therapies: Essential fatty acids, Aerobic exercise (30+ mins mod intensity 3–5d/wk), and bright light therapy.

Breastfeeding and antidepressants

Data is available on mother and infant serum levels of medication and active metabolites. These are usually below the level of accurate detection for sertraline, paroxetine, and nortriptyline. Adverse effects have been reported in breast-fed infants of mothers taking SSRIs (e.g., fluoxetine and citalopram). Current recommendations: www.toxnet.nlm.nih.gov.

Untreated PPD may resolve spontaneously within several months or linger for over a year. Women who have had PPD are at risk for relapse following all subsequent pregnancies and at higher risk for MDD independent of childbirth. Note that all MDD in the postpartum period is Identified as PPD, whether or not it had its onset prior to parturition.

Recommended further reading

1 O'Hara, M.W., et al. (2000). Efficacy of interpersonal psychotherapy for postpartum depression, Arch Gen Psychiatry **57**, 1039–45.

2 Appleby, L. et al. (1997). A controlled study of fluoxetine and cogntive behavioural counselling in the treatment of postnatal depression, BMJ. **314**, 932–936.

Postpartum depression scale

Edinburgh Postnatal Depression Scale (EPDS)[1]

As you have recently had a baby, we would like to know how you are feeling. For each of the following 10 questions, please indicate on the following scale the answer which comes closest to how you have felt IN THE PAST 7 DAYS, not just how you feel today:

Answer Scale: As much as I always could/Not quite so much now/Definitely not so much now/Not at all

  1. I have been able to laugh and see the funny side of things.
  2. I have looked forward with enjoyment to things.
*3. I have blamed myself unnecessarily when things went wrong.
  4. I have been anxious or worried for no good reason.
*5. I have felt scared or panicky for not very good reason.
*6. Things have been getting on top of me.
Yes, most of the time I haven't been able to cope at all/
Yes, sometimes I haven't been coping as well as usual/
No, most of the time I have coped quite well/
No, I have been coping as well as ever
*7. I have been so unhappy that I have had difficulty sleeping.
*8. I have felt sad or miserable.
*9. I have been so unhappy that I have been crying.
*10. The thought of harming myself has occurred to me.

Response categories are scored 0, 1, 2, and 3 according to increased severity of the symptoms.
    0 As much as I always could
    1 Not quite so much now
    2 Definitely not so much now
    3 Not at all
Items marked with an asterisk (*)(e.g.: 3, 5, 6, 7, 8, 9, 10) are reverse scored (i.e., 3, 2, 1, and 0).

A total score of 12 or higher is usually regarded as significant, although cutoffs ranging from 10–13 are also used.

Look at the answer to question #10 specifically. For any answer except "never" additional information by interview is required.

A printable version of this scale can be found on line to distribute to patients to self-administer at:
http://www.state.nj.us/health/fhs/ppd/screeningtool.shtml

Recommended further reading

1 Cox, J.L., Holden, J.M., Sagovsky, R. (1987). Detection of postnatal depression. Development of the 10-item Edinburgh Postnatal Depression Scale. *BJP* **150**, 782–786.

Postpartum psychosis

Postpartum psychosis refers to an acute psychotic episode in the mother, usually occurring within one month of birth, with peak occurrence at two weeks postpartum. Incidence is 1.5/1000 live births. The etiology is unknown, but may relate to reduction of estrogen (leading to DA super-sensitivity), cortisol levels, or postpartum thyroiditis.

Symptoms

Three common clinical presentations:

- Prominent affective symptoms (80%) mania or depression with psychotic symptoms.
- Schizophreniform disorder (15%).
- Acute organic psychosis (5%).

Common features

These include insomnia for several nights, agitation, expansive or irritable mood, bewilderment and disorientation, and avoidance of the infant. Delusions or hallucinations often involve the infant and may include auditory hallucinations "telling" the mother to kill her infant.

Management

Postpartum psychosis is a psychiatric emergency due to the risk of the mother harming herself or her baby (or both). Admit to an inpatient unit for treatment with antipsychotic agents and mood stabilizers. At the time this chapter was written, there were no mother-baby psychiatric units in the United States, so the mother and baby will be separated whether or not this is clinically indicated.

Risk factors

- Personal or family history of major psychiatric disorder.
- Lack of social support.
- Single parenthood.
- Previous postpartum psychosis (30% risk of psychosis; 38% risk of PPD).

Prescribing during pregnancy

For up-to-date guidelines, see: www.toxnet.nlm.nih.gov

Overview

- Data is limited (and often conflicting) regarding the safety of psychotropic drugs in pregnancy. Older agents are often preferred because there is more data on these compounds.
- The risks of in utero exposure to a given medication must be balanced against the benefits of psychiatric treatment for the mother. The risks of untreated psychiatric illness on both the mother and the fetus must be considered. Possible risks include, but are not limited to teratogenicity, miscarriage, neonatal withdrawal symptoms, neonatal adaptation problems, neurobehavioral effects, maternal relapse if dosing is inadequate, and any possible risk of self-medication of untreated or undertreated illness with licit or illicit drugs, alcohol and/or tobacco.
- Prior to initiation of any medication during pregnancy or lactation, have a discussion with the patient (and when possible, other family members) regarding the risks, benefits, and alternatives of treatment for both the pregnant woman and her baby. Document this discussion of informed consent. In evaluating any given medication consider: alternative nonpharmacological and pharmacological options, the woman's prior response to medication, family history of response, side-effect profile and relevance to the individual woman, functioning level of the woman without the medication, risks to the fetus, interactions with concurrent medications, and whether a woman plans to breastfeed.
- Avoid abrupt discontinuation of medication upon learning of a patient's pregnancy. There can be serious effects on the mother and possibly the fetus with abrupt discontinuation, including an increased incidence of maternal suicidal ideation and maternal and fetal withdrawal effects. Decisions regarding discontinuation of psychotropic treatment during pregnancy should involve well-documented discussion between the pregnant woman, her psychiatrist, and her obstetrician.
- Recommendations may vary based on trimester. The first trimester is when most organ development takes place. Often women do not realize they are pregnant until at least halfway through the first trimester. Therefore, it is important to discuss both contraception and the risks of taking medication while pregnant before prescribing medication to any reproductive age woman.
- Maternal and fetal physiology change greatly during pregnancy, and after delivery. These changes may require adjustments in the dose and/or timing of medication administration to avoid overdosing while preventing relapse.
- Immediately following birth (with the severing of the umbilical cord) the infant must begin to metabolize the medication and its metabolites itself. Premature and/or sick infants are at high risk for metabolic difficulties, as are infants who continue to be exposed to the drug via breast milk. Manifestations can include neonatal sedation, irritation,

cyanosis, and floppiness. To minimize these effects, tapering psycho-tropic medication(s) down and/or discontinuing prior to delivery may be considered by a patient's psychiatrist in consultation with the pregnant woman and her obstetrician.

Antidepressants

SSRIs are the current treatment of choice for depression in pregnancy. Fluoxetine is the most studied in pregnancy and is currently recommended in the absence of other factors influencing choice. Sertraline is less well studied in pregnancy, but may be preferred due to its safety record in lactation when the mother plans on breastfeeding. There is little data suggesting teratogenicity, except for a small amount of evidence for first trimester paroxetine. SSRI exposure in the second half of pregnancy is associated with a risk of persistent pulmonary hypertension (the absolute risk remains low at 6–12:1000 exposed infants). Late pregnancy SSRI exposure is associated with increased risk of neonatal behavioral syndrome, which resolves spontaneously in a few days to weeks.

Benzodiazepines

Neonatal respiratory depression, hypothermia, hypotonia ("floppy baby syndrome") and withdrawal syndromes may occur when benzodiazepines are used close to delivery. Despite earlier reports of an increased risk of facial clefts, the current expert consensus is that these medications are not teratogenic. Short-term use and minimum effective dose are advised if benzodiazepines are necessary, particularly close to delivery. Clonaze-pam or lorazepam are generally preferred over alprazolam or diazepam.

Mood stabilizers

Lithium has a lower risk of cardiac defects than anticonvulsants, and no increased risk of neural-tube defects. It has been associated with an increased risk (1:1000) of Epstein's anomaly. This is much less than the 3% incidence found in early studies. Fetal echocardiography is indicated at 18–20 weeks.

Valproate and to a lesser extent carbamazapine are associated with neural tube defects. Hence folic acid supplementation is recommended prophylactically at 4mg/day for women of child-bearing potential taking anticonvulsants—although evidence for the benefit is inconclusive. Check B_{12} level before prescribing high-dose folate. Detailed ultrasonography should be carried out at 16–18wks, and maternal serum alpha-fetoprotein (AFP) levels measured. Little data is available for gabapentin, lamotrigine, or other newer anticonvulsants and the risk/benefit needs to be carefully considered.

Antipsychotics

All antipsychotics carry a moderate risk and should be used with caution. Little evidence re: teratogenicity or long-term effects of most compounds, except for possible increased malformation risk with the phenothiazines. Conventional antipsychotics usually preferred because more available data. Depot formulations should be avoided as gradual withdrawal prior to delivery is complicated (and neonatal withdrawal may be more severe).

Prescribing during lactation

For up-to-date guidelines, see: www.toxnet.nlm.nih.gov, "LactMed" link.

General concerns

- All psychotropic medications transfer into breast milk, to varying degrees.
- Levels of most psychotropic drugs in breast milk are relatively low (although in some cases they are higher than maternal serum levels). Infant blood levels may be undetectable.
- Infant exposure from breast milk may be much lower than the in utero exposure (if mother was taking medication during pregnancy). There are still developmental risks of from exposure and withdrawal.
- Monitoring of the infant varies from medication to medication. In many cases, it involves no more than routine pediatric examinations to ensure development is within normal parameters. In other cases it may include biochemical testing such as renal and liver function tests and/or behavioral measures.

Decision-making in lactation

As in pregnancy, the possible risks and benefits to mother and infant of treatment with psychotropic medications must be weighed. There are few randomized and/or large trials of the effects of maternal medication on breastfed infants. Most guidelines are based only upon laboratory studies and case reports. Even when evidence may be lacking for specific risks, use caution.

Possible risks

- Infant exposure to psychotropic medications could result in immediate drug toxicity, withdrawal, and/or in as yet, undetermined long-term effects.
- Untreated maternal psychiatric conditions have effects both directly on the mother and indirectly to the infant through decreased efficacy of parenting and maternal attachment.

Possible benefits

- Treatment and/or prevention of maternal psychiatric condition.
- Infant receives the benefits of breast milk.
- Strengthening of infant-mother bonding and attachment through breastfeeding.

Overall, the benefits of breastfeeding and maternal treatment may be greater than the potential risks of exposure to certain safer psychotropic medications.

Treatment in nursing mothers

- Where possible, consider nonpharmacological treatments.
- If medication is necessary, the lowest effective therapeutic dose should be used, the safest choices should be closely considered and polypharmacy should be avoided.
- Work in consultation with the patient's and the infant's treatment team (e.g., PCP, pediatrician, OB/GYN, therapist).

Antidepressants

SSRIs are usually the first-line antidepressants when breastfeeding; they have not been shown to have major adverse effects on the infant. Sertraline is the current first choice when breastfeeding. Fluoxetine is the best studied SSRI, and is not preferred due to the long half-life of its metabolite norfluoxetine. Current recommendations are to continue using fluoxetine if it was effective in pregnancy. The most evidence exists for the TCAs (especially imipramine and nortriptyline), and no adverse effects have been documented. There is little data on SNRIs and other antidepressants so they should not be used, unless the mother has taken them during the pregnancy. Do not use MAOIs.

Benzodiazepines

Use cautiously and in low doses due to possible sedation and withdrawal in infants. Use medications with no active metabolites (e.g., clonazepam, lorazepam).

Mood stabilizers

Lithium and breastfeeding are not compatible due to accumulation of lithium in breast milk and infant serum. Carbamazepine and valproate may be used cautiously when necessary, preferably given as a single dose in slow-release form. This recommendation is based on multiple and consistent reports that show small to unquantifiable levels of these medications in breast milk. However, there is no evidence regarding the long-term effects of these medications on breastfed infants.

Antipsychotics

Do not use clozapine. There is little safety information available on the use of these drugs in lactation, therefore breastfeeding is usually not recommended. If the woman nevertheless chooses to breastfeed, use the lowest effective dose and monitor the infant closely. Actively psychotic women should not breastfeed, and should be supervised at all times when with their baby.

Strategies to minimize infant exposure

- Breastfeeding should be avoided at the time when breast milk and/or serum levels in the mother are likely to be at their peak (check drug information for these values).
- If practical, breast milk may also be expressed when medication levels are at their lowest levels and used later.

Contraindications

Breastfeeding should be avoided when the mother is concurrently taking MAOIs, lithium, or clozapine. Use extreme caution when there is evidence in the infant of renal, hepatic, cardiac, or neurological disorders.

Sexual function

Normal sexual function

There are no widely accepted guidelines of normal sexual function. Normal function also changes with experience, age, the availability and novelty of suitable partners, and the expectations and standards that are characteristic of the individual's social, cultural, ethnic and/or religious affiliation(s).

Sexual dysfunction

Criteria for a diagnosis of sexual dysfunction include:
- Inability to participate in a preferred sexual relationship.
- Presence of the sexual dysfunction on (almost) all occasions.
- Duration of at least six months.
- Significant stress or interpersonal difficulties.
- Not accounted for by a physical disorder, drug treatment (or use), or other mental or behavioral disorder.
- Sexual dysfunction is only a problem when the patient and/or his or her partner finds it to be a problem.
- Frequency: 43% of women, 31% of men. 50% of American couples have some type of sexual dysfunction.

Sexual dysfunction is common in the general population with lifetime prevalence in young adults, estimated as shown in Table 12.1.

Table 12.1 Lifetime prevalence of sexual dysfunction

Problem	Male	Female
Reduced libido	30%	40%
Arousal difficulties	50%	60%
Reaching orgasm too soon	15%	10%
Failure to have orgasm	2%	35%
Dyspareunia	5%	15%

Psychological factors (either within an individual or within a relationship), are a common etiology for sexual dysfunction. These can occur concurrently with a general medical condition, medication side-effects, and drug abuse.

All phases of the sexual response cycle and associated practices such as sexually arousing acts and intercourse are interrelated. Therefore, function in one phase usually requires function in previous phases. Anticipation of problems in a later phase can lead to problems in an earlier phase. Although a person may receive more than one DSM IV diagnosis related to a sexual disorder, often these diagnoses are all rooted in a single problem.

Masters and Johnson "Phases of Sexual Response"[1]

The following "Phases of Sexual Response" were published by Masters and Johnson in the 1960s. It has since been expanded (e.g., sexual response phases in women likely overlap and are not always sequential). Knowledge of the basic phases allows for vocabulary during discussion of sexual function and dysfunction.

- Sexual Desire: Fantasies about sexual activity and a desire to have sexual activity.
- Sexual Excitement: A subjective sense of sexual arousal and pleasure with accompanying physiological changes.
  - Females: pelvic vasocongestion, vaginal lubrication and expansion, swelling of external genitalia. Males: penile tumescence and erection.
- Orgasm: A climax of sexual pleasure with accompanying rhythmic contractions and the release of sexual tension.
  - Females: vaginal contractions. Female orgasm can be, but is not necessarily, associated with release of fluid. Males: sensation of ejaculatory inevitability, followed by the ejaculation of semen.
- Resolution: A sense of general relaxation, well-being and muscular relaxation.
  - Females: may be able to respond to additional stimulation almost immediately with further excitement and orgasm. Males: are physiologically refractory to further erection and orgasm for a highly variable period of time (seconds to hours). There are no DSM-IV disorders related to this phase.

Recommended further reading

1 Masters, W.H., Johnson, V.E. *Human Sexual Response*. Toronto; New York: Bantam Books, 1966.

Taking a sexual history

Sexual history is an important part of every medical history. When sexual dysfunction involves a couple, ideally the sexual history is done together, and then with each partner alone. To facilitate a sense of comfort and a feeling of safety in self-disclosure, the interviewer should strive to:
- Take an empathic, nonjudgmental approach.
- Provide support and encouragement.
- Avoid leading questions.
- Proceed from open-ended questions to specific, detailed questions about practices and response.
- Request clarification with direct questions.
- State the medical reason for the inquiries.
- Do not make any assumptions (especially regarding experience, orientation, practices, number of partners).
- When appropriate, acknowledge that sexual problems can be a difficult topic to discuss and/or that sexual problems are common and usually treatable.

Common barriers to discussing sexual issues
- Embarrassment of interviewer and/or patient.
- Terminology: Explain the terms you are using, and/or use simpler terms. If the patient's terminology is vague, ask for clarification. With the patient's permission, pictures of external male and female anatomy may be useful.
- Differences between interviewer and patient in culture, socioeconomic level, age, gender, and/or race can lead to embarrassment and/or more difficulty in discussing of these issues.
- Insufficient privacy, or a patient's inadequate knowledge of confidentiality rules.
- If a patient does not see sexuality as a psychiatric issue, they may be very reluctant to discuss sexual issues or problems with a psychiatrist.

Common triggers for sexual problems

Psychological: relationship problems; life stressors; anxiety/depression; low self-esteem; sexual performance anxiety; excessive self monitoring of arousal; feelings of guilt; fear of pregnancy/STDs; lack of knowledge about sexuality/"normal" sexuality; previous significant negative experience.

Environmental: (fear of) interruptions/physical discomfort.

Physical: drugs/alcohol/medication side-effects; pain/discomfort due to illness; feeling tired/run down; recent childbirth.

Factors related to the partner: sexual attractiveness (gender, physical characteristics); novelty; evidence of disinterest; criticism, inconsideration, and/or inability to cope with difficulties (especially sexual); sexual inexperience/poor technique; preference for sexual activities that are unappealing to the partner.

Taking a sexual history to assess for and to diagnose sexual disorders

Questions and issues for the couple or individual

- Describe the problems in your own words.
- Why are you seeking help at this time?
- Are these problems present in all situations?
- If there are multiple problems, which is most troubling? Which one do you want to focus on first?
- Specifically explore the couple's emotional intimacy, degree of sexual communication, activities prior to sexual activity, when and where they are sexually active (including amount of privacy and fatigue level), sexual knowledge, expectations for fertility or details of birth control used (type, safety, satisfaction with method), risk of STDs.
- How was your sexual response prior to the problems? How is it now when problems do not occur?
- How have you reacted to these problem (sexually, behaviorally, and emotionally)?
- Have you sought help for or advice about this problem before? If no, what got in the way? If yes, were there any recommendations? Did you try them? Did they work?

Questions to assess for each person alone if possible

- What do you think is causing this problem?
- Do you respond sexually when you self-stimulate? To sexual fantasies or sexual thoughts?
- What past sexual experiences have you had? What did you like and dislike about these experiences?
- Were you emotionally close to anyone growing up? Were you treated with love, respect, and physical affection? Were there losses or traumas? Were you physically and/or sexually abused as a child? Later in life?
- Have you ever felt hurt or threatened in the current relationship? If yes, do you want to share more about that?
- How is your physical health? Ask specifically about any difficulties with fatigue, impaired mobility, or self-image.
- Are you taking any medications? Ask specifically about common medications with known sexual side-effects including SSRIs, beta-blockers, antiandrogens, GnRH agonists, OCPs.
- How does your mood correlate with your sexual problems?

Sexual dysfunction (1)—desire and arousal

Hypoactive sexual desire disorder (DSM-IV-TR)

This is characterized by a persistent or recurrent deficiency or absence of sexual fantasies and desire for sexual activity. A clinician judges whether this disorder is present while taking into account factors that may affect sexual functioning such as age and life events.

The American Urological Association (AUA) definition includes a lack of "responsive desire" e.g., desire triggered during the sexual encounter. Data show that women in sexually satisfactory, established relationships do not necessarily have desire prior to the initiation of sexual activity.

Sexual aversion disorder

Strong negative feelings, fears, or anxieties that arise regarding the prospect of sexual interaction. This revulsion is often focused on a particular aspect of sexual experience (e.g., vaginal penetration, genital secretions). However, some individuals experience a generalized aversion to all sexual activity. When a sexual opportunity occurs, an individual feels fear, disgust, and/or anxiety.

Lack of subjective arousal (AUA, not in the DSM-IV)

* Combined arousal disorder: characterized by absent or markedly reduced mental feelings of sexual arousal from any type of stimulation. Reflexive genital sexual arousal (vulval swelling and lubrication) is also absent or impaired.
* Subjective arousal disorder: characterized by absent or markedly reduced mental feelings of sexual arousal from any type of stimulation. However, reflexive genital sexual arousal (vulval swelling and lubrication) occurs and one is aware of this.

Female sexual arousal disorder (DSM-IV-TR)

"Persistent or recurrent inability to attain, or to maintain until completion of the sexual activity, an adequate lubrication-swelling response of sexual excitement."

The AUA adds that subjective arousal can be present from nongenital stimuli (kissing, erotica, stimulating one's partner, etc.). It is the absence of or impairment of sexual arousal specifically to genital stimuli that characterizes this disorder.

Male erectile disorder (DSM-IV-TR)

This occurs when a man is unable to attain or to maintain an erection adequate for penetration and/or intercourse. This can happen at any point in the sexual encounter: from inability to initially attain an erection, loosing an erection when attempting to penetrate, or during thrusting. Some men are only able to have an erection when masturbating or while sleeping. If an individual does not have erections during masturbation or on awakening, then a general medical condition, medication side-effect, or drug abuse is a likely cause.

Specify type
- lifelong type v. acquired type;
- generalized type v. situational type;
- due to psychological factors v. due to combined factors.

Sexual dysfunction (2)—orgasm and intercourse

Female orgasmic disorder (DSM-IV-TR)

This disorder is characterized by a persistent or recurrent delay or absence of orgasm after a normal sexual arousal phase. It has been a controversial disorder due to misconceptions regarding the normal frequency and "type" of female orgasm. Women have a wide variation in orgasmic capacity and in the type and intensity of stimulation that triggers orgasm. This diagnosis should only be given when orgasmic function is less than would be expected given an individual's age, experience, degree of stimulation, etc. Note: a women's orgasmic capacity tends to increase with age and sexual experience.

It is also important to differentiate this from the arousal disorders, as women with arousal disorders rarely or never experience orgasm and are often misdiagnosed with orgasmic disorder.

Arousal disorders are subjective, and it is difficult to determine their prevalence.

Male orgasmic disorder (DSM-IV-TR)

Defined as a persistent or recurrent delay or absence of orgasm following a normal sexual excitement phase. This disorder can be situational, where ejaculation can occur only in response to specific stimuli. It can involve a prolonged delay, when ejaculation occurs during intercourse but only after very prolonged and intense noncoital activity. This diagnosis should be made only when orgasmic functioning is less than would be expected given the stimulation and the individual's age. Unlike in women, in men orgasmic capacity tends to decline with age.

Premature ejaculation (DSM-IV-TR)

Defined as the inability to control ejaculation sufficiently to allow both partners to enjoy the sexual interaction. Ejaculation may occur before, on, or immediately after penetration, or in the absence of an erection. This is most common in young and sexually inexperienced men. It is affected by the duration of the excitement phase, the novelty of the situation and/or sexual partner, and how long it has been since the man's last orgasm. Psychological stressors and organic impairment (such as pain) can also cause premature ejaculation. It is common for men with this disorder to have greater control over ejaculation during self-masturbation than during intercourse.

Dyspareunia (DSM-IV-TR)

Defined as pain during intercourse (not due to a general medical condition). This can occur in both men and women.

In women the pain may be felt superficially (at the entrance of) or deep within the vagina. Refer to a gynecologist or primary care practitioner for a physical examination to exclude physical causes of pain such as infection, tender episiotomy scar, endometriosis, and vaginal obstruction from growths or the hymen.

Pain during intercourse in men usually has a physical cause (e.g., urethral infection, scarring secondary to STD, tight foreskin) and should be evaluated by a urologist or a PCP.

Where deep pain is experienced after intercourse in either women or men, this may be due to pelvic congestion syndrome (with physical symptoms similar to premenstrual syndrome) caused by accumulation of blood during arousal without occurrence of orgasm. Achieving orgasm (by intercourse, masturbation, or use of a vibrator) may help to alleviate this congestion.

Vaginismus (DSM-IV-TR)

Defined as involuntary constriction of the muscles of the outer third of the vagina that interferes with sexual intercourse, a gynecological exam, or causes physical discomfort (not due to a general medical condition). In most cases, sexual intercourse is possible but painful/uncomfortable. The woman is usually not aware of the vaginal spasms. Complaints of physical discomfort during sexual intercourse are common. This diagnosis is not made when it is caused exclusively by organic factors or when it is symptomatic of another Axis I mental disorder. Vaginismus is usually related to anxieties or fearful thoughts e.g., fear of pain on penetration, previous sexual assault, belief that sex is wrong or sinful, anticipatory fear of pain at first coitus, and/or fear of pregnancy. Since vaginismus may lead to pain during intercourse, it can reinforce these beliefs. It can also be an unconscious form of nonverbal protest when a woman feels mistreated by or is abused by her partner.

Treatment

Referral to a specialist is usually advised for education on specific strategies to achieve penetration (e.g., self-exploration, Kegel exercises, use of graded trainers, sensate focus exercises, involvement of partner, graded attempts at intercourse, reassurance for the partner).

Sexual dysfunction (3)—evaluation and treatment

Psychiatric evaluation of sexual dysfunction is done via a complete sexual history (see earlier in chapter).

A physical examination is also part of the complete evaluation of all sexual dysfunction. If a patient has not already had sufficient workup to strongly suggest a pure psychiatric etiology, then you should refer to a PCP, gynecologist, or urologist prior to initiating treatment.

Treatment

Psychological Interventions: men and women:

- Cognitive behavior therapy (CBT): this focuses on identifying factors that contribute to sexual dysfunction (such as unreasonable expectations, maladaptive thoughts, insufficient genital or nongenital stimulation, and specific behaviors that decrease one's partner's interest and/or trust). Ways of modifying these factors are suggested and tried.
- Sex therapy of couples: this focuses on similar issues to CBT and also includes sensate focus techniques that begin with nonsexual physical touch and progressing to sexual touch. Partners are encouraged to discuss what is pleasurable. This is particularly helpful when a performance goal, such as orgasm, has been overprioritized. A combination of CBT and sex therapy, typically lasting three to six sessions, can also be used.

There is data to support both of the above approaches. There is no evidence to support short-term psychotherapy.

Education

General sexual education regarding arousal and physical stimulation (including specific issues of "normal" time before ejaculation occurs). To dispel myths, understand "normal" physiology, the effects of alcohol. Reduction of "performance anxiety." Learn varied intercourse positions, relaxation techniques and Kegel exercises. Use self-help guides/exercises.

Specific exercises for sexual dysfunction:

(Refer to references or to specialty texts for details.)

"Sensate focus." A series of specific exercises for couples (essentially a form of *in vivo* "desensitization" to reduce sexual anxiety), initially encouraging each partner to take turns in paying increased attention to their own senses.

"Stop-start" technique (Semans' technique). This increases the sensory threshold of the penis and is effective in up to 90% of cases of premature ejaculation.

"Squeeze technique." If control does not develop using the "stop-start" technique, this method may be used to inhibit the ejaculatory reflex.

Pharmacologic and mechanical treatment
Women
The only FDA-approved medication to treat sexual dysfunction in women is estrogen therapy. This can treat dyspareunia related to genitourinary atrophy.

Multiple drugs are used off-label for treatment. However there is minimal data regarding their effectiveness. These drugs include sildenafil, buproprion, and multiple hormonal preparations. There is some evidence that for women who have undergone surgical menopause and are on estrogen replacement, adding testosterone may increase sexual desire and response, and reduce distress. This is an investigational therapy only. There is no evidence regarding the safety or efficacy of long-term androgen use.

Oral and transdermal estrogens in postmenopausal women have not been proven to be effective for sexual dysfunction, and they are associated with multiple other risks. Antidepressant use is associated with sexual dysfunction in from 20–60% of women. SSRIs have the highest rates, and buproprion the lowest rate. Adding buproprion to an SSRI may be beneficial. Drug holidays (halting the use of short-acting SSRIs over the weekend) may be beneficial, but are not recommended due to possible decrease of compliance and to withdrawal symptoms. A clitoral suction device, the EROS Clitoral Therapy Device, is FDA-approved to treat female sexual arousal disorder. It works by drawing blood to the clitoris to trigger arousal and to enhance orgasms. It is available by prescription only.

Men
Sildenafil; training in self-administration of papaverine or prostaglandin E_1 into the penis prior to intercourse; use of a vacuum constriction device; surgical implantation of semirigid or inflatable penile prostheses.

For all sexual dysfunctions, consider referral to a specialist, especially for complex cases such as those with vague or intermittent problems, associated secondary sexual or psychiatric problems, or when initial treatment is unsuccessful.

Paraphilias (1)—diagnosis

Paraphilias are Axis I disorders in which an individual is sexually aroused by inappropriate stimuli. These can range from nearly normal behavior to behavior destructive to oneself, to other individuals or to the community. Paraphilias are legally significant when they involve nonconsenting partners. The term *paraphilia* replaces the older terms of *perversion* and *sexual deviation*.

Definition

DSM-IV-TR defines each paraphilia as involving at least six months of recurrent, intense, sexually arousing fantasies, sexual urges, or behaviors involving a particular inappropriate act or object. These can involve non-human objects or children, or the suffering or humiliation of oneself, a partner or partners, or a nonconsenting person(s). All paraphilias are clinically significant if they cause significant personal distress or impairment in social functioning. Pedophilia, frotteurism, voyeurism, exhibitionism, and sexual sadism are also clinically significant if the person has acted on them, regardless of distress or impairment.

Classification

Many different objects and acts may be the focus of paraphilias (see Table 12.2). Many of the defined categories are extreme forms of fantasies, urges, and behaviors that are common parts of "normal" sexual activity.

Epidemiology

It is difficult to estimate the prevalence of these disorders. Many individuals do not present for help and may not admit to sexually deviant arousal in surveys. The prevalence of paraphilias is likely to be significantly higher than the cases diagnosed (based on the large market in paraphilic paraphernalia and pornography). There is a wide range of sexual practices in the "normal" population, and the diagnosis is limited to those whose arousal meets the criteria above.

Paraphilias are more common in males than females (perhaps 30 times more common). More than 50% have onset before age 18, and the prevalence of paraphilias peaks between ages 15 and 25. Many individuals have multiple paraphilias, in series and/or in parallel, which is sometimes defined as "polymorphous perversity."

Etiology

Physiological factors

These may include genetic factors, prenatal influence of hormones in utero, hormonal abnormalities in adults, and perhaps brain abnormalities. For most, causality versus association has not been determined.

Psychological theories

This may be a conditioned response, where nonsexual objects, situations, or people become sexually arousing when they are paired with a sexually pleasing activity such as masturbation. Psychoanalytic theory postulates that paraphilias develop from failure to resolve the oedipal crisis. They are an outlet to cope with the sexual and aggressive drives associated with the anxiety of separation from the mother and castration by the father.

Table 12.2 DSM IV-TR classification of paraphilias

Type	Sexually arousing object or act
Fetishism	Nonliving object (e.g., clothing, shoes, rubber) that is not designed for tactile sexual stimulation (e.g., unlike a vibrator).
Transvestic fetishism	Cross-dressing (often involves a complete outfit, perhaps with wig and make-up). Clear association with sexual arousal distinguishes from transsexual tranvestism. However, may be an early phase in some transsexuals. Specify if with gender dysphoria: a persistent discomfort with gender role or identity.
Exhibitionism	Exposure of genitals to strangers.
Voyeurism	Watching others who are naked, disrobing, or engaging in sexual acts.
Pedophilia	This specifically refers to the sexual act with a prepubertal child by a person five or more years older than the child *and* at least 16 years old. May be specified as attracted to males, females, or both, as limited to incest, and as exclusive (attracted only to children) or nonexclusive.
Sexual masochism	Being humiliated, beaten, bound, or made to suffer.
Sexual sadism	Psychological or physical suffering of others.
Frotteurism	Touching and rubbing against nonconsenting person.
Paraphilia not otherwise specified	Paraphilias that do not meet any of the above criteria. Includes telephone and computer scatalogia (obscene phone calls or computer communications), necrophilia (corpses), partialism (exclusive focus on part of body), zoophilia (animals), coprophilia (feces), urophilia (urine), klismaphilia (enemas), autoerotic asphyxia (self-asphyxiation).

Paraphilias (2)—assessment and treatment

Assessment

Why is the person presenting now?

May present due to own concerns, or due to the influence of a partner/family member when this behavior is discovered or starts to cause problems in relationships. Presentation may occur after committing a legal offence. Occasionally paraphilias present as sexual dysfunction, with disorder of preference coming to light on further assessment.

Is there another psychiatric, neurological, or medical disorder?

Some medical or psychiatric disorders may influence individuals to engage in inappropriate sexual behaviors. These may or may not be in individuals who have experienced fantasies but not acted on them previously. When a significant change from prior sexual expression is reported, it is important to rule out another disorder, especially if there are signs and symptoms of neurological and/or endocrine disorders. In addition to a full psychiatric history and MSE, and possibly a neurological examination, consider referral to a PCP and/or specialist to rule out endocrine, brain, and other medical abnormalities. Also evaluate for reactions to medications and use of licit or illicit drugs.

Does the person want treatment, and if so what do they want from it?

- Do they want help at all or have they been forced into treatment (by spouse, legal system, etc.)?
- Do they want to adapt better to the behavior without changing it?
- Do they want to change the focus of their sexual arousal and/or desist from the overt behavior?
- Are they motivated to engage in treatment?

Treatment

General issues

Treatment should not be imposed on people who do not want it. Most treatments will take considerable effort on the patient's part and the aims of treatment should be clear from the beginning. There are three possible broad aims:

- Better emotional acceptance of one's paraphilia(s) without behavioral change.
- Cessation of overtly problematic behavior while retaining paraphilic arousal.
- Changing the focus of the arousal.

Where treatment is aimed at change, some or all of the following may need to be addressed:

- Development of "normal" relationships.
- Addressing feelings of or actual sexual inadequacy (some sexual dysfunction approaches can be useful).
- Development of interests, activities, and relationships that fill the time previously taken up by fantasizing about, preparing for, and taking part in paraphilic activity.

- Decreasing masturbation to paraphilic fantasies, and encouraging masturbation to more normative fantasies.

Specific treatment modalities
- CBT, which can include social skills training, cognitive restructuring, trigger avoidance and development of victim empathy.
- Modified aversive behavioral therapy may also be used.
- Addressing cognitive distortions regarding sex, women, or children may also be important.
- Insight-oriented psychotherapy.
- Treatment of co-morbid conditions such as depression and substance abuse.
- Reduction of sexual drives with antiandrogens such as medroxyprogesterone acetate.
- SSRIs are now being tried as treatment.
- External control mechanisms: elimination of opportunities by peers, family, and legal controls such as prison in the case of crimes.

Gender identity disorder (1)

Gender identity refers specifically to an individual's identification with either the male or female gender; their gender's physical characteristics; and the expected gender role within their society.

Gender identity *does not* refer to one's sense of sexual orientation. Sexual orientation is determined by whether one is sexually attracted to members of the same sex, the opposite sex, or both sexes.

The more complex gender identity disorder may often be due more to society's intolerance for the grey areas of gender identity rather than to a problem inherent to the individual. There is wide variability of gender traits among individuals; acceptability of gender traits within a society may vary over time, setting, and culture. Caution must be used when applying this diagnosis; a very high threshold must be set before giving this diagnosis.

> Terms: diagnostic terms are used in the medical field, but understanding slang terms is useful for working with patients. A few examples are provided below.
> Gender identity disorder: transsexual, drag queen (when particularly flamboyant).
> Sexual orientation: lesbian, bisexual, homosexual, gay, queer.

Diagnosis

Gender identity disorder has slightly different requirements in children and adults. Diagnosis can be particularly difficult in children due to the following reasons:

- They are often not able to verbally express discomfort or distress. Therefore, an adult may mistakenly interpret the presence or absence of distress.
- Gender identification can change with age, or vary based on developmental stage.
- Distress regarding gender-related behaviors may involve the parent's expectations and not the child's.

This disorder in childhood is beautifully portrayed in the movie *Ma Vie en Rose*, Columbia TriStar Home Video, © 1998.

The DSM-IV diagnostic criteria are given on the next page.

DSM-IV diagnostic criteria

A. A strong, persistent cross-gender identification (not merely a desire for perceived cultural advantages of being of the other sex).

In children, four out of five criteria must be met:
1) An individual must repeatedly state the desire to be, or the insistence that he or she is, the other sex.
2) In boys, a preference for cross-dressing or simulating female attire; in girls, insistence on wearing only stereotypically masculine clothing.
3) Strong and persistent preferences for cross-sex roles in make-believe play or persistent fantasies of being the other sex.
4) Intense desire to participate in the stereotypical games and pastimes of the other sex.
5) Strong preference for playmates of the other sex.

In adolescents and adults, this is manifested in symptoms such as a stated desire to be the other sex, frequently passing as the other sex, desire to live as or to be treated as the other sex, or the conviction that he or she has the typical feelings and reactions of the other sex.

B. Persistent discomfort with his or her sex or sense of inappropriate-ness in the gender role of that sex.

In children this can be manifest by any of the following: Boys: stating that his penis or testes are disgusting or will disappear, stating it would be better not to have a penis, aversion to rough-and-tumble play and rejection of male stereotypical toys, games, and activities. Girls: rejec-tion of urinating in a sitting position, assertion that she has or will grow a penis, stating that she does not want to grow breasts or menstruate, marked aversion toward normative female clothing.

In adolescents and adults: manifested by symptoms such as preoccupa-tion with getting rid of primary and secondary sexual characteristics (e.g., request for hormones, surgery, or other procedures to physically alter sexual characteristics to simulate the other sex) or belief that he or she was born the wrong sex.

C. The disturbance is not concurrent with a physical intersex condition.

D. The disturbance causes clinically significant distress or impairment in social, occupational, or other important areas of functioning.

Specify:

Based on current age: gender identity disorder in children and gender identity disorder in adolescents or adults.

For sexually mature individuals, specify if sexually attracted to males, females, both, or neither.

Gender identity disorder (2)

Etiology

Most people with gender identity disorder report that their beliefs about their gender were present from early childhood. Karyotype and phenotypic development are normal. Gonadal, genital, and hormonal abnormalities as well as the sex one is reared as are not consistently related to gender identity disorder. Some evidence that the bed nucleus of the stria terminalis in the brain of male-to-female transsexuals (MTFs) follows a female pattern.

Epidemiology

There is a 3:1 M:F prevalence internationally. Prevalence within a society ranges from 1:10,000 to 1:30,000 for male-to-female (MTF) transsexuals and from 1:30,000 to 1: 100,000 for female-to-male (FTM) transsexuals. One-third to 2/3 of cases eventually report homosexual orientation, though this is more frequently reported in males than females.

Differential diagnosis (DSM-IV)

- Transvestic fetishism (see paraphilias): wearing clothes of the opposite sex for sexual arousal. Not associated with a core belief of incorrect gender found in the transsexual).
- Schizophrenia: occasionally associated with the delusion that the patient is the wrong sex or is changing sex.
- Gender identity disorder not otherwise specified: sexual identity disorders that are not classified as a specific gender identity disorder. Examples include:
  - Intersex conditions accompanied by gender dysphoria (ruled out by normal karyotyping, and normal primary and sexual characteristics for the birth sex).
  - Transient, stress-related cross-dressing behavior.
  - Persistent preoccupation with castration or penectomy, without a desire to acquire the sex characteristics of the other sex.

Co-morbidity

Common co-morbidities are impaired social and occupational functioning due to a person's desire to act in their desired gender role and depression, often due to feelings of hopelessness regarding gender reassignment.

Presentation and assessment

Transsexuals usually come to psychiatric attention, not because they wish to change their feelings about their gender, but to gain the psychiatrist's support for undertaking hormonal treatment and/or sex reassignment surgery (SRS). Many such patients arrive with their diagnosis and preferred treatment option (hormones or sex reassignment surgery). The aim of assessment is to establish the diagnosis with certainty. Contraindications to treatment are psychotic illness, major depression, substance misuse, and personality disorder. Assessment should be by a specialist in gender identity disorders. The aim is to make the diagnosis of gender identity disorder, to treat co-morbid disorders, to offer alternative treatments, to provide supportive psychotherapy, and to supervise the real-life test.

Treatment

Multiple treatments are available to align a person's physical identification with their psychologically congruent gender. Sex reassignment surgery is a definitive treatment. Because it is irreversible and expensive, a careful, standardized protocol precedes this surgery to ensure that only appropriate patients are treated. Treatments and therapies should only be completed by specialists in gender identity disorders. Each step of the following protocol may also be a form of treatment.

- Thorough assessment.
- Real-life test: A trial of cross-gender living for at least three months, sometimes up to a year. The patient attempts to live as the other gender by changing their name, their dress, and interacting with all people (friends, family, co-workers, etc.) as a member of their preferred gender.
- Hormonal treatments: These induce secondary sexual characteristics. Estrogen treatment in MTF transsexuals produces diminished libido and erectile function, some breast and hip development, and skin softening. There is no effect on voice pitch; speech therapy may produce a female vocal pattern. Androgen treatment in FTM transsexuals causes muscle development, some lowering of vocal pitch, male body hair pattern, and amenorrhea. Many transsexuals (estimated at >50%) like the changes these treatments make and do not have surgery.
- Sex reassignment surgery: This is a controversial procedure. Outcome studies are variable, but approximately 70% MTF and 80% FTM patients report satisfaction. Unsatisfactory psychological results are correlated with a pre-existing mental disorder.
  - MTF surgery: orchidectomy and penectomy with vaginoplasty using penile skin. Cosmetic results can be good, although candidates vary in their ability to be orgasmic postsurgery.
  - FTM surgery: bilateral mastectomy, hysterectomy, and bilateral salpingo-oopherectomy. Phalloplasty is undertaken in less than half of patients as current techniques are neither cosmetically acceptable or functional for penetration.

For recent, detailed protocols for hormonal reassignment of gender, including the specifics of hormonal treatment, follow a link through the Tom Wadell Clinic, San Francisco Department of Public Health: http://www.dph.sf.ca.us/chn/HlthCtrs/transgender.htm

Sexual disorder

Excessive sexual behavior

This is the inability to control sexual impulses that results in repetitive, continued sexual behaviors despite negative consequences, yet does not meet the other DSM disorders described earlier in this chapter.

These consequences can include clinical distress, social or relational impairment, physical disease, disability, etc. More precise terms include sexual addiction, compulsive sexual behaviors, hypersexuality and excessive sexual desire disorder, but these are not currently in the DSM-IV-TR.

"Excessive sexual behavior" is historically referred to as nymphomania (women) or satyriasis (men). It can manifest with the characteristic elements of an addictive disorder, an impulse control disorder, and/or an obsessive-compulsive disorder. There is dispute about whether it should be a subclassification of one or all of these disorders or its own separate disorder. There are no boundaries to distinguish diseased sexual behavior patterns from behaviors within society's norms. For some people the thoughts, urges, and behaviors are ego-dystonic and for others ego-syntonic. The epidemiology is not well delineated. These disorders appear to be more common in men than in women, to co-occur with impulse control disorders, and to be associated with histories of sexual abuse. Etiology, except in some cases in which the disorder is secondary to neurological disorders, is not understood.

Compulsive sexual behaviors

Can be paraphilic (see 📖 *pp. 522–23*) or nonparaphilic. (Paraphilic behaviors are those outside the conventional range of sexual behaviors). Non-paraphilic behaviors involve common sexual practices in a given culture such as compulsive masturbation, excessive use of pornography, Internet sexual behaviors, and engagement in extramarital affairs. If there are no adverse consequences, then the disorder may not be present. Possible consequences of compulsive sexual behaviors: higher risk of STDs and for physical injuries due to repetitive sexual practices; loss of time and productivity; associated financial losses; legal consequences; destruction of interpersonal relationships due to deception, secrecy, and violations of trust that may accompany these behaviors; shame and guilt; stigmatization.

Excessive and compulsive sexual behaviors can present as a sign or symptom of other disorders, including substance abuse, mania, dementia, temporal-lobe seizures, or frontal-lobe tumors, or a side-effect of medication use (dopamine agonists). Sexual behaviors return to normal when the underlying condition is treated.

Treatment

Psychosocial

The most widely available treatment is a 12-step program such as Sex Addicts Anonymous (see www.sexaa.org for further information).

Other treatment options include inpatient, intensive outpatient, and individual psychotherapy. Cognitive behavior therapy and psychodynamic psychotherapy are commonly used, with the first focused on identifying triggers to sexual behaviors and reshaping cognitive distortions about these sexual behaviors. Psychodynamic psychotherapy explores the core conflicts that drive dysfunctional sexual expression. Family and couples therapy are often used in treatment. There are little data to document the outcomes of these treatments.

Pharmacotherapy

There are no FDA-approved medications for excessive or compulsive sexual behaviors. SSRIs are commonly used, and theoretically decrease the urges, cravings, and preoccupation. They may work by treating co-occurring disorders. Mood stabilizers are efficacious for co-occurring bipolar disease. Naltrexone, an opiate antagonist used to treat addictions, has been evaluated and is promising. Case studies and open-label studies show promise for anti-androgen medications. There are no randomized controlled trials yet.

Personality disorders

Introduction

Personality disorders are diagnosed on Axis II in DSM-IV-TR and are thus distinguished from psychopathology on Axis I. This distinction is due to the concept that personality by definition is stable and enduring over one's lifetime while disorders on Axis I may wax and wane. Although there are clear diagnostic criteria, the term is sometimes used as a pejorative label for patients. Diagnostic reliability is poor—half of patients diagnosed with a personality disorder do not show diagnostic stability over one year.[1] Moreover, the validity of the concept has been criticized for being medicalization of socially unacceptable behavior.

Further complicating the issue is the overlap of many personality disorder criteria with Axis I disorder criteria. There are some in psychiatry who propose that character pathology is more accurately a spectrum of features within the major Axis I disorders. This allows for the treatment of symptoms within the framework of the medical model. Therefore, some psychiatrists question the utility of making Axis II diagnoses if it is assumed the key features are stable and maladaptive traits unamenable to intervention. They argue that:

• Personality is by definition unchangeable.
• There is little evidence that psychiatric care is very helpful.
• Some Axis II-labeled patients may be disruptive and impinge negatively on the treatment of other patients.
• Some Axis II-labeled patients are not ill and are responsible for their behavior.
• Psychiatry is being asked to deal with something that is essentially a social problem.

On the other hand, others in psychiatry see certain Axis I disorders as possible subtypes of dysfunctional personalities (e.g., bipolar II disorder, cyclothymia). They believe that the concept of personality disorder is valid and, therefore, falls within the realm of psychiatric treatment, arguing:

• People with personality disorder suffer from the symptoms of their disorder.
• They have high rates of suicide, other forms of premature death, and of other mental illness.
• There are treatment approaches which are effective.
• Their opponents are rejecting patients because they dislike them or do not have the proper training to recognize and treat these disorders.
• Traditional psychiatric services do not provide the type of approach and services that are necessary to help these patients.

Clearly, the diagnosis of a personality disorder does not lessen the suffering that patients experience. These disorders are debilitating and impact patients in almost every aspect of their lives. Advances in both basic neuroscience and in various treatment modalities have changed our

---

1 Maj, M., Akiskal, H.S., Mezzich, J.E., Okasha, A. (eds.). *Personality Disorders*. West Sussex.: John Wiley & Sons, 2005.

perception of these patients as merely "difficult" to that of deserving the care afforded to all those who suffer from mental illness. The focus of this chapter is on the clinical assessment and management of people with personality disorders. The place of personality disorder in mental health legislation and personality disorder and offending are discussed in Chapters 17 and 18.

The concept of personality disorder

Key features

Personality refers to enduring patterns of cognition, emotion, motivation, and behavior that are activated in particular circumstances[1]. This definition emphasizes two aspects of personality: first, personality is dynamic, characterized by continuous interaction of mental and behavioral processes and environmental events, and second, the potential of flexibility and variation within the personality under particular circumstances. Another way of viewing personality that helps us understand personality disorder is by considering its functional aspects. The major function of personality is to solve major life tasks-the problems that affect individuals in everyday life, such as developing the capacity for fulfilling relationships and establishing meaningful goals. We all recognize, among people we know well, some who manifest certain characteristics more than others: shyness, confidence, anger, generosity, tendency to display emotions, sensitivity, and being rigid, to name but a few. When these enduring characteristics of an individual are such as to cause distress or difficulties for themselves or in their relationships with others, then they can be said to be suffering from personality disorder. Personality is separate from illness, although the two interact.

Definition

The following definition is based on DSM-IV-TR. Personality disorders are enduring (starting in childhood or adolescence and continuing into adulthood), persistent and pervasive disorders of inner experience and behavior that cause distress or significant impairment in social functioning. Personality disorders manifest as problems in cognition (ways of perceiving and thinking about self and others), affect (range, intensity, and appropriateness of emotional response), and behavior (interpersonal functioning, occupational and social functioning, and impulse control).

Personality disorders could be defined as the failure to achieve adaptive solutions to life tasks. The adaptive failures involve one or more of the following: failure to establish stable and integrated representations of self and others, interpersonal dysfunction as indicated by the failure to develop the capacity for intimacy and to function adaptively in terms of attachment. From that theory, the overall goal of treating personality disorders is to improve adaptation. To diagnose personality disorders the manifest abnormalities should not be due to other conditions (such as psychosis, affective disorder, substance abuse, or general medical condition) and should be out of keeping with social and cultural norms.

---

1 Westen, D. (1995). A clinical-empirical model of personality: life after the Mischelian ice age and the NEO-lithic era, *Journal of Personality*, 63(3): 495–524.

Development of the concept[2]

The development of clinical concepts of conditions that would today be recognized as personality disorder started in the early 19th century, at a time when the main two groups of mental conditions acknowledged by psychiatrists were insanity and idiocy. It became clear that there were individuals who were neither insane (not suffering from delusions or hallucinations) nor clearly idiots, imbeciles, or morons (to use the then contemporary terminology for mental retardation), but who nevertheless manifested abnormalities in their behavior.

The term *moral insanity* was introduced by Prichard in 1835. *Moral* meant "psychological" (rather than the modern meaning concerning ethics), and among the patients described were people who had affective disorders as well as people who were personality disordered.

Kraeplin (1896) and Schneider (1923) introduced classification systems that can be seen as forerunners of the current categorical approaches in DSM-IV and ICD-10. The concept first became codified in DSM I in 1952. The initial classification delineated four cardinal personality types, four pathological traits, and four personality disorders in relation to societal norms. This last group contained those with addictions and sexual deviations. There were no diagnostic criteria; merely brief clinical descriptions. Only with the advent of DSM III in 1980 were diagnostic criteria introduced. The approach was polythetic, meaning that only a subset of the criteria is adequate grounds for a diagnosis. Subsequent editions of the DSM added and eliminated subtypes culminating in the 10 categories of DSM-IV-TR.

Key contributions to the development of concepts related to personality disorder

1809	Pinel describes "manie sans délire."
1812	Rush describes "perversion of the moral faculties."
1835	Prichard describes "moral insanity."
1838	Ray describes "moral mania."
1891	Koch describes "psychopathic inferiority."
1896	Kraepelin describes and categorizes "psychopathic personalities."
1919	Kretschmer suggests relationship between body types and personality.
1923	Schneider describes and categorizes "psychopathic personalities."
1930	Partridge describes "sociopathy."
1939	Henderson describes "psychopathic states."
1941	Cleckley publishes "Mask of Sanity" describing psychopaths.
1968	Category "Antisocial personality disorder" introduced in DSM-II.

---

2 Coolidge, F. and Segal, D. (1998). **Evolution of personality disorder diagnosis in the** *Diagnostic and statistical manual of mental disorders. Clinical Psychological Review*, **8**, Iss. 5, pgs 585–599.

Theory and development of personality (1)

Personality may be thought of as a dynamic interaction of biological, social, and psychological forces that forges the person each of us becomes in life. Defining "normal personality" has been a much debated topic. One approach has been defining normality in its opposition to the "disordered" personality, while other approaches view normality as representing a statistical majority of behavioral patterns in the population. Regardless of the definition of normal personality, most view the development as a process begun in the earliest stages of life.

Throughout the history of psychiatry, there have been various theories to describe this process starting with Hippocrates' "humoral" (choleric, sanguine, melancholic, and phlegmatic) theory. Much of the first half of the twentieth century was dominated by the psychodynamic perspective while more recently "psychobiological" models have been more widely accepted.

Psychodynamic approach

Much of this approach owes its origins to the work of Sigmund Freud and the development of psychoanalysis as a tool to understand psychopathology. Later contributions were made by Anna Freud and her elaboration on defense mechanisms. The concept of personality is seen as a reflection of the development of the ego and subsequent utilization of defenses based upon its level of maturity. Successful navigation through the key psychosexual stages, i.e., resolution of the Oedipal Complex, would determine the formation of the ego (personality) and the level of its psychic defenses. Immature defenses are characteristic of weak ego strength and utilize splitting and projection. Intermediate level defenses, so-called neurotic, utilize repression and undoing. Mature defenses, seen as representing the "healthy personality" are suppression, altruism, sublimation, and humor. Critics of this approach point out that the use of defense mechanisms is unstable over a person's life—one may utilize a range of defenses depending upon stressful life events or particular interpersonal interactions. See 📖 p. 988 for more detail.

Psychobiological approaches[1]

Also known as dimensional, these view a variable number of traits as continuous scales along which each person will have a particular position; the positions on all the traits represent a number of dimensions that describe personality. Examples include: Eysenck's three-factor theory (neuroticism, extraversion, psychoticism) or Costa and McCrae's five-factor model (neuroticism, extraversion, openness, agreeableness, conscientiousness). Cloninger's seven-factor model (Fig. 13.1) is a comprehensive view to personality development informed by modern understanding of genetics

---

1 Cloninger, C.R. (1999). A new conceptual paradigm for the genetics and psychobiology for the science of mental health. *Australian and New Zealand Journal of Psychiatry* **33** (2), 174–186.

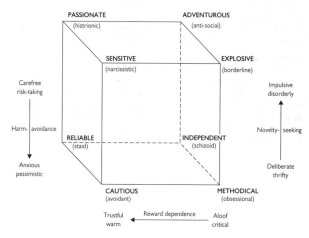

Fig. 13.1 Cloninger's Temperament Cube, from Maj, M., Akiskal, H.S., Mezzich, J.E., Okasha, A. (eds.) (2005). *Personality Disorders*. West Sussex: John Wiley & Sons.

and neuroscience. This model sees personality as dimensions of temperament (novelty seeking, harm avoidance, reward dependence, persistence) and character. Genetic differences account for 50% of the variance seen in temperament traits. Temperament is viewed as basic emotions that condition how one responds to the environment. Different temperamental traits may be associated with specific neurotransmitter systems, i.e., novelty seeking with dopmaninergic system. Normal individuals are characterized as having different scores on the dimensions of each temperament, thereby giving rise to individual personality styles. Thus normal personality in this model would represent statistical normal distribution in the score of each dimension. Those at the outliers may represent disordered personality.

Character represents higher cognitive functions and the conceptual core of personality. It, unlike temperament, is a conscious representation of the self and involves volition. Character is made up of secondary emotions that dictate how one views oneself in the world and in relation to others. It is comprised of the dimensions of self-directedness, cooperativeness, and self-transcendence.

Personality then, in the psychobiological model, is the interplay between temperament and character. The strength of this model is that it posits a cohesive model in conceptualizing both normal and abnormal personality—everyone may be represented on these dimensions, those with disorders simply representing the dimensional extremes. While the dimensional approach may have more explanatory power for disorders, the categorical method, represented by DSM-IV-TR, may represent a more useful and convenient approach to those in clinical psychiatry.

Is personality stable?

Are there traits that are persistent and predict a person's behavior over time in a number of situations? Situationists have argued that the situation was a stronger determinant of behavior than personality traits. However, more recent research has demonstrated the long-term stability of a number of personality traits and, perhaps unsurprisingly, most now agree that both the situation and personality traits are important in determining behavior.

Classification of personality disorders (1)

As outlined in the previous section it is largely accepted that normal personality is best described and classified in terms of dimensions or traits. Although this also applies to personality disorder, our current psychiatric classifications are categorical. The DSM-IV-TR divides the personality disorders into three distinct clusters based upon fundamental behavioral repertoire. The clusters may represent an analogous organization to temperament/character dimensions.

Cluster A

These disorders are viewed as personalities with odd, aloof, or eccentric features. These are typically individuals who seek little interaction with others and lack the desire for meaningful relationships. In the dimensional model, these are people who are low in the temperamental trait of reward dependence (social sensitivity) and low in the character trait of cooperativeness (empathy).

Cluster B

Cluster B disorders are compromised of individuals who are dramatic and erratic. These are people who have stormy interpersonal relationships and impulsive behavior. This is the most likely cluster to come to the attention of the mental health or legal system based upon maladaptive patterns of behavior (suicidal acts, criminality). The temperamental trait of high novelty seeking (pleasure/reward motivation) maps well onto this cluster as do low scores on the trait of cooperativeness.

Cluster C

These disorders include those who are fearful and anxious. These are individuals who often cannot obtain meaningful, bidirectional relationships with people. Their behavioral repertoire is rigid and limited. Dimensionally, they score high in traits of harm avoidance (inhibited behavior) and low in self-directedness (self-sufficiency).

Each of the individual personality disorder categories falls within one of the three clusters. There are a number of important points to bear in mind when using standard categorical approaches in the diagnosis of personality disorders:

- Due to their heterogeneous origins, there is overlap between the criteria for some categories.
- It is more common for individuals to meet the criteria for more than one category of personality disorder than to meet only the criteria for a single category.
- When making a diagnosis one should use all the categories for which a person meets the criteria.

- If a person meets criteria for more than one category, then they do not suffer from more than one actual disorder. A person has a personality and this may or may not be disordered. If it is disordered it may have various features that are rarely described adequately by a particular category.
- Clinically, it is more important to understand and describe the specific features of a person's personality than it is to assign them to a particular category.

DSM-IV-TR and ICD-10

The personality disorder categories in DSM-IV-TR and ICD-10 are set out opposite to each other. The two schemes are similar, but there are categories that appear in one but not the other and for some categories different terms are used. Each category has a list of features, a number of which should be present for the person to be diagnosed as manifesting that particular aspect of personality disorder. DSM III (and subsequent editions) placed personality disorder on a separate Axis (along with other developmental disorders in Axis II) from mental illness (Axis I). See p. 14.

DSM-IV-TR and ICD-10 classifications of personality disorder

DSM-IV-TR*	ICD-10	Description
Paranoid	Paranoid	Sensitive, suspicious, preoccupied with conspiratorial explanations, self-referential, distrust of others.
Schizoid	Schizoid	Emotionally cold, detachment, lack of interest in others, excessive introspection and fantasy.
Schizotypal	(Schizotypal disorder classified with schizophrenia and related disorders)	Interpersonal discomfort with peculiar ideas, perceptions, appearance, and behavior.
Antisocial	Dissocial	Callous lack of concern for others, irresponsibility, irritability, aggression, inability to maintain enduring relationships, disregard and violation of others' rights, evidence of childhood conduct disorder.
—	Emotionally unstable— impulsive type	Inability to control anger or plan, with unpredictable affect and behavior.
Borderline	Emotionally unstable— borderline type	Unclear identity, intense and unstable relationships, unpredictable affect, threats or acts of self-harm, impulsivity.
Histrionic	Histrionic	Self-dramatization, shallow affect, egocentricity, craving attention and excitement, manipulative behavior.
Narcissistic	—	Grandiosity, lack of empathy, need for admiration.
Avoidant	Anxious (avoidant)	Tension, self-consciousness, fear of negative evaluation by others, timid, insecure.
Obsessive-compulsive	Anankastic	Doubt, indecisiveness, caution, pedantry, rigidity, perfectionism, preoccupation with orderliness and control.
Dependent	Dependent	Clinging, submissive, excess need for care, feels helpless when not in relationship.

* DSM-IV uses three broader clusters to organize the categories of personality disorder—
Cluster A (odd/eccentric)—paranoid, schizoid, schizotypal.
Cluster B (flamboyant/dramatic)—antisocial, histrionic, narcissistic, borderline.
Cluster C (fearful/anxious)—avoidant, dependent, obsessive-compulsive.
Although this may seem sensible, there is no particular validity to this clustering.

Classifications of personality disorders (2)

Clusters

As outlined in the previous section it is sometimes clinically useful to think of personality disorders as "clusters." At times in the past, these groupings were felt to lack a basis in any identifiable etiologic comparison; however, there is now evidence to support at least some of these groupings. As mentioned on 📖 *p. 542*, the different personality disorders fall generally within the following clusters:

- Cluster A: paranoid, schizoid, schizotypal (evidence linking these presentations to family members with schizophrenia or other primary psychotic disorders).
- Cluster B: borderline, narcissistic, histrionic, antisocial (evidence supporting a shared genetic basis of these disorders in lab animals with different social exposures).
- Cluster C: obsessive-compulsive, avoidant, dependent, personality disorder NOS (close relationship to family members with depressive and anxious disorders).

Paranoid personality disorder

Key features

These are distrustful individuals who are frequently suspicious of seemingly innocuous events, and who can become angry and hostile when they feel slighted. They can be found in the person of jealous spouses, racists, and the frequently litigious. These patients can appear tense, overly mannered, and initially quite logical. The overarching trait in these individuals is a belief that they will be harmed or in some way exploited by others.

- **DSM diagnosis:** Pervasive distrust/suspiciousness leading to the interpretation of others' motives as malevolent. Should have four or more of the following occurring separate from an acute psychotic episode related to schizophrenia, mood disorder with psychosis, or general medical condition: suspicious of harm/exploitation, preoccupation with trustworthiness and loyalty of others, reluctance to confide in others, reads hidden threats or insults into benign remarks/events, persistent grudges, quick to react angrily to perceived attacks, and recurrent suspicions of fidelity without justification.
- **Epidemiology:** 0.5–2.5% prevalence, onset in early adulthood, men>women, possibly higher in the deaf and in minority groups.
- **Defense mechanisms:** Projection.
- **Treatment and prognosis:** Primarily psychotherapy; also may consider standard pharmacologic treatments for anxiety (clonazepam, temazepam) or even short-course treatment with antipsychotics if thinking approaches delusionality. Prognosis can vary from full remission to the development of schizophrenia. Most patients remain symptomatic for their lives and always have relational difficulties.

Schizoid personality disorder

Key features

These individuals seem to derive little joy from life and seem distant from others. They can be found in the person of night-shift workers or other solitary jobs, pet "collectors," or mathematic theoreticians.

- **DSM diagnosis:** Pervasive detachment from social relationships and restricted range of emotions. Should have four or more of the following outside the context of a primary psychotic illness, psychosis related to a mood disorder, pervasive developmental disorder, or general medical condition: does not desire or enjoy close relationships, chooses solitary activities, little interest in sexual activities with others, takes pleasure in few activities, lacks close friends, indifferent to praise or criticism, and emotional coldness/detachment/flattened affect.
- **Epidemiology:** Up to 7.5% prevalence, onset in early childhood, unclear but likely male > Female.
- **Defense mechanisms:** Fantasy.
- **Treatment and prognosis:** Primarily psychotherapy as these patients can be very introspective once they become comfortable with the therapist. Depending on individual symptoms, low-dose SSRIs and antipsychotics have both been found to be effective. Prognosis may include an unknown relationship to schizophrenia or eventual resolution of symptoms.

Schizotypal personality disorder

Key features

These individuals display much of the social discomfort associated with schizoid personality disorder, but with the addition of bizarre thinking and behavior. They may have ideas of reference, persecutory beliefs, or thoughts that they have special mind powers.

- **DSM diagnosis:** Pervasive pattern of social and interpersonal deficits with cognitive and perceptual distortions and eccentricities. Should have five or more of the following outside the context of schizophrenia or another primary psychotic disorder or a mood disorder with psychotic features: ideas of reference, odd beliefs or magical thinking that influence behavior and are not consistent with subcultural norms, unusual perceptual experiences, odd thinking and speech, suspiciousness or paranoid ideation, inappropriate affect, odd/eccentric/peculiar behavior, lack of close friends, and excessive social anxiety associated with paranoia.
- **Epidemiology:** 3% prevalence, no male-female difference, onset in early adulthood.
- **Defense mechanisms:** Distortion, fantasy.
- **Treatment and prognosis:** Primary psychotherapy with particular sensitivity to the patient's beliefs. Antipsychotics and antidepressants may also be used based on symptoms. Prognosis may range from the development of schizophrenia to persistent PD with high function.

Classifications of personality disorders (3)

Borderline personality disorder

Key features

These individuals are characterized by very unstable self-image, interpersonal relationships, and mood/affect as well as impulsive, self-destructive behaviors. They may always appear to be in crisis and self-mutilation and suicide attempts are common. Another observed feature is the micropsychotic episode—a short-lived period of psychotic features.

- **DSM diagnosis:** Pervasive pattern of instability of interpersonal relationships, self-image, and affects with marked impulsivity. Should have five or more of the following: frantic efforts to avoid real or imagined abandonment, pattern of unstable/intense interpersonal relationships with extremes of idealization and devaluation, identity disturbance, impulsivity in at least two self-damaging areas (not including suicidal or self-mutilating behavior), recurrent suicidal behaviors or threats or self-mutilation, affective instability, chronic feelings of emptiness, inappropriate/intense anger, and transient stress-related paranoia or severe dissociation.
- **Epidemiology:** 1–2% prevalence, female:male = 2:1, onset in early adulthood, frequent history of childhood abuse.
- **Defense mechanisms:** Splitting, acting out, projective identification (leading to strong counter-transference), dissociation.
- **Treatment and prognosis: Dialectical behavior therapy** (DBT) is the treatment of choice. In this treatment, patients are taught to recognize maladaptive behaviors and to substitute more skillful ones. Pharmacologically, multiple drug classes can be used to target specific symptoms although this frequently results in patients on large amounts of medication with little effect. Prognosis is for the disorder to continue throughout the life course with some tendency to "burn out" in later life.

Narcissistic personality disorder

Key features

These individuals have a marked sense of entitlement that derives from heightened self-importance and lack of empathy. They frequently handle criticism poorly and exaggerate their own accomplishments. These patients are very ambitious, but are often thwarted by interpersonal difficulties and occupational problems.

- **DSM diagnosis:** Pervasive pattern of grandiosity, need for admiration, and lack of empathy. Should have five or more of the following: grandiose sense of self-importance, preoccupied with fantasy of unlimited success/power/beauty/brilliance, believes self to be "special" and should only associate with other special high-status people, requires excessive admiration, sense of entitlement, interpersonally exploitative, lacks empathy, often envious or believes others to be envious, and shows arrogant behaviors/attitudes.

- **Epidemiology:** <1% prevalence, male>female, onset in early adulthood, frequently familial.
- **Defense mechanisms:** Acting out, idealization, symbolization.
- **Treatment and prognosis:** Best practice is unclear although insight-oriented psychotherapy and group therapy are frequently utilized. Pharmacotherapy consists of lithium for mood swings and serotonergic antidepressants for the often-accompanying depressive symptoms. Symptoms tend to worsen as the patient ages given the increasing number of blows to their self-esteem.

Histrionic personality disorder

Key features

These individuals are frequently seen as dramatic and extroverted. They can display flamboyant, seductive behavior and have difficulty maintaining long-lasting relationships. They have difficulty recognizing their true feelings and motivations.

- **DSM diagnosis:** Pervasive pattern of excessive emotionality and attention seeking. Should have five or more of the following: uncomfortable when not the center of attention, interactions often inappropriately sexual or seductive, rapidly shifting and shallow expression of emotions, uses physical appearance to draw attention, excessively impressionistic speech lacking details, self-dramatization/theatricality/exaggerated emotion, suggestible, and considers relationships to be more intimate than they actually are.
- **Epidemiology:** 2–3% prevalence, women>men, onset in early adulthood.
- **Defense mechanisms:** Dissociation, repression.
- **Treatment and prognosis:** Psychodynamic psychotherapy can help these patients to better understand their motivations for behavior. Pharmacotherapy has limited effectiveness, but can be used to target specific symptoms. Prognosis is for symptoms to decrease with age.

Antisocial personality disorder

Key features

These individuals (sometimes referred to as sociopaths) treat others poorly, frequently breaking laws, lying, and using others to achieve their own ends. This is typically done without regard for safety and without remorse. Despite these things, these patients can come across as charming and seductive.

- **DSM diagnosis:** Pervasive pattern of disregard for and violation of the rights of others occurring since at least 15 years of age with the individual now being **at least 18 years old**. Should have three or more of the following outside of the context of schizophrenia or mania: failure to conform to social norms (performing acts that are grounds for arrest), deceitfulness, impulsivity, irritability and aggressiveness, reckless disregard for safety of self/others, consistent irresponsibility, and lack of remorse.
- **Epidemiology:** 2% prevalence (as high as 75% in prison population), male:female = 3:1, frequently begins in youth as oppositional defiant disorder and then progresses to conduct disorder and then to Antisocial PD. May sometimes be familial in nature.

- **Defense mechanisms:** Conversion.
- **Treatment and prognosis:** Group and milieu therapy have shown to be helpful while individual psychotherapy has limited effectiveness. Limit-setting is a must. Antiepileptics (carbamazepine, valproate) have been tried to improve impulsivity with mixed results. Patients tend to peak in early adulthood and symptoms can remit as the patient ages.

Classifications of personality disorders (4)

Obsessive-compulsive personality disorder
Key features
These individuals are defined by their perfectionism and lack of flexibility. This can make them stubborn, indecisive, overconscientious, and unable to delegate. Lack of control can lead to an increase in anxiety. They have a marked attention to detail and can frequently be successful in methodical, detail-oriented jobs.

- **DSM diagnosis:** Pervasive pattern of preoccupation with orderliness, perfectionism, and mental/interpersonal control, at the expense of flexibility, openness, and efficiency. Should have four or more of the following: preoccupied with details/rules/lists/order/schedules and losing sight of the major point of the activity, perfectionism interferes with task completion, excessively devoted to work to exclusion of friendship and leisure, inflexible about matters of morality/ethics/values (not due to culture or religion), unable to discard worthless or worn-out objects, reluctant to delegate, adopts miserly spending style, and shows rigidity and stubbornness.
- **Epidemiology:** 1% prevalence, male > female, more frequent in oldest children.
- **Defense mechanisms:** Isolation.
- **Treatment and prognosis:** These patients frequently seek treatment due to their recognition of things being amiss personally and professionally. They respond well to individual psychotherapy, but may actually benefit more from groups with behavioral approaches. For patients with breakthrough symptoms of obsessive-compulsive disorder (specific, recurring obsessions with accompanying compulsions), consider clomipramine, fluoxetine, or other serotonergic agents.

Avoidant personality disorder
Key features
These individuals are very sensitive to criticism and rejection. They tend to feel inadequate and present as timid. Despite a strong desire for human companionship, they tend to be fearful of relationships. They will often take jobs with little opportunity for advancement or personal recognition.

- **DSM diagnosis:** Pervasive pattern of social inhibition, feelings of inadequacy, and hypersensitivity. Should have four or more of the following: avoids occupational activities requiring significant interpersonal contact due to fear of disapproval or rejection, unwilling to get involved with people unless certain to be liked, shows restraint within intimate relationships (fears being shamed), preoccupied with criticism or rejection socially, inhibited by feelings of inadequacy in new interpersonal situations, views self as inept and inferior, and reluctant to take personal risks due to possible embarrassment.
- **Epidemiology:** 1–10% prevalence, male = female, onset likely in childhood but recognizable in adolescence.
- **Defense mechanisms:** Introjection.

- **Treatment and prognosis:** Individual psychotherapy that cautiously approaches the patient's fear of rejection may be helpful. Assertiveness training or other behavior therapies can also have benefit. Antidepressants and anxiolytics may be useful depending on symptoms. β-blockers have also been effective in some patients when approaching new situations. Prognosis can be excellent if the patient remains in a supportive environment, but may progress to social phobia, anxiety, or depression.

Dependent personality disorder
Key features
These individuals display extreme submissiveness and a need to be cared for. They have difficulty making decisions without extra support and so tend to avoid responsibility. Relationships can be very long-lasting.

- **DSM diagnosis:** Pervasive and excessive need to be taken care of leading to submissive behavior and fear of separation. Should have five or more of the following: difficulty making everyday decisions without excessive advice/reassurance, needs others to assume responsibility for most major areas of life, difficulty expressing disagreement due to fear of loss of approval, difficulty initiating projects or doing things on his/her own due to lack of self-confidence, goes to excessive lengths to gain support, feels uncomfortable or helpless when alone, urgently seeks another relationship when a close one ends, and is unrealistically preoccupied with fears of caring for self.
- **Epidemiology:** Women > men, more common in younger individuals, associated with childhood chronic physical illness.
- **Defense mechanisms:** Identification.
- **Treatment and prognosis:** Insight-oriented psychotherapies have been very successful as have CBT based models. There is a danger that the patient will become dependent on the therapist. Anxiolytics and serotonergic antidepressants can be utilized when symptoms warrant. Prognosis is for long-term occupational and social decline but is greatly influenced by those whom the patient depends upon.

Personality disorder NOS
Key features
This is the category for those individuals who share features with more than one personality disorder but don't fill criteria for any one. It also includes some well-defined subtypes that are not considered to be categorical personality disorders such as passive-aggressive, depressive, sado-masochistic, and sadistic.

- **Passive-aggressive type:** These individuals are felt to display passive behaviors (procrastination, resisting performance demands, finding fault with others) that reflect underlying aggression. They have rocky interpersonal relationships that are full of manipulation. They tend to have low self-confidence, feel misunderstood, focus on the fortunes of others, and have a pessimistic view of the future. Psychotherapy should be primarily supportive and focus on consequences of behaviors, and medication has very limited utility.

- **Depressive type:** These individuals show a lifelong pattern of anhedonia, dysthymia, and self-doubt. In the past, they've been called melancholic. They are at a higher lifetime risk of developing a major mood disorder. Long-term, insight-oriented psychotherapy has proven to be useful as has the use of serotonergic antidepressants and psychostimulants.

Etiology of personality disorder

While there is no single, convincing theory explaining the genesis of personality disorder, the following observations are suggestive of possible contributing factors.

Genetic

This has been the most widely studied component of personality in recent years. There is now good evidence supporting the link between schizophrenia and schizotypal personality disorder based upon family studies. Antisocial personality has been associated with variability in neurotransmitter systems such as allelic differences in the MAO-A gene, while there is no good evidence for relationship between XYY genotype and sociopathy. Borderline personality disorder has been associated with heritability of mood disorders. Relatives of those with borderline PD have an increased risk for developing Axis I mood disorders.

Biologic

Much of the recent research has focused on the various neurotransmitter systems. The serotonin system has been implicated in the regulation of emotion and aggressive behaviors. Low levels of CSF 5-HIAA, a metabolite of serotonin has been a consistent finding in borderline patients and violent individuals. Psychotic symptoms have been associated with increased dopaminergic activity in schizotypal disorder as evidenced by increased plasma and CSF levels. Imaging studies in individuals with personality disorders have shown that hyper-responsiveness of amygdala and other limbic structures may be related to affective instability.

Childhood development

Difficult infant temperament may proceed to conduct disorder in childhood and personality disorder, attention-deficit-hyperactivity disorder (ADHD) may be a risk factor for later antisocial personality disorder; insecure attachment may predict later personality disorder (particularly disorganized attachment); harsh and inconsistent parenting and family pathology are related to conduct disorder, and may, therefore, be related to later antisocial personality disorder; severe trauma in childhood (such as sexual abuse) may be a risk factor for borderline personality disorder and other cluster B disorders.

Psychodynamic theories

Freudian explanations of arrested development at oral, anal, and genital stages leading to dependent, obsessional, and histrionic personalities; "borderline personality organization" described by Kernberg (diffuse unfiltered reaction to experience prevents individuals from putting adversity into perspective leading to repeated crises); narcissistic and borderline personalities seen as displaying primitive defense mechanisms such as splitting and projective identification; some see antisocial personalities as lacking aspects of superego, but a more sophisticated explanation is in terms of a reaction to an overly harsh superego (representing internalization of parental abuse).

Cognitive-behavioral theories

There are maladaptive schemata (stable cognitive, affective, and behavioral structures representing specific rules that affect information processing). These schemata represent core beliefs that are derived from an interaction between childhood experience and preprogrammed patterns of behavior and environmental responses. Schemata are unconditional compared with those found in affective disorders (e.g., "I am unlovable" rather than "If someone important criticizes me, then I am unlovable") and are formed early, often preverbally.

Dialectical behavioral model (📖 p. 1022)

Innate temperamental vulnerability interacts with certain dysfunctional ("invalidating") environments leading to problems with emotional regulation. Abnormal behaviors that are manifested represent products of this emotional dysregulation or attempts to regulate intense emotional states by maladaptive problem solving.

Epidemiology of personality disorder[1]

The measurement of the prevalence of personality disorder of any type and of specific categories of personality disorder in any population has a number of problems: in earlier studies, personality disorder and other mental disorders were mutually exclusive, not allowing for the recording of co-morbidity; studies differ in the method used to make a diagnosis (interviews/case-notes/informants, clinical diagnosis versus research instruments, emphasis on current presentation or on life history); and in some studies subjects were only allowed to belong to one category of personality disorder.

Furthermore, cultural perspectives need to be considered. For instance, cluster C disorders appear more prevalent in Scandinavian epidemiologic studies as compared to North America.

Personality disorder of any type

Community

Rates of personality disorder in the community have been found to be 2–18% (the generally accepted approximate is 10%). It is more prevalent in younger adults, and may be more prevalent in males.

Primary care

20–30% of patients presenting to a primary care physician meet the criteria for a personality disorder.

Psychiatric patients

30–40% of outpatients and 40–50% of inpatients have a personality disorder, not usually as a primary diagnosis. A primary diagnosis of personality disorder occurs in about 5–15% of inpatients.

Other populations

5–75% of prisoners have a personality disorder. Antisocial personality disorder is most prevalent, but many prisoners fulfill the criteria for more than one diagnostic category, and many personality disordered prisoners do not meet the criteria for the antisocial category.

1 Sperry, L. Handbook of diagnosis and treatment of DSM-IVTR personality disorders. New York: Brunner-Routledge, 2003.

Specific categories of personality disorder

The prevalence rates of the categories of personality disorder in the general population are approximately:

DSM-IV	Prevalence
Paranoid	0.5–4.5%
Schizoid	0.5–7.5%
Schizotypal	0.5–5%
Antisocial	2–3.5%
Borderline	1.5–2%
Histrionic	2–3%
Narcissistic	0.5–1%
Avoidant	0.5–5%
Dependent	0.5–2.5%
Obsessive-compulsive	1–2%

Co-morbidity between personality disorder and other mental disorders

The current state of classification and understanding of the etiology and pathogenesis of mental disorders is such that most psychiatric diagnoses are based on descriptive criteria. It is common to find that an individual meets the criteria for an Axis I disorder along with a personality disorder. At one extreme, both may be a manifestation of the same underlying condition; at the other, they may represent two completely separate etio-pathogenic entities.

DSM-IV-TR allows for the designation of Axis II as the reason for presentation to a mental health professional indicated by principal diagnosis on the multi-axial formulation. This facilitates the understanding of the case by indicating that the disordered personality is the focus of clinical attention and thus allows for a more detailed approach to the patient. Nonetheless it is more common than not that individuals with Axis II disorders suffer from co-morbid Axis I disorders. The issue becomes complex when criteria for the Axis II disorder overlap with Axis I criteria. Specifically, DSM-IV-TR cautions against the diagnosis of personality disorders when patients are experiencing current symptoms of an Axis I disorder.

Borderline personality disorder

Much of the literature on co-morbidity has focused on borderline personality disorder (BPD) due to the prevalence of this disorder within the psychiatric population and the overlap in diagnostic criteria with other Axis I disorders.

Mood disorders

From a strict criteria perspective, BPD shares many criteria with mood disorders (i.e., moodiness, irritability/anger, emptiness, impulsivity, and suicidal behavior). Current studies estimate that 75% of patients with BPD have a co-morbid mood disorder (61% major depressive disorder, 41% dysthymia, 5% bipolar). The degree of overlap between mood disorders and BPD has lead some to feel that BPD represents a subtype on the spectrum of mood disorder, namely bipolar disorder. Although this relationship is still under research, it underscores the need for careful diagnosis and the understanding of the longitudinal course of psychiatric illness.

Anxiety disorders

There is a strong association between BPD and anxiety disorders with PTSD receiving the most attention. Many have postulated early childhood sexual trauma as fundamental in the development of later BPD. Current studies estimate that 58% of BPD patients meet criteria for PTSD while 90% suffer from some form of anxiety disorder.

Substance disorders

Over 60% of BPD patients have a substance use disorder. This is crucial in recognizing in both as a target for treatment and a barrier to therapy.

Co-morbidity between other personality disorders and specific mental disorders[1]

Strong associations

- Avoidant personality disorder and social phobia (possibly because they both describe a group of people with the same condition).
- Substance misuse and cluster B personality disorders.
- Eating disorders and cluster B and C personality disorders (particularly bulimia nervosa and cluster B).
- Anxiety disorders and cluster C personality disorders.
- Somatoform disorders and cluster B and C personality disorders.
- Substance use disorders and impulse disorders and cluster B personality disorders.

Moderate associations

- Schizotypal personality disorder and schizophrenia (also a weaker association between schizophrenia and antisocial personality disorder).
- Depression and cluster B and C personality disorders.
- Delusional disorder and paranoid personality disorder.

Impact of personality disorders on manifestation, treatment, and outcome of other mental disorders

As the above associations indicate it is important to recognize that personality disorders have an impact on the presentation, treatment, and outcome of Axis I disorders, and it is therefore useful to recognize such co-morbidity from a clinical perspective.

Presentation

The presentation of Axis I disorders may be distorted, exaggerated, or masked by the presence of an underlying personality disorder.

Treatment and outcome

The presence of co-morbid personality disorder will usually make treatment more difficult and worsens the outcome of Axis I disorders. This may be due to problems in the following areas: help-seeking behaviors, compliance with treatment, coping styles, risk-taking, lifestyle, social support networks, therapeutic alliance, alcohol and substance abuse.

---

1 Tyrer, P. (2000). Co-morbidity of personality disorder and mental state disorders. In *Personality disorders: diagnosis, management and cause* (ed. Tyrer P). Oxford: Butterworth Heinemann.

Assessment of personality disorder (1)[1,2]

Potential pitfalls

There are a number of potential pitfalls in the assessment and diagnosis of personality disordered patients:

- Relying on diagnoses made by others (unstructured clinical interviews often do not take into account all of the necessary diagnostic criteria).
- Failing to recognize co-morbidity.
- Misdiagnosing personality disorder as an Axis I disorder and vice versa.
- Inadequate information. Patients may have distortions of perception, insight, and presentation making diagnosis difficult.
- Negative counter-transference (basing diagnosis on your negative reaction to a patient rather than on an objective assessment). Negative feelings toward an individual should not be the primary basis for a diagnosis of personality disorder.
- Applying DSM-IV-TR categories without a broader assessment of personality.
- Differential prevalence rates leading to gender biases in diagnosis.

Making the diagnosis of personality disorder

- A clinical diagnosis of personality disorder should be based on an accurate assessment of a person's enduring and pervasive patterns of emotional expression, interpersonal relationships, social functioning, and views of self and others when they are not suffering from another mental disorder.

- Information from sources other than the patient is important. These include: clinical interviews, observation, previous records (medical, prison, school, social work), independent accounts (from several sources such as relatives and other professionals).

- Information from the psychiatric history (childhood and adolescence; work record; forensic history/other aggression or violence; relationship history; psychiatric contact/self-harm) will give an indication of a person's personality and whether it may be disordered. Personality traits, by definition, should originate in childhood, adolescence, or early adulthood.

- Specific inquiry can be made regarding the following aspects of personality: interests and activities, relationships, mood/emotions, attitudes (religious, moral, health), self-concept, coping with difficulties, specific characteristics or traits (perhaps based on personality disorder categories), including both positive and negative aspects.

1 Gunn, J. Personality disorder: A clinical suggestion. In *Personality disorders: diagnosis, management and cause* (ed. Tyrer P). Oxford: Butterworth Heinemann, 2000.
2 Widiger, T.A. and Samuel, D.B. (2005). Evidence-based assessment of personality disorders. *Psychological Assessment* **17**(3), 278–287.

- In describing personality and personality disorder, first the features of a person's personality should be described. Then a decision should be made about whether the degree of distress and disruption due to personality traits indicates the presence of personality disorder. Then the features that are pathological should be described. If one wants to make categorical diagnoses, then the category or categories for which the criteria are met should be stated.

- Developmental history includes: parental and family relationships, reactions to key developmental events and transitions, significant losses or separations including relocations, preliminary assessments of incidents of trauma and deprivation, peer relationships, and important memories. Attention to process is an extremely important part of the assessment since it establishes the conditions for treatment and forges positive expectations about treatment, initiates therapeutic alliance, and prepares patients for therapy. Evaluating the three patterns of personality disorders is essential:

  - Emotional dysregulation with its core traits affective lability and anxiousness.
  - Inhibition with its traits of intimacy problems and restricted expression.
  - Dissocial behavior: callousness and rejection.

Other areas of assessment include parasuicidal and suicidal behaviors, perceptual and cognitive symptoms, dissociation, neuropsychological symptoms, quality of object relations, and psychological mindedness, which is the capacity to understand and utilize psychological explanations to behavior. Patients with a low level of psychological mindedness have difficulty using psychological interventions and require a more focused behavioral approach.

Assessment of personality disorder (2)

Instruments to assess personality disorder

There are a number of instruments available for assessing personality disorder. Such instruments are mainly used in research and are rarely seen in clinical practice. Most require training and some take a considerable amount of time to complete.

Self-report questionnaires
- Millon Clinical Multiaxial Inventory (MCMI).
- Personality Disorder Questionnaire (PDQ-IV).
- Wisconsin Personality Inventory (WISPI).

Structured clinical interviews with patient only
- Structured Clinical Interview for DSM-IV Personality Disorder (SCID-II).
- Diagnostic Interview for DSM-IV Personality Disorders (DIPD-IV).

Structured clinical interviews with informant only
- Standardized Assessment of Personality (SAP).

Structured clinical interviews with patient and/or informant
- Personality Assessment Schedule (PAS).
- Structured Interview for DSM-IV Personality Disorders (SIDP-IV).
- International Personality Disorder Examination (IPDE).

Instruments assessing specific personality disorders
- Schedule for Interviewing Borderlines (SIB).
- Diagnostic Interview for Borderline Patients (DIB).
- Borderline Personality Disorder Scale (BPD-Scale).
- Psychopathy Checklist-Revised (PCL-R).
- Psychopathy Checklist-Screening Version (PCL-SV).
- Schedule for Schizotypal Personalities (SSP).

Diagnostic instruments including an assessment of antisocial personality disorder
- Diagnostic Interview Schedule (DIS).
- Feigner Diagnostic Criteria.

Functional assessment

The functional assessment of personality and associated problems has been proposed as a useful clinical approach that can produce a formulation identifying issues to be addressed in management. Elements of the functional assessment include:

List abnormal personality traits
- Thoughts about self and others (e.g., identity problems, paranoia, grandiosity, magical thinking, exaggerating, suggestibility, preoccupation with death, obsessionality, self-esteem).
- Feelings and emotions (e.g., depression, elation, mood instability, callousness, loneliness, anger, irritability).
- Behavior (e.g., stubbornness, quarrelsomeness, sadism, self-destructiveness, compliance, impulsivity, theatricality, attention seeking).

- Social functioning (e.g., social isolation, controlling others, dependence on others, mistrust of others, inviting rejection, forming unstable intense relationships, manipulating and using others).
- Insight (including the ability to understand and integrate one's thoughts, feelings and actions).

Describe associated distress and co-morbid Axis I disorders
Describe interference with functioning

- Occupational.
- Family and relationships.
- Offending/violence.

Management of personality disorder (1)—general aspects

It is generally felt that personality disorders are challenging to treat. Patients often present at a time of crisis and/or when they develop a co-morbid Axis I disorder.

Principles of successful management plans

Four strategies are considered as a part of the general therapeutic strategies and they include: building and maintaining a collaborative relationship, maintaining a consistent treatment process, establishing and maintaining a validating treatment process, and building and maintaining motivation for change. A successful management plan in personality disorder is tailored to the individual's needs and explicitly states jointly agreed and realistic goals. The approach to patients should be consistent and agreed across the services having contact with the patient. Plans should take a long-term view, recognizing that change, if it comes, will only be observable over a long period.

Possible management goals

Potential management goals include: psychological and practical support; monitoring and supervision, intervening in crises, increasing motivation and compliance, increasing understanding of difficulties, building a therapeutic relationship, limiting harm, reducing distress, treating co-morbid Axis I disorders; treating specific areas (e.g., anger, self-harm, social skills), and giving practical support (e.g., housing, finance, child care).

Managing co-morbid Axis I disorders

It is important to recognize and treat co-morbid Axis I pathology in patients with personality disorders. Standard treatment approaches should be used, taking into account aspects of the patient's personality (e.g., impulsivity and an anti-authoritarian attitude may lead to noncompliance with medication).

Understanding and managing the relationship between the patient and staff [2]

Rejection for treatment of patients with personality disorders is often due to the intense negative feelings patients may engender and the disruptive and uneasy relationships they form with those who try to help them. Just as they do in many of their interpersonal relationships, patients with personality disorders display disordered attachment in their relationships with staff (whether with individuals or with a service). When dealing with such patients, this needs to be recognized, acknowledged, and managed. An understanding of these dynamics is a necessary part of the therapeutic alliance. Any behaviors related to these dynamics should be addressed assertively in a therapeutic manner, and be considered part of the treatment process.

Admission to hospital

Patients with personality disorder benefit little from prolonged admissions to conventional psychiatric units. Admission to such units may be necessary when there is a specific crisis (usually in the short term) or the patient presents with an Axis I disorder. Longer-term admission for the treatment of personality disorder could be undertaken in a therapeutic community. Involuntary long-term hospitalization of patients with personality disorder primarily to prevent harm to others where there is little prospect of clinical benefit to the patient is ethically concerning. Indications for inpatient admission include the following: danger to others, high risk of suicide or other high-risk behaviors that cannot be managed in a different setting, transient psychotic episodes, and severe dissociative states. Many patients have a tendency to regress in inpatient settings, and there are serious risks associated with inpatient treatment. For this reason, admission should be brief. Moreover, there is also no evidence that long-term admission is useful in treating patients with personality disorder.

Managing crises (ensuring safety)

Individuals with personality disorder often present in crisis. This may follow life events, relationship problems, or occur in the context of the development of co-morbid mental illness. In some cases the crisis may follow what appears to the outside observer to be a relatively minor or nonexistent stressor. Clinical features of crisis states and episodes of acute behavioral disorganization include:

- Affective dysregulation such as anxiety and panic, rapid mood changes, anger and rage, generalized dysphoria, severe depression.
- Behavioral disorganization and dyscontrol such as suicidal and parasuicidal behavior, impulsivity, regression, dissociation.
- Cognitive disorganization such as transient psychotic episodes, impaired information processing with reduced coping capacity and problem solving.

Crises are best managed by using a continuum of interventions, beginning with containment strategies, cognitive behavioral interventions, and medications to control and reduce symptoms and promote affect regulation followed by less structured interventions that address the cognitive, affective, and interpersonal processes leading to symptoms and maladaptive behavior. Always evaluate suicide risk during crisis, which includes change in suicide intent, level of impulsivity, and level of control such as change in consciousness related to alcohol or drugs and dissociative behavior. When patients repeatedly present in crisis, it can be helpful for the various professionals involved to plan what the response should be in such situations. A consistent response is important, but there should be sufficient flexibility to deal with changes in circumstances.

- For example, when a patient repeatedly presents with self-harm it may be appropriate for outpatient treatment to continue following any necessary medical treatment. However, if this patient presents threatening suicide following the death of a partner, then it may be appropriate to arrange admission to hospital.

Recommended further reading

1 Davison, S.E. (2002). Principles of managing patients with personality disorder. *Advances in Psychiatric Treatment* **8**, 1–9.
2 Adshead, G. (1998). Psychiatric staff as attachment figures. Understanding management problems in psychiatric services in the light of attachment theory. *BJP* **172**, 64–9.

Management of personality disorder (2)—specific treatments[1-4]

Specific treatments should address regulation and control that include affects, impulses, trauma, dissociative behavior, and interpersonal problems.

Role of medication[3]

The main indication for medication in patients with personality disorder is the development of co-morbid mental illness. There is little evidence that medication has any effect on personality disorders themselves. The positive findings from studies have been short-term, and probably due to the effects of medication on co-morbid disorders rather than on the personality disorder itself. Symptom-targeted pharmacotherapy can be helpful with psychotherapy representing the primary or core treatment for personality disorders especially borderline personality disorder. Bearing this in mind, the following have been suggested:

Antipsychotics

These may be of some benefit in cluster B (particularly borderline) and cluster A (particularly schizotypal and perhaps paranoid) disorders.

Antidepressants

These may be of benefit in impulsive, depressed, or self-harming patients (particularly borderline), and in cluster C (particularly avoidant and obsessive-compulsive) disorders. Fluoxetine in combination with olanzapine led to substantial improvement in clinician-rated depression and impulsive aggression in borderline personality disordered patients.

Anticonvulsants and lithium

These have been suggested where there is affective instability or impulsivity. Divalproex sodium has shown some benefits for patients with borderline personality disorder and for patients with cluster B personality disorders who demonstrate impulsive aggression.

Therapeutic community

A therapeutic community is a consciously designed social environment and program within a residential or day unit, in which the social and group process is harnessed with therapeutic intent. It is an intense form of psychosocial treatment in which every aspect of the environment is part of the treatment setting, in which interpersonal behavior can be challenged and modified. The main principles are:

- Democratization.
- Permissiveness.
- Communalism.
- Reality confrontation.

There are various interactions between patients and staff both individually and in groups, particularly in the daily community groups, which contribute toward achieving these principles. There is some evidence that such treatment is effective with some patients with personality disorders.

Specific therapies that may be useful with personality disorders

Dialectical behavior therapy (📖 p. 1022)

A combination of individual and group therapy lasting at least 12 months. In stage 1, individual therapy focuses on a detailed cognitive-behavioral approach to self-harm and other "therapy interfering" behaviors. Internal and external antecedents are explored, and alternative problem-solving strategies are developed. Group therapy focuses on tolerance of distress, emotional regulation and interpersonal skills. "Mindfulness training" based on Eastern meditation techniques is a key part of this.

In stage 2, patients are helped to process previous trauma, but only when stage 1 skills are developed. In stage 3, the focus is on developing self-esteem and realistic future goals. Another aspect of DBT is that patients may contact therapists by telephone between sessions to help them apply skills when difficulties arise. There is evidence that DBT may be an effective therapy for outpatients with **borderline personality disorder**. DBT has also been shown to be effective for borderline symptoms, not substance use, in patients with co-morbid borderline personality disorder and substance abuse.

Cognitive behavior therapy (📖 p. 1016)

Schema-focused therapy concentrates on identifying and modifying early maladaptive schemas and related behaviors. Patients are educated about schemas and led to expect that they will be difficult to change (for example, patients will distort new information to fit in with their existing schemas). "Empathic confrontation" is used to help patients to repeatedly and persistently challenge their core beliefs about themselves and others. Issues related to interpersonal schemas may arise in the therapeutic relationship and be used as "data" for dealing with these schemas.

There are other models used in cognitive behavior therapy to treat personality disorder, but all have in common: the goal-directed problem-solving approach; the teaching of specific skills; a longer time-scale than the relatively brief length of therapy for most other disorders; emphasis on developing, maintaining, and utilizing the therapeutic relationship; a focus on underlying core beliefs (schemas) regarding self and others; and, a longer-term historical perspective in therapy as opposed to the here-and-now focus with many other disorders.

Psychodynamic therapy (📖 p. 1022)

Classic Freudian or Jungian psychoanalysis is of no proven benefit for patients with personality disorder, and is probably contraindicated in patients with severe personality disorders. However, psychodynamic concepts are extremely useful in understanding personality disordered patients and the reactions they provoke in others, including ourselves. Modified psychodynamic approaches for patients with borderline and narcissistic personality disorders have been developed.

Other therapies are being piloted for borderline personality disorders such as interpersonal therapy, systems training for emotional predictability and problem-solving (STEPPS), comprehensive validation therapy (CVT), and a cognitive behavioral systems-based form of time limited group treatments for patients with borderline personality disorder.

Recommended further reading

1 Davidson, K. and Tyrer, P. Psychosocial treatment in personality disorder. In *Personality Disorders: Diagnosis, Management and Cause* (ed. Tyrer P). Oxford: Butterworth Heinemann, 2000.
2 Deary, I. and Power, M. Normal and abnormal personality. In *Companion to Psychiatric Studies* (eds. Johnstone EC, Freeman CPL, Zeally AK). Edinburgh: Churchill Livingstone, 1998.
3 Tyrer, P. Drug treatment of personality disorder. In *Personality Disorders: Diagnosis, Management and Cause* (ed. Tyrer P). Oxford: Butterworth Heinemann, 2000.
4 Markovitz, P.J. (2004). Recent trends in the pharmacotherapy of personality disorders. *Journal of Personality Disorders.* **18**(1), 90–101.

Outcome of personality disorder[1,2]

Morbidity and mortality

High rates of accidents, suicide, and violent death, particularly where cluster B features are prominent. There are high rates of co-morbidity with other mental disorders (see 📖 p. 560).

Outcome of other disorders in patients with personality disorder

The outcome of mental illness and physical illness is generally worse in patients with personality disorders.

Persistence of personality disorder

Some contend that personality disorder is by definition life-long and, therefore, has a poor prognosis. The evidence for this is far from conclusive.

Comparison between different age groups

Personality disorder is diagnostically less prevalent in older adults than younger adults, particularly for cluster B disorders. In terms of "normal" personality, compared with young adults, the elderly are more likely to be cautious and rigid and less likely to be impulsive and aggressive. Although pathology and symptoms may improve over time, the underlying personality traits tend to be enduring and lead to continued maladaptive behavior over a lifetime.

Follow-up of individuals over time

Borderline

A third to a half of patients fulfilling the criteria for borderline personality disorder meet criteria when followed up after 10–20 years. About a third continue to have borderline personality disorder and others have other predominating personality disorders. Poor prognostic indicators are severe repeated self-harm and "co-morbid" antisocial personality.

Schizotypal

Generally, these patients have poorer prognosis than borderline patients. About 50% may develop schizophrenia.

Obsessional

May worsen with age. More likely to develop depression than OCD.

Clusters

There is some evidence that cluster A traits worsen with age, cluster B traits improve, and cluster C traits remain unchanged.

Recommended further reading

1 Tyrer, P. and Seivewright, H. Outcome of personality disorder. In *Personality disorders: diagnosis, management and cause* (ed. Tyrer P). Oxford: Butterworth Heinemann, 2000.

2 Paris, J. (2005). Outcome and epidemiological research on personality disorders: Implications for classification. *Journal of Personality Disorders.* **19**(5), 557–562.

Geriatric psychiatry

Our aging population

Introduction

In developed countries such as the United States, Canada, and Western Europe, over the last century, the population of older adults has been increasing steadily. In the United States, by the year 2000, those aged 65 and older had increased more than 10-fold, compared to 1900, totaling approximately 35 million. Those aged 75 and older increased nearly 19-fold, and the number of people 85 and older increased nearly 38-fold.[1]

This trend is largely attributed to the decline in infant mortality, control of infectious diseases, and improvement in sanitation, living standards, and nutrition, as well as a declining birth rate. The implications of an increased number of older adults in society include a drop in the proportion of the working population, an increase in overall disability and health needs, and a corresponding increase in the need for both health and social services.

In terms of psychiatric disorders, it is well known that certain disorders increase in frequency with advancing age. For example, 5% of people older than 65 suffer from moderate to severe dementia and the prevalence increases to over 30% for those over 85.[2] Fifteen to twenty percent of older adults have significant depressive symptoms.[3] The prevalence of other disorders in people >65 yrs is approximately 1.1% for schizophrenia and 7.3% for generalized anxiety disorder.[4]

The rates of mental disorders increase as individuals move from the community to assisted living and nursing home settings. For example, the rate of depression of older adults residing in assisted living facilities has been estimated at 13%. Even if not diagnosed with depression, 25% express significant symptoms of depression.[5] In nursing home residents, depression has been estimated to occur at rates of 17%,[6] with rates of depressive symptoms estimated at 44%.[7] Finally, it is regrettably the case that psychiatric disorders are commonly either undiagnosed or misdiagnosed at the primary care level. Having said this, research has demonstrated a marked improvement over the last decade in both diagnosis and management at this level.

Geriatric psychiatry: a response to our aging world

The specialty of geriatric psychiatry was born and developed over the past 60 years both in response to demographic changes and to keep pace with the developments in geriatric medicine. Geriatric psychiatry was also inspired by the "social psychiatry" movement and growing emphasis on the care and welfare of vulnerable sectors of the population.

Psychiatric illnesses in older people include:
• Pre-existing psychiatric disorders in the aging patient.
• New disorders related to the specific stresses and circumstances of older age (e.g., bereavement, chronic medical illnesses, loss of independence, sensory deficits, social isolation).
• New disorders related to the changing physiology of the aging brain, as well as psychiatric and behavioral complications of neurological and systemic illnesses.

Psychiatric problems often coexist with physical problems such as cardiac disease, pulmonary conditions, and persistent pain (e.g., arthritis and fibromyalgia). Treatment strategies need to account for:
- These co-morbid medical conditions.
- The altered pharmacokinetics and frequent polypharmacy often present in older adults.

Cognitive assessment and physical examination are always essential parts of psychiatric management of the older person. Cognitive impairment and dementia are two of the main areas of interest in geriatric psychiatry. However, the discipline is also concerned with the assessment and treatment of depressive illnesses, late-life anxiety, paranoia and other psychotic conditions, delirium, caregiver burden, and other social and developmental problems of late life.

Because older people are often dependent on others, consideration of the role, needs, and level of burden of family members and caregivers are important to the practice of geriatric psychiatry. To effectively diagnose, treat, and maintain treatment progress in older adults, the system in which our patients live must be understood. In addition, the psychiatric care of older adults often interfaces with a range of services, both state and independent (e.g., social services, housing and welfare services, the legal system, charity organizations, and religious institutions). Knowledge of the legal entitlements and service opportunities facilitates the care of this often vulnerable population.

The role of the geriatric psychiatrist

- Diagnose and treat affective, anxiety, psychotic, and cognitive disorders of late life.
- Collaborate (often in a leadership role) with other mental health practitioners to develop multidisciplinary treatment plans.
- There are relatively few geriatric psychiatrists compared to the overwhelming need for their expertise. Thus, geriatric psychiatrists improve the quality of psychiatric care for older adults by teaching their nonpsychiatric colleagues about diagnosing and treating older adult patients with psychiatric conditions.
- Work proactively as promoters of healthy living and preventative interventions to reduce the incidence of new psychiatric disorders in older adults.
- Given the frequent complexity of the psychiatric conditions that affect older adults, geriatric psychiatrists have the opportunity to be innovative in their approach to care.
  - For example, individuals working in this area have the opportunity to be creative in developing appropriate services and new age-specific treatments.
- The nature of psychiatric problems in older adults demands that geriatric psychiatrists collaborate with internists, home-care nurses, and lay people in the community, hospitals, and other institutions to optimize treatment plans.

Recommended further reading

1 Commerce UDo. *We the American Elderly*. Washington, D.C.: U.S. Department of Commerce, Economics and Statistics Administration, Bureau of the Census; 1993.

2 Jorm, A.F., Korten, A.E., Henderson, A.S. (1987). The prevalence of dementia: a quantitative integration of the literature.[see comment]. *Acta Psychiatrica Scandinavica.* **76**(5), 465–479.

3 Gallo, J.J., Lebowitz, B.D. (1999). The epidemiology of common late-life mental disorders in the community: themes for the new century. *Psychiatric Services.* **50**(9), 1158–1166.

4 Aartjan, T. F., Beekman, M.A.B., Dorly, J.H., Deeg, Anton, Van Balkom, J. L. M. Van Balkom, Smit, H., De Beurs, Edwin, Van Dyck, Richard, Van Tilburg, Willem. (1998). Anxiety disorders in later life: a report from the longitudinal aging study Amsterdam. *International Journal of Geriatric Psychiatry.* **13**(10), 717–726.

5 Watson, L.C., Garrett, J.M., Sloane, P.D., Gruber-Baldini, A.L., Zimmerman, S. (2003). Depression in assisted living: Results from a four-state study. *American Journal of Geriatric Psychiatry.* **11**(5), 534–542.

6 Smalbrugge M, Jongenelis L, Pot A, Beekman A, Eefsting J. (2005). Co-morbidity of depression and anxiety in nursing home patients. *International Journal of Geriatric Psychiatry.* **20**(3), 218–226.

7 Jongenelis K, Pot AM, Eisses AM, *et al.* (2003). [Depression among older nursing home patients. A review]. *Tijdschrift voor Gerontologie en Geriatrie.* **34**(2), 52–59.

Normal aging

Neurobiology of normal aging

In most normally aging individuals the weight and volume of the brain decrease by 5% between the ages of 30 and 70, by 10% by the age of 80, and by 20% by the age of 90. There is a proportionate increase in the size of the ventricle and size of the subarachnoid space. Although the reductions are generalized, the frontal lobes are usually more affected.

Approximately 30–50% of older adults show no evidence of cortical atrophy, cell loss, senile neuritic plaques, or neurofibrillary tangles. In many individuals, however, there is some nerve cell loss and reductions in dendritic processes in the cortex, hippocampus, substantia nigra, and Purkinje cells of the cerebellum. The cytoplasm of nerve cells may accumulate a pigment (lipofuscin), and there may be changes in cytoskeletal components. Demyelination in subcortical and periventricular brain structures is frequently observed in older adults.

Senile plaques appear in the neocortex, amygdala, hippocampus, and entorhinal cortex but are usually not associated with significant distortion of the surrounding neuropil (the fibrous network of delicate unmyelinated nerve fibers interrupted by numerous synapses found in the CNS). They are referred to as diffuse plaques as opposed to the mature neuritic plaques seen in Alzheimer's disease (AD). Diffuse plaques are common in normally aged individuals and are not thought to have pathological significance. Neurofibrillary tangles are also observed in normally aging adults, usually in the cells of the hippocampus and entorhinal cortex. Lewy bodies may occur in the substantia nigra and the locus ceruleus. Hirano bodies (rod-shaped actin) occur in new hippocampal pyramidal cells.

Psychology of normal aging

- IQ is thought to peak at 25 years of age, plateau through 60–70, and then decline.
- In general the abilities related to previously learned ("crystallized") skills tend to decline to a lesser degree than those involved with acquiring new ("fluid") information.
- Peripheral sensory deficits (e.g., visual and auditory) can confound cognitive deficits observed in older adults.
- Information processing speed (central and perceptual) tends to be slower with older age.
- Decline in free recall memory is usually more pronounced than in recognition. Short-term memory is more affected than working memory or long-term memory. Episodic memory (e.g., autobiographical memory, the explicit memory of events) is more impaired than semantic memory (memory of meanings, understandings, and other knowledge). Nonverbal memory is more susceptible to older age than verbal memory.
- Divided attention (also known as "cocktail party phenomenon") is more impaired than focused or selective attention.
- Problem-solving ability deteriorates. Cognitive assessment is often complicated by physical illness or sensory deficits.

Social challenges of normal aging

Older adults face a number of social losses that include status, independence, spouse/partner, friends, and financial income. Facing these losses, one of the main challenges in late-life is to maintain mental activity and social engagement and avoid isolation, marginalization, depression, and stigmatization. Beneficial activities to be recommended would include church attendance, outings to restaurants, cinemas, sports games, playing cards, gardening, cooking, shopping, volunteering, and exercise. Both group and individual activities are encouraged.

Recommended further reading

1 Cabeza R. (Jul 2001). Cognitive neuroscience of aging: contributions of functional neuroimaging. *Scand J Psychol.* **42**(3), 277–286.
2 Moss M, Albert M. Neuropsychology of Alzheimer's Disease and related disorders. In: Albert M, Moss M, eds. *Geriatric Neuropsychology.* New York: Guilford Press; 1988: 1451–1472.
3 Byrum C., Moore, S., CM, H. Neuroanatomy, neurophysiology, and neuropathology of aging. In: D.G. Blazer, D.C. Steffens, E.W. Busse (eds.) *The American Psychiatric Publishing Textbook of Geriatric Psychiatry.* 3 ed. Arlington, VA: American Psychiatric Publishing, 2004: 53–81.

Multidisciplinary assessment

Older adults suffering from mental health problems often have a range of psychological, physical, and social needs. This implies that individual assessment, management, and follow-up require collaboration between health, social, and voluntary organizations and families. Assessment of the older patient with mental illness includes the following:

- Full history from the patient, family, and caregivers.
- Full physical and neurological examination.
- Mental status examination, including full cognitive assessment.
- Functional assessment (evaluation of ability to perform activities of daily living [ADLs] and instrumental activities of daily living [IADLs]).
- Social assessment (appropriateness and safety of residence; need for increased level of care such as home health services and/or nursing; financial, legal, and testamentary issues; social and leisure activities).
- Assessment of the needs and level of burden of caregivers.

The ideal place for performing an assessment is in the patient's home. A home visit has the advantage of being more convenient and relaxing for the patient and it provides the geriatric psychiatrist with an opportunity to assess living conditions, social activities, and medications kept in the house. In addition, family members, neighbors, and caregivers may be available for interviewing. However, the majority of assessments are conducted in clinics or the private office setting. Sending a letter about your assessment and treatment plan to the referring physician or therapist is crucial to facilitate coordinated care.

Sometimes brief admission is indicated, especially if the older adult has pressing physical or psychiatric needs, or if support is unavailable (or the support desperately needs respite). A full inpatient assessment may involve doctors, nurses, physical and occupational therapists, psychologists, social workers, voluntary workers, legal professionals, clergy, and others involved with older adults. Many geriatric inpatient units dedicated to caring for older adults are called Geriatric Evaluation and Management (GEM) units. Their use of comprehensive geriatric assessment with interdisciplinary team care and management of medical, rehabilitation, and psychosocial issues contributing to geriatric syndromes has been shown to improve functioning, improve placement, and prolong survival.[1] In obtaining a thorough history it is important to allow the patient to tell his/her own story. One needs to inquire about the presenting problem and how it has evolved, whether it is a new or longstanding problem, and whether the individual has a personal or family history of psychiatric conditions. In addition, it is important to inquire about losses, social history, and social circumstances (housing, income, social activities, etc), medical problems and medications, alcohol and illicit drug history, as well as the presence or absence of family support. It is particularly important to assess activities of daily living such as level of independence, ability to cook, shop, pay bills, maintain the home, and manage hygiene, toilet, laundry, etc.

The mental status exam should include an assessment of sight and hearing as well as determining the presence or absence of anxiety or mood symptoms, likeliness of suicide, abnormal beliefs or perceptions, and cognitive impairment.

Cognitive assessment must include: orientation; fund of knowledge; memory; concentration and attention; language, praxis; simple calculation; insight; and judgment. A mini mental state examination (MMSE) will incorporate some of these elements. Be certain to ask the highest level of education attained. There is a wide range of rating scales for assessing depression, anxiety, cognitive performance, activities of daily living, and caregiver burden—see Burns and Lawlor[2] for an overview.

Key questions for family members and caregivers

- Relationship to the patient (spouse, adult child, close friend).
- Their awareness of support or voluntary organizations.
- What expectations they have from services.
- Amount and types of care provided (psychological support, assistance with shopping, bathing, toileting).
- Degree of stress or psychological burden they experience as a result of providing care for the older adult (depression, anger, resentment, personal fulfillment).
- What forms of assistance are appropriate and acceptable (counseling, support groups, visiting nurse, recommendation that the older adult be moved to a facility that can provide a higher level of care).
- Understanding and knowledge of the patient's illness (ability and/or capacity to grasp how depression or dementia affects behavior).

Recommended further reading

1 Lavizzo-Mourey, R.J., Hillman, A.L., Diserens, D., Schwartz, J.S. (1993). Hospitals' motivations in establishing or closing geriatric evaluation management units: diffusion of a new patient-care technology in a changing health care environment. *Journal of Gerontology*. **48**(3), M78–83.

2 Burns A., Lawlor B., Craig S. (Feb 2002). Rating scales in old age psychiatry. *Br J Psychiatry*. **180**, 161–167.

3 Butler R. and Pitt, B. Assessment. In: R. Butler and B. Pitt (eds.) *Seminars in Old Age Psychiatry*. England: Gaskell, 1998.

Cognitive disorders

Epidemiology

- Cognitive disorders are the most prevalent psychiatric disorders of later life.
- AD is the most common cause of dementia among people 65 years or older.
- AD is the fourth leading cause of death due to disease for people 65 years and older.
- The prevalence of AD rises exponentially with age, from 5% in people aged 65 to 74 years to almost 50% in people aged >85 years.
- Advancing age and family history are the most potent risk factors.
- Most cases are of late onset (after 65 years) and most of late-onset cases are sporadic.
- Risk factors for early-onset AD include presenilin 2 gene (chromosome 1), presenilin 1 gene (chromosome 14), and amyloid precursor protein gene (chromosome 21).
- The Apolipoprotein E (apoE) genotype (specifically the ε4 allele) increases the risk of late-onset AD.
- Vascular dementia (VaD), dementia with Lewy bodies (DLB), frontotemporal dementias (FTDs), dementia secondary to alcohol dependence, and other (unknown) causes account for the rest.
- The annual treatment cost of AD in the United States is approximately $100 billion, $200,000 per patient.
- More than 70% of people with AD live at home, where family and friends provide most of their care. As the disease progresses, there may be tremendous physical, emotional, and financial stress on caregivers as they assume growing responsibilities that may include meeting physical needs, managing daily routines, and making important medical and legal decisions.

Clinical features

Dementia is a syndrome in which individuals lose independence of daily functioning because of acquired cognitive dysfunction. Cognitive dysfunction that does not substantially interfere with daily functioning may also occur. This latter condition is currently referred to as mild cognitive impairment. Both mild cognitive impairment and dementia may be caused by AD, VaD, other dementias, or a combination of pathologies (see Chapter 5).

The central feature of the dementia syndrome is acquired memory impairment. In addition, at least one of the following cognitive deficits must be present:

- Aphasia (language impairment secondary to disrupted brain function).
- Apraxia (inability to perform complex motor activities despite intact motor abilities).
- Agnosia (failure to recognize or identify objects despite intact sensory function).
- Disturbance in executive functions (i.e., difficulties with planning, sequencing, organizing, and abstracting).

General features of dementia

- AD has an insidious onset, with gradual progression of cognitive deficits ranging from 3–20 years.
- VaD often progresses in a stepwise manner, reflecting new episodes of cerebral infarction.
- Patients with dementia due to alcohol use often show meaningful improvement when they abstain from drinking for sustained periods of time.
- Social disinhibition may be prominent in FTD.
- Visual hallucinations and extreme sensitivity to the motor side-effects of antipsychotics are common in DLB.
- Behavioral problems, such as verbal and physical agitation, occur in 86% and 55%, respectively, of community-dwelling persons with dementia.
- Behavioral problems occur at higher rates among nursing home residents with dementia.
- Early symptoms of dementia include social withdrawal, apathy, depression, and paranoid delusions. Changes of diurnal rhythms and anxiety are often present before diagnosis. Irritability, agitation, socially unacceptable behavior, and wandering frequently occur during the first year after diagnosis. Geriatric psychiatrists are frequently called upon to manage these behavioral symptoms.

Pathophysiology

It is hypothesized that the loss of cholinergic neurons in the cortex is responsible for much of the cognitive changes of AD. The histopathological changes of AD, prominent in the hippocampus and neocortex include:

- Neuritic plaques.
- Neurofibrillary tangles.

Lewy bodies are present in the cytoplasm of substantia nigra cells of Parkinson's disease (PD) patients. Patients with DLB have:

- Lewy bodies in the limbic and neocortical areas.
- Modest amounts of neuritic plaques and neurofibrillary tangles.

FTD is notable for:

- Frontotemporal atrophy (visualized by brain imaging or at autopsy).
- Neuronal cell loss, gliosis, and the presence of massed cytoskeletal elements called Pick bodies.
- Abnormal function of the cytoskeletal protein tau ("tauopathy").

Management

Pharmacological

There are four cholinesterase inhibitors approved for the treatment of mild to moderate AD (arbitrarily defined as a MMSE of 10–24). These medications are tacrine, donepezil, rivastigmine, and galantamine, and have been shown to:

- Slow the progression of the disease.
- Increase the amount of time patients receive home care versus nursing-home placement.

- Reduce the frequency and intensity of problem behaviors such as agitation.
- Decrease the need for additional psychotropics such as antipsychotics and benzodiazepines (BDZs).

Memantine, an uncompetitive antagonist with moderate affinity for NMDA receptors, is approved for the treatment of moderate to severe AD.

Problem behaviors such as crying, yelling, asking repetitive questions, pacing, hitting, and extreme fear, may be treated with SSRI antidepressants. Low dose atypical antipsychotics (e.g., olanzapine, risperidone) have demonstrated efficacy, but are associated with increased risk of stroke and mortality when used in this population.

Psychosocial
Reminiscence and life review
- Facilitates recall of past experiences to promote intrapersonal and interpersonal functioning and thereby improve well-being.

Reality Orientation (RO) is a general philosophy of inpatient treatment. RO posits that confusion and agitation may be reduced through:
- Mental stimulation.
- Social interaction.
- Adjusting behavioral contingencies (i.e., if a patient perseverates about wanting to go home, changing the subject or offering to take him/her for a walk may reduce this behavior).
- Other interventions include:
- Maintaining consistent daily routines.
- Assuring adequate lighting.
- Promoting a normal sleep/wake cycle.

Recommended further reading

1 Gauthier, S., Reisberg, B., Zaudig, M., *et al.* (Apr 15, 2006). Mild cognitive impairment. Lancet. **367**(9518), 1262–1270.

2 Knopman, D.S. (Feb 2006). Dementia and cerebrovascular disease. *Mayo Clinic Proceedings.* **81**(2), 223–230.

3 Ropacki, S.A., Jeste, D.V. (Nov 2005). Epidemiology of and risk factors for psychosis of Alzheimer's disease: a review of 55 studies published from 1990 to 2003. *American Journal of Psychiatry* **162**(11), 2022–2030.

4 Livingston, G., Johnston, K., Katona, C., Paton, J., Lyketsos, C.G. (nov 2005). Old Age Task Force of the World Federation of Biological P. Systematic review of psychological approaches to the management of neuropsychiatric symptoms of dementia. *American Journal of Psychiatry.* **162**(11), 1996–2021.

5 Desai, A.K. and Grossberg, G.T. (Jun 28, 2005). Diagnosis and treatment of Alzheimer,s disease. *Neurology* **64**(12 Suppl 3), S34–39.

6 Tariot, P.N., Farlow, M.R., Grossberg, G.T., *et al.* (Jan 21, 2004). Memantine treatment in patients with moderate to severe Alzheimer disease already receiving donepezil: a randomized controlled trial. *JAMA* **291**(3), 317–324.

7 Seltzer, B., Zolnouni, P., Nunez, M., *et al.* (Dec 2004). Efficacy of donepezil in early-stage Alzheimer disease: a randomized placebo-controlled trial.[erratum appears in Arch Neurol. **62** (May 2005)(5): 825]. *Archives of Neurology* **61**(12), 1852–1856.

8 Volicer, L. and Hurley, A.C. (Sept 2003). Management of behavioral symptoms in progressive degenerative dementias. *Journals of Gerontology Series A-Biological Sciences & Medical Sciences.* **58**(9), M837–845.

Depression (1)

Epidemiology

Rates of depression in older adults differ depending on the setting:

- 0.5–1.5% in the community,.
- 6–9% of outpatients.
- 10–12% of inpatients.
- 15–30% of those in residential and nursing homes.

About 2% of the older adult population has dysthymia and 4–13% has minor depression. Minor depression appears to be a risk factor for developing major depression, and 25% of these patients develop major depressive disorder (MDD) within two years. (Note: minor depression, also known as "depressive disorder NOS" or "subclinical depression," is defined by at least two weeks of depressive symptoms but with fewer than the five items required for the diagnosis of MDD.)

Other risk factors for late-life depression include past history of depression; incompletely treated previous episodes of depression; spousal death; marital separation or divorce; low socioeconomic status; limited social support; neurotic personality traits; serious medical illness (malignancies, chronic pain), neurological diseases (PD, AD), endocrine disorders (hypothyroidism), cardiovascular disease (coronary artery disease, congestive heart failure); presence of disability; and care-giving for an older adult with serious medical, neurologic, or psychiatric illness.

Of note, 50% of patients who had a myocardial infarction or underwent cardiac catheterization experienced either minor or major depression. Gender differences in prevalence appear to diminish with advancing age. Recurrence rates vary from 50 to 90% within 2–3 year period if effective treatment is not provided. Recurrent episodes occur more frequently and may last longer. Late-onset depression often has a worse prognosis than early-onset depression. Poor outcome is associated with severity of the initial illness, psychotic symptoms, the presence of suicidal ideation, physical illness, poor medication compliance, and severe life events during the treatment and follow-up periods.

Clinical features

Depressed older adults often report symptoms similar to younger adults. However, some symptoms are more common in this population. Severe psychomotor retardation or agitation occurs in up to 30% of depressed older adults. Cognitive complaints and deficits are more common and are related to attention, concentration, speed of processing, and executive dysfunction. Recent work has shown that most older individuals who are cognitively impaired during a depressive episode remain impaired when their depression remits. In addition, a substantial proportion of older depressed individuals who are cognitively intact when depressed are likely to be impaired one year later, although their depression has remitted.[1]

Somatic preoccupations are common and may be the main complaints in some older depressed patients. Depression can present as social withdrawal and irritability without sadness. It is important to assess for hopelessness as it is strongly associated with suicidal ideation. When depression has associated delusional symptoms, hospitalization is usually required as these patients are at a higher risk of suicide. The content of delusions is often poverty, guilt, physical illness, nihilism, jealousy, and paranoia.

Depression in older adults is associated with hypercortisolemia, increased abdominal fat, decreased bone density, increased risk for type 2 diabetes, hypertension, and mortality from coronary artery disease (perhaps due to platelet hypercoagulability and/or altered heart rate variability).

Distinguishing between early-onset (before age 60) and late-onset (60 and older) depression in older adults can help with both treatment planning and prognosis. Patients who had their first depressive episode before age 60 (early-onset) may have stronger genetic loading while late-onset depression is often associated with chronic medical illness. In addition, older adults with late-onset depression are hypothesized to have a vascular component to their depression. This may be especially true for those patients who have risk factors for cardiovascular and cerebrovascular disease such as hypertension, diabetes, hypercholesterolemia, and smoking.

Neurologic conditions with high depression co-morbidity include dementia, PD, and stroke. It is likely a combination of brain pathology and functional disability that contributes to the depression in these conditions. All older adults with medical and neurological conditions that have impacted their quality of life or level of functioning should be assessed for depression.

Pathophysiology

Although a positive family history may be less relevant in late-life depression, heredity still accounts for 18% of the variation in depressive symptoms. Genetic factors that have been suggested to be associated with late-life depression include serotonin 2A receptor gene promoter A/A genotype, allele ε4 of apolipoprotein E, and the C677T mutation of the enzyme methylene tetrahydrofolate reductase. There is also evidence that allelic variation (ll genotype) of the serotonin transporter gene (SLC6A4) promoter region (5-HTTLPR) may contribute to the variable initial response of patients treated with a selective serotonin reuptake inhibitor.[2]

Structural and functional brain imaging show abnormalities in the frontostriatal pathways (e.g., dorsolateral cortex, putamen, caudate nucleus, anterior cingulate and corpus callosum), hippocampal formation, and amygdala. Other physiologic abnormalities include increased adrenocortical activity, impaired T-cell response, and increased inflammatory activity.

Recommended further reading

1 Bhalla, R.K., Butters, M.A., Mulsant. B., et al. (May 1, 2006). Persistence of Neuropsychologic Deficits in the Remitted State of Late-Life Depression. *Am. J. Geriatr. Psychiatry* **14**(5), 419–427.

2 Pollock, B.G., Ferrell, R.E., Mulsant, B.H., et al. (2002). Allelic variation in the serotonin transporter promoter affects onset of paroxetine treatment response in late-life depression. *Neuropsychopharmacology* **23**(5), 587–590.

3 Alexopoulos, G.S. (Jun 4–10, 2005). Depression in the elderly. *Lancet* **365**(9475), 1961–1970.

4 Reynolds, C., Alexopoulos, G., Katz, I. (2002) Geriatric depression: Diagnosis and treatment. *Generations* **26**, 28–31.

Depression (2)

Assessment and differential diagnosis

A complete history and exam are essential. Standardized rating scales may be useful in assessing depression and they include the Hamilton Rating Scale for Depression (HAM-D), the Beck Depression Inventory (BDI), and the Geriatric Depression Scale (GDS).

Assessing both co-morbid medical diseases and medications that could be contributing to depression is critical. Some of these medical conditions include: infection, thyroid or parathyroid abnormality, Cushing's disease, leukemia, lymphoma, pancreatic cancer, cerebrovascular disease (lacunar infarcts, stroke, vascular dementia), myocardial infarction, B_{12} deficiency, and malnutrition. Among the medications that can induce depression are: methyldopa, long-acting BDZs or BDZs with active metabolites, reserpine, steroids, anti-Parkinsonian drugs, β-blockers, cimetidine, clonidine, hydralazine, progesterone, tamoxifen, vinblastine, vincristine, and dextropropoxyphene.

Psychiatric differential diagnoses include bipolar disorder, dysthymic disorder, minor depression, adjustment disorder with depressed mood, personality disorder, anxiety disorder, dementia with depressed mood, substance use disorder, and bereavement.

Management

- Treat any underlying illness and remove any offending agent.
- If the patient is actively abusing or is dependent on alcohol or other substances (e.g., opioid analgesics), this must be treated, or the depression will likely not improve.
- Antidepressants, psychotherapy or combination treatments are the preferred methods of care in late-life depression. For maintenance treatment, psychopharmacology may be sufficient.[1]
- SSRIs (e.g., escitalopram, sertraline) and SNRIs (e.g., venlafaxine, duloxetine) are the first choice antidepressants. If these are ineffective, after a 6–8-week trial at an optimized dose, switching to mirtazapine, bupropion, nortriptyline, or desipramine are options.
- Cognitive therapy, supportive psychotherapy, problem-solving therapy, and interpersonal therapy are the preferred psychotherapies.
- For those patients who exhibit a partial response to treatment with a SSRI or SNRI, augmentation with bupropion, lithium, or triiodothyronine is indicated.
- Consider ECT for treatment-resistant depression, for severe depression with suicide risk, malnutrition or psychosis.
- Add an antipsychotic to an antidepressant for psychotic depression or for depression with agitated features.
- Although antidepressants dosages should be low initially, they should be titrated up to doses as high as in younger adults.
- After successful response, maintenance treatment for 2 years reduces recurrence.

Other key points about late-life depression

- For older adults with recurrent depression, the relative risk of recurrence over the course of two years is 2.4 times higher for those patients receiving placebo versus active medication.[1]
- Among older adults with recurrent depression, the Number Needed to Treat (NNT) with paroxetine to prevent one recurrence is four.[1]
- Combined pharmacotherapy and interpersonal psychotherapy (IPT) has also been shown to be a superior treatment in preserving remission/recovery.[2]
- In the Prevention of Suicide in Primary Care Elderly (PROSPECT) study, patients were randomized to receive either depression treatment tailored for the elderly with associated care management versus usual care. Patients who received "depression care management" had a more favorable course of depression in both degree and speed of symptom reduction and reduction in suicidal ideation than patients who received usual care.[3]
- Complicated grief (key components include searching, yearning, preoccupation with thoughts of the deceased, crying, disbelief regarding the death, feeling stunned by the death, and lack of acceptance of the death) appears to be distinct from depressive symptoms. Complicated grief is associated with enduring impairment in functioning, mood, sleep, and self-esteem.[4]
- The combination of medication and psychotherapy is associated with the highest rate of treatment completion for older adults experiencing major depression in the wake of a serious life stressor such as bereavement.[5]

Recommended further reading

1 Reynolds, C.F., 3rd, Dew, M.A., Pollock, B.G., et al. (2004). Maintenance treatment of major depression in old age. *New England Journal of Medicine* **354**(11), 1130–1138.

2 Reynolds, C.F., 3rd, Frank, E., Perel, J.M., et al. (1999). Nortriptyline and interpersonal psychotherapy as maintenance therapies for recurrent major depression: a randomized controlled trial in patients older than 59 years. *JAMA* 281(1), 39–45.

3 Bruce, M.L., Ten Have, T.R., Reynolds, C.F., 3rd, et al. (2004). Reducing suicidal ideation and depressive symptoms in depressed older primary care patients: a randomized controlled trial. *JAMA* **291**(9), 1081–1091.

4 Prigerson, H.G., Frank, E., Kasl, S.V., et al. (1995). Complicated grief and bereavement-related depression as distinct disorders: preliminary empirical validation in elderly bereaved spouses. *American Journal of Psychiatry* **152**(1), 22–30.

5 Reynolds, C.F., 3rd, Miller, M.D., Pasternak, R.E., et al. (1999). Treatment of bereavement-related major depressive episodes in later life: A controlled study of acute and continuation treatment with nortriptyline and interpersonal psychotherapy. *American Journal of Psychiatry* **156**(2), 202–208.

Anxiety disorders

Epidemiology

Anxiety disorders are thought to be among the most prevalent disorders in older age, with community prevalence rates up to 10.2%, and higher rates in older patients with medical co-morbidities or living in long-term facilities. Generalized anxiety disorder (GAD) is the most frequently diagnosed with prevalence rates as high as 11.5%. Other disorders diagnosed in older adults include specific phobias, panic disorder, social phobia, obsessive-compulsive disorder (OCD) and post-traumatic stress disorder (PTSD). Although studies report mild decreases in prevalence rates in the middle and oldest geriatric population, there is concern that these rates are underestimates. Reasons for this include:
- Underreporting by older adults who do not want to be seen as complainers,
- Acceptance of symptoms as a normal part of aging.
- Difficulty in diagnosing anxiety disorders when medical and mood disorders are co-morbid.

Of note, functionally impairing anxiety symptoms that do not meet criteria for a disorder are quite prevalent, up to 20%, which raises the question of whether the current diagnostic criteria are optimal for use with older patients.

Clinical features

Some unique features in the manifestation of anxiety disorders in older adults include the minimization of psychological complaints, an increase in somatic complaints, and an amplification of external obstacles (i.e., difficulty with transportation, concerns about finances, and fears for the health of family members). GAD often presents as restlessness, irritability, fatigue, insomnia, and muscle tension. The more common phobias of late life include fears of driving, traveling, and falling.

Pathophysiology

A speculated neuroanatomical model for anxiety disorders suggests increased activity in the "imbic system" (e.g., anterior temporal cortex and the posterior medial orbitofrontal cortex) and related subcortical structures (e.g., nucleus accumbens). This model includes increased activity in the prefrontal cortex in an attempt to suppress subcortically mediated anxiety. Neurochemical studies suggest abnormalities in the serotonergic, noradrenergic and GABAergic systems.

Psychosocial factors that may contribute to the development of new-onset anxiety symptoms in older adults include major life events and losses, physical illness, feelings of loneliness, impaired self-care, persistent pain, and increased dependence.

Differential diagnosis

Diagnoses to be considered include physical illness, mood disorders, and substance misuse disorders.

Management

After addressing any physical or psychosocial etiological factors, both pharmacological and psychosocial treatments should be considered. Combination treatment is often most effective in achieving remission and maintaining recovery.

If pharmacotherapy is selected, treatment should follow the "start low, go slow, but go all the way" rule. This is especially important because the medications that are most efficacious for the long-term treatment of anxiety disorders (SSRIs and SNRIs) can exacerbate the anxiety symptoms initially. The target dosages should be as high as needed and tolerated, but within the recommended range.

BDZs are the most commonly prescribed psychotropics for older adults with anxiety. Although short trials are usually efficacious, both short- and long-term use carry the risk of serious side-effects including increased risk of falls, impaired ability to drive, and cognitive impairment. SSRIs and SNRIs are usually the preferred agent considering their safer side-effects profiles and their efficacy, especially for GAD. Buspirone is usually well tolerated but its therapeutic response has been inconsistent.

Psychotherapeutic interventions should be included because:
- They work.
- Many older adults would rather not take another medication.
- The skills learned may generalize to improve the individual's sense of self-efficacy.

Cognitive behavior therapy (CBT) is an empirically validated treatment for GAD and panic disorder. CBT has been shown to be effective in group settings as well as when delivered individually.

The components of CBT include:
- Psycho-education about anxiety.
- Identifying and restructuring cognitive distortions.
- Behavioral relaxation.
- Desensitization techniques.

Older adults with cognitive deficits may not be able to fully engage in CBT. Another psychotherapy, problem solving therapy (PST), may be more amenable for anxious older adults. Collaboration with primary care providers is critical for effective treatment.

Recommended further reading

1 Jeste, D.V., Blazer, D.G., First, M. (Aug 15, 2005). Aging-related diagnostic variations: need for diagnostic criteria appropriate for elderly psychiatric patients. *Biol Psychiatry* **58**(4), 265–271.

2 Wetherell, J.L., Lenze, E.J., Stanley, M.A. (Dec 2005). Evidence-based treatment of geriatric anxiety disorders. *Psychiatr Clin North Am* **28**(4), 871–896, ix.

Bipolar disorder

Epidemiology

The prevalence of older adults with bipolar disorder presenting for psychiatric care is 5–19%. Among inpatients older than 55, 8–10% have bipolar disorder. Five percent of all patients with bipolar disorder have the illness onset after the age of 50. Late-onset bipolar disorder is believed to be associated with lower rates of positive family history—although some studies found higher rates—and with more medical and neurologic co-morbidities. Female to male ratio is ~3:2. An older person with presenting bipolar disorder/mania has, on average, a 20-year history of affective symptoms.

Clinical features

Manic episodes are believed to be less intense in severity but longer in duration and hospital stay. This could be due to medical co-morbidities. The interepisodes of euthymia are thought to be shorter. Psychosis is present in about 64% of manic episodes, similar to younger adults. Bipolar older adults patients often have persistent cognitive deficits. Mean duration between onset of depression and mania in older adults could be up to 15 years. Bipolar disorder is associated with high morbidity and mortality, less than in schizophrenia but more than in late-life depression.

The prevalence of co-morbid substance use disorders is lower in older than younger adults with bipolar disorder (25–29% v. 61%). Other common co-morbidities include anxiety and personality disorders.

Pathophysiology

Brain imaging studies report increases in ventricle: brain ratio, sulcal widening, and frequency and size of white-matter lesions. However, it is not clear if these changes are secondary to the bipolar disorder or to other co-morbid conditions such as (untreated) hypertension.

Management

- Lithium remains one of the treatments of choice. Lithium is indicated in the treatment of manic episodes of bipolar disorder. Maintenance therapy with lithium prevents or diminishes the intensity of subsequent episodes in those bipolar patients with a history of mania. Important side-effects to watch for and ask about in older adults are sedation, confusion, tremors and hypothyroidism. Older adults are at risk of dehydration in hot weather or if he/she are ill. If an older patient becomes dehydrated while taking lithium, they can rapidly develop lithium toxicity, which can lead to cardiac arrhythmias, renal failure, and death.
- Valproic acid is an alternate first choice. Valproic acid is indicated for the treatment of acute manic or mixed episodes associated with bipolar disorder, with or without psychotic features. Side-effects include sedation, nystagmus, gait disturbances, weight gain, hair loss, and thrombocytopenia.

- While lithium and valproic acid are approved for both the acute and maintenance phases of treatment, lamotrigine is at present only indicated for the maintenance treatment of bipolar I disorder.
- Lamotrigine helps to delay the time to recurrence of mood episodes (depression, mania, hypomania, mixed episodes) in patients treated for acute mood episodes with standard therapy, and appears to have antidepressant qualities.
- ECT is indicated for use in treatment-refractory bipolar depression or in bipolar mania in which the patient is putting his/herself at risk by dangerous, impulsive behaviors or via overactivity.
- Carbamazepine is considered a second line choice. Adverse reactions include hematological, cardiovascular, and possibly cognitive abnormalities.

Recommended further reading

1 Depp, C.A and Jeste, DV. (Oct 2004). Bipolar disorder in older adults: a critical review. *Bipolar Disord* **6**(5), 343–367.

2 Gildengers, A.G., Butters, M.A., Seligman, K., *et al.* (Apr 2004). Cognitive functioning in late-life bipolar disorder. *Am J Psychiatry* **161**(4), 736–738.

3 Young, R.C.(Dec 2005). Evidence-based pharmacological treatment of geriatric bipolar disorder. *Psychiatr Clin North Am.* **28**(4), 837–869, viii.

Psychotic disorders

Epidemiology

Prevalence of paranoia in older adults ranges between 4–6%; however, prevalence of new onset schizophrenia after the age of 45 years is 0.6%. Community prevalence rates for schizophrenia in older adults range from 0.1% to 0.5%. Women are more represented in late-onset schizophrenia. Many may have had premorbid cluster A personality disorders.

Clinical features

Most of the symptoms of late-onset schizophrenia are similar to those of early-onset. However, some of the more common symptoms include catatonia, confusion, nonauditory hallucinations, paranoia, and persecutory delusions. Less common symptoms include formal thought disorder, flat affect, and other negative symptoms.

In late-onset schizophrenia, patients appear to have less occupational and psychosocial impairment compared to early-onset patients.

Older chronic schizophrenic patients are those who developed schizophrenia at a young age and were impaired by their symptoms throughout their adult lives. These patients tend to have less positive symptoms than when they were younger and more negative, apathetic, and depressive symptoms.

Pathophysiology

As in early-onset schizophrenia, etiology is unknown.
MRI studies report:
- Both increased ventricle-to-brain ratio and third ventricle volume.
- Reductions in left temporal lobe and superior temporal gyrus volumes.
- Areas of high signal intensities and infarcts for which cerebrovascular disease may account.

Functional imaging studies show:
- Decreased activity in the frontal and temporal lobes.

Neuropsychological testing shows impairment in:
- Executive functions,.
- Verbal learning.
- Motor skills.

Sensory deficits, especially hearing impairment, have been associated with late-onset schizophrenia and paranoia.

Differential diagnosis

Differential assessment should be the same as in early-onset schizophrenia. Additional disorders that need to be carefully considered include dementia with psychotic features, psychotic disorders secondary to medical conditions, substance-induced psychosis, and chronic delirium (secondary to medication or medical illness).

Management

Refer also to Psychopharmacology section (📖 *p. 228–254*). Treatment trials in older adult with schizophrenia are scarce. Both conventional and atypical antipsychotics are FDA approved for treatment of schizophrenia.

Older adults are more susceptible to the side-effects of conventional (first generation) antipsychotics. These side-effects include extrapyramidal symptoms such as tardive dyskinesia (TD) and parkinsonism. Other side-effects such as sedation, constipation, micturition difficulties, orthostatic hypotension, and impaired cognition are also concerns of using conventional antipsychotics. Atypical antipsychotics are considered first-line treatment. This is based mainly on extrapolation from adult age studies.

Psychosocial interventions include

- Social skills training.
- Family education.
- Cognitive retraining.
- Housing and financial support.
- Addressing sensory deficits.

Psychotherapeutic techniques which utilize a cognitive behavioral approach attempt to

- Modify the meaning of delusions.
- Improve sense of control over hallucinations.

Recommended further reading

1 Howard, R., Rabins, P.V., Seeman, M.V., Jeste, D.V. (Feb 2000). Late-onset schizophrenia and very-late-onset schizophrenia-like psychosis: an international consensus. The International Late-Onset Schizophrenia Group. *Am J Psychiatry.* **157**(2), 172–178.

2 Hassett, A. (2001). Psychotic disorders in older persons. *Current Opinion in Psychiatry.* **14**(4), 377–381.

3 Jeste, D.V., Dolder, C.R., Nayak, G.V., Salzman, C. (2005). Atypical antipsychotics in elderly patients with dementia or schizophrenia: review of recent literature. *Harv Rev Psychiatry.* **13**(6), 340–351.

Substance use in older adults (1)

Refer to Substance use disorders for general information ([image] Chapter 15).

The prevalence of alcohol use disorders in older adults is generally accepted to be lower than in younger people, but rates may be underestimated because of underdetection and misdiagnosis. Diagnosing substance use disorders in older adults is limited because:

- Older adults may be less likely to disclose a history of excessive alcohol intake.
- Physicians have a lower degree of suspicion when assessing older people for alcohol use.
- Physicians are less likely to refer older adults for specialist treatment.
- Physicians may perceive alcohol use disorders in older people as being understandable in the context of poor health and changing life circumstances.

Alcohol

Epidemiology

- Community based 1-year prevalence rates for alcohol abuse and dependence is 2.75% in older men and 0.51% in older women.
- 11–33% develop late-onset alcohol use disorders.
- More women than men start drinking heavily at an older age.
- The National Institute on Alcohol Abuse and Alcoholism recommends no more than a standard drink per day for persons older than 65 years of age.
- Co-morbidity between depression and alcoholism is more common in older adults than younger adults and risk of suicide in older adults increases if there is a current or past history of heavy alcohol drinking. Heavy drinking is also a risk factor for depression, dementia, falls and confusion in older adults.

Screening

- Use the CAGE (see Substance use chapter [image] p. 626) to screen for alcohol-related problems. Remember, one positive response indicates a positive screen.
- The Short Michigan Alcoholism Screening Test-Geriatric Version (SMAST-G) is another screening tool that was designed specifically for older adults.

Presentation

- Persistent falling.
- Confusion.
- Malnutrition.
- Depression.
- Anxiety.
- Symptoms of withdrawal.

Alcohol-related dementia is characterized by:
• Ataxia.
• Peripheral neuropathy.
• Cognitive deficits (which classically do not include anomia).
• The cognitive deficits tend to stabilize and sometimes improve with abstinence.

Treatment
• Motivational techniques within the context of brief interventions have been shown to be effective in older adults.
• Brief interventions (e.g., 10–15 minutes of counseling followed up by phone calls) are effective in reducing the amount of drinking at 12-months follow-up.
• Disulfiram usually is avoided in older adults because of potential side-effects (i.e., vomiting if alcohol is ingested).
• Naltrexone has been shown to be safe and efficacious in reducing relapse to heavy drinking in older adults. Naltrexone reduces the pleasure associated with drinking alcohol.
• Acamprosate is a promising newer agent. Acamprosate is a glutamate receptor modulator that reduces the physiological and psychological distress during the postacute withdrawal period.
• Abstinence success and compliance rates are better in older adults than younger adults.
• Improvement in ADLs and level of independent living has been reported with abstinence.

Recommended further reading

1 O'Connell, H., Chin, A.V., Cunningham, C., Lawlor, B. (2003). Alcohol use disorders in elderly people—redefining an age old problem in old age. *BMJ.* **327**(7416), 664–667.

Substance use in older adults (2)

Tobacco

Epidemiology

15.2% of community-dwelling individuals age 65 to 74 and 8.4% of those aged 75 and older are smokers. Older smokers are at greater risks from smoking because they:
- Have smoked longer (an average of 40 years).
- Tend to be heavier smokers.
- Are more likely to suffer from smoking-related illnesses.
- Are also significantly less likely than younger smokers to believe that smoking harms their health.[1]

Treatment

Quitting and abstinence success rates increase with older age. Depression co-morbidity increases the risk of relapse. If a patient is depressed, that is not the time to recommend that they stop smoking. Treat the depression first.

Quitting smoking has proven health benefits, even at a late age. When an older person quits smoking[2]:
- Circulation improves immediately.
- The lungs begin to repair damage.
- In one year, the added risk of heart disease is cut almost in half.
- Risk of stroke, lung disease, and cancer diminish.

Behavioral interventions include motivational techniques which focus on the five As
- Asking about smoking.
- Advising to quit.
- Assessing willingness to quit.
- Assisting in quitting.
- Arranging follow-ups.

Pharmacological techniques include
- Nicotine replacement therapy may be used on a short-term basis to assist in the process of withdrawal. In older adults, it is important to monitor for signs of nicotine excess, such as nausea, tachycardia, or dizziness, and to lower the dose if necessary. The FDA has approved the use of nicotine replacement agents for up to 6 months of therapy, although many patients have continued to use these agents for extended periods of time with no apparent adverse effects.
- Buproprion SR is also indicated as an aid to smoking cessation treatment

It is important to remember that relapse is common. This should be treated as a temporary setback, not a failure.

Benzodiazepines

11.4% of older adult outpatients are reported to be dependent on BDZs.

The typical continuous users of BDZs, of at least once daily for four months or longer, are:

- Older females.
- Taking other psychotropic medications.
- Having multiple medical problems, especially cardiovascular and rheumatologic.

There is a high correlation between alcoholism and prescription drug abuse.

The Beers Criteria for Potentially Inappropriate Medication Use in Older Adults[3] recommends the following guidelines when using BDZs with older adults:

- Avoid any use of diazepam, flurazepam, chlordiazepoxide,
- Doses the following short-acting agents no greater than: lorazepam 3mg, oxazepam 60mg, alprazolam 2mg, temazepam 15mg, or triazolam 0.25mg.

Opioids

Most older adults who are opioid dependent (i.e., actively seeking medications or illegal drugs to ingest, inhale, or inject) developed their dependence at a younger age.

Older adults who suffer from persistent pain (e.g., cancer, musculoskeletal, neuropathic) often are prescribed opioid analgesics. It is rare for older adults who have chronic pain to become truly addicted to opioid analgesics prescribed by their physicians. True addiction is psychological dependence, in which the addict compulsively seeks the drug without regard to negative social, physical, and financial consequences. Although psychological dependence is rare, older adults often become physically dependent on opioids. In this case, abruptly stopping the drug results in symptoms of withdrawal. These symptoms can be avoided (if the drug is to be discontinued) by decreasing the drug dosage gradually over days to weeks.

Recommended further reading

1 Rimer, B.K., Orleans, C.T., Keintz, M.K., Cristinzio, S., Fleisher, L. (1990). The older smoker. Status, challenges and opportunities for intervention. *Chest.* **97**(3), 547–553.

2 Taylor, D.H., Jr., Hasselblad, V., Henley, S.J., Thun, M.J., Sloan, F.A. (2002). Benefits of smoking cessation for longevity.[erratum appears in *Am J Public Health* 2002 Sep; **92**(9), 1389]. *American Journal of Public Health.* **92**(6), 990–996.

3 Fick, D.M., Cooper, J.W., Wade, W.E., Waller, J.L., Maclean, J.R., Beers, M.H. (2003). Updating the Beers criteria for potentially inappropriate medication use in older adults: results of a U.S. consensus panel of experts. [erratum appears in *Arch Intern Med.* 2004 Feb 9;**164**(3), 298]. *Archives of Internal Medicine.* **163**(22), 2716–2724.

4 Patterson, T.L., Jeste, D.V. (Sept 1999). The potential impact of the baby-boom generation on substance abuse among elderly persons. *Psychiatr Serv.* **50**(9), 1184–1188.

5 Oslin, D.W. Evidence-based treatment of geriatric substance abuse. (Dec 2005). *Psychiatr Clin North Am.* **28**(4), 897–911, ix.

Psychopharmacology in older adults (1)

Pharmacokinetics

The physiological changes associated with aging result in altered pharmacokinetics:

- Absorption could be reduced due to changes in gastric pH, reductions in intestinal and splanchnic blood flow, and reductions in intestinal motility.
- Distribution of lipid-soluble drugs (e.g., antidepressants) can increase due to decreased muscle mass and increased adipose tissue which leads to an increased elimination half-life. The volume of distribution of water-soluble drugs (e.g., lithium) may decrease due to decreased intravascular space. Free concentrations of drugs in plasma can be affected as well by increased concentration of α1-acid glycoprotein and decreased plasma albumin.
- Metabolism is reduced due to decreased blood flow to the liver, decreased liver size, and decreased efficiency of liver microsomes.
- Excretion is reduced with the decrease in renal clearance.

Pharmacodynamics

Pharmacodynamic changes in the older adult include:

- Increased sensitivity to anticholinergic effects of medications (via antimuscarinic action). This may result in tachycardia, constipation, urinary retention, dry mouth, and confusion.
- Increased susceptibility to extrapyramidal side-effects of antipsychotic medications. This could be related to decreased dopaminergic function in older adults as suggested by decreased levels of the dopamine transporter and several dopamine receptors. Older adult women with mood disorders are at increased risk of developing tardive dyskinesia if treated with antipsychotic medication.
- Increased susceptibility to adrenergic and noradrenergic side-effects including orthostatic hypotension, hypertension, dry mouth, tachycardia, increased risk of congestive heart failure, insomnia, and tremor.
- Multiple changes in the central serotonergic system, particularly decreases in 5-HT_{2A} receptor levels.
- Decreased activity of the growth hormone axis, testosterone, and dihydroepiandrosterone; declining estrogen in women; and declining allopregnolone in men.
- Increased susceptibility to the syndrome of inappropriate antidiuretic hormone (SIADH), which results in hyponatremia. SSRIs are associated with SIADH in older adults. Risk factors for its development in older adults include older age, low sodium when the SSRI is initiated, female gender, and concomitant use of thiazide diuretics.
- Decrease in cholinergic innervations throughout the brain.

Other pharmacodynamic factors to be considered in the older adult include:

- Increased probability of drug-drug interactions: the average older. American takes three prescription drugs and four over-the-counter medications daily.
- Difficulties with adherence—this is especially true for older adults with cognitive impairment or confusing medication regimens.

Antidepressants

- SSRIs and SNRIs are preferred over TCAs and MAOIs.
- SSRIs are equally efficacious and well-tolerated in older adults.
- Citalopram, escitalopram, and sertraline are favored by experts in geriatric psychiatry because of short-half lives (1–3 days), linear kinetics across therapeutic range, and minimal drug-drug interactions.
- SSRIs have also been shown beneficial in the treatment of
  - Anxiety disorders in older adults.
  - Behavioral disturbances associated with dementia, especially when the behaviors are irritability and agitation.

Psychostimulants

- Methylphenidate and dextroamphetamine are used to treat apathy and anergia, especially in the physical rehabilitation setting.
- These agents are usually well tolerated. However, risks include exacerbation of anxiety, psychosis, weight loss, hypertension, and tachycardia. Methylphenidate can also increase the bleeding time in patients who are co-prescribed warfarin.

Recommended further reading

1 Lotrich, F.E., Pollock, B.G. (2005). Aging and clinical pharmacology: implications for antidepressants. *J Clin Pharmacol.* **45**(10), 1106–1122.

Psychopharmacology in older adults (2)

Antipsychotics

- Second-generation antipsychotics (risperidone, olanzapine, quetiapine, ziprasidone, aripiprazole) are preferred over conventional antipsychotics (haloperidol, chlorpromazine, perphenazine) mainly because of a better motor side-effect profile.
- Older adults are more susceptible to side-effects, including sedation, EPS, and gait disturbances.
- Metabolic changes such as weight, body mass index, blood pressure, lipid panel, and fasting blood glucose should be routinely monitored.
- The use of atypical antipsychotics in the treatment of behavioral symptoms in patients with dementia has been associated with increased risk of mortality. The most often reported cause of death associated with these medications in this population is stroke. They are also associated with increased morbidity, most frequently from cardiac-related events or infections such as pneumonia. Similar risks have been reported for conventional antipsychotics. When using these agents in patients with dementia who exhibit behavior problems, be certain to weigh the risk/benefit ratio and alternative pharmacological and psychosocial interventions first.
- Clozapine is of use to some older adults, especially those with Parkinson's disease with psychosis for whom other atypical antipsychotics are ineffective. Clozapine, at daily doses of 50mg or less, has been shown to be safe and significantly improves drug-induced psychosis without worsening Parkinsonism. However, older adults may be more susceptible to risks of sedation, hypersalivation, seizures, and agranulocytosis.

Mood stabilizers

- Limited data is available on the use of mood stabilizers in older adults.
- Lithium is the most commonly used despite increased risk of toxicity with age-associated reductions in renal clearance and total body water. Target serum levels in older adults are usually 0.4–0.8mEq/L.
- Older adults are more susceptible to lithium-related neurologic side-effects which may be because of increased blood-brain barrier permeability or changes in sodium-lithium counter-transport.
- Because of increased risk of lithium-induced hypothyroidism, it is recommended to check TSH every six months.
- Valproic acid is also used in older adults for bipolar disorder and behavioral agitation. Side-effects of particular relevance to old age include thrombocytopenia, liver toxicity, hyerammonemia, pancreatitis, increased bone turnover, reduction in serum folate, and elevation in plasma homocysteine. Because of drug-drug interactions and variable albumin level, free drug levels are recommended.
- Carbamazepine is usually avoided in older adults because of complex drug-drug interactions although it was found to be efficacious in treating agitation and aggression in nursing home residents.

- Gabapentin is used in older adults because of its favorable side-effect profile, modest anxiolytic effect, and analgesia for neuropathic pain. It is
  - Not metabolized.
  - Not protein-bound.
  - Eliminated by renal excretion.

Older adults are susceptible to its side-effects including sedation, ataxia, and disorganized thinking.

- Lamotrigine is relatively well tolerated in older adults based on epilepsy literature. Stevens-Johnson syndrome is the most serious side-effect and it should be discontinued at the first sign of rash or hypersensitivity.

Anxiolytics

- SSRIs and SNRIs are preferred for treatment of anxiety disorders.
- Among BDZs those ones with intermediate half-lives are preferred over the long or very short acting ones.
- BDZ use is associated with falls, hip fractures and cognitive impairment.
- Many BDZs are metabolized by cytochrome P450 isozymes (phase I oxidation) the activity of which decline with age and is affected by other drugs. This can result in relatively long and variable half-lives.
- Temazepam, oxazepam and lorazepam are the preferred BDZs in older adults because they are metabolized by glucuronide conjugation (phase II), and therefore their half-lives do not change with age.
- Buspirone is well tolerated in older adults and carries a lower risk of sedation. Its efficacy has been shown in GAD but not in panic disorder or OCD. Its use is limited by the fact that it takes several weeks for onset of action.

Cognitive enhancers

- The four approved cholinesterase inhibitors in the U.S. are tacrine, donepezil, rivastigmine, and galantamine. They have been shown to have modest effect on cognition and function in patients with AD of mild to moderate severity.
- Tacrine is no longer recommended because of hepatic toxicity.
- The main side-effects of these agents are related to peripheral cholinergic action, especially gastrointestinal distress.
- Donepezil and galantamine are metabolized by liver cytochromes.
- Rivastigmine level is affected by renal clearance.
- Memantine is another cognitive enhancer that is approved for moderate to severe AD. This agent has a unique mechanism of action; it is a noncompetitive NMDA receptor antagonist. Memantine has been shown to slow the deterioration of AD, as well as to temporarily enhance cognition and ADLs in combination with donepezil.
- Memantine has minimal drug-drug interactions and is renally excreted.

Recommended further reading

1 Jeste, D.V., Dolder, C.R., Nayak, G.V., Salzman, C. (2005). Atypical antipsychotics in elderly patients with dementia or schizophernia. *Harv Rev Psychiatry*, **13**(6): 340–51.
2 Lotrich, F.E., Pollock, B.G. (2005). Aging and clinical pharmacology: implications for antidepressants. *J clin Pharmacol*, **45**(10): 1106–1122.

Personality problems

Personality refers to an individual's habitual ways of relating to other people, interacting with the environment, and thinking about oneself.[1] Personality traits such as cautiousness, introversion, dependence, and obsessionality often become more prominent and rigid in old age. Personality disorders, however, have a lower prevalence in older than younger adults,[2] with community rates estimated at 5–10%.[3] The natural history of personality development in later life is affected by both the medical and neurological changes associated with aging, as well as the changes in support networks and degree of independence.

A common feature of dementing disorders is a change in personality or an exacerbation of pre-existing characteristics. In some cases increasing paranoia in a cognitively impaired individual may be mistaken for a paranoid psychotic state such as delusional disorder.

Depression is the most commonly reported co-morbid psychiatric condition of personality disorders in older adults.[4] The association is higher for early-onset, recurrent depression than for late-onset depressive disorders.[4,5]

Personality problems may be associated with Diogenes syndrome[6] (also called senile squalor syndrome), in which eccentric and reclusive individuals become increasingly isolated and neglect themselves, living in filthy, poor conditions. They are often oblivious to their condition and resistant to help, necessitating intervention.[7] Personality characteristics associated with this disorder include being aloof, suspicious, emotionally labile, aggressive, and reality-distorting (e.g., cluster C).[7]

Treatment issues

- Treat co-morbid affective illness or psychosis.[8]
- Focus psychosocial interventions on targeting specific symptoms which discomfort, threaten, or endanger patients or their caregivers.
- Educate caregivers that changes in personality may not be under full volitional control because of changes in the brain.

Recommended further reading

1 APA. *Diagnostic and Statistical Manual of Mental Disorders.* 4th, Text Revision ed. Washington, DC: American Psychiatric Association Press, 2000.

2 Agronin, M.E., Maletta, G. Personality disorders in late life. Understanding and overcoming the gap in research. (2000). *American Journal of Geriatric Psychiatry* **8**(1), 4–18.

3 Agronin, M. (1994). Personality disorders in the elderly: An overview. *Journal of Geriatric Psychiatry* **27**(151–191).

4 Devanand, D.P., Turret, N., Moody, B.J., *et al.* (2000). Personality disorders in elderly patients with dysthymic disorder. *American Journal of Geriatric Psychiatry* **8**(3), 188–195.

5 Fava, M., Alpert, J.E., Borus, J.S., Nierenberg, A.A., Pava, J.A., Rosenbaum, J.F. (1996). Patterns of personality disorder co-morbidity in early-onset versus late-onset major depression. *American Journal of Psychiatry* **153**(10), 1308–1312.

6 Rosenthal, M., Stelian, J., Wagner, J., Berkman, P. (1999). Diogenes syndrome and hoarding in the elderly: case reports. *Israel Journal of Psychiatry & Related Sciences* **36**(1), 29–34.

7 Clark, A.N., Mankikar, G.D., Gray, I. (1975). Diogenes syndrome. A clinical study of gross neglect in old age. *Lancet* **1**(7903), 366–368.

8 Kunik, M., Mulsant, B., Rifai, A. (1993). Personality disorders in elderly inpatients with major depression. *American Journal of Geriatric Psychiatry* **1**(38–45).

Suicide

Epidemiology

Advanced age is a risk factor for suicide. It is estimated that approximately 20% of all suicides occur in older adults. There is a male predominance of 2:1 in this age group, as suicide rates tend to increase with age in men.

Predictors of suicide in older adults

- Increasing age.
- Male.
- Physical illness (35–85% cases).
- Social isolation.
- Widowed or separated.
- Alcohol abuse.
- Depressive illness, current or past (80% cases).
- Recent contact with psychiatric services.

Suicidal behaviors and statements

Older adults tend to use highly lethal means to commit suicide. In 1988, nearly 80% of suicides committed by men 65 years of age and older and involved use of a firearm. Hanging and poisoning are also frequent suicide methods used by older adults. All suicidal behaviors should be taken seriously. It is possible that what appears to be "parasuicide," (i.e., suicidal gesture or a suicide attempt which does not result in death) may actually be a failed suicide attempt with the intent to die. It is important to diagnose depression, understand personality structure and coping skills, and assess the current support system. Of patients who exhibit nonlethal parasuicidal behavior:

- 60% are physically ill.
- 50% have been previously admitted to a psychiatric hospital.
- 8% go on to complete a suicide within three years of nonlethal suicidal behavior.

Elder abuse

Elder abuse is often overlooked because its screening is not routine. When suspected or discovered, its remedy requires an integrated response from multiple disciplines and agencies, including health and social services, the criminal justice system, and government.

Elder abuse is an all-inclusive term representing all types of mistreatment or abusive behavior toward older adults:
* Physical abuse—inflicting, or threatening to inflict, physical pain or injury on a vulnerable elder, or depriving him/her of a basic need.
* Emotional abuse—inflicting mental pain, anguish, or distress on an elderly person through verbal or nonverbal acts.
* Sexual abuse—nonconsensual sexual contact of any kind.
* Exploitation—illegal taking, misuse, or concealment of funds, property, or assets of a vulnerable elder.
* Neglect—refusal or failure by those responsible to provide food, shelter, health care or protection for a vulnerable elder.
* Abandonment—the desertion of a vulnerable elder by anyone who has assumed the responsibility for care or custody of that person.

Epidemiology
Elder abuse occurs in both domestic and institutional settings:
* Domestic setting: approximately 4–6% of community dwelling older adults report incidents of abuse or neglect in domestic settings. The most common forms of abuse are verbal abuse and financial exploitation by family members and physical abuse by spouses. Gender distribution (of victims) is equal and neither economic status nor age is related to the risk of abuse. Of concern is the underreporting of elder abuse— 450,000 older adults in domestic settings were abused, neglected, or exploited in the United States during 1996, of which only 70,000 were self-reported.
* Institutional settings: one survey of nursing-home staff disclosed that 36% of staff had witnessed at least one incident of physical abuse in the preceding year, while 10% admitted having committed at least one act of physical abuse themselves.

The main risk factors for elder abuse include:
* Dependency and social isolation of the victim.
* Caregiver has psychiatric or substance misuse problems.
* Absence of a suitable guardian.

Addressing the problem
Effectively responding to elder abuse requires both a multidisciplinary approach and a proactive system of assessment of suspicious cases. An integrative response via prevention is the best approach, and a number of measures have proved effective:
* Providing training and/or counseling to caregivers and reducing their level of caregiving burden.
* Reducing the isolation of elders by engaging community support programs.

- Periodic respite care (i.e., employing a home health aid, attending a day program, or living for a period of time at a skilled nursing facility).
- Visits by home-care nurses.

Federal laws on child abuse and domestic violence fund services and shelters for victims, but there is no comparable federal law on elder abuse. However, all 50 states and the District of Columbia have enacted legislation authorizing the provision of adult protective services in cases of elder abuse. In most jurisdictions, these laws pertain to abused adults who have a disability, vulnerability, or impairment as defined by state law, not just to elderly people.

Additionally, all states and the District of Columbia have laws authorizing the Long Term Care Ombudsman Program (LTCOP), to advocate on behalf of long-term-care-facility residents who experience abuse, violations of their rights, or other problems.

If a vulnerable adult is in immediate danger, the police should be notified right away. If elder abuse is suspected, or there is concern about the well-being or safety of an older person, information and referral is available from the national Eldercare Locator, a public service of the U.S. Administration on Aging (1-800-677-1116).

More information is available from the Web site of the National Center on Elder Abuse (www.elderabusecenter.org).

Recommended further reading

1 Wolf, R.S. (Mar 1, 1999). Suspected abuse in an elderly patient. *Am Fam Physician.* **59**(5), 1319–1320.
2 Payne, B. (2002). An integrated understanding of elder abuse and neglect. *Journal of Criminal Justice* 30, 535–547.
3 Benbow, S.M., Haddad, P.M. (Oct 1993). Sexual abuse of the elderly mentally ill. *Postgrad Med J* **69**(816), 803–807.

Sexual problems in older adults

Physiologic changes that occur in normal aging:
- Decrease in testosterone levels in men and women (which is associated with decreased libido).
- Menopause for women.
- Decreased penile and pelvic blood flow.
- Narrowing and shortening of the vagina.
- Decreased lubrication and atrophy of urogenital tissue.
- Fewer and less functional sperm.
- Erections require more tactile stimulation, take longer to achieve, are less rigid, and are more difficult to sustain.
- Decreased clitoral sensitivity.
- Orgasm requires more tactile stimulation and takes longer to achieve. Ejaculation and vaginal contractions are less forceful.
- Longer refractory periods.

The sexual disorders encountered by older adults include disorders of sexual desire, arousal, orgasm, and sexual pain disorders. Sexual dysfunction in older adults is often multifactorial, and includes medical (cardiac disease, COPD, diabetes, incontinence), psychiatric (depression), psychological (low self-esteem, fears of self-injury or death during sex because of medical conditions) and medication-related (antiandrogens, antidepressants, anticholinergics, antihypertensives).

Erectile dysfunction (ED) is the most common sexual disorder in older men affecting 20–40% of men in their 60s and 50–70% of men in their 70s and 80s.

Hypoactive sexual desire (50% in late 60s and 70s), inhibited orgasm and dyspareunia are the most common sexual disorders in older women.

The majority of individuals older than 60 years are sexually active. More men than women report having regular sexual partners or masturbating if there is no partner.

In general, although the frequency of sexual intercourse may decrease with older age, other forms of sexual intimacy may continue, including hugging, kissing, caressing, oral sex, and masturbation.

Among nursing home residents ~10% report being sexually active in the past month and ~20% report the desire to be sexually active. Privacy should be ensured in long-term facilities.

Sexually transmitted diseases have much lower prevalence rates in older than younger adults. However, 10% of AIDS patients are older than 50. This proportion will likely increase as the life span of people diagnosed with AIDS earlier in their life continues to increase. Diagnosis in later life is problematic, because this translates to later initiation of treatment. HIV tends to progress faster in older adults, so screening for HIV in older patients who engage in high-risk behaviors is crucial, so early treatment can be started.

If possible, sexual orientation should be explicitly addressed in a non-judgmental manner. Older gay and lesbian patients often face the challenge of both ageism and homophobia, so providing a safe, supportive atmosphere will help to improve the doctor-patient relationship, facilitating their psychiatric and medical treatment.

Sexual behavior may be altered in dementia. Sexually inappropriate behavior (SIB) occurs in up to 25% of residents on dementia units.

Hypersexuality, defined as a persistent, uninhibited sexual behavior directed at oneself or other people, is rare. It typically involves inappropriate behavior in relation to others. However, not every SIB is secondary to hypersexuality. A behavior could appear inappropriate because it occurs in the wrong place at the wrong time.

Assessment of a sexual problem should include a detailed history and exam. Involvement of the partner leads to more successful results. The workup may include blood tests (testosterone, prolactin, thyroid function tests, and prostate specific antigen [PSA]). For men, penile tumescence testing and penile duplex ultrasonography may also be performed.

Treatment

Several treatment options used in younger adults can be used in older adults. These include cognitive-behavioral sex therapy, testosterone cream, penile intracavernosal self-injecting agent and implants, oral phosphodiesterase type 5 inhibitors, and vacuum constriction devices. Estrogen replacement therapy (ERT) may help improve sexual arousal and comfort in women. The use of a vibrator can improve clitoral stimulation and inhibited orgasm in women.

Treatment should also involve reassurance and education, especially about forms of sexual intimacy other than intercourse (e.g., foreplay). Minimizing the contribution of specific medical illnesses to sexual dysfunction may improve the quality of the older adult's sex life. For example, if shortness of breath is interfering with sex, consider recommending minimal exertion or β-agonist inhalers prior to sex. Similarly, if joint pain, immobility, or weakness is a problem, recommending a warm bath or analgesic use before sexual activity may be helpful.

Consider alternate medications if sexual side-effects are suspected.

It is important to treat co-morbid psychiatric disorders. Libido can be negatively affected by depression.

When a SIB is identified, it is important to characterize it within the context of its occurrence. Many times the appropriate response to such behavior may be modifying the environment and providing the resident with privacy. Other times responses can be gentle verbal or physical redirection. The staff should avoid reinforcement of the SIB such as laughing at an inappropriate joke or teasing the resident.

In general, unless SIB are present, it is not necessary to assess sexual history in advanced dementia. The pharmacology used to reduce the frequency and intensity of SIB include progesterones (e.g., medroxyprogesterone), anti-androgens (e.g., cyproterone acetate), anticonvulsants (e.g., valproic acid), and antidepressants (e.g., ecitalopram).

Recommended further reading

1 Tsai, S.J., Hwang, J.P., Yang, C.H., Liu, K.M., Lirng, J.F. (Jan 1999). Inappropriate sexual behaviors in dementia: a preliminary report. *Alzheimer Dis Assoc Disord* **13**(1), 60–62.

2 Agronin, M. Sexual Disorders. In: D.G. Blazer, D.C. Steffens, E.W. Busse (eds.). *The American Psychiatric Publishing Textbook of Geriatric Psychiatry.* 3rd ed. Arlington, VA: American Psychiatric Press, 2004, pp. 303–318.

Legal issues in geriatric psychiatry

Competence (📖 p. 830)

Competence refers to the ability to perform either a specific task or a range of tasks. All adults are presumed competent until declared otherwise. This is a legal concept and only judges can adjudicate incompetence.

Competence can be either general or specific to a particular domain. General competence refers to the ability to perform all personal affairs, and may be questioned in cases of severe dementia. Specific competence refers to a specific task (e.g., competence to make a decision about medical treatment or financial concerns). Incompetence may be time-limited.

Capacity (📖 p. 946)

This reflects the assessment of the clinician, and should be specific to a certain decision or action. Thus, two types of capacity can be distinguished: decisional (e.g., executing a will) and functional (e.g., driving a car). The four key components of capacity include:

• Understanding of the facts of the condition and the options available.
• Appreciation of the significance of these facts and options.
• Reasoned consideration of the facts and options based on personal and cultural preferences and values.
• Expression of choice based on above.

Guardianship (📖 p. 830)

Guardianship is determined by a judge. Guardianship can be for:

• A person (affects issues about medical care and residence).
• An estate (affects financial concerns).
• A plenary (this type of guardianship is for both person and estate).

The goal of guardianship is to protect a vulnerable person's health, well-being, and financial interests.

Advance directive

The term Advance Directive describes two types of legal documents that enable patients to plan for and communicate end-of-life issues in the event they are unable to communicate:

• A living will allows patients to document their wishes concerning medical treatments at the end of life.
• A medical power of attorney (or health care proxy) allows patients to appoint a person they trust as their health care agent (or surrogate decision maker), who is authorized to make medical decisions on their behalf. This directive becomes active should the patient become incapacitated.

Do-not-resuscitate (DNR) order

DNR is an order that prohibits the use of cardiopulmonary resuscitation in the event of cardiac arrest. Advanced directives do not need to include a DNR order, and the patient does not need an advanced directive to have a DNR order.

Recommended further reading

1 Kapp, M.B. Decisional capacity in theory and practice: legal process versus "bumbling through". *Aging Ment Health.* Nov 2002; **6**(4), 413–417.

End-of-life care

(see also 📖 p. 982)

In the United States, 80% of deaths occur in older adults. The vast majority of people die in hospitals.

Palliative care aims at reducing suffering during the dying process without attempting to prolong life. Palliative care is directed toward the patient and his or her loved ones. Palliative care can extend to beyond the patient's death when it involves support and bereavement care to the family.

Discussing end-of-life care should be started early during a life-threatening illness.

The primary aim is to understand the patient's perspective on his or her illness. This facilitates understanding his or her values system within the context of his or her culture.

Other treatment goals include:

• Understanding what "dying with dignity" means to the patient.
• Maintaining an alliance with the patient and family to foster trust and ease fear of abandonment.
• Expressing empathy and maintaining timely and appropriate communication.

End-of-life syndromes on which geriatric psychiatrists collaborate

• Pain: Routinely assess pain as the "fifth vital sign" by direct inquiry. Altered mental status, irritability, or pain behaviors (grimacing, moaning, restricting movement) are nonverbal cues that pain is causing problems. Aim at eliminating pain unless it is not the wish of an informed patient. Use fixed dosages of analgesics and prn medications for breakthrough pain. While not perfect, the WHO analgesic ladder is a useful was to initiate analgesia:
  • Acetaminophen and NSAIDS.
  • Oxycodone and codeine.
  • Morphine.

Other agents include steroids, bisphosphonates, and calcitonin for bone pain; as well as TCAs, and anticonvulsants for neuropathic pain. Non-pharmacological treatments include anesthesia, surgical interventions, physical rehabilitation, transcutaneous electrical nerve stimulation, hypnosis, acupuncture, massage, cognitive-behavioral psychotherapy, meditation, guided imagery, and relaxation.

• Depression: Diagnosing depression in a dying patient may be challenging since many vegetative symptoms can be caused by co-morbid medical conditions. The psychiatrist should focus on the affective and cognitive symptoms of depression. It may be difficult to distinguish acceptance of dying and thoughts about death in a dying patient from hopelessness and suicidality secondary to depression. Remember that treating depression often reduces the severity of pain, and treating pain may improve some symptoms of depression.
• Anxiety: Anxiety symptoms are common and distressing in dying patients. BDZs are commonly used. Longer-term treatment would comprise antidepressants or buspirone. If the time, motivation, and

cognitive abilities allow, the dying patient may benefit from cognitive behavioral psychotherapy to reframe symptoms and their stage in the life course as less anxiety provoking.

- Delirium: Delirium may be difficult to treat in a dying patient because the underlying cause is untreatable (or has been chosen to not be treated) or because the offending agent is used for palliative care (e.g., opioids). Weighing the risks and benefits of determining the etiology and/or intervening should be discussed with the patient and family. Many times palliative care would just consist of treating the associated anxiety, psychosis and agitation.
- Psychosocial issues: The geriatric psychiatrist often finds herself dealing with issues related to the patient's relationships with family members and loved ones. Addressing these issues may facilitate the resolution of long-standing conflicts as well as prevent bereavement related depression or traumatic grief.

Physician assisted suicide (PAS)

PAS is defined as a person killing him- or herself by using medications or a device provided by a physician for that explicit purpose. Euthanasia is defined as the physician-ordered intentional killing of a patient, typically a lethal dose of a medication administered by the physician or designee, such as a nurse. Euthanasia is illegal throughout the United States.

In Oregon, PAS is sanctioned, but each case has to meet several prerequisites including the absence of depression.

Issues to consider in educating patients and families at the end of life

- The family or patient may request to withdraw or withhold a treatment if it is perceived as noncompatible with an acceptable quality of life. To help them make informed choices, the psychiatrist can assure they understand both the prognosis and the compatibility of this prognosis with the patient's views on acceptable quality of life and dignity.
- There is a lack of evidence that tube feeding prolongs or improves end-of-life quality in patients with advanced dementia.
- With some patients it is difficult to achieve an acceptable quality at the end of life because of pain or agitation. Consequently, the physician, with the family's consent, can pursue terminal sedation, keeping the patient unconscious until he/she dies from the underlying disease. BDZs, opioids and anesthetics are often used for that purpose. Even though the side-effects of these medications may hasten the death process, the explicit goal of their use is to alleviate pain and suffering. This is referred to as the "doctrine of double effect."

Recommended further reading

1 Lyness, J.M. (Sep–Oct 2004). End-of-life care: issues relevant to the geriatric psychiatrist. *Am J Geriatr Psychiatry* **12**(5), 457–472.

Substance use disorders

Introduction

The concept of substance use disorders (SUDs) historically has been complicated by how the society views individuals who engage in addictive behaviors. Philosophical issues of whether SUDs are seen as a medical condition or a moral failing determine the impact on addiction and recovery from addiction. The long-held mistaken beliefs about people with SUDs as morally weak or as having criminal tendencies have also been held by their families, their communities, and the health care professionals who work with them. If viewed as an illness, SUD will be treated. Recent overwhelming scientific research provided strong evidence that not only do drugs interfere with normal brain functioning, but they also have long-term effects on brain metabolism and activity. At some point, changes occur in the brain that can turn drug abuse into addiction, a chronic, relapsing illness influenced by biological, social, and psychological factors. Alcohol and drug abuse and dependence are common problems in our society. Overall, an estimated 22.5 million Americans aged 12 and older were classified with substance abuse or dependence (9.4% of the population) according to the 2003 data from the National Survey on Drug Use and Health (SAMSHA, 2004). Alcohol and drugs are frequent causes of major family dysfunction, including domestic violence and child abuse, and are major causes of both work-related and non-work-related accidents. Alcohol and drug use is associated with violent crime. The economic costs of drug and alcohol use are substantial. It is estimated that the total yearly costs to the U.S. economy from alcohol and drug abuse and dependence are $238 billion. Of this, $34 billion are attributed to direct health care costs of hospitals, health care services, and treatment centers.

Clinical practice and outcome studies confirm that effective treatment for SUDs is available. Despite the serious and costly sequelae of untreated SUDs, treatments with demonstrated efficacy, cost effectiveness, and cost benefit have not penetrated fully into mainstream medicine. Controlled studies have shown that with proper diagnosis and treatment, abstinence rates ranging from 50 to 90% can be achieved on a long-term basis in recovery from SUDs and treatment is cost-effective. Studies on health care utilization find significant savings in total health care costs when treatment for SUDs is available. For all these reasons, it is imperative that clinicians correctly assess, diagnose, and aggressively treat SUDs in their patients.

This chapter discusses the common aspects of SUDs and then examines issues pertinent to specific drug classes, followed by treatment interventions. It then presents a review of pregnancy and SUDs, co-occurring disorders (CODs), levels of care, and other nonsubstance addictions. It concludes with most current street names of drugs, and offers a list of suggested readings and Internet resources.

Diagnostic criteria (DSM-IV-TR)

Substance abuse

A maladaptive pattern of substance use leading to clinically significant impairment or distress, as manifested by one (or more) of the following, occurring within a 12-month period:

- Recurrent substance use resulting in a failure to fulfill major role obligations at work, school, home (e.g., repeated absences or poor work performance related to substance use; substance-related absences, suspensions, or expulsions from school; neglect of children or household).
- Recurrent substance use in situations in which it is physically hazardous (e.g., driving an automobile or operating a machine when impaired by substance use).
- Recurrent substance-related legal problems (e.g., arrests for substance-related disorderly conduct).
- Continued substance use despite having persistent or recurrent social or interpersonal problems caused or exacerbated by the effects of the substance (e.g., arguments with spouse about consequences of intoxication, physical fights).

The symptoms have never met the criteria for substance dependence for this class of substance.

Substance dependence

A maladaptive pattern of substance use, leading to clinically significant impairment or distress, as manifested by three (or more) of the following, occurring at any time in the same 12-month period:

1. tolerance, as defined by either of the following:
   - a need for markedly increased amounts of the substance to achieve intoxication or desired effect,
   - markedly diminished effect with continued use of the same amount of substance,
2. withdrawal, as manifested by either of the following:
   - the characteristic withdrawal syndrome for the substance,
   - the same (or a closely related) substance is taken to relieve or avoid withdrawal symptoms,
3. the substance is often taken in larger amounts or over a longer period than was intended,
4. there is a persistent desire or unsuccessful efforts to cut down or control substance use,
5. a great deal of time is spent in activities to obtain the substance, use the substance, or recover from its effects,
6. important social, occupational or recreational activities are given up or reduced because of substance use,
7. the substance use is continued despite knowledge of having a persistent or recurrent physical or psychological problem that is likely to have been caused or exacerbated by the substance (e.g., continued drinking despite recognition that an ulcer was made worse by alcohol consumption).

Course specifiers

With physiological dependence

This specifier should be used when substance dependence is accompanied by evidence of tolerance (criterion 1) or withdrawal (criterion 2).

Without physiological dependence

This specifier should be used when there is no evidence of tolerance (criterion 1) or withdrawal (criterion 2). In these individuals, substance dependence is characterized by a pattern of compulsive use (at least three items from criteria 3–7).

Early full remission

No criteria for dependence or abuse have been met for at least 1 month, but less than 12 months.

Early partial remission

One or more criteria for dependence or abuse have been met (but the full criteria for dependence have not been met) for at least 1 month, but less than 12 months.

Sustained full remission

None of the criteria for dependence or abuse have been met at any time during a period of 12 months or longer.

Sustained partial remission

Full criteria for dependence have not been met for a period of 12 months or longer; however, one or more criteria for dependence or abuse have been met.

On agonist therapy

Specifier if patient is on prescribed agonist medication, such as methadone, and no criteria for dependence or abuse have been met for that class of medication for at least the past 1 month.

In a controlled environment

Specifier used if the individual is in an environment where access to alcohol and controlled substances is restricted, and no criteria for dependence or abuse have been met for at least the past 1 month (e.g., jail, locked hospital unit).

Substance intoxication

The development of a reversible substance-specific syndrome due to a recent ingestion of (or exposure to) a substance.

Clinically significant maladaptive behavioral or psychological changes that are due to the effect of the substance on the central nervous system (e.g., belligerence, mood lability, cognitive impairment, impaired judgment, impaired social or occupational functioning) and develop during or shortly after use of the substance.

The symptoms are not due to a general medical condition and are not better accounted for by another mental disorder.

Substance withdrawal

The development of a substance-specific syndrome due to the cessation of (or reduction in) substance use that has been heavy and prolonged.

The substance-specific syndrome causes clinically significant distress or impairment in social, occupational, or other important areas of functioning.

The symptoms are not due to a general medical condition and are not better accounted for by another mental disorder.

Social context and epidemiology

Five primary sources provide insights into the epidemiology of alcohol and drug dependence in the United States. They are the following:

- The National Survey on Drug Use and Health.
- The Epidemiological Catchment Area Survey (ECA).
- The National Comorbidity Survey (NCS).
- The Drug Abuse Warning Network (DAWN).
- The National Epidemiological Survey on Alcohol and Related Conditions (NESARC).

The National Survey on Drug Abuse Use and Health showed consistent substantial levels of illicit drug use in the United States. The results are the following:

- 19.5 million Americans (8.2%) used illicit drugs in 2003.
- 6.2 million marijuana users; 2.3 million cocaine users; 119,000 heroin users; 4.7 million users of pain relievers for non-medical purposes (Office of Applied Studies, 2004a).
- More than 21 million individuals (9.1%) met criteria for a diagnosis of current alcohol and/or drug dependence.

The data from the Substance Abuse and Mental Health Services Administration indicate that the nonmedical use of pain relievers has been increasing gradually in the United States among people aged 18 to 25. In 1992, the rate of such drug use among young adults was 6.8% and in 2004, it has increased to 24.3%.

An estimated 17.6 million American adults (8.5%) meet standard criteria for an alcohol use disorder and approximately 4.2 million (2%) meet criteria for a drug use disorder. Overall, about one-tenth (9.4%) of American adults or 19.4 million persons meet clinical criteria for SUD-either an alcohol or drug use disorder or both-according to results from the 2001-2002 NESARC.

Data from the ECA surveys showed that the estimated annual incidence of Diagnostic Interview Schedule (DIS)-defined alcohol disorders among men was highest for the youngest age group (those aged 18 to 29). For women, incidence also decreased with age.

In the NCS, the lifetime prevalence of drug abuse without dependence was found to be 5.4% among males and 3.5% among females. The estimates for lifetime prevalence for dependence were 9.2% among males and 5.9% for females.

The Drug Abuse Warning Network monitors admissions to emergency rooms in major metropolitan areas. The results are the following:

- More than 670,000 drug abuse-related emergency episodes during 2002.
- Over 10,000 drug-related deaths occurred in these areas in 2002 (Office of Applied Studies, 2004b).
- Totaling deaths both directly and indirectly caused by use of substances shows that alcohol use resulted in 105,000 and other drug use (exclusive of tobacco) in 39,000 deaths in 1995.

- In 2003, decedents aged 35 to 54 years accounted for more than half of the drug misuse deaths in 30 metropolitan areas and three fourths of such deaths in Detroit; Milwaukee; and Washington, DC. The consequences of this shift in use to older adults will present more challenges to health care providers.

According to a survey of 49,000 students in 400 secondary schools nationwide, the use of illegal drugs among adolescents continues to decline modestly, but abuse of some prescription drugs is increasing. The Office of National Drug Policy Control reported a sharp drop in methamphetamine and steroid use among young people in 2001. The most common substances used by youth are alcohol, tobacco, and marijuana. Alcoholism and prescription drug abuse in the elderly are common problems and often not diagnosed or treated.

In general, the national household surveys of drug use find higher rates of current illicit drug use by blacks than by whites or Hispanics. When epidemiological analyses of drinking by racial/ethnic groups include ethnic origin, pronounced differences are observed within racial groups as well as across racial groups. People of Hispanic and Native American origin are less likely to drink than whites of European heritage, but they consume more per drinking occasion. Asian drinkers, in particular those from non-Japanese origin, have the most moderate drinking patterns of all racial and ethnic groups. The rate of violent victimization due to/related to alcohol use among Native Americans is well above that for other U.S. racial/ethnic subgroups. Among all racial/ethnic groups, Native Americans seem to be the most likely victims when the perpetrator has been drinking. Alcohol-related problems are highly associated with intimate partner violence among blacks and whites but not among Hispanics.

The epidemiological findings highlight the importance of treatment and prevention strategies that address the general needs of the community, as well as the special needs of important subgroups.

Costs and consequences of SUDs

Overall societal costs related to alcohol use reached $148 billion and $98 billion for drug use (1992 data). The alcohol-related costs were relatively constant over the prior 20 years and the drug-related costs showed a pattern of escalation. Costs of crime are noticeable. For example, with regard to heroin addiction alone, the estimated costs to society in 1996 reached $21.9 billion, including $11.5 billion in lost productivity, $5.2 billion for crime, and $5 billion for medical care. High health care costs for drug users are related in part to the numerous medical conditions caused by this activity. Heavy alcohol use can potentially damage nearly every organ system. Cocaine and marijuana can cause acute and chronic lung injury. Cocaine can also cause myocardial ischemia and cardiac arrhythmias, seizures, and strokes. Medical problems common in the injection drug users include pneumonia, sexually transmitted diseases, endocarditis, CNS infections, viral hepatitis, and HIV infection. Drugs users also have higher rates of psychiatric disorders that require interventions.

In summary, SUDs are common and associated with significant morbidity, mortality, and considerable societal costs.

Neurobiology

Our knowledge of the neurobiology of addiction has expanded significantly recently based on decades of animal studies and advances in human neurosciences. Addiction has been cogently conceptualized as a disease of brain reward centers involved in the survival of organisms and species. By dysregulating neurotransmitters in the reward and stress systems, addictive drugs essentially hijack brain circuitry leading to progressive loss of control over drug intake in the face of medical, interpersonal, occupational, and legal consequences. There is even recent evidence that denial may be associated with drug-induced dysfunction in the prefrontal cortex. The impaired control over substance use behavior is both the hallmark of addiction and the source of societal stigma.

- The acute reinforcing effects of drugs of abuse initiate the cycle of addiction (drug euphoria) and the withdrawal, craving, and hedonic dysregulation maintain the addictive process (relapse).
- The changes in the reward and stress systems convey the vulnerability for development of dependence.
- Neurotransmitters such as dopamine (DA) and opioid peptides mediate acute reinforcing effects of drugs in a specialized basal forebrain superstructure called the "extended amygdala" (central nucleus of the amygdala, the bed nucleus of the stria terminalis, and the transition zone in the shell of the nucleus accumbens).
- The changes also include decreased dopaminergic activity in the mesolimbic system (hypofrontality and low D2/reduced gray matter density).
- There is also recruitment of the stress pathways that become dysregulated.
- Craving is a complicated phenomenon that can be enhanced by cues that have become associated with drugs through conditioned learning. Neuroimaging studies have demonstrated a link between cue-induced craving, considered to be the most persistent clinical component of addiction, and brain function (activation of limbic structures on PET and fMRI).
- In addition, genetic and environmental factors can also contribute to the dysregulation in the prefrontal cortex.
- The existence of bidirectional interactions between different drugs of abuse such as opioids and cannabinoids, provides further findings to support the common neurobiological substrate for the addiction process.

The neurobiology of addiction clearly supports a brain-disease concept. Recent advances in addiction research, if disseminated to the public, would potentially facilitate changes in policy to improve treatment and access to care.

Genetic and family studies

Addictive disorders are complex genetic diseases in which genetic factors interact with environmental factors to affect risk. There is no one gene in which variation inevitably leads to the disease; rather, variations in many different genes, acting together with variations in the environment, affect an individual's risk for the disease. Addictions are in fact very much like other complex genetic diseases such as type II diabetes, or hypertension, in which genes, behaviors, and exposure affect vulnerability. The findings on SUDs were identified through adoption studies, twin studies, linkage studies, and association studies (protective genes, genes involved in neurotransmitters, pharmacogenetics).

Environmental factors may play a larger role in initiation, experimentation, and early stages of use, whereas genetic factors take precedence in individuals who move from use to dependence. Multiple physiological pathways are involved in the genetic aspect of SUDs. Genetic variation may influence response to psychosocial treatment and medication. Familial factors play a major role in vulnerability to SUDs. A family history of substance abuse is one of the strongest risk factors for development of a SUD. One of the strongest predictors for presence of a SUD is the presence of another SUD. There is a general drug abuse vulnerability factor with genetic, family, and nonfamily environmental components that is shared all across drugs of abuse, in addition to some specific factors that appear to be unique for individual classes of substances.

Screening and assessment of substance use disorders (1)

Screening stage

Screening is defined as the use of specific procedures to identify individuals with substance use problems or those who are at risk for developing a SUD. It is crucial to understand the difference between screening and assessment. The goal of screening is to detect individuals with possible substance use problems or those at risk for developing such problems. The goal of assessment is to gather more detailed information in order to formulate a diagnosis and evaluate a treatment process. Screening tools should be incorporated into the social history including smoking history and caffeine use. Maintaining nonjudgmental and empathic attitude, asking initially open-ended questions, using direct questions, and challenging rationalizations are important skills used in the assessment.

The spectrum of "at risk drinking" includes:
- "Risky use" is defined as more than seven standard drinks (a standard drink is approximately 12 to 14g of ethanol, which corresponds to 5oz of wine, 12oz of beer, or 1.5oz of 80-proof liquor) per week or more than three per occasion for women and more than 14 standard drinks per week or more than four per occasion for men; there are no alcohol-related consequences, but the risk of future physical, psychological, and social harm increases with increasing levels of consumption,
- "Problem drinking" refers to the use that is accompanied by alcohol-related consequences but not meeting DSM-IV-TR or ICD-10 criteria for a SUD.
- Alcohol abuse as per DSM-IV-TR.
- Alcohol dependence as per DSM-IV-TR.

Alcohol screening tests
- Has your use ever caused problems for you?
- Have you ever been concerned about your drinking?

CAGE

Consists of four questions. It does not assess current problems, levels of alcohol use, or binge drinking. It is better at detecting dependence. It is not recommended when screening to identify hazardous drinkers for risk reduction. The CAGE is often adapted to drug use, as well. Two affirmative answers predict seven times more likelihood to have an alcohol problem.
- Have you felt the need to Cut down on your drinking? (Most sensitive)
- Have you ever felt Annoyed by someone criticizing your drinking?
- Have you ever felt bad or Guilty about your drinking?
- Have you ever had a drink the first thing in the morning (Eye opener) to steady your nerves and get rid of a hangover? (Most specific)

AUDIT

The Alcohol Use Disorders Identification Test contains 10 questions that cover quantity and frequency of alcohol use, drinking behaviors, adverse psychological symptoms, and alcohol-related problems.

AUDIT-C consists of only the first three quantity-frequency questions:
- How often do you have a drink containing alcohol?
  - (never = 0; monthly or less = 1; two to four times/month = 2; two to three times/week = 2; more than four times/week = 4).
- On a typical day when drinking, how many drinks do you have?
  - (one to two drinks = 0; three to four drinks = 1; five to six drinks = 2; seven to nine drinks = 3; more than ten drinks = 4).
- How often do you have six or more drinks on one occasion?
  - (never = 0; less than monthly = 1; monthly = 2; weekly = 3; daily or almost daily = 4).

AUDIT and AUDIT-C were designed to identify hazardous drinking and harmful drinking and focuses on recent drinking behaviors (current to past year). The AUDIT 10-item questionnaire uses a 0–5 score for each question. A score of 8 or above out of 40 has reasonably good sensitivity in detecting an alcohol use disorder. Each question in the AUDIT-C is scored from 0 to 4 and a total score of >4 for men or >3 for women is considered to be a positive result.

The single question test

"When was the last time you had more than four drinks (women) or five drinks (men) in one day?" A positive answer within the past three months detected 86% of individuals with recent hazardous drinking or current alcohol use disorder.

Once these steps are taken, the next step is a full assessment and a detailed review of alcohol or drug-related complications.

The drug abuse screening test

This is a self-report measure that is brief and easy to score. The Drug Use Screening Inventory profiles the frequency of substance use behavior in conjunction with severity of disturbances in 10 spheres of functioning.

Screening and assessment of substance use disorders (2)

Assessment and drug use history

Establish diagnosis along the continuum

The continuum of use → abuse → dependence uses the criteria of DSM-IV-TR. Ask specifically about each class of substances, use slang or terms that patient will understand.

- What is your drug of choice?
- Why?
- When was your first use of that drug, of any drug?
- Quantity and frequency of use?
- Duration of heavy use period?
- Has your use increased or decreased since then?
- Have you ever tried to quit?
- What is your longest clean time off a particular drug?
- What was your longest clean time off all drugs?
- Have you had to use progressively more amounts of drug to get same effect?
- Do you ever have withdrawal symptoms?
- Have you stopped for long enough periods to feel withdrawal?
- Have you had any medical complications of withdrawal (i.e., loss of consciousness, delirium tremens, seizures, gastrointestinal bleeds, head injuries, hospital admissions, ER visits, and accidents)? Assess severity of withdrawal.
- Have you been in trouble with the law because of drug use?
- Difficulties at work/school because of drug use?
- Conflicts with family or friends because of drug use?

Assess patient's readiness to change

It is not appropriate to assume that everyone presenting for treatment is equally motivated to make changes in his or her substance use behavior. The patient's motivation for behavior change will contribute to his/her readiness to change. The transtheoretical model of change provides a conceptual framework within which motivation to change substance use behavior may be placed. Individuals progress through a series of stages in deciding to change their substance use behavior. "Meeting the patient where he/she is" helps identify treatment approach to the individual's stage of change. As one moves through the stages, commitment to change is increased and ambivalence is resolved. The stages are the following:

- Precontemplation—individual sees no need for change and surely not for treatment. Focus on moving the patient to contemplative stage.
- Contemplation—individual knows a problem exists, weighing the costs and benefits of continuing to use at the current level, also weighing pros and cons of stopping or reducing use.
- Preparation—perceived need for change outweighs the desire to continue using and the individual makes a commitment to facilitate the change.

- Action—individual is implementing change strategies in environment, activities, and acquaintances.
- Maintenance—individual has made the desired changes and is working on relapse prevention.

Assess relapse factors

These include high-risk situations, self-efficacy to change substance use, coping skills, outcome expectations, spirituality, religiosity, craving, twelve-step affiliation, and support system. Also assess for co-morbid psychopathology and neurocognitive impairment. Assess for co-morbid medical problems such as hepatitis C and HIV.

Assess prior treatment

- What treatment have you sought in the past?
- How many times have you been in treatment?
- Did you complete treatment or how long did you participate?
- What was the outcome of treatment?
- What was your experience with previous treatment?
- What type of treatment do you believe worked best for you?
- What type of treatment are you seeking now?
- Assess history of prescribed medications, current and past, including patterns of adherence.

Physical examination

- Head and neck: jaundice, smell of alcohol or strong mouthwash on breath, strong aftershave/perfume (masking alcohol), nasal irritation (cocaine), perioral irritation (inhalants), red conjunctiva (smoking), parotid gland enlargement (alcohol).
- Cardiovascular system: tachycardia (cocaine, amphetamines, inhalants).
- Pulmonary system: chronic cough or wheeze (smoking, inhalants), black sputum (crack).
- Abdomen: hepatomegaly, epigastric/abdominal tenderness, gynecomastia.
- Extremities: tremor, stained/burned fingers/nails (smoking, inhalants).
- Genitals: testicular atrophy.
- Skin: scars, abscess, cellulitis from skin popping, track marks, spider angiomata (alcohol), diaphoresis, bruises/abrasions/cuts.
- Musculoskeletal system: muscle atrophy, gout.
- Neurological system: decreased concentration and attention, incoordination, ataxia, slurred speech, unsteady gait, nystagmus, stupor.
- Vitals: hypertension/labile blood pressure (alcohol withdrawal), tachycardia.
- Psychiatric: mood lability, depression, anxiety.

Laboratory studies

Laboratory studies can be useful for patient assessment in known or suspected patients with SUDs but need to be used selectively. Biomarkers of heavy drinking will be discussed in a later section. Most labs use immunoassay for detection, then confirmation with gas chromatography-mass spectroscopy. Time to detection: breath (minutes) > saliva (hours) > urine (hours to days) > hair and nails (months).

Substances detectable on urine drug screen	Approximate detection times
Propoxyphene	6–48 hours
Amphetamines-methamphetamine	48–72 hours
Heroin	36–72 hours, longer-acting opiates 1–2 days
Cocaine	6–8 hours (metabolites detected for up to 3 days)
LSD	24 hours
Benzodiazepines	3–7 days (depends on half-life)
PCP	8 days
Cannabis	3 days–4 weeks (depends on use)
Methadone	7–9 days
Barbiturates	1–16 days (depends on half-life)

Source: *Principles of Addiction Medicine.* A.W. Graham, T.K. Schultz, M.F. Mayo-Smith, R.K. Ries (eds.). Maryland: ASAM, 2003.

Substance	Possible cause of false positive on urine drug screen
Opiates	quinolones, rifampin, poppy seeds
Cannabis	efavirenz (Sustiva®), NSAIDS, dronabinol (Marinol®)
PCP	dextromethorphan, diphenhydramine, thioridazine, venlafaxine
Benzodiazepines	sertraline (Zoloft®), oxaprozin
Amphetamines	bupropion (Wellbutrin SR®, Zyban®, and Wellbutrin XL®), selegiline (Eldepryl®), OTC decongestants (pseudoephedrine), trazodone, chlorpromazine, ranitidine, desipramine, amantadine
Barbiturates	phenytoin
LSD	amitriptyline, chlorpromazine, doxepin, fluoxetine, haloperidol, metoclopramide, risperidone, sertraline, thioridazine, verapamil
Propoxyphene	cyclobenzaprine, diphenylhydramine, doxylamine, imipramine, methadone

Source: *Principles of Addiction Medicine.* A.W. Graham, T.K. Schultz, M.F. Mayo-Smith, R.K. Ries (eds.). Maryland: ASAM, 2003.

Alcohol (1)

Epidemiology

According to 2004 National Study on Drug Use and Health, 50% of Americans reported drinking alcohol in the past year. Approximately 22% endorsed binge drinking, defined as five or more drinks on one occasion during the past month. Approximately 7% reported heavy drinking, defined as five or more drinks on the same occasion for five or more days of the past month. Rates of both binge (41.2%) and heavy drinking (15.1%) are highest in 18–25 years old, peaking at age 21. Underage alcohol use is common, with 28.7% of 12–20 year olds endorsing alcohol use in the past month. Rates of past-month binge and heavy drinking are all slightly higher in full-time college students compared to those enrolled part time or not at all. Males are more likely to binge drink, engage in heavy drinking, and drive under the influence of alcohol. An epidemiologic survey of the general population in the United States documented a prevalence of alcohol abuse and alcohol dependence estimated to be between 7.4% and 9.7%. The lifetime prevalence is estimated to be even higher.

Diagnosis

Screen and assess for use, abuse, and dependence in all patients, utilizing screening tools and DSM-IV-TR. There appear to be two "types" of alcoholism:

- Type 2 alcoholism accounts for about 25%, characterized by onset in teens, increased rates in sons of type 2 drinkers, drinking for the "high" and antisocial (criminal) behavior,
- Type 1 alcoholism, approximately 75%, is characterized by adult onset, drinking to relieve anxiety and guilt and fear about drinking.

Biomarkers of heavy drinking can be used clinically for screening, to develop the differential diagnosis, and to monitor for relapse. Current biomarkers lack the specificity to detect heavy alcohol use in the general population but may be used as indicators of heavy use in known or suspected alcoholics.

Elevated GGT (gamma-glutamyl transferase) is the most widely used biomarker of alcohol abuse. GGT rises with heavy prolonged alcohol use (~70 drinks/week for several weeks) and returns to normal within two to six weeks of abstinence. It is useful as an indicator of chronic heavy use, but not episodic use. Elevated GGT has many false positives including chronic liver disease, diabetes, hypertension, obesity, hypertriglyceridemia. In addition, sensitivity is only ~50%.

Carbohydrate-deficient transferrin (CDT) is another indicator of heavy alcohol use and requires >60g/day use for two to three weeks for elevation. CDT returns to normal after two to four weeks of abstinence. CDT and GGT have similar sensitivities but CDT is more specific than GGT; false positives are rare.

Elevated transaminases (AST, ALT) are indicators of liver damage, which may be due to alcohol use or other acute/chronic liver disease. An AST: ALT ratio of 2:1 is characteristic of alcoholic liver damage.

Elevated erythrocyte macrocytic volume (MCV) is often found in alcoholic patients, but the utility of this finding is low. It has a low sensitivity and slowly returns to normal after abstinence. Testing more than one biomarker is more useful for screening purposes.

Pharmacology

Alcohol is a CNS depressant with actions at numerous neurotransmitter systems, including GABA, glutamate, opioid, serotonin (5-HT) and DA. Alcohol enhances inhibitory neurotransmission at $GABA_A$ receptors and reduces excitatory neurotransmission at glutamate NMDA receptors. The reinforcing effects of alcohol are thought to be mediated through the resultant effect on the mesolimbic dopaminergic system. In addition, alcohol increases both opioid and cannabinoid activity. Alcohol's inhibitory effect on glutamate receptors results in an upregulation of glutamate receptors. This is theoretically responsible for the increased neuroexcitability and thus, increased potential for seizures, upon alcohol withdrawal.

Clinical features

Intoxication

There is great individual variability in the effects of alcohol on mood, ranging from euphoria to anger to depressant. Slurred speech, unsteady gait, nystagmus, lack of coordination, attention and memory deficit, decreased reaction time, nausea/vomiting, poor judgment, labile mood, and memory lapses. At higher levels, depressant-sedative effects predominate, however sleep quality is poor and REM sleep decreased. Delirium may occur during intoxication. Both the quantity and rate of rise of blood alcohol level (BAL) determine the level of intoxication. Blackouts are periods of amnesia without other neurological impairment that may occur during a rapid rise in BAL.

Withdrawal syndromes

Withdrawal symptoms begin 6–24 hours after the last drink and can occur before the BAL has returned to zero. The first symptoms of withdrawal include anxiety, anorexia, nausea, headache and insomnia. There may also be signs of autonomic instability (tachycardia, hypertension, diaphoresis, fever). Tremors, evaluated best in outstretched hands or tongue, begin 8–12 hours after last drink and peak at 24–36 hours. Alcohol withdrawal may be accompanied by perceptual disturbances, such as auditory, visual or tactile hallucinations or illusions. These are transitory and usually develop within 48 hours from cessation of drinking called "alcohol hallucinosis" (the person knows that the perceptions are caused by alcohol).

Alcohol withdrawal seizures are most common within the first 24–48 hours. Delirium tremens (DTs) are more likely to develop if the patient had an alcohol withdrawal seizure or a concomitant medical disorder such as an infection, hepatitis, or pancreatitis. Onset is usually two to three days after cessation of alcohol and usually lasts three to seven days, but can be prolonged. It is more common in older people, after decades of alcohol dependence and a prior episode of DTs is a risk factor. DTs may begin after the individual has started showing signs of improvement in early withdrawal. Signs and symptoms include agitation, tachycardia, hypertension or labile blood pressure, nausea, vomiting, diaphoresis, gross tremor, difficulty concentrating, sweating, and possibly fever and hallucinations. Withdrawal and seizures can occur at BAL in the 100s and in chronic users whose BAL has quickly fallen from 400s. DTs have a mortality rate of 5–15% and must be considered a medical emergency.

Alcohol (2)

Clinical features (cont'd)

Medical complications

- Wernicke's encephalopathy (WE) is a neurological emergency, characterized by oculomotor disturbance (nystagmus and gaze paralysis, classically sixth nerve palsy), ataxia, and cognitive disturbance (confusion, drowsiness, apathy). WE is due to thiamine deficiency from intestinal malabsorption. Prevalence rates data have come primarily from necropsy studies, with rates of 1 to 3%. Prevalence at autopsy exceeds recognition in life. All patients presenting with any of these symptoms should be treated immediately with thiamine 50mg IV and 50mg IM. Thiamine should always be given before IV glucose is given because increased brain glucose metabolism could precipitously exhaust the B vitamin stores, resulting in an acute Wernicke's encephalopathy. All patients with alcohol use history should be given 50–100mg po thiamine supplementation.
- Korsakoff's dementia/psychosis (alcohol amnestic disorder) is a late manifestation of Wernicke's syndrome that is characterized by anterograde amnesia. Confabulation may or may not be present. The development of Korsakoff's dementia from Wernicke's encephalopathy is not well understood. It is treated with thiamine 100mg/day for at least three months. Mortality is 15% when left untreated. Only one-third of treated patients with complete memory impairment will actually have clinically relevant improvement.
- Seizures are most common in the first two days of withdrawal, are usually generalized, and lead to a higher risk for subsequent withdrawal seizures. Magnesium deficiency can lower seizure threshold.
- Toxic polyneuropathy The most common neurological consequence of chronic alcohol dependence is a toxic polyneuropathy, which results from inadequate nutrition, mainly deficiency of thiamine and other B vitamins. Signs and symptoms include stocking-glove peripheral neuropathy, weakness and atrophy of distal muscles, and dysfunction of autonomic fibers.

Neurological	Wernicke's encephalopathy, Korsakoff's dementia, seizures, toxic polyneuropathy, stroke, alcoholic coma
Gastrointestinal	GI bleeds, peptic ulcer, glossitis, stomatitis from malnutrition, Mallory-Weiss tears, esophageal strictures, fatty liver (steatosis), hepatitis, irreversible fibrosis, cirrhosis, portal hypertension, cancers
Cardiovascular	cardiomyopathy, berberi, holiday heart syndrome, hypertension, hyperlipidemia
Hematologic	pancytopenia, folic acid and B_{12} deficiency
Respiratory	lung cancer
Musculoskeletal	muscle wasting, osteoporosis
Renal	renal failure, hepatorenal syndrome
Endocrine	testicular atrophy, sexual disorders, menstrual irregularities
Pregnancy	low birth weight, morphologic abnormalities, developmental delays

Alcohol (3)

Treatment

Detoxification (detox) can occur in an outpatient or inpatient setting.

- Outpatient detox is appropriate for patients with a stable home environment and intact support system providing close monitoring. Outpatient detox generally involves daily visits to a treatment program or physician's office, often in conjunction with other supports, such as Alcoholics Anonymous (AA) or other cessation groups. Treatment programs are variable and may be intensive (entire day programs) or brief (short visit with take-home medications).

- Indications for inpatient detox include severe hypertension, fever, extreme agitation, marked tremor, hallucinations, DTs, seizure (current or history), history of severe withdrawal symptoms, signs of Wernicke's encephalopathy, inability to take oral medication due to nausea/vomiting, medical conditions (severe or acute liver disease, severe cardiovascular disease), pregnancy, lack of medical or social support system to allow safe outpatient detoxification. Inpatient detox enables 24-hour monitoring and treatment of withdrawal, evaluation and monitoring of medical conditions, and a safe, stable environment in which patients can receive individual and group counseling.

Benzodiazepines (BDZs) are first-line medication for alcohol detoxification, although there is some evidence for anticonvulsants for treatment of alcohol withdrawal. Long half-life benzodiazepines (i.e., diazepam (Valium®) or chlordiazepoxide (Librium®) should be used, as they are self-tapering. Oxazepam (Serax®) or lorazepam (Ativan®) are safer to use in patients with liver disease because of minimal biotransformation in the liver.

Detoxification is safest when medications are given early in the course of withdrawal. Symptom-triggered or as needed scheduling is preferable to a fixed-schedule regimen of medication with tapering occurring over several days.

The Addiction Research Foundation Clinical Institute Withdrawal Assessment for Alcohol (CIWA-Ar 🕮 p. 638) has been widely used as a tool for rating and monitoring alcohol withdrawal. It assesses 9 withdrawal symptoms (nausea/vomiting, tremor, sweats, anxiety, agitation, tactile disturbance, auditory disturbance, visual disturbance and headache) on a scale of 0 to 7 and one symptom (orientation) on a scale of 0 to 4, with maximum possible score of 67. Patients with scores less than 10 generally can be monitored without pharmacologic treatment medication can be used on an as needed basis. Patients with scores of 14 or greater should receive pharmacologic treatment for withdrawal. For scores between 10 and 14, clinical judgment should be used regarding the need for medication and close monitoring for worsening withdrawal should continue. Anti-convulsants such as phenytoin have not been demonstrated to reduce withdrawal seizures better than benzodiazepines do. Of the antiepileptic drugs, carbamazepine (Tegretol®) and Divalproex (Depakote® and Depakote ER®) are sometimes used for alcohol detoxification. To date, the vast majority of evidence supports BDZs as the safest treatment for alcohol withdrawal and their use is recommended until further research is done to clarify details of anticonvulsants use. All patients presenting with an alcohol dependence history, especially those requiring alcohol detoxification should be given thiamine 100mg, folate 1mg and a multivitamin because of the risk of vitamin deficiency.

Alcohol (4)

CIWA-Ar
NAUSEA & VOMITING
Ask, "Do you feel sick to your stomach? Have you vomited?"
- 0 no nausea/vomiting.
- 1.
- 2.
- 3.
- 4. intermittent nausea with dry heaves.
- 5.
- 6.
- 7. constant nausea, frequent dry heaves and vomiting.

TACTILE DISTURBANCES
Ask, "Do you have any itching, pins and needles sensations, any burning, any numbness or do you feel bugs crawling on or under your skin?"
- 0. none.
- 1. very mild itching, pins and needles, burning or numbness.
- 2. mild itching, pins and needles, burning or numbness.
- 3. moderate pins and needles, burning or numbness.
- 4. moderately severe hallucinations.
- 5. severe hallucinations.
- 6. extremely severe hallucinations.
- 7. continuous hallucinations.

TREMOR
Arms extended and fingers spread apart.
- 0. no tremor.
- 1. not visible, but can be felt fingertip to fingertip.
- 2.
- 3.
- 4. moderate, with patient's arms extended.
- 5.
- 6.
- 7. severe, even with arms not extended.

AUDITORY DISTURBANCES
Ask, "Are you more aware of sounds around you? Are they harsh? Do they frighten you? Are you hearing anything that is disturbing you? Are you hearing things you know are not there?" Observation.
- 0. not present.
- 1. very mild harshness or ability to frighten.
- 2. mild harshness or ability to frighten.
- 3. moderate harshness or ability to frighten.
- 4. moderately severe hallucinations.
- 5. severe hallucinations.
- 6. extremely severe hallucinations.
- 7. continuous hallucinations.

PAROXYSMAL SWEATS
- 0. no sweat visible.
- 1. barely perceptible sweating, palms moist.
- 2.
- 3.
- 4. beads of sweat obvious on forehead.
- 5.
- 6.
- 7. drenching sweats

VISUAL DISTURBANCES
Ask, "Does the light appear to be too bright? Is its color different? Does it hurt your eyes? Are you seeing anything that is disturbing to you? Are you seeing things you know are not there?"
- 0. not present.
- 1. very mild sensitivity.
- 2. mild sensitivity.
- 3. moderate sensitivity.
- 4. moderately severe hallucinations.
- 5. severe hallucinations.
- 6. extremely severe hallucinations.
- 7. continuous hallucinations.

ANXIETY
Ask, "Do you feel nervous?"
- 0. no anxiety, at ease.
- 1. mildly anxious.
- 2.
- 3.
- 4. moderately anxious, or guarded, so anxiety is inferred.
- 5.
- 6.
- 7. equivalent to acute panic as seen in severe delirium or acute schizophrenic reactions.

HEADACHE, FULLNESS IN HEAD
Ask, "Does your head feel different? Does it feel like there is a band around your head?" Do not rate for dizziness or lightheadedness.
- 0. not present.
- 1. very mild.
- 2. mild.
- 3. moderate.
- 4. moderately severe.
- 5. severe.
- 6. very severe.
- 7. extremely severe.

AGITATION
- 0. normal activity.
- 1. somewhat more than normal activity.
- 2.
- 3.

- 4. moderately fidgety and restless.
- 5.
- 6.
- 7. paces back and forth during most of interview, or constantly thrashes about.

ORIENTATION & CLOUDING OF SENSORIUM
Ask, "What day is this? Where are you? Who am I?"
- 0 oriented and can do serial additions.
- 1 cannot do serial additions or is uncertain about date.
- 2 disoriented for date by no more than 2 calendar days.
- 3 disoriented for date by more than 2 calendar days.
- 4 disoriented for place and/or person.

Alcohol (5)

Psychosocial treatment

Brief advice, Motivational Enhancement Therapy based on an adaptation of Motivational Interviewing (Project MATCH), and cognitive behavior therapy (Project MATCH) have been shown to be effective for reducing alcohol use among problem drinkers and patients with alcohol dependence. Self-help groups, in particular, regular AA attendance has been shown to be associated with better long-term outcomes and functioning.

Pharmacotherapy for alcohol relapse prevention

Both naltrexone and acamprosate have been shown to be effective in producing abstinence at least over a course of four to six months in randomized controlled trials and meta-analyses. Disulfiram has not been shown to increase sobriety but may be helpful in some individuals who are highly motivated, have solid social support and do not have serious medical complications of alcoholism.

The FDA has recently approved naltrexone for extended-release injectable suspension, 380mg (Vivitrol®) for the treatment of alcohol dependence. This monthly IM injectable medication is indicated for alcohol-dependent patients who are able to abstain from drinking in an outpatient setting and are not actively drinking when initiating treatment. Treatment with Vivitrol should be used in combination with psychosocial support.

Topiramate (Topamax®) facilitates GABA function and antagonizes glutamate, which theoretically should decrease mesocorticolimbic DA after alcohol use and decrease cravings. Decreased drinking, decreased craving, and greater abstinence have been seen with use of topiramate, however, topiramate is not FDA approved for alcohol dependence.

Selective serotonin reuptake inhibitors (SSRIs) have not been found to be effective in producing abstinence in patients without co-morbid depression or anxiety, but may benefit some patients with co-morbid anxiety or depression.

Medication	Dosing	Mechanism	Contra-indications	Side-effects
Acamprosate (Campral®)	666mg po tid, start after alcohol withdrawal while abstinent	enhances GABA transmission & inhibits glutamate transmission	Severe renal impairment	Diarrhea; flatulence; nausea; abdominal pain; headache
Naltrexone (ReVia®)	50mg po daily, best if abstinent for 5–7 days	opiate antagonist	Opiate use, consider UDS for opioids before prescribing; acute hepatitis, liver failure	Nausea; abdominal pain; constipation; headache; anxiety; fatigue; drowsiness
Disulfiram (Antabuse®)	start 500mg/d × 1–2 weeks, then maintenance dose 125–500mg/d	inhibits aldehyde dehydro-genase, when taken with alcohol results in accumulation of acetaldehyde, manifest by nausea, vomiting dyspnea, diaphoresis, chest pain, palpitations, hypotension	Diabetes, emphysema, seizures, liver or renal disease, coronary artery disease, pregnancy, drug interactions	Contact with or ingestion of any alcohol containing product (i.e., cough medicine) or topical (i.e., perfume, aftershave) can trigger a disulfiram-ethanol reaction (DER)

Sedative-hypnotics and benzodiazepines (1)

Including, barbiturates, and other non-BDZ hypnotic drugs with addiction potential (Ambien®, Sonata ®, Lunesta®).

Epidemiology

The 2004 National Study on Drug Use and Health estimates a lifetime prevalence of ~12.4% illicit use of sedatives or tranquilizers. In 2002, 100,784 emergency room visits were related to BDZs, with nearly half due to suicide attempts. These drugs are often abused in those dependent on other substances and less often a primary addiction. Opioid dependent patients sometimes use barbiturates and BDZs to self-medicate for opioid withdrawal and some have reported a heightened euphoric effect with opioids. Rates of BDZ use are also much higher in those who are alcohol dependent. This class of drugs should be avoided or used with high caution in those with history of substance dependence due to the high risk of addiction.

Diagnosis

Recent use of BDZ and barbiturates is detectable in routine urine drug screens. It is important to recognize that many patients take BDZs for anxiolytic effects or insomnia without developing dependence. Dependence typically occurs in patients who abuse other substances. Abuse may be unintentional (those who started taking BDZs as prescribed for anxiety or insomnia and began taking more than prescribed) or intentional (those who use to alleviate withdrawal or supplement highs from other substances). Sometimes BDZs are taken 2 hours after methadone to augment "high" or to alleviate withdrawal or side-effects from cocaine and alcohol. Diazepam (Valium®), lorazepam (Ativan®), and alprazolam (Xanax®) have been reported as subjectively providing the greatest high by BDZ users.

It is imperative to distinguish between normal physiologic dependence, which can occur in patients legitimately taking BDZs for anxiolytic or hypnotic indications, and addiction/substance dependence. Addiction is defined by a loss of control regarding drug use and compulsive drug-seeking behavior. Some patients will "shop" for numerous prescriptions from multiple providers. When in doubt or when patients report high doses or multiple prescription drugs from same class, obtain consent and call patient's pharmacy or doctor's office to verify prescriptions.

Pharmacology

All drugs in the class are agonists at $GABA_A$ receptors, the predominant inhibitory receptor in the CNS. BDZs facilitate the action of GABA at its ion channel receptor, causing an increase in the duration of channel opening. Barbiturates both enhance GABA binding and directly activate the ion channel. Zolpidem (Ambien® and Ambien CR®), eszopiclone (Lunesta®), and zaleplon (Sonata®) are selective agonists at $GABA_{A1}$ receptors and have more favorable side-effect profile, faster onset and shorter duration of action.

Factors that dictate abuse potential are half-life, speed of onset, and offset. Speed of onset is the primary factor, with faster onset giving more rapid and greater euphoric effect. A short half-life causes the desired effect to end faster, resulting in repeated dosing. Metabolism is decreased in the elderly, resulting in longer-half lives and a greater potential for accumulation with daily dosing.

Clinical features

Intoxication
Slurred speech, ataxia, incoordination similar to alcohol intoxication. Stupor, respiratory depression and coma may develop in severe intoxication and overdose. In older adults, a paradoxical agitated confusion and delirium can occur. There is cross-tolerance between the sedative-hypnotics and with alcohol, so alcohol and sedative-hypnotic dependent patients may require much higher doses of sedatives for anesthesia or sedation. Withdrawal symptoms overlap with alcohol withdrawal, including tachycardia, hypertension, agitation, anxiety, insomnia, tremor, nausea, diarrhea, and sensory disturbances. Severe withdrawal can result in delirium, seizures and death.

Tolerance
Tolerance develops to the sedation and psychomotor impairment of BDZs but not to the short-term memory loss and anxiolytic effect. When BDZs are used in moderate doses for short periods (less than 2 weeks), there is usually no tolerance, dependence, or withdrawal.

Withdrawal syndrome
This includes:
- Anxiety.
- Agitation.
- Insomnia.
- Paresthesias.
- Irritability.
- Sensitivity to light and sound.
- Muscle cramps and twitches.
- Fatigue.
- Headache.
- Dizziness.
- Decreased concentration.
- Nausea.
- Loss of appetite.
- Confusion.
- Seizures.

Withdrawal is more severe in patients who have been on higher doses for longer periods of time. Alprazolam in particular can cause an immediate, severe withdrawal syndrome and should always be tapered. It can be difficult to differentiate between relapse of anxiety and true withdrawal symptoms. True withdrawal will occur within days after BDZs stopped (depending on drug half-life), including objective signs of withdrawal (tremors, paresthesias, light/sound sensitivity, muscle twitches, and/or seizures) and will lessen over time. Relapse of anxiety will occur more than a week after discontinuation and will worsen over time.

Withdrawal is influenced by:
• Length of use.
• Dose.
• Half-life; shorter half-lives have more severe and faster onset of withdrawal.

There is a greater risk of withdrawal seizures in patients who also abuse alcohol. Barbiturate withdrawal tends to be more severe and carries greater risk for seizure than BDZ withdrawal.

Sedative-hypnotics and benzodiazepines (2)

Generic	Brand	Equivalent dose (mg)	Onset of action	Half-life (hours)	Active metabolite
Alprazolam	Xanax®	1	Intermediate	6–20	Y (little activity)
Lorazepam	Ativan®	2	Intermediate	10–20	N
Triazolam	Halcion®	0.25–0.5	Intermediate	2–3	Y (little activity)
Clonazepam	Klonopin®	0.5	Intermediate	18–50	N
Oxazepam	Serax®	15–30	Slow	3–21	N
Temazepam	Restoril®	30	Intermediate	10–12	N
Chlordia-zepoxide	Librium®	25	Intermediate	5–200	Y
Clorazepate	Tranxene®	15	Rapid	30–200	Y
Diazepam	Valium®	10	Rapid	30–200	Y
Flurazepam	Dalmane®	30	Rapid	0.5–120	Y
Buspirone	Buspar®	15–30	Slow	2–11	Y
Zaleplon	Sonata®	10	Rapid	2.5	N
Zolpidem	Ambien®	10	Rapid	1	N
Eszopiclone	Lunesta®	2	Rapid	6	
Secobarbital	Seconal®	100			
Butalbital	Fiorinal®	100			
Phenobarbital		30			
Methaqualone	Quaalude®	300			
Carisoprodol	Soma®	700			
Chloral Hydrate	Noctec®	500			

Source: *Principles of Addiction Medicine.* A.W. Graham, T.K. Schultz, M.F. Mayo-Smith, R.K. Ries (eds.). Maryland: ASAM, 2003.

Medical complications

The major complication of acute intoxication/overdose is respiratory and CNS depression. Use caution in prescribing BDZs to patients with COPD or sleep apnea because significant respiratory impairment can occur. Flumazenil (Romazicon®), a competitive BDZ antagonist, can be used to reverse life-threatening BDZ overdose. Flumazenil 0.2mg IV can be given in emergency situation where BDZ overdose is known or suspected. If there is no response within 30 seconds after first dose, follow with 0.3mg IV, and 0.5mg IV q 60 seconds for up to 3mg total dose. Flumazenil may induce withdrawal, including seizure, in BDZ dependent patients or in overdoses with multiple substances. In the elderly, studies have shown that sedative-hypnotic use is associated with an increased risk of fall and hip fracture, which carries a high mortality rate. Elderly patients should be prescribed half of the usual starting dose of sedative-hypnotics given the potential for oversedation and adverse events.

Treatment

There are several scenarios in which a reduction or discontinuation of benzodiazepines may occur:

- Patients who are taking BDZs as prescribed for anti-anxiety/insomnia indication in whom a trial off the medication is warranted.
- BDZ-dependent patients utilizing supratherapeutic doses.
- Polysubstance dependent patients, in whom the degree of tolerance is unclear.

Patients with chronic sedative-hypnotic use should not be stopped abruptly because of the potential for uncomfortable and potentially dangerous withdrawal. There are two approaches to detoxification: gradual tapering or substitution and tapering.

Gradual tapering

This is appropriate in the outpatient setting, in patients dependent on therapeutic doses, and those dependent only on BDZs. Decrease dose by 10% (or 5mg diazepam equivalents) each week or decrease 50% within first few days, 25% over next week and then last 25% over several weeks. Expect the first 50% reduction to be smoother and the final 25% with more withdrawal symptoms. If withdrawal occurs, increase dose slightly until symptoms resolve, hold the taper for a few days until patient is stable, and then taper again at slower rate.

Substitution with longer-acting benzodiazepine and tapering

Substitute long-acting BDZ (chlordiazepoxide, clonazepam) or pheno-barbital at equivalent dose. Oxazepam is a good substitute in patients with liver disease. Lorazepam is generally not considered a good substitute because of high abuse potential. Split the equivalent dose over 3–4x daily dosing (2–3 doses/day for clonazepam). Can give additional as needed doses for withdrawal symptoms first week only and use this to guide dosing. Taper gradually as described above. Only prescribe enough medication until next visit and schedule frequent or daily visits. Be suspicious of lost and stolen medications and evaluate case by case whether you should replace them or not.

Pentobarbital tolerance testing

This can be used to determine degree of tolerance when it is not clear in polysubstance dependent patients or those with a variable use history. Once an initial dose is established, a tapering regimen should be utilized. Pentobarbital is used because of rapid onset of action, short half-life, and its ease of monitoring signs of toxicity (sedation). In patients who are unable to discontinue BDZs, either because of psychological dependence, severe rebound anxiety, repeated failed discontinuation attempts, the benefit of continuing a lowest efficacious dose BDZ may outweigh the risk.

Opioids (1)

Opioids, such as heroin and morphine, are available in a variety of forms. Morphine has many derivatives, including hydrocodone (Vicodin®), oxycodone, sustained-release oxycodone (OxyContin®). The substances are frequently used intravenously, especially heroin. They are also used intranasally and orally. Methadone, a long-acting opioid agonist, while typically used as a treatment for opioid dependence, is sometimes used illicitly.

Epidemiology

Heroin use has a lifetime prevalence of 1–1.5% in the U.S. In the past year, between 300,000 and 400,000 individuals used heroin. Most users were older than the age of 26. Use is becoming more common among females, with this group representing a larger proportion of those seeking treatment. Furthermore, use is more prevalent amongst Latinos than other ethnic groups. Abuse of narcotic analgesics such as OxyContin has also dramatically increased from 1994 to 2002, as indicated by the incidence of emergency departments visits (SAMHSA, 2004). Approximately 1% of the adult population is using narcotic medications without a prescription or in excess of the prescribed amount at a given time. The highest use tends to be in young adults between the ages of 18 and 25. In 2002, 20% of teens (4.7 million) reported that they had used prescription painkillers without a doctor's prescription and 40% of 12th graders did not see great risk in using heroin once or twice.

Diagnosis

Diagnosis of opioid use can be made by a careful clinical history and physical exam, with particular emphasis placed on the features of intoxication or withdrawal, discussed below. Furthermore, heroin and other opioids are typically part of a routine urine drug screen. Heroin will typically produce a positive result on a urine drug screen from 1 to 3 days after last use, while methadone and other longer-acting opiates, such as sustained release oxycodone, may give a positive result for several days to over one week.

Pharmacology

Opioids, such as heroin and morphine, exert their effect via binding to the mu opioid receptor. Heroin, or diacetylmorphine, is absorbed best intravenously, but can also be used intranasally and orally. It has a very rapid onset of action with a fairly short half-life.

Clinical features

Intoxication

Mild to moderate opioid intoxication results in feelings of euphoria and alterations in consciousness/sedation. Severe intoxication is an emergent situation, typically manifested by decreased or absent respirations, pinpoint pupils, central nervous system depression/unconsciousness, and cardiopulmonary arrest. In patients with such a presentation, obtaining collateral history is extremely important if available. A known history of drug use would raise suspicion for an opioid overdose. Other clues include track marks on the patient's extremities or markings suggestive of "skin-popping," that is, areas where an individual may be injecting under the skin but not into a vessel.

Tolerance

Individuals using opioids on a chronic basis, whether for recreational or medicinal purposes, typically do develop tolerance to the substances. As a result, more of the substance is generally required to produce the same effect as use continues.

Withdrawal

During acute withdrawal, the patient typically develops a variety of symptoms, which may last from several hours to several days. Although often quite uncomfortable, opioid withdrawal is typically not life threatening. Symptoms and signs include dysphoric mood, lacrimation or rhinorrhea, pupillary dilation, piloerection or sweating, nausea or vomiting, diarrhea, muscle aches, yawning, fever, and insomnia. Tachycardia and hypertension are sometimes also observed. The time period of withdrawal is highly variable, varying largely by the type of drug used (i.e., short-acting versus long-acting). Heroin withdrawal typically begins within four to six hours of last use, whereas withdrawal from methadone may not start for one to two days. Similarly, the length of the withdrawal period is also highly variable, often lasting three to four days, but sometimes lasting upward of two weeks. Both subjective and objective scales should be used in assessing opioid withdrawal. Scales currently in use include the Subjective Opiate Withdrawal Scale (SOWS), Objective Opioid Withdrawal Scale (OOWS), and the Clinical Opiate Withdrawal Scale (COWS).

Medical complications

Opioid use, especially intravenous, has a variety of medical complications. Of particular concern, especially amongst those who use dirty needles for injection, are HIV, hepatitis B, and hepatitis C. Indeed, the co-occurrence of intravenous heroin use and these diseases is extremely high. Over one-third of individuals with HIV have reported intravenous substance use, and nearly one in five individuals who use substances intravenously has a diagnosis of HIV or AIDS. Further, one half or more of individuals who use intravenous substances have a diagnosis of hepatitis C. Abscesses and other bacterial infections are relatively common. Endocarditis and other infections of the heart and its components may occur. Emboli may result from the injection of impurities in the mix of heroin, such as talc. These clots may stop up vessels in the liver, kidney, lungs, and brain, resulting in considerable organ damage. Other infections, such as tuberculosis, may result given the generally poor health of individuals who use opioids. Arthritis and other rheumatologic problems are also not uncommon in individuals who use opioids.

Opioids (2)

Treatment

Management of severe opioid intoxication or opioid overdose follows the basic principles of basic life support and advanced cardiac life support, with attempts to open the patient's airway and support ventilation if needed. Intubation may be necessary. Naloxone, an opioid antagonist available as the brand Narcan®, can also be administered. Typical dose is 0.4 to 0.8mg intravenously, intramuscularly, or subcutaneously. Administration can be repeated at approximately two-minute intervals. Other causes of unconsciousness, respiratory depression or arrest, and cardiac arrest should be considered, including hypoglycemia and electrolyte abnormalities. Patients who have overdosed on longer acting opioids, such as sustained-release oxycodone, may need to be placed on a naloxone drip (i.e., continuous intravenous administration).

Acute withdrawal is typically treated symptomatically with the goal of making the patient more comfortable. As the subjectively uncomfortable withdrawal symptoms often lead patients to leave the hospital prematurely, assisting patients during this difficult time may better facilitate ongoing treatment. Trazodone at a starting dose of 50mg or other sleep aids may be considered for insomnia. Loperamide may be used for abdominal cramping and diarrhea, while hydroxyzine 25mg by mouth every four to six hours may help with anxiety and restlessness. Clonidine is used by some practitioners to ameliorate withdrawal symptoms, typically at dose of 0.1mg by mouth every four to six hours.

Another treatment strategy involves placing patients in acute withdrawal on methadone (given in increments of 5mg until withdrawal signs subside) then tapering the dose down by 10 to 20 percent per day. Buprenorphine, a partial agonist at the mu receptor and a newer treatment for opioid maintenance therapy, may also be used for detoxification, with data on efficacy regarding the rapidity of detoxification via this mechanism being highly variable.

Longer-term opioid dependence maintenance treatment may be initiated with a variety of pharmacologic approaches. Methadone, a long acting opioid agonist with a peak plasma concentration at two to four hours following administration has a considerably longer half-life than most opioids typically approximately 24 hours. The slower onset of action makes it less likely for patients to obtain the euphoria that is typically experienced with heroin, morphine, and other opioids. Methadone, when used for opioid detoxification or maintenance therapy on an outpatient basis, may only be administered at approved sites. It may not be obtained via prescription at a pharmacy, nor can it be dispensed at a physician's office, making access somewhat limited. However, studies of individuals who use methadone in place of heroin show a dramatic decrease in the reduction of infectious diseases, such as hepatitis C and HIV. Furthermore, some of the illegal behaviors that occur to procure heroin, such as stealing, also decrease when individuals are switched from heroin to methadone.

Buprenorphine, available as the brand Subutex® and Suboxone® (buprenorphine combined with naloxone), is a relatively new treatment option for opioid maintenance therapy. The medication is a partial agonist at the mu receptor, and it is available as a sublingual tablet. Naloxone was added to the combination form of the pill to discourage illicit use of the buprenorphine (i.e., attempting to use the medication intravenously to achieve a "high"). As a partial agonist, the danger of overdose on buprenorphine is limited. Furthermore, given its improved safety over methadone, it is available in an office-based setting. Access to care for opioid maintenance treatment has been expanded as a result, especially to those individuals who fear the stigma of going to a methadone clinic or whose schedules do not permit daily visits to such a clinic. Buprenorphine can be prescribed by physicians with a special waiver, generally obtained by extra training in the use of the medication.

Naltrexone, a long-acting opioid antagonist is also used as a maintenance agent for people with opioid abuse or dependence. The medication is typically started around 7 to 10 days after the acute withdrawal period with an average daily dose of 50mg. Because the medication blocks the opioid receptors, the patient does not obtain a "high" from using heroin. However, most studies indicate a relatively small treatment retention rate.

A number of well-studied psychosocial interventions are also available for treatment of opioid dependence. These will be discussed at length elsewhere in this chapter (📖 pp. 673–677).

Cocaine, methamphetamine and other stimulants (1)

Cocaine is a stimulant available for use as either a base or a salt. The base typically vaporizes at a relatively low temperature, and is, therefore, used most frequently via inhalation. The smoked form of cocaine is typically called "crack." The salt form is highly soluble and is often used for injection. It can also be used for snorting. Methamphetamine is used intranasally, orally, and intravenously. It can also be smoked, similar to cocaine. A variety of other stimulants are available either over the counter or by prescription, including pseudoephedrine, methylphenidate, and phenteramine. Sometimes these tablets are crushed to allow for intranasal use.

Epidemiology

Slightly over six million people or 2.6% of people, in the United States used cocaine in the past year. Approximately one percent of the population used cocaine in the past month. Use is more common in persons between the ages of 18 and 25. Males were over two times as likely to use as females. Cocaine is the second most widely used illicit drug.

In 2004, approximately 1.5 million persons used methamphetamine, whereas nearly 600,000 had used methamphetamine in the past month. The average age of first use was 22 years. Although methamphetamine use was initially more common in rural areas, it is becoming more and more widespread, with a considerable amount of use in urban and suburban areas. Use in urban areas is becoming more prevalent amongst gay-identified males. Furthermore, amphetamine use is growing amongst individuals with co-occurring eating disorders, given the propensity of such use to suppress appetite.

Diagnosis

Individuals using stimulants may present to the emergency department or other setting with symptoms suggestive of schizophrenia or another psychotic disorder. Persons intoxicated on cocaine may differ from patients with acute psychosis in that there are generally fewer, if any delusions, and the delusions are often not as bizarre as they are in schizophrenia. Further, there is less evidence of a thought disorder. Tactile hallucinations are particularly common. Cocaine is generally included in a urine drug screen and is detectable for up to 96 hours after the last use.

Methamphetamine is also typically found in urine drug screens with a detectable level existing through approximately three days after last use.

Pharmacology

Stimulants work at multiple sites with activity in both the central and peripheral nervous systems. This class of drugs works to increase monoamine activity, via DA, norepinephrine (NE), and 5-HT. Some members of this class work at the reuptake sites; some enhance presynaptic release. Stimulants typically reach the brain in less than 10 seconds when use via inhalation. Intranasal and oral have an onset of action that is usually between 30 and 45 minutes.

Clinical features

Intoxication

Stimulant use typically results in increased energy, hypersexuality, euphoria, decreased need for sleep, decreased appetite. Effects may progress to anxiety, irritability, panic attacks, paranoia, and hypervigilance. Some individuals may develop hallucinations or other psychotic symptoms. Often, tachycardia, hyperventilation, mydriasis, tremulousness, and diaphoresis are seen. These effects do not typically warrant medical attention. In rare cases, generally seen with higher doses of cocaine, potentially life-threatening complications may occur. Such events include myocardial infarction, arrhythmia, hypertension, stroke, and hyperthermia.

Tolerance

Chronic exposure to stimulants results in tolerance to the effects of use, such as tolerance of appetite suppression and tolerance to cardiovascular effects. Tolerance to these effects generally subsides after one to two weeks.

Withdrawal

Withdrawal from cocaine is not life threatening and hospitalization to treat withdrawal is rarely indicated. Symptoms typically involve low mood, difficulty concentrating, fatigue, increased need for sleep, and increased appetite. The withdrawal period from stimulants can last for several hours to several days. These symptoms, particularly increased need for sleep and hypersomnolence, are often referred to as a "crash."

Medical complications

Long-term use of stimulants leads to poor nutrition, given the combination of poor appetite and poor self-care. Weight loss, often considerable, is common amongst individuals who use cocaine. Furthermore, poor dentition is not uncommon and is often referred to as "meth mouth" (dirty or missing teeth, very friable or bleeding gums, dental abscesses). In addition, stimulant use can result in cardiac and pulmonary complications.

Stimulant-associated chest pain is observed with some regularity in this patient population. It is thought that the chest pain is secondary to coronary vasospasm. The overwhelming majority of individuals who use stimulants and present with chest pain will not go on to develop a myocardial infarction. Given the low sensitivity of an electrocardiogram, especially in this patient population, an EKG is not always helpful. Serial troponin studies are currently the best available method for diagnosing acute myocardial infarction. Use of beta-blockers should be avoided in this patient population. Rhabdomyolysis is also a cause for concern, given the high degree of activity that can result from stimulant intoxication. As with other substances in which intravenous use occurs, users of stimulants via this method are at high risk for hepatitis C and HIV. Long-term neurological and psychiatric sequelae are common amongst users of stimulant drugs. Other medications that enhance catecholamine activity, such as monoamine oxidase inhibitors, should also be avoided in persons who use stimulants. In addition, given the possibility of arrhythmias with both tricyclic antidepressants (TCAs) and stimulants, TCAs should not be used in persons who use stimulants.

Cocaine, methamphetamine and other stimulants (2)

Treatment

Treatment of severe agitation or anxiety in persons with stimulant intoxication can generally be accomplished with benzodiazepines. Lorazepam 1–2mg po, IM or IV, is the recommended starting dose. If an antipsychotic is necessary to control psychosis, consider haloperidol 2.5 to 5mg po, IM, or IV. Physical restraint should be avoided as much as possible given the possibility of rhabdomyolysis and hyperthermia in this already at-risk population.

Hospitalization is generally not indicated to control stimulant withdrawal. No notable trials comparing pharmacologic treatments to general supportive care exits (i.e., ensuring food and fluid intake). BDZs or medications such as trazodone or hydroxyzine may be considered on an as needed basis for individuals with persistent anxiety or sleep disturbances during withdrawal.

On a long-term basis, drug counseling, motivational strategies and contingency management, as detailed elsewhere in this chapter, are used to treatment stimulant abuse and dependence. The Matrix Model incorporates multiple strategies and provides a framework for engaging patients who abuse stimulants in treatment and helping them achieve abstinence. Although some studies are underway, there is no role for pharmacologic approaches for maintenance treatment of stimulant use at this time. As with all substance use, treating co-morbid depression or other psychiatric conditions plays an important role in successfully managing stimulant use.

Cannabis

Tetrahydrocannabinol (THC) is the main psychoactive ingredient found in marijuana. Marijuana is the most commonly used illicit substance. It is available in multiple forms, but is most commonly smoked in the form of a joint. Use of a pipe for smoking, also known as a bong, is also a popular method of administration. THC has been proposed for use for both appetite stimulation, especially in patients with cancer or AIDS, and also for treatment of chronic pain. Dronabinol, sold as the brand Marinol®, is a schedule III drug marketed for antiemetic use. Other more controversial indications include chronic pain and spasticity, such as from multiple sclerosis.

Epidemiology

Nearly 15 million people in the United States used marijuana in the month prior to being studied in a 2004 survey by the Substance Abuse and Mental Health Services Administration. Sixty-four percent of first-time users were under the age of 18. Studies suggest higher usage amongst black or Latino individuals, with perhaps a slightly higher prevalence amongst men compared to women.

Diagnosis

Persons using marijuana will often present with deficits in attention, fatigue, and generally slowed responsiveness. Depending on degree of use, cannabis will result in a positive drug screen for three days to several weeks following last use.

Pharmacology

Tetrahydrocannabinol acts in both the central and peripheral nervous systems. The effects of cannabis result from THC binding to the CB1 receptor, which is found mostly in the central nervous system.

Clinical features

Intoxication

Use of marijuana may result in impaired ability to make decisions, with slowed reaction time and impaired short-term memory. Individuals using the drug may also have dry mouth, red eyes, tiredness, and increased appetite. Paranoia can result, in addition to hallucinations. There is typically a mild euphoria when using the substance.

Tolerance

Some degree of tolerance does develop to the pharmacologic effects of cannabis. Some studies have shown a down-regulation of cannabinoid receptors after extensive use; however, these results have not been well replicated.

Withdrawal

Withdrawal is sometimes observed in individuals who frequently use marijuana. Withdrawal is not life threatening and is self-limited, with typical resolution in one to five days. Symptoms include insomnia, suppressed appetite, irritability, low mood, and mild tremulousness. The withdrawal syndrome is not recognized in DSM-IV-TR.

Medical complications

The most common complication associated with marijuana use is pulmonary dysfunction, secondary to smoking. Individuals who chronically use marijuana develop complications similar to cigarette smokers, including frequent wheezing and coughing, chronic bronchitis, and reduced performance on pulmonary function tests. There is also an increased risk of lung cancer, especially in individuals who concurrently smoke tobacco.

Marijuana use may also lead to a decline in immune functioning, possibly making dronabinol a poor choice in treating appetite suppression or pain in individuals with AIDS or cancer. In some individuals, marijuana use may result in orthostatic hypotension and tachycardia. These effects are not likely to be of clinical significance in generally healthy, young individuals. Furthermore, cannabis use has also been shown to induce galactorrhea and cause disruption of the menstrual cycle.

Treatment

Treatment of marijuana intoxication should be generally supportive and can typically be done without medication. The patient should be placed in a low-stimulus environment.

Marijuana withdrawal is also generally self-limited and can be treated supportively. Pharmacologic intervention is typically unnecessary.

Long-term treatment of marijuana abuse and dependence may be accomplished with motivational or cognitive-behavioral strategies. There are no medications available for maintenance treatment of individuals with marijuana dependence.

Hallucinogens and club drugs

A broad range of synthetic and naturally occurring substances that alter perception, including MDMA, LSD, PCP, ketamine, GHB, psilocybin & psilocin (some mushrooms), and mescaline (peyote). The method of ingestion is typically eating (transmucosal absorption via colorful or cartoon printed papers placed in the mouth) or smoking. PCP can be smoked with marijuana or tobacco but can also be eaten, injected, or inhaled nasally.

Epidemiology

According to the 2004 National Study on Drug Use and Health, ~14% of the U.S. population over age 12 endorses hallucinogen use at some point in their life, with 1–2% having used in the past year. Highest rate of use is in the 18–25 years old adults. Lifetime use is highest for LSD, followed by mushrooms and MDMA.

Diagnosis

Consider evaluating for hallucinogen use in patients, especially young adults, who present with confusion, paranoia, psychoses or obtundation. PCP is detectable in urine and is included in most routine urine drug screens. MDMA and LSD are detectable in urine but not routinely included in drug screens.

Pharmacology

Partial or full agonists at $5HT_2$ receptor and other serotonergic receptors (MDMA, LSD, psilocybin and psilocin, mescaline) or antagonists at NMDA receptors (PCP, ketamine).

Clinical features

Intoxication

Acute intoxication includes hypertension, tachycardia, sweating, blurred vision, tremor, pupil dilation, poor coordination, perceptual disturbances and they can be mild to severe. A "bad trip" refers to the experience of marked anxiety, depression or paranoia, fear of losing one's mind, accompanied by frightening hallucinations or synesthesias (sensation in one modality triggering a sensation in another modality, i.e., seeing a sound, smelling a color); it is usually resolved within 12 hours.

PCP can also cause dysarthria, increased muscle tone and hyperactive reflexes. Patients with PCP intoxication may become combative and/or psychotic. PCP overdose can cause seizures, respiratory depression, stupor, coma and death. Posthallucinogenic perception disorder—rare, repeated experience of perceptual disturbance (i.e., flashbacks of prior trips).

Tolerance

Develops rapidly but resolves after several days of abstinence.

Withdrawal

Does not occur.

Medical complications

• Accidental or self-inflicted injury due to agitated/psychotic behavior.
• Rhabdomyolysis and renal failure can result from PCP use.

Treatment

Isolate patient in nonstimulating environment until PCP clears and then talk down the patient. For acute agitation, use benzodiazepines such as lorazepam (Ativan®) 1–2mg IM. For agitation and psychosis, use an antipsychotic that does not have potent anticholinergic effects such as haloperidol (Haldol®), as PCP itself has anticholinergic actions. Urine acidification may increase the drug clearance, but can also increase risk of renal failure.

Tobacco (1)

Epidemiology

29.2% of Americans 12 and older report past month use in 2004, most cigarettes (89%). Highest use is seen among 18–25 year old individuals (44%). Smoking rates decline with education level and employment.

Diagnosis

Assessment of past or present smoking history should be part of every patient assessment. Nicotine has a half-life of approximately 2 hours and is metabolized by the liver into cotinine. Cotinine has a half-life of 18 hours, but detection is mainly utilized in research studies as a marker of recent smoking.

Pharmacology

Nicotine binds to nicotinic acetylcholine receptors, which results in the release of a number of neurotransmitters, including DA, NE, 5-HT, and opioids. Chronic nicotine administration results in an increase in the number of nicotinic receptors and a concomitant desensitization. Within seconds, a cigarette delivers anywhere between 1–3mg of nicotine to the brain via the extensive pulmonary vasculature, chew/snuff delivers 2–3mg via the highly vascular oral mucosa.

Clinical features

Acute effects

Activation of nAchR has a mild stimulatory effect, increases attention and alertness, and decreases appetite.

Overdose

There is minimal potential for overdose via cigarettes and chewing tobacco, especially in chronic users. Overdose usually occurs in children who have ingested cigarettes or are exposed to nicotine patches. Symptoms of overdose include nausea, vomiting, diarrhea, weakness, and dizziness.

Withdrawal

Many users experience strong cravings, irritability, dysphoria, anxiety, difficulty concentrating, restlessness, insomnia, and increased appetite. These symptoms peak in the first four days and wane over the course of a week to one month after cessation, except for increased appetite and weight gain, which can linger for several months postcessation.

Medical complications

Smoking is one of the major preventable causes of death and disability. The leading causes of death due to smoking occur from cardiovascular disease, COPD and lung cancer. Smoking cessation significantly reduces morbidity and mortality.

- Cutaneous—aging, discoloration, wrinkling of skin.
- Head/neck—cataracts, periodontal disease, squamous cell carcinoma, oropharyngeal cancer.
- Pulmonary—COPD, lung cancer, respiratory infections
- Cardiovascular—CAD, PVD, thromboangiitis obliterans, aortic aneurysms.
- Gastointestinal—esophageal, pancreatic, stomach, colorectal, anal cancers, PUD, GERD.

- Renal—renal insufficiency, renal carcinoma, renovascular disease.
- Genitourinary—bladder and cervical cancer, sexual dysfunction.
- Neuromuscular—stroke.

Treatment

Tobacco dependence is a chronic condition that often requires repeated intervention. Effective treatments can produce long-term or even permanent abstinence. The patients who are willing to try to quit tobacco should be provided treatments that work. Patients who are unwilling to quit tobacco use should be provided a brief intervention designed to enhance their motivation to quit. There is a strong dose-response relation between the intensity of tobacco counseling and its effectiveness. Cessation should be the goal of treatment. There is little evidence that decreasing the number of cigarettes or switching to lower tar cigarettes results in better health outcomes. Three types of counseling were found to be effective and they include problem-solving/skills training, intratreatment social support, and extra-treatment social support. Hypnosis and acupuncture have been investigated in RCT and meta-analyses and have not been shown to be effective.

Pharmacotherapies

All Nicotine Replacement Therapies (NRT) significantly increase cessation rates 1.5 to 2 times over placebo. There is no significant evidence for one NRT over another and thus, choice depends on patient's preference, side-effects, presence of medical conditions, and previous success/failure with a particular NRT (summarized in table 📖 *p. 665*).

Multiple studies have shown increase in efficacy for a combination of sustained and intermittent nicotine delivery systems (i.e., patch and gum, or nasal spray) over single NRT. No significant adverse events have been reported with proper use of combination therapy, however this treatment is not FDA approved.

Sustained-release bupropion (Zyban®) is the only FDA approved non-NRT for smoking cessation and is first-line pharmacotherapy. Its mechanism is via blockade of DA and NE reuptake and antagonism of nicotinic acetylcholine receptors. Bupropion reduces withdrawal symptoms and reduces/delays weight gain. Side-effects are insomnia, dry mouth, and sleep disturbances.

Nortriptyline (Pamelor®) is a second line agent for smoking cessation because of its less favorable side-effect profile. It has comparable efficacy to bupropion but can cause bothersome side-effects, including blurry vision, dry mouth, constipation, and orthostatic hypotension. It acts by blocking NE and 5HT reuptake.

Clonidine is another second-line agent. It acts via sympathetic blockade at alpha2-adrenergic receptors in locus coeruleus. Clonidine can cause hypotension.

A medication that was just recently approved by the FDA, varenicline (Chantix®), may help significantly higher percentage of patients quit smoking compared to bupropion. The drug is a novel selective nicotinic receptor partial agonist that helps ease withdrawal craving and blocks the nicotine effect of smoking. The label recommends not combining it with bupropion or nicotine patch.

Tobacco (2)

Principles of smoking cessation counseling

ASK	Include smoking status (current, past or no use) in every adult and child substance use assessment. Positively reinforce nonsmoking or quit patients, especially in adolescents.
ASSESS	Determine the level of willingness to quit so that a targeted approach to quitting can be matched to the patient's stage of change (pre-contemplation, contemplation, action, maintenance, relapse). Remember that people in all stages of change can be helped.
	Success is progressing through the stages, not just quitting.
	Relapse is a not a failure, but a common stage in the process.
ADVISE	Every encounter should include a clear, strong, supportive and non-confrontational cessation message.
	Personalize the statement with references to current illness, life events, social and economic costs and impact on others in the household.
	Use motivational interventions (5 Rs) to help patients identify their own key issues.
	Relevance—help the smoker determine why quitting is important to them.
	Risks—identify negative consequences of use.
	Rewards—identify benefits of quitting.
	Roadblocks—identify specific obstacles to quitting.
	Repetition—reinforce the motivational message often and reassure that repeated quit attempts are often necessary.
ASSIST	Precontemplation– Advise that you/healthcare professionals are able to help when ready to quit. Provide smoking cessation material. Try to explore barriers to quitting using motivational interventions.
	Contemplation—Above, plus, encourage patients to talk about the quitting process. Provide smoking cessation support materials.
	Action—Help plan a quit plan (set date, anticipate challenges, tell family/friends, remove tobacco products). Encourage total abstinence. Review previous attempts for what helped/did not help in reducing use.
	Maintenance—Congratulate success, encourage abstinence, reinforce the importance. Use open-ended questions to identify triggers and explore feelings surrounding relapse/cessation.
	Relapse—Ask what precipitated relapse. Identify strategies to overcome barriers. Reaffirm the ability to quit. Encourage them to set another quit date.
ARRANGE	Follow-up on patients' progress when considering quitting, planning to quit, recently quit or relapsed. Follow-up in person or by phone, with physicians, nurses, or other healthcare workers can all be effective.

Source: Anderson JE, et al.

Treatment	Advantage	Dosing	Directions	Side-effects	Contraindications
NRT					
Nicotine gum	least expensive; can control your own dose	1 piece q1–2 hours daily for at least 1–3 months <20cigs/day–2mg >20cigs/day 4mg	chew slowly and tuck in between gum and cheek	hiccups, nausea, heartburn	TMJ, dentures, oral problems exacerbated by chewing
Nicotine lozenge	delivers 25% more nicotine over the gum; can control your own dose	1 lozenge q1–2 hours for 2–4 weeks, then taper to 1 lozenge q2-4 hours	allow lozenge to slowly dissolve in the mouth, do not bite or chew	sore throat, irritated gums, heartburn, nausea	phenyl-ketonuria
Transdermal nicotine	easy to use; little to no evidence of withdrawal after cessation	various doses 10+ cigs/day use highest dose patch, reduce dose after 6 weeks	apply in a.m. and remove at bedtime or in the next a.m.	headaches, dizziness, nausea, blurred vision, skin irritation	skin conditions exacerbated by the patch/ adhesive

Treatment	Advantage	Dosing	Directions	Side-effects	Contraindications
Intranasal Nicotine nasal spray (Rx only)	acts quickly to relieve cravings and most closely resembles the pharmacokinetics of smoking a cigarette; can control your own dose	1 spray q nostril per hour (not to exceed 5 doses/hour or 40 doses per day)	taper gradually; do not use for >3 months	nasal irritation	sinusitis, nasal polyps, rhinitis
Nicotine inhaler (Rx only)	most closely resembles the act of smoking; can control your own dose	continuous puffing for 20 minutes delivers 4mg of nicotine (only 2mg are absorbed)	use 6–16 inhalers daily for up to 24 weeks	irritation of oral mucosa	asthma, respiratory disease
Non-NRT					
Bupropion (Zyban®) (Rx only)	easy to use, reduces urge to smoke	150mg qam x 3 days, then 150mg bid, start 1–2 weeks before quitting		disturbed sleep, dry mouth	seizure disorder (not absolute), eating disorder, MAOIs
Varenicline (Chantix®)	easy to use, reduces cravings, blocks effects of nicotine	0.5mg daily x 3 days, then 0.5mg bid x 4 days, then 1mg bid; start ~1 week prior to quit date		nausea, insomnia, constipation, headache	

Anabolic-androgenic steroids

Including oral forms (danazol: Danocrine®; methandrostenolone: Diana-bol®; stanozolol: Winstrol-V®) and IM injections (nandrolone: Deca® Durabolin IM® and Durabolin IM®; testosterone cyprinate: Virilon IM®) and transdermal patch includes testosterone.

Epidemiology

More than 1 million current or former users in 1995, median age of use is 18 years old. In one study of high school football players, prevalence was 6.3%.

Diagnosis

Ask about use in all body builders and athletes, especially high school football players. Note the presence of androgen-induced side-effects such as high blood pressure and rapid weight gain in men:

- Alopecia.
- Severe acne.
- Testicular atrophy.
- Impotence.
- Infertility.
- Gynecomastia.
- Painful penile erections.
  In women:
- Hoarse voice.
- Hirsutism.
- Dysmenorrha/amenorrhea.
- Increased appetite.
- Decreased breast size.
- Clitoral hypertrophy.

Be aware of "stacking"—using more than one steroid preparation and "pyramiding"—gradually increasing dose and then tapering.

Pharmacology

Steroids promote skeletal muscle growth and increase lean body mass.

Clinical features

Single doses of testosterone have no acute effect, but with chronic use total body weight increases (partially due to salt and water retention) and lean body mass increases. Severe mood swings and increased aggressiveness, referred to "roid rage," paranoid thoughts, and impulsivity can be seen.

Tolerance

Evidence supporting the development of tolerance is not strong.

Withdrawal

There is little evidence of physical dependence on anabolic-androgenic steroids.

Medical complications

Androgen-induced side-effects listed above including liver disease and cardiovascular disease (case reports). The use of steroids is associated with an increased risk of developing liver tumors with the potential for liver failure. Heart attacks and cardiac arrests have been reported. A number of complications can arise from injection steroid use because of needle-sharing practices, such as hepatitis B, C, and HIV infection.

Treatment

No specific treatment; counseling and psychosocial interventions as with other drugs of abuse, monitor for psychiatric manifestations such as:
- labile affect,
- depression,
- suicidal ideation,
- psychosis,
- delirium.

Inhalants

A large, pharmacologically diverse group of substances that share a common route of intoxication includes volatile solvents (paint thinners, gasoline, nail polish remover, glue, rubber cement), nitrites (amyl, butyl, alkyl), and volatile anesthetics (nitrous oxide). Nitrites are known as "poppers" because of the small glass vials containing the substance that are popped open. Ingestion occurs via sniffing, or "huffing" the substances from the container or a cloth soaked with the substance.

Epidemiology

Estimates from NSDUH 2004, of U.S. population age 12 and older, lifetime use of inhalants 9.5%, past month use approximately 1%. Highest lifetime use is in 18–25 year old individuals but increasing use in 12–18-year-old individuals. Highest rate of use in past month is in 12–18-year-old individuals (1.2%).

Diagnosis

Suspect in patients, especially teenagers and young adults who present with constellation of symptoms consistent with intoxication or overdose.

Pharmacology

Solvents are highly lipophilic, thereby reaching high concentration in the brain, heart, liver, and muscles, and requiring hours to days to clear. Onset occurs in minutes, effects last 30 minutes to hours, and they are detected in the blood for only 4–10 hours.

Clinical features

Intoxication

Is similar to alcohol or sedative-hypnotics with symptoms of:
- Mild euphoria.
- Belligerence.
- Aggression.
- Impaired judgment.
- Impulsivity.
- Ataxia.
- Confusion.
- Disorientation.
- Slurred speech.
- Dizziness.
- Decreased reflexes.
- Nystagmus.

In overdose, inhalants can cause delirium and seizures. Poppers may be used to enhance sexual arousal via vasodilation, which also produces light-headedness and euphoria.

Tolerance and withdrawal

Little is known about the development of tolerance to and dependence on inhalants. In general they do not appear to be significant features.

Medical complications

Death can occur from suffocation, aspiration of vomit, cardiac arrhythmias or myocardial infarction. Toxic effects can cause permanent brain damage even after the first dose, liver damage, kidney damage, bone marrow suppression, peripheral neuropathy, and immunosuppression. Sudden death cases related to cardiac arrhythmias have been reported. A major danger of inhalant use lies in the possibility of asphyxiation, when an air-proof bag held over the nose and the mouth administers the substance.

Treatments

Short-term treatment of intoxication is supportive medical care (fluids, monitor vital signs).

Treatments (1)

General principles of SUDs treatment

Formal treatment can have a compelling force for change, however, informal help (such as AA, a family friend, physician or member of the clergy) and ongoing social resources tend to play a powerful and enduring role. Recovery from SUDs, that is sustained after treatment is not simply due to treatment but also affected by the same sets of factors that maintain the resolution of the problems without treatment. This issue calls for a change in the way interventions are delivered. Treatment addressing and improving the individual's life circumstances (environmental factors) are likely to be beneficial.

Neurocognitive impairment in patients with SUDs could affect their ability to utilize treatment effectively. Patients seeking formal treatment are usually more impaired, have more severe problems, and more difficult life contexts. Common social and cognitive processes underlie the process of problem resolution that occurs in formal treatment, informal care, and "natural" recovery. Studies have shown that duration and continuity of care are more closely associated with better treatment outcome than the sheer amount of treatment. For example, drug-dependent patients with longer episodes of residential or outpatient care experience better substance use and crime-related outcomes.

Patients treated by substance abuse and mental health specialists experience better outcomes (less substance use, less likely to have psychiatric symptoms, and more likely to be employed) than do comparable patients seen only in the general medical center. Common aspects of treatment could have a significant impact. Empathic style and ability to establish therapeutic alliance are associated with engagement in treatment and better treatment outcomes. On the other hand, confrontational interventions elicit resistance and withdrawal from treatment. Treatment settings and counselors oriented toward personal growth goals and setting structure and clarity in treatment tend to promote positive substance use outcomes. A challenging issue regarding SUDs treatment is about how to integrate evidence-based practice with the humanitarian recovery-based model that values the patient's personal experiences, responsibility, choice, and empowerment. Incorporating patient's preferences in terms of treatment options would be helpful in clinical decision making.

It is important to realize that a patient with SUD copes with his/her feelings in a very intense and complex way. This can provoke disconcerting and confusing feelings in the physician/therapist, who may not be emotionally ready to deal with them. Patients with SUD may be involved in delinquent and criminal acts. However, the person experiences an internal conflict made of powerful and intense inner experiences, which is not what a person with antisocial personality disorder experiences. This is very important to identify since it helps understand what patients with SUD go through to avoid, regulate, or escape these painful internal conflicts through self-medication with substances. Physicians'/therapists' personal values, opinions, attitudes, and counter-transference reactions toward the patient with SUD need to be identified and acknowledged and worked through so they do not interfere negatively with the therapeutic work.

Brief interventions and motivational interviewing (MI)

To a significant extent, motivation for change is transactional and depends very highly on the interpersonal interaction. Analyzing verbal transactions occurring in the therapeutic process have identified five themes that occur in behavior change conversations, reflecting:

- Desire.
- Ability.
- Reasons.
- Need.
- Commitment to change.

Of these, only commitment language seems to predict subsequent behavior change. Motivation for change is enhanced by an empathic and accepting approach rather than by confrontation. Reaching a decision and making a commitment may be a final pathway to change, having both interpersonal and intrapersonal factors. There is solid scientific evidence for the efficacy of brief interventions for alcohol problems. What accounts for the impact of brief interventions? Six components are often present in effective brief counseling with problem drinkers and are summarized in the acronym FRAMES:

- Feedback regarding personal status, relative to norms of drinking and its consequences.
- Responsibility for change is left with the patient, emphasizing personal autonomy.
- Advice and encouragement to reduce or stop drinking.
- Menu of options for how to change drinking behavior.
- Empathic style that listens to the patient.
- Support for self-efficacy, hope, and optimism about the possibility for change.

Brief interventions do not include education, confrontation, or teaching skills. Brief physician advice has been found to help with smoking cessation. The counseling style of MI shares many of these attributes. MI is a brief person's-focused psychotherapeutic intervention for helping patients change addictive behaviors.

MI strategies include two phases, building the patient's motivation to change, and strengthening the patient's commitment to change. The principles of MI are the following:

- Express empathy.
- Develop discrepancy; between the patient's goals and current problem behavior.
- Roll with resistance: ambivalence is normal. Reflect back the patient's own ambivalence and confusions about his or her drug or alcohol use.
- Support self-efficacy; enhancing self-confidence based on hope and optimism about the possibility for change.

Typically, the MI therapist uses a variety of techniques to help increase intrinsic motivation for change. These techniques are divided into two categories: microskills and strategies. The microskills function to initiate and facilitate engagement and open discussion with the patient about problem areas. They include the use of open-ended questions, reflective listening, using affirmations, and summarizing the patient's statements in a balanced manner. This is essential to the creation of an empathic and collaborative atmosphere to start discussing patient's ambivalence about changing his or her use of substances. MI strategies involve increasing directive techniques for building intrinsic motivation for change, particularly when the microskills are limited in their effect. The strategies include constructing decisional matrices to elicit the patient's perceptions of the costs and benefits of remaining the same or trying to change. Through the use of these skills, the clinician attempts to move the patient from a position of establishing the patient's motivation for change to strengthening commitment to attempt the change.

The therapist clearly does not pressure patients with SUDs to subscribe to a goal of complete abstinence nor required to attend self-help meetings or other groups. "Denial" is not confronted nor "broken down" before meaningful change can occur.

Treatments (2)

Cognitive-behavioral therapies

These include contingency management models, cognitive behavior therapy, family and social network interventions. They have been generally shown to be effective across the major classes of SUDs. This has a clinical implication since the norm is mostly polysubstance use syndromes. Furthermore, the targets of these approaches are the commonalities across the many types of SUDs. Another important issue is the strong support for their efficacy for treating psychiatric disorders, which are highly co-morbid with SUDs. Overall good outcomes with these therapies are seen in patients who have less severe or less chronic SUDs with good support system, fewer psychiatric problems, less involvement with the criminal justice system, and less medical co-morbidity. These different models share common principles of behavior change. Behavioral therapies help patients achieve better behavioral control and interrupt and change learned pathways. Contingency management models focus on changing reinforcement contingencies so that abstinence is facilitated and rewarded through interpersonal support, delivery of tangible incentives, increased emphasis on and access to other reinforcers and alternatives to substance use and introduction of normative comparisons. For example, patients involved in treatment in a methadone maintenance program who continue to use cocaine will reduce their use when offered tangible incentives such as "take-home" doses or access to employment, contingent on producing drug-free urines.

Cognitive-behavioral models encourage behavior change through exposure to and practice of coping behaviors, interventions that minimize the risk of relapse (relapse prevention). They include coping with craving and cues that trigger craving, dealing with negative emotional states, addressing early warning signs of relapse, helping patients identify high-risk situations and develop cognitive and behavioral coping responses to manage them, helping patients improve communication skills, relationships, and develop recovery social network, and helping patients identify and correct cognitive distortions that increase relapse risk.

Family approaches such as behavioral couples therapy has been described as one of the top empirically supported treatments for alcohol problems. They have a positive effect on substance use and also lead to improvement in couple's adjustment. In addition, they reduce intimate partner violence and improve emotional and behavioral functioning on the part of the children in the family. Involvement of nonsubstance abusing family members and significant others promotes help seeking and fosters better retention in treatment. Generally family-involved treatment may facilitate positive treatment outcomes and families should be involved in the treatment process.

To summarize, behavioral therapies in combination with pharmacotherapy target one or two major goals: improving impulse control and reducing craving. These interventions are complex and multidimensional (social, cognitive, behavioral, and neurobiological).

Group therapy/self-help groups

The specific ways in which groups can help initiate abstinence and maintain it as well as making lifestyle changes needed to support recovery, include providing education on addiction, recovery, and relapse; resolving ambivalence and enhancing motivation to change; instilling hope and optimism for change; providing opportunity to give and receive feedback from peers; teaching recovery skills; understanding and resolving problems contributing to addiction; creating an experience of positive membership in a recovery-oriented group; preparing the patient to be involved in long-term treatment; and facilitating the patient's interest in participating in self-help groups. There are different types of group therapies including: milieu groups, psycho-educational groups, skill groups, and therapy or counseling groups. They are selected depending on the treatment context and stages of change. All clinicians should support group therapies because they play a major role in treatment of SUDs. Patients participating in group therapies often benefit from pharmacotherapy. The combination of individual therapy and group therapy is optimal. Therapy groups are different from self-help programs in that they are designed to help patients explore psychological issues in an atmosphere of support and empathy in which self-disclosure is promoted.

Spiritual mutual help groups such as AA have strong scientific support. The AA's ability to reduce problem drinking is comparable to that for other ambulatory interventions. With regard to outcomes such as self-esteem and psychiatric symptoms, AA appears to have some benefit on average, but at a lower level than it has on drinking. Narcotics Anonymous (NA) and Cocaine Anonymous (CA) participation appears to predict decreased drug use. Among the mediators of the effects of 12-step groups are increased self-efficacy, greater commitment to abstinence, greater acceptance of alcoholic identity, and increased abstinent-specific social support from friendship networks. The patients who engage in spending more time helping others recover and doing other "12-step work" are the most likely to achieve long-term sobriety in AA.

Pharmacological treatments

The role of pharmacotherapy played in the treatment of SUDs depends on the drug of abuse. For example, pharmacotherapy is a mainstay of treatment of nicotine dependence, which typically incorporates little behavioral interventions, however, the main treatment of cocaine and amphetamine dependence is behavioral and pharmacotherapy has currently no role (no FDA-approved medications).

FDA-approved medication therapies are now available for the treatment of nicotine, alcohol, and opiate use disorders. Pharmacotherapies for SUDs address two major objectives: initial attainment of abstinence after treating withdrawal and prevention of relapse (anticravings). Behavioral interventions in combination with pharmacological therapies can increase adherence to medications and retention.

Pregnancy and SUDs

Prevalence

59% of women admitted to consumption of alcohol during pregnancy, 11% using illegal substances and cocaine is the primary drug in 75% of substance-using pregnant women. Women of low socioeconomic status are usually at increased risk of using substances during pregnancy. Rates for black and white women are identical. Studies have shown little difference in the prevalence of drug and alcohol use in public and private settings.

Screening and recognition

Early recognition is crucial. Health history can elicit risk factors for SUDs. The most common psychiatric disorder among addicted women is personality disorders. Family history of substance abuse should alert the physician. Always it is important to elicit information about a history of SUD in the patient's significant other. Screening tools for alcohol use include T-ACE and TWEAK (T-ACE: T is for tolerance: how many drinks does it take to get high?; A for annoyed: have people annoyed you by criticizing your drinking?; C for cut down: have you felt you ought to cut down on your drinking?; E for eye opener: have you ever had a drink first thing in the morning to steady your nerves or get rid of a hangover?. A positive answer to the tolerance question or two positive answers to the other three questions indicate an increased likelihood that the woman is drinking at a level that may be harmful to the fetus.). T-ACE is derived from CAGE but emphasizes tolerance. TWEAK can be used to detect a range of drinking levels (T for tolerance, W for worry, E for eye-opener, A for amnesia, and K for cut down: one point for each except tolerance 2 points for two or more drinks: with 3 or more points indicating that the woman is more likely to be engaged in problematic levels of alcohol use). Urine toxicology could help with screening process. A history of recurrent cellulites and/or endocarditis should raise suspicion about possible drug abuse.

Assessment

Ambivalence is a major issue, many addicted women are aware of the risks of substance use. The use of motivational strategies could be very helpful to engage the patient and address ambivalence. Practical problem solving is also important. Addressing factors that can interfere with treatment such as guilt, shame, lack of support, and uncertainty about the success of treatment is crucial. Collaboration between obstetrical service and addiction treatment program is a key to success.

Maternal withdrawal syndromes

Alcohol and sedative-hypnotic drugs

It is important to assess the symptoms of withdrawal that could overlap with pregnancy symptoms. The treatment should be inpatient. Any medication with cross-dependence could be used, and it is always better to err on the side of slightly over- rather than undermedicating (same scales mentioned above could be used). Advanced withdrawal should be treated aggressively. BDZs can affect the fetus; however, the risk to both the mother and the fetus from untreated withdrawal is greater than the potential risk to fetus from exposure to these medications in a controlled setting. The following symptoms are common to pregnancy and withdrawal: restlessness, insomnia, nausea and vomiting, hypertension, tachycardia, tachypnea, and seizures. The following manifestations are common to withdrawal but not pregnancy: impaired memory, agitation, tremor, fever, diaphoresis, distractibility, and hallucinations.

Stimulants

Withdrawal is more subtle and complex. Abrupt discontinuation does not cause gross physiological sequelae. The use of BDZs is indicated for severe agitation.

Opioids

Opioid withdrawal can lead to fetal distress and premature labor. Medical withdrawal is not recommended because of high rates of relapse and the increased risk to the fetus of intrauterine death. Methadone is used to treat withdrawal. Titration of the dose is important (total score for all 10 symptoms is determined: the severity of 10 symptoms is graded on a scale of 0 to 2 points: 0 point if symptom is absent, 1 point if the symptom is present, and 2 points if severe; the total score for all 10 symptoms is determined and each point is equivalent to 1mg of methadone. The patient should be evaluated and the symptom score totaled every 6 hours for the first 24 hours and after 24 hours, the total dose given is computed; this dose is equivalent to the dose the patient was taking. The symptoms include pupillary dilation; lacrimation; rhinorrhea; piloerection; nausea; vomiting; diarrhea and abdominal cramps; chills; hot flashes; myalgias; arthralgias; yawning; irritability and restlessness. Naloxone should not be given except as a last resort because of risk of spontaneous abortion. Methadone maintenance is the treatment of choice for opioid dependent pregnant women. It allows for a consistent blood level in contrast to wide fluctuations, it reduces the use of illicit opioids, it decreases criminal activities and disruption of maternal-child unit, and enhances the ability of the woman to engage in treatment. The dose of over 60mg daily is most effective. Women can breastfeed if not using any other drugs and are not HIV+ or have hepatitis C. Infants with known and suspected intrauterine drug should be monitored for withdrawal syndrome and treated appropriately. The criminal prosecution of pregnant substance-abusing women should not be supported.

Tobacco

The use of tobacco during pregnancy has been linked to adverse birth outcomes and should be a target of prenatal screening and intervention.

Co-occuring disorders

Prevalence

Epidemiological surveys and studies of clinical populations have shown high rates of co-occurring SUDs and psychiatric disorders. NIMH/ECA showed that 37% of patients with alcohol use disorders and 72% of those who used drugs had at least one psychiatric co-morbidity. More than half of patients with severe mental illness were dually diagnosed: 55% with schizophrenia and 62% with bipolar disorder. Bipolar disorder consistently displays the highest rate of SUD. Co-occurring disorders are associated with increased service use, worse treatment outcomes, more severe course of illness, especially for antisocial personality disorder, bipolar disorder, and schizophrenia, higher health care utilization, increased risk of violence/trauma/suicide/child abuse/neglect/involvement in criminal justice system, higher health care costs, and more medical co-morbidities such as HIV and hepatitis C infections. People who seek treatment for either a mental illness or SUD are more likely to have a co-morbid disorder than people who do not seek treatment. In summary, co-occurring disorder is a dominant clinical entity in most treatment settings.

What accounts for the co-morbidity?

- Secondary psychopathology models (increased co-morbidity due to substance use causing psychiatric disorders in vulnerable individuals).
- Secondary substance abuse models: psychiatric disorders causing SUDs in vulnerable patients. These models include the self-medication hypothesis and supersensitivity model.
- Common factor models: it means that another underlying variable independently increases the risk (genetic, familial, social).
- Bidirectional models: different factors related to SUDs and psychiatric disorders can contribute to the onset and maintenance of co-morbidity. Research has indicated that PTSD is associated with the subsequent development SUD that in turn exacerbates PTSD.

There is a lack of support for any single one of these models or a meta-model of co-morbidity.

Treatment

Parallel or sequential treatment approaches are ineffective. Integrated treatment is associated with better outcomes; however, interventions need to be matched not only to diagnosis but also to phase of recovery, stage of treatment, and stage of change. A variety of interventions include individual, group, residential, and pharmacological modalities. Phases of recovery start with acute stabilization (engagement, using MI) then prolonged stabilization (active treatment and relapse prevention) then rehabilitation and recovery.

Assessment of CODs

Longitudinal and integrated structured assessments are needed. Probing for negative consequences of SUD not just focusing on quantity, because small amounts of ingested drug can exacerbate psychiatric problems.

Tracking caffeine and nicotine use is a crucial part of the assessment. Patterns of SUDs and psychiatric symptoms as well as treatment experiences including medications help formulate a better treatment plan.

The principles of pharmacological treatment
- Treat clear symptom clusters.
- Consider safety and side-effect profiles and avoid medications with abuse liability and addiction potential.
- Choose strategies that enhance adherence to medications.
- Be aware of potential interactions between psychotropics and substances of abuse.

Clinical evidence support the use of atypical antipsychotics as first line treatment in psychotic disorders and schizophrenia; SSRIs may be more effective than other antidepressants in reducing alcohol consumption; anticonvulsants and especially valproate is superior to lithium for bipolar disorder; use of benzodiazepines beyond detoxification is not generally indicated; SSRIs and SNRIs, and atypical antipsychotics are safe and effective alternatives in treating anxiety disorders; stimulants are beneficial once sobriety is achieved, longer acting with lower abuse liability and diversion potential are preferable; Atomoxetine is nonaddictive but effective trials in SUDs are lacking.

The principles of psychosocial interventions
- Develop a supportive therapeutic alliance and focus on MI in the engagement phase.
- Integrate evidence-based treatment for addictions such as MI, relapse prevention, 12-step facilitation with evidence-based mental health treatment.
- Help the patient achieve abstinence, coping and recovery skills.
- Encourage establishing social support network including 12-step meetings.
- Utilize short-term case management approach during vulnerable periods to help with adherence to medications and maximize retention.

Psychosocial approaches could include dialectical behavior therapy (DBT) in individuals with co-morbid borderline personality disorder and SUD, incorporating individual, group, pharmacotherapy, case management, phone consultation, and therapist consultation. Newer approaches emphasize skills training, trauma treatments, and adherence interventions, substance-abuse domestic-violence treatment, and combinations of many approaches such as contingency management, CBT, and MI.

ASAM criteria

American Society of Addiction Medicine (ASAM) Levels of Care/ASAM Patient Placement Criteria (ASAM PPC-2R)

ASAM has developed criteria for placement of patients requiring treatment of substance use disorders. There are five basic levels of care. Within each level, a decimal number is used to indicate gradations of intensity required.

Level 0.5: early intervention
- Individuals who are at risk of developing substance-related problems.

Level I: outpatient treatment
- Organized, non-residential services.
- Professional personnel provided evaluation, treatment, and recovery services.

Level II: intensive outpatient treatment/partial hospitalization
- Organized outpatient service delivering treatment during the daytime, typically before or after work or school, in the evenings, or on weekends.
- Essential education and treatment components.
- Medical and psychiatric consultation.
- Medication management.
- 24-hour crisis services.

Level III: residential/inpatient yreatment
- Organized staff services by addiction and mental health professionals.
- Planned regimen of care in 24-hour inpatient or residential setting.
- Self-help groups meet regularly on-site.

Level IV: medically managed intensive inpatient treatment
- Mental health and substance-related problems are of sufficient severity to require medical, psychiatric, and nursing care 24 hours per day.
- Full resources of a general medical or psychiatric hospital are available.
- Addiction-credentialed physicians and other mental health professionals.

Opioid maintenance therapy
- Can be provided at any level of care.
- Generally provided at level I.

Other addictions/impulse control disorders

Pathological gambling currently exists in the DSM-IV-TR as an impulse control disorder. Certainly, however, it shares a variety of characteristics with other addictions. Other addictions include sexual addiction and internet addiction.

Pathological gambling

Persistent and recurrent maladaptive gambling behavior as indicated by five (or more) of the following:

- Preoccupied with gambling (e.g., preoccupied with reliving past gambling experiences, handicapping or planning the next venture, or thinking of ways to get money with which to gamble).
- Needs to gamble with increasing amounts of money in order to achieve the desired excitement.
- Has repeated unsuccessful efforts to control, cut back, or stop gambling.
- Is restless or irritable when attempting to cut down or stop gambling.
- Gambles as a way of escaping from problems or of relieving a dysphoric mood (e.g., feelings of helplessness, guilt, anxiety, depression).
- After losing money gambling, often returns another day to get even ("chasing" one's losses).
- Lies to family members, therapist, or others to conceal the extent of involvement with gambling.
- Has committed illegal acts such as forgery, fraud, theft, or embezzlement to finance gambling.
- Has jeopardized or lost a significant relationship, job, or educational or career opportunity because of gambling.
- Relies on others to provide money to relieve a desperate financial situation caused by gambling.

The gambling behavior is not better accounted for by a manic episode.

Epidemiology

The prevalence of pathological gambling is not well known, however, estimates range from one to three percent—three to nine million Americans. Furthermore, approximately one-quarter of individuals with pathological gambling were found to have co-morbid alcohol or substance abuse or dependence. The disorder is more common amongst men, with a ratio of three males to one female. Furthermore, it is more common among younger adults.

Assessment and treatment

Several screening tools are available for the diagnosis of pathological gambling, including the South Oaks Gambling Screen and the National Opinion Research Center DSM Screen for Gambling Problems (NODS). Limited evidence is available on the efficacy of treatments for pathological gambling. Similar to Alcoholics Anonymous, Gamblers Anonymous follows a 12-step, self-help model. Cognitive behavior therapy may be the most efficacious treatment. There are no medications shown to be effective as a primary treatment for the condition.

Sexual addiction

Sexual addiction can involve a variety of thoughts and behaviors. Addictive sexual behaviors can usually be classified into one of three major DSM-IV categories: paraphilia, impulse control disorder not otherwise specified (NOS), or sexual disorder NOS. These behaviors may begin as frequent or excessive masturbation and/or extensive use of pornography, with progression to increasingly dangerous or risky behaviors. Similar to other addictions, the desire for sexual fulfillment or engaging in sexual behaviors becomes more time consuming. It may reach a point where it interferes with the multiple spheres of functioning, including life at home, work, or school. Further, someone with a sexual addiction may wish to stop and make efforts to do so, but will often fail in decreasing such activity. Concerning behaviors may include sex in public, anonymous sexual encounters, forcing others to have sex, spending excessive time searching for sex (i.e., via the Internet, at bookstores). Sexual addiction also has contributed significantly to the spread of HIV.

Epidemiology
One of the first studies of sexual addiction in the 1980s indicated a prevalence of sexual addiction of 8% amongst males and 3% amongst females. Follow-up studies indicate that these numbers may be an over-estimate.

Treatment
Sex Addicts Anonymous is a 12-step, self-help program available for individuals with a sexual addiction disorder. Cognitive, behavioral, and cognitive-behavioral approaches have been used to treat sexual addiction. There is some evidence for the use of SSRIs in treating such addiction, but further studies are still needed.

Internet addiction

As usage of the Internet becomes more widespread, so do problem behaviors associated with Internet usage. Though not a diagnosis contained in the DSM, certainly behaviors associated with addiction can be seen with Internet use. Such behaviors might include spending increasing amounts of time on the Internet to the point that use interferes with functioning in other spheres of life. Reliable prevalence data are not available, but the pattern of computer and Internet use suggests that younger individuals would be more likely to development problematic behavior.

Street names/slang

Amyl nitrate: poppers, aimes, amys, pearls

Cannabis: pot, weed, 420, Africane, airplane, bammy, bash, black gold, blunt, joint, chronic, Don Juan, doobie, hash, MJ, roach, ash, skunk

Cocaine: base, beam, big C, big flake, blow, C, C-dust, candy C, Charlie, coca, cola, crack, dust, powder, white, nose candy, rock, snow, snow white, sugar

Flunitrazpam (Rohypnol): forget me drug, forget pill, R-2, roachies, roapies, roofies, wolfies, rope, ruffles

Gamma-Hydroxybutyrate (GHB): cherry meth, G, G-riffic, GHB, grievous bodily harm, jib, liquid E, liquid G, liquid X, sleep, vita-G, Georgia home boy

Heroine: Big H, black pearl, black tar, china white, dirt, dope, dust, fix, junk, mother pearl, smack, snow, whack

Ketamine: black hole, K-hole, special K, Vitamin K, super C, Cat killer, ket, kit kat, jet

Lysergic Acid Diethylamide: acid, big D, blotter cube, conductor, contact lens, ghost, mind detergent, zen

Methamphetamine: crank, blade, crystal, crystal meth, ice, meth, poor man's coke, rock, speed, tina

Methylenedioxymethamphetamine (MDMA, ECSTASY): 007s, 69s, batmans, cloud nine, E, elephants, letter biscuits, Mercedes, Mitsubishi, rave energy, red devils, Rolls Royce, smurfs, tom and jerries, wafers, white diamonds, Z-pills, X, Adam

Methylphenidate (Ritalin): Rits, west coast, R, vitamin R

Morphine: dreamer, first line, God's drug, M, MS, Miss Emma, morf, morpho

Nitrous Oxide: laughing gas, buzz bomp, whippets

Oxycontin: 40, 40-bar, 80, cotton, hillbilly heroin, kicker, OC, ox, oxy

Phencyclidine (PCP): angel dust, star dust, magic dust, glitter

Steroids: gym candy, stacking, weight trainers, pumpers, juice

Recommended further reading

1 Anderson, J.E. *et al.* (2002). Treating tobacco abuse and dependence: an evidence-based clinical practice guideline for tobacco cessation. *Chest* **121**, 932–941.

2 Bouza, C, *et al.* (2004). Efficacy and safety or naltrexone and acamprosate in the treatment of alcohol dependence: a systematic review. *Addiction* **98**, 811–828.

3 Graham, A.W., Schultz, T.K., Mayo-Smith, M.F., Ries, R.K. (eds.). *Principles of Addiction Medicine*. Chevy Chase, Maryland: ASAM, 2003.

4 Grant, B.F., Dawson, D.A., Stinson, F.S., Chou, S.P., Dufour, M.C., & Pickering, R.P. (2004). The 12-month prevalence and trends in DSM-IV alcohol abuse and dependence: United States, 1991-1992 and 2001-2002. *Drug & Alcohol Dependence* **74**(3), 223–234.

5 Grant, B.F., Hasin, D.S., Chou, S.P., Stinson, F.S., & Dawson, D.A. (2004). Nicotine dependence and psychiatric disorders in the United States: results from the national epidemiologic survey on alcohol and related conditions. *Archives of General Psychiatry* **61**(11), 1107–1115.

6 Grant, B.F., Stinson, F.S., Dawson, D.A., Chou, S.P., Dufour, M.C., Compton, W., *et al.* (2004). Prevalence and co-occurrence of substance use disorders and independent mood and anxiety disorders: results from the National Epidemiologic Survey on Alcohol and Related Conditions. *Archives of General Psychiatry* **61**(8), 807–816.

7 Grant, B.F., Stinson, F.S., Dawson, D.A., Chou, S.P., Ruan, W.J., & Pickering, R.P. (2004). Co-occurrence of 12-month alcohol and drug use disorders and personality disorders in the United States: results from the National Epidemiologic Survey on Alcohol and Related Conditions. *Archives of General Psychiatry* **61**(4), 361–368.

8 Griffiths, R.R. and Johnson, M.W. 2005. Relative Abuse Liability of Hypnotic Drugs: A conceptual framework and algorithm for differentiating among different compounds. *Journal of Clinical Psychiatry* **66** [suppl 9], 31–41.

9 Johnson, B, Ruiz, P, and Galanter, M. *Handbook of Clinical Alchoholism Treatment*. Philadelphia: Lippincott, Williams & Wilkins, 2003.

10 Johnson, BA, *et al.* (2003). Topiramate for treatment of alcohol dependence: a randomized controlled trial. *Lancet* **361**, 1677–1685.

11 Keifer, F, *et al.* (2003). Comparing and combining naltrexone and acamprosate in relapse prevention of alcoholism. *Archives of General Psychiatry* **60**, 92–99.

12 O'Brien, CP. (2005). Benzodiazepine Use, Abuse, and Dependence. *Journal of Clinical Psychiatry*, [suppl 2], 28–33. www.niaaa.nih.gov http://oas.samhsa.gov/nsduh/2k4nsduh/

13 Rastegar, D.A. and Fingerhood, M.I. *Addiction Medicine: An Evidence-Based Handbook*. Philadelphia: Lippincott, Williams & Wilkins, 2005.

14 Ziedonis, D.M., Smelson, D., Rosenthal, R., *et al.* (2005). Improving the care of individuals with schizophrenia and substance use disorders: Consensus recommendations. *Journal of Psychiatric Practice* **11**, 315–339.

Child and adolescent psychiatry

Pediatric mental health treatment

Treatment of pediatric patients has the potential for large impact

Children and adolescents are constantly learning from the environment, integrating what they see and experience in the context of rapid cognitive, social, emotional, and neurobiological development.

Mental health problems can limit the inherent potential in this process. Clinicians who assess and treat pediatric mental health concerns can help influence the developmental trajectory of pediatric patients and their families in order to maximize social, emotional, academic, and vocational development. The potential impact can be rewarding, but there are important challenges posed by working with rapidly developing children and their families.

Children and adolescents are dependent on their caretakers

Mental health is influenced by environment. This is quite clear when working with children, adolescents, and their families. Pediatric patients are dependent on their care providers for food, clothing, and developmental support. Each child brings his or her personal temperament to this environment and the development of the child is dependent on the match of temperament, as well as how caregivers and children navigate any mismatches.

Level of development impacts behavior

Behaviors that are considered normative in one developmental stage may be a source of concern in another. For example, stranger anxiety is expected to occur at around nine months, but if a nine-year-old had significant stranger anxiety it would significantly impair the ability to engage with their environment at home and school.

Special considerations are needed for building treatment alliance

A strong treatment alliance with both the young patient and their family is essential for the provision of effective mental health care. Because pediatric patients are most often brought into treatment by their adult caregivers, development of this an alliance with the identified patient can be complex. Cognitive development also impacts ability to engage in treatment. Traditionally, professionals who work with pediatric patients have utilized play and/or informal methods in order to engage children and adolescents as participants in treatment.

Widespread use of evidence-based treatments is not the norm

The widespread use of evidence-based treatments require well-defined phenomenology and a solid evidence base for treatments that work in controlled conditions and the community. Very few conditions in child and adolescent psychiatry have an evidence base that fulfill all of these conditions. Although there are a number of therapeutic interventions that have proven useful in very controlled environments, some have failed to reach the general population of care providers and patients in a consistent, effective manner. In addition, pharmacologic treatments tend to be used in a manner that outpaces the evidence base. Ultimately the choice of treatment should be a combination of evidence-based recommendations, and the specific needs of the pediatric patient and family.

Evaluation and formulation

The goals of evaluaton

- Identify precipitants of referral. Attempt to discern both the chief complaint and the reason why it rose to the level of referral at *this time.*
- Identify the goals of the child and family.
- Obtain an accurate picture of the nature and extent of the child's behavioral difficulties, functional impairment and/or subjective distress.
- Understand the child's developmental strengths and limitations in all domains—cognitive, language, motor, behavioral, ability to form relationship, etc.
- Identify the potential individual, family, or environmental factors that may account for, influence, or ameliorate these difficulties.
- Acquire the information necessary to create a responsive biopsychosocial treatment plan that is patient centered, family focused, family driven, and culturally competent.

Clarify the role of the care providers

Before beginning any evaluation it is important to clarify the nature of the treatment relationship. This includes the relationship with the family and patient as well as any referring provider. Whatever the formal relationship (consultant or collaborator) it is important to clarify the treatment relationship. Some specific issues include:

- Who will make recommendations?
- Who will implement recommendations?
- How will the family return for follow-up if problems ensue?

There are also specific rules of confidentiality that must be considered and made clear to patients and their families for forensic evaluations, custody evaluation and school referrals, just to name a few examples.

Confidentiality and release of information

Confidentiality has always been of utmost concern in the mental health field, but it has come under close scrutiny recently in the United States as new laws to protect privacy have been established. It is important to obtain releases to speak to all members of the treatment team. Many mental health institutions require formal written releases. Specific considerations must be taken for children and adolescents in the care of someone other than their adoptive or biological parents. Laws also vary from state to state regarding the treatment of minors without parental consent and commitment to psychiatric hospital. In all settings, it is important to inform your patient that confidentiality will be superseded in the face of danger of harm to self or others.

Components of the evaluation

Evaluation includes assessment and treatment planning for a child and family. It can be complex and requires multiple components that a traditional adult process does not include. In some venues components of this process may be performed and/or augmented by different members of the treatment team. This section will include brief information on the key components of assessment and treatment that are provided by a mental health provider.

Parent/guardian interview

Inclusion of each parent or guardian in the process of assessment and treatment planning is ideal for several reasons:
- Each guardian may have different viewpoints, which will help to create a thorough assessment.
- The presence of entire family unit together at least once will help evaluate the dynamics of the family system.
- Family history can usually be more accurately obtained by interviewing each parent, because not everyone shares their entire personal and/or family mental health history with their partner.

Parents are often the only source of accurate information about history of pregnancy, developmental history, temperament, and shifts in behavior. Parents can also give excellent information about overt behaviors such as hyperactivity and oppositionality.

Child/adolescent interview

The child and adolescent interview is an essential part of the evaluation. Pediatric patients are often the best source of information about internal mood states—e.g., feeling down or worried. Traditionally "play" has been used as a way to access the internal mood states of pediatric patients who have difficulty verbalizing their internal mood states because of their developmental stage or resistance. Children and adolescents will frequently either understate or inflate their oppositional and/or behavioral problems. The child and adolescent interview is also a way to assess the ability of a pediatric patient to talk to a stranger, and separate from their parents.

Other sources of information

As mentioned in the previous section, information can be gleaned from many members of the child or adolescent's life. Checklists and formal instruments can be used for the pediatric patient, parents, teachers and guardians. Informal discussions with other members of the treatment team can be very helpful. Teachers are often an invaluable source of information about a child's behavior in both a structured and unstructured environments, and often can serve as a gauge to help compare the child's behavior to other classmates his or her age.

Formulating the case and plan

Case formulation

Formulation of the case (bio-psycho-social assessment and plan) should be an ongoing component of the treatment planning process. The clinician should share the formulation with the family and consider how the formulation affects the family-centered treatment goals.

Diagnostic considerations

Because mental illness in pediatric patients is often in a state of evolution, it is important to help the family understand what mental health conditions are being considered. Families may choose to begin educating themselves about all of the possibilities at this point, or may simply want information about "what to look for." Work with the family's individual needs and requests, and be certain to address comprehensive risks, benefits, and alternatives of all treatment options.

Prioritizing co-morbidity

Co-morbidity is often the rule in child and adolescent psychiatry. In addition, children and their families often have multiple needs when they come for evaluation. One method of formulating a hierarchy is to consider issues that threaten the safety of the child or others first, then those that threaten the continuity of the therapy and treatment. Then, focus therapeutics on interventions that will be most likely to improve functionally outcome and return the child to a normal developmental trajectory. It is important to recognize these needs, and make recommendations that address the long-term and short-term priorities of the child and family. It may also be important to understand the needs of the community in these decisions.

- For example, if a young child with bipolar disorder and violent behavior at school seems to be having increased difficulties because of family discord, it is not appropriate to simply refer the family for family counseling without addressing the immediate safety of the child and community, as well as the possibility that a manic episode may have been triggered.

Evaluation in practice

Parent/guardian interview
- It is essential to establish rapport with child and family members.
- Define needs of child and family.
- Obtain family psychiatric, medical, and social history. A genogram can be helpful (🕮 p. 47).
- Inquire about sexual behavior/ HIV risk/ pregnancy, development, sibling relationships, friendships, temperament, shifts in behavior.
- Observe family functioning and interactions. Note: patterns of communication, degree of warmth, power dynamics, alliance.

Child/adolescent interview
- First establish rapport and gain child's confidence. Play can be helpful.
- Begin with subjects well away from the presenting problem/s (e.g., interests and hobbies, friends and siblings, school, holidays).
- Progress to enquiring about child's view of the problem, worries, fears, sleep and appetite, mood, self-image, peer and family relationships, experiences of bullying or teasing, abuse, persistent thoughts, fantasy life, abnormal experiences, suicidality, etc. (It may take several interviews to obtain a full picture.)
- Observe: levels of activity and attention; physical and mental level of development; mood and emotional state; quality of social interaction.

Other sources of information
- Obtain consent to contact school for meeting or report from teachers, school psychologists, etc. Consider asking teacher to complete a behavior rating scale (e.g., Child Behavior Checklist; Connors' Teacher Rating Scale).
- Obtain consent and consult other caregivers, medical professionals who have treated the child, and social agencies that have been involved with the child and/or family.
- Psychological tests: may include IQ, personality, and developmental assessments.
- Investigations: hematology, chromosome studies, EKG, EEG, CT, etc.

Assessment principles
- Identify the problem behavior/s—obtain a full description (from parents, child, teachers, etc.) of the problem behavior/s. This should include the evolution of the behavior, a chronology of the child's typical daily activities, the setting in which the problem behavior occurs, the effects of it on family, school, relationships, etc, and attitudes of others to the behavior/s. It is always appropriate to speak to the child alone (if possible) to establish his/her views, desires, and mental state.
- Determine the parental strategy—it is important to find out how the parents deal with the behavior/s. This includes information about their expectations, philosophy of parenting, interpretation of the behavior/s, moral, religious, and cultural views on parenting, etc. Also;
  - How do the parents react or respond to the behavior/s?
  - How do they discipline or punish?

- What do they tolerate?
- Are they permissive or restrictive?
- Are they overprotective or uninvolved?
- Do they feel empowered or impotent, helpless, and incompetent as parents?
- How do they manage their frustrations, anger, etc?
- What coping mechanisms do they have?
- Family history and dynamics—as well as gathering a full family history of health, psychiatric problems, social and cultural circumstances, and support structures, it is also important to assess parental and sibling relationships, the presence of any significant stressors or losses, and how the problem behavior interacts with family dynamics.
- Social behavior—the evolution of the child's social behavior, including social developmental, attachment behavior, imaginary play, reading of social cues, relationships, and language use.
- School behavior—attendance, changes in school, separation issues, socialization, performance, peer and teacher interactions, and responses, friendships, bullying, etc.
- Child's health and development—pregnancy, birth, and developmental milestones. Was the child planned, wanted? How did siblings react? How did parents and siblings cope? Any postpartum problems? Were there supports? Also, child's temperament, illnesses, treatment, etc.
- Direct observation of parent-child interaction—during the interview/s it is important to note how the child behaves and how parents respond and interact with the child. If siblings can be present their behavior and interactions can also be evaluated. A home and/or school visit may add additional information about the behavior in these settings.
- Collateral information—teachers, extended family, and social services may be able to provide important input, and permission should be sought to contact and involve them where appropriate.

Formulation of the case (bio-psycho-social)

- Consider predisposing, precipitating, perpetuating, and protective factors.
- Formulate a multiaxial diagnosis. See Chapter 2 for details.

Create a feasible plan

- Determine goals for child and family. *Goals should be specific and target specific behaviors, performance, and domains.* For example: "Johnny should do better with his homework" may translate into "Johnny will turn in completed homework 90% of the time."
- Determine the methods to meet the goals. Medication can be one method, although often inadequate alone. Behavioral modification, school intervention, family therapy, individual therapy can be other essential methods.
- Determine who will be responsible for helping the child and/or adolescent meet each of their goals. Decide which health care providers prescribe medication or perform therapy. It is important that family members are prepared and able to take on roles in the implementation of treatment plan.

Formulating a differential diagnosis

Clinical pearls

- The interpretation of behavior is contextually, culturally, and developmentally dependent. Almost all behaviors listed below have the potential to be considered normal in the correct context.
- Multiple determinants of behavior is the rule.
- Co-morbidity is common.
- Genetic predisposition confers potential for many behaviors and psychiatric diagnosis, but environment always has the potential to modulate behavior.
- Parents often bring their children concerned about one specific behavior or cluster of behaviors, but the key to diagnostic formulation is maintaining a wide differential diagnosis while assessing resilience and risk factors within the context of the pediatric patient's specific context.

Diagnostic considerations

The following list contains some examples of diagnostic considerations when evaluating chief complaints in the field of pediatric mental health. The following is a list of chief complaints and potential psychiatric diagnoses.

- Hyperactivity—ADHD, oppositional and conduct disorders, anxiety disorders, depression, mania, autism spectrum disorders, substance abuse, sexual abuse, post-traumatic stress disorder.
- Inattention—ADHD, oppositional and conduct disorders, learning disorders, autism spectrum disorders mood disorders, anxiety disorders, substance abuse, sexual abuse, language processing disorders, hearing deficit.
- Separation problems—attachment disorders, anxiety, depression, developmental delay, sexual abuse, post-traumatic stress disorder.
- Social problems, avoidance—depression, anxiety, social phobia, autism-spectrum disorders, sexual abuse, post-traumatic stress disorder.
- Aggression, hostility—oppositional and conduct disorders, ADHD, mania, psychosis, depression, anxiety, developmental disorders, learning disorders, autism spectrum disorders, substance abuse, sexual abuse, post-traumatic stress disorder.
- Regression—depression, anxiety, developmental problems, learning disorders, autism spectrum disorders, substance abuse, sexual abuse.
- Sexually inappropriate behaviors—sexual abuse, learning disorders, autism spectrum disorders, conduct disorders, substance abuse, mania, psychosis, learning disorders, autism spectrum disorders.
- Somatic symptoms—anxiety, depression, learning disorders, autism spectrum disorders, psychosis, sexual abuse.
- Tantrums—oppositional and conduct disorders, ADHD, depression, anxiety, learning disorders, autism spectrum disorders, sexual abuse, physical problems, mania, psychosis.
- Ritualistic behaviors— anxiety, obsessive-compulsive disorder, learning disorders, autism spectrum disorders, psychosis.

Team approach

Identify the "team" in the child's life

A care provider who attempts to understand all members of a patient's team will be best prepared to clarify treatment goals and respond when goals are not being met.

Each member of the team brings their own strengths and limitations, as well as viewpoints. Each member has the potential to take on different roles. Pediatric patients exist in a biological, genetic, and psychosocial context. Striving to include all members of the child's care team will improve the ability to understand that context and be more responsive. Possible members of the treatment team can include: parents, grandparents, coaches, clergy, teachers, school administrators, kin, and other social supports. This list is not merely limited to traditional medical providers! Identifying all potential members of a child's natural treatment team will help expand the treatment options, and identify the key participants in the formal treatment planning process. The formation of a formal child and family team is often not mandated until a family system has reached a breaking point. Thus, encouraging the family to be inclusive and seek social support, as well as to be a source of information to clinicians, can be very helpful throughout the treatment process.

Utilize the entire treatment team

As an evaluation occurs, and treatment planning begins, it is important to keep in mind that there are many ways that members of the formal treatment team, as well as the "informal team" can be utilized. It can often be helpful to try to identify who is and who isn't worried about the child and why. Each member of a child (and the family's) life will bring his or her own viewpoints, strengths and limitations. Some states mandate formal "child and family teams" when treatment goals have consistently not been met and the child's situation is threatening their placement in the community. At this point, goals can often seem reactive and the number of formal health care professionals involved can sky rocket. These situations can often be avoided with successful use of a natural "team" early in the evaluation and treatment planning process. When first evaluating psychosocial and mental health complaints, it can be much easier to focus on strengths of the child and their family system. Also, getting information from members of the system when they are not in crisis usually provides a better understanding of the perceived strengths in the child, which can be utilized to the advantage of the child later. Finally, the identifying members of the "natural team" and developing a healthy support system that capitalizes on their strengths can help the child and family meet their initial goals and move toward recovery.

Attention deficit hyperactivity disorder (ADHD) (1)

ADHD is among the most commonly diagnosed and treated pediatric mental health problems, and is increasingly being diagnosed in adults as well. The hallmark symptoms of ADHD are a persistent pattern of inattention and/or hyperactive/impulsive behaviors that are developmentally inappropriate, chronic, and interfere with function. DSM-IV-TR specifies that some symptoms must have been present before seven years of age, although some studies have suggested that a large number with the "inattentive" subtype may have a later onset.[1] To fulfill diagnostic criteria, the ADHD behaviors should also adversely affect at least two functional domains (e.g., academic, familial, social, occupational) and have persisted for at least six months.

Clinical features of ADHD

Inattention symptoms may include: poor attention to details or tendency to make careless mistakes; easy distractibility; difficulty sustaining attention; poor listening; poor task completion; disorganization; avoidance of tasks requiring sustained attention; tendency to lose things necessary for tasks; and forgetfulness.

Hyperactivity/impulsive symptoms may include: fidgetiness; inability to stay seated; running or climbing inappropriately; noisiness in play; seeming "on the go" or "driven like a motor"; excessive talkativeness; prematurely blurting out answers; inability to take turns; and interrupting others.

Three different subtypes are described: a predominantly inattentive subtype with at least six inattentive symptoms, a predominantly hyperactive/impulsive subtype with at least six hyperactive/impulsive symptoms, and a combined subtype with at least six symptoms from both inattentive and hyperactive/impulsive categories.

Epidemiology

The prevalence of ADHD is reported in community studies of children and adolescents in the United States to be 3–5%, whereas in the United Kingdom a lower rate of 1% is reported. Such differences are thought to be due to differences in ascertainment, and have not persisted in studies in which similar diagnostic methods with the same structured interviews were used.[2] There is a male predominance of 3:1 in youths. The inattentive subtype is the most common in community settings, whereas in psychiatric clinical settings, the combined subtype is the most common. A similar rate of ADHD has been reported in a large community sample of adults, and the disorder is generally thought to be underdiagnosed in that age range.

Etiology[3,4,5,6]

Genetics

Heritability in ADHD is among the highest of psychiatric disorders. Fifty percent rate of concordance in MZ twins; there appears to be separate heritability for different components of ADHD; 2x increased risk in other siblings; increased rates of conduct disorders, depression, and substance abuse in parents.

Neurological

Functional imaging suggests abnormalities in the prefrontal cortex regardless of stimulant use.[3]

Catecholamine hypothesis

Attributes ADHD to dysregulations of dopamine or norepinephrine activity in the central or peripheral nervous system.

Co-morbidity

Approximately 50–80% of youths with ADHD have co-morbid disorder, including specific learning disorders (60%); CD and ODD (40%); depression (15–32%); anxiety disorder (25%); and BD (5–10%).[4] In adults, high rates of co-morbidity are also noted, including mood and anxiety disorders, antisocial personality disorders, and substance abuse. Substance abuse is higher in older adolescents and adults with ADHD, though this co-morbidity is due to the high co-occurrence with conduct disorders and antisocial personality disorders rather than because of ADHD itself or its pharmacological treatment.[5]

Outcome

Impulsive and hyperactive symptoms may remit with maturity, while inattentive symptoms often persist. Increasing evidence suggests that youths with ADHD continue to have symptoms of the disorder into adulthood and these are associated with substantial impairment in multiple domains.[6] Adult patients with ADHD overall have higher arrest rates, and greater risks of fatal car accidents, marital problems, and occupational or academic underachievement. Approximately 30% of youths who go on to have ADHD as adults have a particular problematic course, with academic and occupational underachievement; progression from ADHD to substance abuse is most common when there is co-morbid conduct disorder.[5]

Assessment[7]

ADHD is a clinical diagnosis with no specific biological or cognitive tests validated. Evaluation should ideally include:

- Interview with parents to evaluate developmental, medical, and family history and assess family functioning.
- Interview with child to evaluate for physical disorder, co-morbid mood disorder, anxiety disorder, externalizing disorder, tic disorder, substance use disorder, developmental disorder, or speech and language problems.
- Patients with ADHD, either youths or adults, tend to underreport their ADHD symptoms so collaborative history helpful.

- Refer to pediatrician for physical examination to rule out medical problems (e.g., endocrinopathy, environmental exposure, or neurological disorder, such as petit mal epilepsy or complex partial seizures), including potential risk factors or medical clearance for various medication options.
- Encourage school to conduct educational testing to rule out a co-morbid learning or language disorder.
- Collateral information from school including teachers' rating scales for ADHD symptoms.
- Specific rating scales for parents and teachers (SNAP-IV-R, Vanderbilt, ADHD Rating Scale, Conners', see below).
- General behavioral rating scales to screen for ADHD symptoms and other psychopathology (e.g., Child Behavior Checklist, Teacher's Report Form).

Assessment scales for ADHD

As with many childhood psychiatric illnesses, ADHD is a diagnosis that occurs in many environments. As such, a combination of the clinical examination and often extensive collaboration is needed to provide the information necessary to obtain a diagnosis. Multiple scales have been developed to aid practitioners in diagnosis, and some are designed to monitor clinical progress. Several scales also assist in screening for potential cormorbid psychiatric disorders. Examples of a few ADHD scales are provided below.

Scale Name	Ratings for	Completed by	Information
SNAP-IV-R	A composite of ADHD, ODD, and aggression	Teachers and parents/ caregivers	Free on line
Vanderbilt ADHD Parent Diagnostic Rating Scale	ADHD, with screens for ODD, CD, Anxiety, and Depression	Teachers and parents/ caregivers	Free on line
ADHD Rating Scale	ADHD severity and improvement with treatment	Teachers and parents/ caregivers.	Free online
Conners' Rating Scale Revised (CRS-R)	ADHD, some ODD/Anxiety; index for monitoring treatment	Teachers and parents/ caregivers.	Copyright only. Self-reports for teens and adults available.

Treatment

The Multimodal Treatment Study for ADHD (MTA) suggested that stimulant medication is a reasonable first-line treatment for most children with ADHD[8] (see ADHD treatment section for details). However, concomitant psychosocial interventions are also useful, especially in patients with co-morbid externalizing or internalizing disorders. In general, ADHD interventions include the following:

- Parent management training (see 📖 *p. 1029*).
- Educational/remedial interventions including evaluation for possible accommodations in the school setting such as preferential seating, un-timed testing in a separate environment with fewer distractions, use of assignment books checked by parents, and an organizational advisor.
- Stimulants: generally the first-line treatment with a 70% response rate, even with most co-morbid disorders. Stimulants include methylphenidate and amphetamine derivatives.
- Nonstimulants: include atomoxetine (Strattera®), bupropion (Wellbutrin®), tricyclic antidepressants (TCAs; desipramine, imipramine, and nortriptyline); and alpha-2 adrenergic receptor agonists (clonidine and guanfacine). All have lower response rates than the stimulants. Often more effective for hyperactive and impulsive symptoms than inattentive symptoms.
- Pharmacological or psychotherapy treatment of co-morbid psychiatric disorders like mood, anxiety or tic disorders sometimes required, and may need to be initiated first, if they are more functionally impairing.

Recommended further reading

1 Applegate, B., et al. (1997). Validity of the age-of-onset criterion for ADHD: a report from the DSM-IV field trials.[see comment]. *Journal Amer Acad of Child & Adolescent Psychiatry* **36**(9), 1211–1221.
2 Anderson, J.C. (1996). Is childhood hyperactivity the product of western culture?. *Lancet* **348**(9020), 73–4.
3 Spencer T.J., Biederman, J., Wilens, T.E., Faraone, S.V. (2002). Overview and neurobiology of attention-deficit/hyperactivity disorder. *Journal of Clinical Psychiatry* **63**(Suppl 12), 3.
4 Pliszka, S.R. (1998). Co-morbidity of attention-deficit/hyperactivity disorder with psychiatric disorder: an overview. *Journal of Clinical Psychiatry* **59**(Suppl 7), 50–58.
5 Wilens, T.E. (2004). Attention-deficit/hyperactivity disorder and the substance use disorders: the nature of the relationship, subtypes at risk, and treatment issues. *Psychiatric Clinics of North America* **27**(2), 283–301.
6 Wilens, T.E., Dodson, W. (2004). A clinical perspective of attention-deficit/hyperactivity disorder into adulthood. *Journal of Clinical Psychiatry* **65**(10): 1301–13.
7 Dulcan, M. (1997). Practice parameters for the assessment and treatment of children, adolescents, and adults with attention-deficit/hyperactivity disorder. *Journal of the American Academy of Child & Adolescent Psychiatry* **36**(Suppl 10): 85S–121S.
8 A 14-month randomized clinical trial of treatment strategies for attention-deficit/hyperactivity disorder (1999). The MTA Cooperative Group. Multimodal Treatment Study of Children with ADHD. *Archives of General Psychiatry* **56**(12): 1073–86.

Attention deficit hyperactivity disorder (2)

Treatment principles of ADHD

Stimulant pharmacotherapy for ADHD—general principles[1,2]

The most effective treatment for ADHD continues to be stimulant medications such as methylphenidate and amphetamine/dextroamphetamine, ideally combined with behavioral treatments. These medications are described in detail at the end of this chapter. Stimulants are not without controversy, however, and practitioners must carefully inform families of the risks, benefits, and alternative treatments.

Important warnings about ADHD stimulants[3]

"An FDA review of reports of serious cardiovascular adverse events in patients taking usual doses of ADHD products revealed reports of sudden death in patients with underlying serious heart problems or defects, and reports of stroke and heart attack in adults with certain risk factors."

Another FDA review of ADHD medicines revealed a slight increased risk (about 1 per 1,000) for drug-related psychiatric adverse events, such as hearing voices, becoming suspicious for no reason, or becoming manic, even in patients who did not have previous psychiatric problems.

The multimodal treatment study of children with ADHD[4]

The MTA was an intensive NIMH funded study included 579 elementary school boys and girls with ADHD. Basically, the subjects were randomly assigned to one of four treatment programs:
(1) Medication management alone.
(2) Behavioral treatment alone.
(3) A combination of both.
(4) Routine community care.
The results of the study indicated that long-term combination treatments and the medication management alone were superior to intensive behavioral treatment and routine community treatment. And in some areas—anxiety, academic performance, oppositionality, parent-child relations, and social skills—the combined treatment was usually superior. Another advantage of combined treatment was that children could be successfully treated with lower doses of medicine, compared with the medication-only group.

Follow-up at 24 months: Effects above were fairly consistent even after 24 months. About 70% of the subjects were still taking medication, and 38% of the behavioral subjects began taking medication.

FDA recommends that children, adolescents, or adults who are being considered for treatment with ADHD drug products work with their physician or other health care professional to develop a treatment plan that includes a careful health history and evaluation of current status, particularly for cardiovascular and psychiatric problems (including assessment for a family history of such problems). This warning included all ADHD stimulants, as well as atomoxetine (Strattera®), a nonstimulant ADHD medication. There are also serious concerns about abuse of stimulants, especially in individual with a previous abuse history. Please refer to the FDA website for the latest updates.

Nonstimulant treatment for ADHD—general principles

Stimulants are the most effective treatment for ADHD. However, nonstimulants may be appropriate when patients have failed or not tolerated stimulants, or have certain co-morbid disorders such as tics, depression, anxiety, or substance abuse (given non-stimulants lack of abuse potential).

Nonstimulant ADHD treatment examples include atomoxetine, bupropion, tricyclic antidepressants (including imipramine, desipramine, and nortriptyline), alpha-2 adrenergic receptor agonists (including clonidine and guanfacine). Refer to the end of this chapter for more details on prescribing in the pediatric ADHD population.

It may be helpful to use agents such as clonidine or guanfacine when children have difficulty sleeping as one of the side-effects of stimulants. These medications may possibly help with other symptoms of ADHD, though this is controversial. However, combining stimulants with alpha-2 adrenergic receptor agonists such as clonidine or guanfacine have been associated with rare reports of sudden cardiac death, and the risks and benefits should be carefully weighed before prescribing such a combination.

Recommended further reading

1 Dulcan, M. (1997). Practice parameters for the assessment and treatment of children, adolescents, and adults with attention-deficit/hyperactivity disorder. American Academy of Child and Adolescent Psychiatry. *Journal of the American Academy of Child & Adolescent Psychiatry* **36**(10 Suppl), 85S–121S.

2 Pliszka, S.R. *et al.* (2000). The Texas Children's Medication Algorithm Project: Report of the Texas Consensus Conference Panel on Medication Treatment of Childhood Attention-Deficit/Hyperactivity Disorder. Part I. Attention-Deficit/Hyperactivity Disorder. *Journal of the American Academy of Child & Adolescent Psychiatry* **39**(7), 908–19.

3 http://www.fda.gov/bbs/topics/NEWS/2007/NEW01568.html

4 http://www.nimh.nih.gov/publicat/adhd.cfm

Oppositional defiant disorder (ODD)

Key features

An enduring pattern of negative, hostile, and defiant behavior, without serious violations of societal norms or the rights of others. Behavior may occur in one situation only (e.g., home) and may lead to social isolation, depression, or substance abuse.

Epidemiology

Onset is between three and eight years old. More common in boys during childhood but equal rates in adolescence. A common condition affecting 15–20 % of children and adolescents.

Etiology

Temperamental factors; sick or traumatized child; power struggle between parents and child (note: differentiate from normal autonomous "struggle" of the young child and adolescent).

Management

- **Parent management training** (PMT) targeting social skills, conflict resolution, and anger management can be highly effective as an intervention (see 📖 Chapter 21). Some children may benefit from home visits or head start programs. Some schools offer prevention programs using these strategies.
- At each step, focus on therapeutic alliance with family and child, cultural sensitivity and consideration of family-specific needs.
- Obtain key information from child and parents/guardians: core symptoms of ODD, age at onset, duration of symptoms, and degree of functional impairment. Consider additional information from outside sources as needed and permitted by the child and parents.
- Utilize rating scales to aid in diagnosis and tracking of ODD symptoms (e.g., Connors' Rating Scale (CRS), Child Behavior Checklist (CBCL)).
- Assess for all possible co-morbid psychiatric conditions, and treat per clinical judgment.
- Develop a team-approach treatment plan using problem solving skills for the child, and family/parent intervention strategies, such as:
  - Reducing positive reinforcement of disruptive behaviors.
  - Increasing reinforcement of prosocial and compliant behavior, using positive reinforcement (e.g., parental attention), and fair and specific punishment (e.g., time out, loss of tokens, and/or loss of privileges).
  - Apply consequences and/or punishment for disruptive behavior.
  - Parental responses are predictable, contingent, and immediate.

Medication usage

- General guidelines: Medication should only be used in combination with psychotherapeutic interventions (use alone is typically *not* effective). Therapeutic alliance with close monitoring is essential. Avoid polypharmacy. If one choice is ineffective, switch classes before adding more medication (see end of chapter for tips on medication management).

- Medication Choice:
  - Medications should be adjunctive to psychotherapeutic treatment. Treatment of co-morbid ADHD symptoms may help with ODD symptoms (see ADHD treatment 📖 *pp. 700–705* and end of chapter).
    - If ODD symptoms are more similar to CD (e.g., highly aggressive), may consider treatment strategies used in CD (see next section)
  - Use least restrictive setting and monitor closely for safety to self and others. Occasionally, more intensive treatment (e.g., day programs, hospitalization, out-of-home placement) may be required. Programs such as boot camps or incarceration are felt to only worsen behaviors, and generally are not recommended.

Outcome

In general 67% do not meet criteria after three years; About 30% continue on to conduct disorder (CD), and 10% continue from there to antisocial personality disorder (ASPD). Earlier onset ODD has a worse prognosis than later onset ODD. Co-morbidities seen more as age increases, and include ADHD (most common), anxiety, and mood disorders. ADHD plus ODD results in worse outcomes, and may facilitate the transition to CD.

DSM-IV-TR Oppositional Defiant Disorder

- A pattern of negativistic, hostile, and defiant behavior lasting at least six months, during which four (or more) of the following are present:
  - Often loses temper.
  - Often argues with adults.
  - Often actively defies or refuses to comply with adults' requests or rules.
  - Often deliberately annoys people.
  - Often blames others for his or her mistakes or misbehavior.
  - Is often touchy or easily annoyed by others
  - Is often angry and resentful
  - Is often spiteful or vindictive.

Note: Consider a criterion met only if the behavior occurs more frequently than is typically observed in individuals of comparable age and developmental level.

- The disturbance in behavior causes clinically significant impairment in social, academic, or occupational functioning.
- The behaviors do not occur exclusively during the course of a psychotic or mood disorder.
- Criteria are not met for CD, and, if the individual is age 18 years or older, criteria are not met for antisocial personality disorder.

Conduct disorder[1,2]

Key features

Conduct disorder (CD) is sometimes referred to as "sociopathy", though this term is rarely used in psychiatry. By definition, CD is a repetitive and persistent pattern of behavior in which the basic rights of others or major age-appropriate societal norms or rules are violated. These violations include aggression or cruelty to people and animals, destruction of property, deceitfulness or theft and serious violation of rules (e.g., truanting or running away). Early sexual behavior, gang involvement, low self-esteem and lack of empathy are also seen. The term "delinquent" is unfashionable and refers to the individual whose behavior leads them into the criminal justice system—"young offender" is the modern term.

CD is important because it is common: it is the cause of great suffering in both the individual and in society; it is a risk factor for adult antisocial behavior; and it is a major burden on public resources. In many countries it constitutes one of the major public mental health problems, making prevention strategies important.

Epidemiology

In North America, CD is a common reason for psychiatric evaluation in children and adolescents. It has an earlier onset and is more common in boys than in girls.

Etiology

A family history of antisocial behavior or substance abuse, possible low CSF serotonin, impaired executive function, high sensation seeking, and diminished conditioning to punishment, low IQ, and brain injury are biological factors associated with risk for CD. Psychosocial risk factors include: parental criminality and substance abuse; harsh and inconsistent parenting; domestic chaos and violence; large family size; low socio-economic status and poverty; early loss and deprivation; lack of a warm parental relationship; school failure; social isolation; and exposure to abuse and societal violence.

Co-morbidity

ADHD; substance abuse; suicidality.

Course and outcome

CD is often chronic and challenging to treat. Adult outcomes include: antisocial personality disorder, criminal activity, substance abuse, and mental disorders. However, less than 50% of CD cases have severe and persistent antisocial problems as adults.

Predictors of poor outcome

Early onset (before 10 yrs), low IQ, poor school achievement, attentional problems and hyperactivity, family criminal history, low socioeconomic status, other siblings with conduct disorder, and poor parenting.

Protective factors
Female gender, high intelligence, resilient temperament, competence at a skill, warm relationship with a key adult, commitment to social values, strong and stable community institutions, increased economic status.

Assessment

- Clarify the purpose of the assessment (clinical, community, forensic).
- Obtain a full history with collateral from school, community, legal system.
- Identify causal risk and protective factors.
- Assess for co-morbidity and make a diagnosis (psychometric testing).
- Formulate the problem and establish management plan.

Management[3]

Multiple strategies are indicated:
- Ensure the safety of the child.
- CBT problem-solving skills—in individual/group setting.
- Parent management training—to improve social exchanges/stability.
- Functional family therapy—combined CBT/systems approach.
- Multisystemic therapy—family–based, including school and community.
- Medication—use only for co-morbid disorders (e.g., ADHD).
- Academic and social support—referral to relevant agencies/groups.
- Some use neuroleptics or lithium to manage extreme aggression.

Prevention strategies and policy implications

- Preschool child development programs—identifying parents and families at risk and instituting home visits and support.
- School programs—identify children at risk and institute classroom enrichment, home visits, and parent and teacher training.
- Community programs—identify children and adolescents through their involvement with social agencies and institute interventions such as enhanced recreation programs, parent training and adult mentoring of youth.
- Social and economic restructuring to reduce poverty and to improve family and community stability.

DSM-IV-TR diagnostic criteria for CD

- A repetitive and persistent pattern of behavior in which the basic rights of others or major age-appropriate societal norms or rules are violated, as manifested by the presence of three (or more) of the following criteria in the past 12 months, with at least one criterion present in the past 6 months:

Aggression to people and animals
  - Often bullies, threatens, or intimidates others.
  - Often initiates physical fights.
  - Has used a weapon that can cause serious physical harm to others (e.g., a bat, brick, broken bottle, knife, gun).
  - Has been physically cruel to people.
  - Has been physically cruel to animals.
  - Has stolen while confronting a victim (e.g., mugging, purse snatching, extortion, armed robbery).
  - Has forced someone into sexual activity.

Destruction of property
  - Has deliberately engaged in fire setting with the intention of causing serious damage.
  - Has deliberately destroyed others' property (other than by fire setting).

Deceitfulness or theft
  - Has broken into someone else's house, building, or car.
  - Often lies to obtain goods or favors or to avoid obligations (i.e., "cons" others).
  - Has stolen items of nontrivial value without confronting a victim (e.g., shoplifting, but without breaking and entering; forgery).

Serious violations of rules
  - Often stays out at night despite parental prohibitions, beginning before age 13 years.
  - Has run away from home overnight at least twice while living in parental or parental surrogate home (or once without returning for a lengthy period).
  - Is often truant from school, beginning before age 13 years.
- The disturbance in behavior causes clinically significant impairment in social, academic, or occupational functioning.
- If the individual is age 18 years or older, criteria are not met for antisocial personality disorder.

Specify type based on age at onset: childhood-onset (before 10), adolescent-onset type (after 10)

Specify severity: mild, moderate, severe.

Recommended further reading

1 Bassarath, L. (2001). Conduct disorder: a biopsychosocial review. *Can J Psychiatry* **46**, 609–616.
2 Waddell, C., Lipman, E., Offord, D. (1999). Conduct disorder: practice parameters for assessment, treatment, and prevention. *Can J Psychiatry* **44**(supp 2), 35s–39s.
3 Kazdin, A.E. (2000). Treatments for aggressive and antisocial children. *Child Adolesc Psych Clinics N America* **9**, 841–858.

Pervasive developmental disorders

Pervasive developmental disorders (PDDs) are defined as spectrum of behavioral problems commonly associated with autism. In fact, "autism spectrum disorders" (ASD) is often used interchangeably with PDD. PDD frequently involve a triad of deficits in *social skills*, *communication/language* and *behavior*. The feature they all have in common is difficulty with social behavior. DSV-IV-TR categorizes PDDs as follows:

- Autistic disorder.
- Asperger's disorder.
- Rett's syndrome.
- Childhood disintegrative disorder.
- PDD-NOS.

PDDs are characterized by either lack of normal development of skills or loss of already acquired skills. There is a gender bias with male > female predominance in all syndromes except Rett's syndrome (female predominance). Prevalence of PDDs ranges from 40–60 cases/10,000, though reports vary.

Assessment of pervasive developmental disorders

The American Academy of Child and Adolescent Psychiatry recommends a multidisciplinary approach involving psychiatrists, psychologists, pediatricians, neurologists, speech therapists, occupational therapists and primary care teams. The efforts of various specialists and consultants should be coordinated and one care provider assumes an overall role as coordinator and liaison with schools and other providers of interventions.

The assessment should include:

- Complete psychiatric assessment that will vary depending on the child's age, history, and previous evaluations. Assessment should include:
  - Pregnancy, neonatal, and developmental history.
  - Medical history.
  - Family and psychosocial factors.
  - Intervention history.
  - Psychiatric examination of the child in observational settings to evaluate overall developmental level and specific problem behaviors.
- Medical examination.
- Neurologic examination including complete audiological and visual examinations and taking a seizure history.
- Diagnostic and laboratory studies; There is no specific laboratory test for autism, but specific studies to search for associated conditions are indicated based on history and clinical presentation. EEG and perhaps MRI, Southern blot testing for Fragile X genetic and Wood's lamp examination for tuberous sclerosis are indicated. The presence of dysmorphic features or other specific findings may suggest obtaining genetic screening for inherited metabolic disorders, specific genetic syndromes, or chromosome analysis.
- Psychological assessment.
  - Developmental/intelligence testing separate estimates of verbal and nonverbal (performance) IQ should be obtained.

- Adaptive skills; Assessment of adaptive skills to document the presence of any associated mental retardation to establish priorities for treatment.
- Other assessments; PDD-specific neuropsychological screening and/or achievement testing may be needed. Examples:
  - Autism Diagnostic Interview-Revised (ADI-R).
  - Autism Diagnostic Observation Schedule (ADOS).
  - Autism Behavior Checklists (ABC).
  - Childhood Autism Rating Scales (CARS).
  - Checklist for Autism in Toddlers (CHAT).
  - Speech-Language-Communication Assessments.
  - Occupational and Physical Therapy Assessments.
- Psycho-education and family and parental support. To the extent possible, involve parents and other family members in the process of assessment. Various parent and family support groups are available and can provide important sources of information and support to parents.
  - National Alliance for Autism Research: http://www.naar.org/
  - International Rett Syndrome Association: http://www.rettsyndrome.org/
  - Childhood Disintegrative Disorder Network: http://www.rarediseases.org/
  - Autism Society of America: http://www.autism-society.org/
  - Aspen of America, Inc. (Asperger's syndrome): http://www.maapservices.org/
  - Cure Autism Now: http://www.cureautismnow.org/
- Differential diagnosis: Other PDDs; childhood schizophrenia; MR; language disorders; neurological disorders (Landau-Klefner syndrome); sensory impairment (deafness or blindness); OCD; psychosocial deprivation.

PDD assessment summary

- Differential diagnosis: childhood schizophrenia; mental retardation; language disorders; neurological disorders; sensory impairment (deafness or blindness); OCD; psychosocial deprivation; reactive attachment disorders.
- A multidisciplinary approach is required, potentially involving a psychiatrist, psychologist, pediatrician, neurologist, speech therapist, occupational therapist, and school team.
- Full clinical evaluation: including physical and mental state as well as specific developmental, psychometric, and educational assessments.
- Possible genetics consultation for fragile X, Rett's (in females), or other genetic disorders.
- Simple rating scales: Autism Behavior Checklist (ABC); Childhood Autism Rating Scales (CARS). In-depth studies: Autism Diagnostic Interview-Revised (ADI-R); Autism Diagnostic Observation Schedule (ADOS).

Autism

History/definition/clinical features

John Haslam in 1809 and Henry Maudsley in 1867 were the first physicians to provide descriptions of children with the clinical features of autism. Leo Kanner named the disorder infantile autism in 1943. Autistic disorder is the prototype of the PDDs defined by qualitative impairments in social interaction, communication and restricted and stereotyped patterns of behavior, interests and activities. Onset of the disorder may be evident by 18 months and to meet the diagnosis must occur before 3 years of age. 30% of autistic children score in the normal intelligence range (high-functioning autism, HFA). About 30% have mild to moderate mental retardation and about 40% have serious to profound mental retardation.

DSM-IV-TR autism criteria

According to DSM-IV-TR criteria, children with autism have to have a total of at least **six** of the following symptoms before age three, with specific numbers from each the three broad categories:
- At least **two** symptoms of **abnormal social relatedness**:
    - impaired nonverbal interactive behaviors (e.g., poor eye contact, inappropriate facial expressions and gestures).
    - failure to develop peer relationships.
    - reduced interest in shared enjoyment.
    - lack of social or emotional reciprocity.
- At least **one** symptom of **abnormal communication or play**:
    - Delayed or lack of spoken language.
    - Difficulty initiating or sustaining conversations.
    - Stereotypic, repetitive, or idiosyncratic language.
    - Lack of imaginative or imitative play.
- At least **one** symptom of **abnormal behaviors**:
    - Stereotyped/restricted, obsessive interests.
    - Rigid adherence to non-functional routines or rituals.
    - Stereotypic/repetitive motor mannerisms (e.g., toe-walking, hand flapping, body rocking).
    - Preoccupation with parts of objects.

Abnormal symbolic or social play or restricted interests or activities

These encompass unusual preoccupations and interests; lack of developmentally appropriate fantasy; adherence to nonfunctional routines or rituals; resistance to change; stereotypies and motor mannerisms (e.g., hand or finger-flapping or body-rocking); and preoccupation with parts of objects.

There are some nonspecific neurological and physiological features that are common to autism, but are not essential or specific features of the disorder, such as seizure disorder, motor tics, large head circumference, abnormal gaze monitoring, increased ambidexterity, hyper- and hyposensitivity to sensory stimuli (loud or high pitched sounds, specific textures, bright lights), abnormal pain and temperature sensation, and altered immune function.

Autistic children also often demonstrate associated, but nonspecific behavioral problems such as poor attention and concentration (60%), hyperactivity (40%), morbid or unusual preoccupations (43–88%), obsessive phenomena (7%), compulsive rituals, anxiety and fear (17–74%), mood lability, irritability, agitation, inappropriate affect (9–44%), sleep problems (11%), or self-injurious behaviors (24–43%).

"**Savants**": persons with obvious mental retardation who exhibit unusually high skill in sharply circumscribed areas, such as visual arts, musical performance, arithmetic skills (calendar calculating, prime numbers). Studies by Hill and Rimland suggest that 0.6% of institutionalized individuals with MR and 9.8% of mentally retarded autistic individuals demonstrate savant skills.

Epidemiology

In 2007 a CDC surveillance network found that an average of 6.7 per 1,000 8-year-olds in 2002 had autism spectrum disorders (ASDs), including pervasive developmental disorder (PDD) and Asperger syndrome. The ratio of males to females with ASDs ranged from roughly 3:1 to roughly 7:1. Autism occurs equally across various races and socioeconomic statuses. At one time, it was more widely diagnosed in higher socioeconomic groups, probably due to referral biases[1].

Etiology

The cause of autism is unknown but it is thought to be a disorder of genetic origins, with a heritability of about 90% with as few as 2 and as many as 15+ genes involved. Neurocognitive studies suggest lack of connectivity may explain many of the cognitive and emotional deficits. Syndromic autism is seen at high rates in various genetic disorders (Tuberous sclerosis, Fragile X, 15q11–q13 duplications, Down syndrome and single gene disorders of metabolism such as adenylate lyase deficiency). However, environmental influences are also important, as concordance in monozygotic twins is less than 100% (36–91% monozygotic twins concordance v. 10% dizygotic twins concordance) and the phenotypic expression of the disorder varies widely. Environmental factors include pre/post-natal infections agents (congenital rubella, CMV), chemical toxins (thimerasol), autoimmune disorders (MMR- anecdotal, not proven), obstetric complications.

Neuropathology

Neuropathology studies show increased cell packing in the limbic system, reduced numbers of Purkinje cells in the cerebellum, age-related changes in the cerebellar nuclei and inferior olives, cortical dysgenesis, and increased brain size, especially in the young autistic child (as measured by head circumference), magnetic resonance image (MRI) brain volume, and postmortem brain weight. Seizures are common.

Neurochemistry

One-third of autistic subjects have elevated whole blood serotonin [5-HT]. Other neurotransmitters (dopamine [DA], norepinephrine, [NE], glutamate, gamma-aminobutyric acid, [GABA]) and neuropeptides (oxytocin, secretin, beta-endorphins) have been implicated, but the evidence is not as reproducible.

Other developmental disorders

Asperger's disorder
History/definition/clinical features
Asperger's disorder is a neurodevelopmental disorder on the autism spectrum, which involves impairments in reciprocal social interactions and restricted repetitive and stereotyped patterns of behavior in the absence of intellectual dysfunction or clinically significant general delay in language. The incidence of Asperger's disorder is conservatively estimated at 2.6/10,000, though this figure varies by source.

High-functioning autism and Asperger's disorder are autism spectrum disorders characterized by cognitive impairments affecting social relatedness and communication, restricted interests/repetitive behaviors, and average or better intelligence. According to the American Psychiatric Association, Asperger's disorder is differentiated from high-functioning autism by the presence of intact basic language and imaginative play abilities.

Rett's disorder
Rett's disorder was first reported on by the Viennese pediatrician Andreas Rett in 1966. A genetic X-linked disorder largely affecting females (7 cases are known to exist in males) with an estimated incidence of 3.8/10,000 based on British Isles survey. There is a period of normal development for the first 5–6 months of life. Head circumference at birth is normal with subsequent deceleration of head growth leading to post-natal microcephaly followed by loss of acquired skills such as purposeful hand function, vocalization, and communication skills, loss of social engagement early in the course (although often social interaction develops later) and appearance of truncal and gait ataxia. Mutations in the MECP2 gene (methyl CpG binding protein 2 gene, Xq 28) account for 80% of patients with classic Rett's disorder. Supportive diagnostic criteria include breathing dysfunction, EEG abnormalities (up to 80% of patients experience epileptic episodes), spasticity, peripheral vasomotor disturbance, scoliosis, and growth retardation. In addition to classic Rett's disorder, some variants have been described presenting some features of the classic form, but displaying differences. Mutations in the X-linked CDKL5 gene (cyclin-dependent kinase-like 5, Xq22) were found in some patients with Rett's disorder variant.

Childhood disintegrative disorder (CDD)
CDD was first described as dementia infantilis by Theodor Heller a Viennese remedial educator in 1908. CDD is defined in DSM-IV as apparent normal development at least until age two followed by clinically significant loss of previously acquired skills (before age 10) in at least two areas: language (expressive or receptive), social skills or adaptive behavior, bowel or bladder control, play, and motor skills. In addition, patients have abnormalities of functioning in at least two of the following areas: qualitative impairment in social interaction by marked regression resulting in autistic features, qualitative impairment in communication or repetitive, restricted and stereotyped behaviors and mentally retarded state (severe to profound MR >60% with IQ<40). Association of seizures or EEG abnormalities has

been documented in about half the cases of CDD (seizures most commonly develop after the onset of CDD). Associated behavioral symptomalogy includes overactivity, affective symptoms/anxiety, deterioration of self-help skills, aggression, agitation, self-injurious behavior, fecal smearing with compulsive behavior. Deterioration in social and self-help skills is more marked than motor skills. The cause is unknown and prognosis poor. Incidence is estimated at 0.2/10,000. Males outnumber females by 4:1. Mean age of onset of 3.36 years. Two types of onset have been seen. More commonly onset is insidious developing over weeks to months and less common over days to weeks.

Pervasive developmental disorder not otherwise specified (PDD-NOS)

Also known as "Atypical autism" this category is used when there is a severe and pervasive impairment in the development of reciprocal social interaction associated with impairment in either verbal or nonverbal communication skills or with the presence of stereotyped behavior, interests and activities, but does not meet criteria for other PDDs, schizophrenia, schizotypal personality disorder, or avoidant personality disorder. Incidence is estimated at PDD-NOS 20.8/10,0000 with a male predominance.

Treatment of pervasive developmental disorders

> **Treatment strategies for PDDs: summary**
>
> - Educational and vocational interventions: most will be eligible for individualized educational plan with accommodations and services to address their special needs.
> - Behavioral interventions: include behavior modification, social skills training, and CBT methods.
> - Family interventions: educational, support, advocacy.
> - Speech and language therapy, occupational therapy.
> - Pharmacotherapy: symptom management, e.g., atypical antipsychotics for stereotypies and aggressive agitation; SSRIs or clomipramine for compulsive and self-harming behaviors, depression/anxiety; stimulants for ADHD symptoms.
> - Treat medical conditions (e.g., epilepsy).

Behavioral treatment

Behavioral/psycho-educational interventions have been used to treat the core symptom features of autism in the realms of communication and social interaction.

- Applied Behavioral Analysis (ABA). A strategy for developing social skills based on the idea that rewarded behaviors will be repeated.
- Treatment and Education of Autistic and Related Communication of Handicapped Children (TEACCH). Structured teaching approach that uses the child's visual and rote memory strengths to improve communication, social and coping skills.
- Picture Exchange Communication System (PECS). Helps nonverbal children express themselves, reduces maladaptive behaviors.
- Play therapy—counseling to help children express themselves through toys.
- Social stories—an intervention to address behavior difficulties.
- Sensory integration—provides controlled sensory input with the goal increased adaptive behaviors/responses and less agitation.
- Speech therapy—teaches how to communicate more effectively— how to hold a conversation, thinking about what the other person in a conversation understands and believes, and tuning in to the meta-linguistic signals of the other person.

Pharmacotherapy

Specific forms of medication treatment have been shown to produce significant improvements in problem behaviors associated with autism in double blind placebo-controlled trials in autistic patients.

- Anxiety symptoms, repetitive behaviors as seen in patients who have obsessions or compulsions, self-injurious behaviors, and perhaps social avoidance/withdrawal have been significantly reduced with the use of

SSRIs (fluoxetine, sertraline, clomipramine, fluvoxamine) and atypical antidepressants (mirtazapine and venlafaxine).
- Neuroleptics have been shown to reduce irritability, hyperactivity (risperidone), aggression (haloperidol low doses and risperidone).
- Stimulants, NMDA antagonists, and alpha-2 noradrenergic receptor agonists have been shown to decrease hyperactivity and inattention (methylphenidate, amantadine, clonidine).

The sometimes exquisite sensitivity of patients who have autism requires careful initiation, titration, and monitoring of any psychopharmacologic/pharmacologic treatments. Treatment of associated disorders such as epilepsy and GI problems should also be carefully monitored.

In 2006, the U.S. FDA approved risperidone for the treatment of irritability associated with autistic disorder, including symptoms of aggression toward others, deliberate self-injuriousness, temper tantrums, and quickly changing moods, in children and adolescents ages 5 to 16 years. This was the first time the FDA has approved any medication for use in children and adolescents with autism.

Language and learning disorders (LLDs)[1]

LLDs comprise a very common set of problems, with estimates that as many as 10% to 20% of children and adolescents have a language and/or learning disorder. The diagnoses of mental retardation, motor skills disorder, ADHD, mood disorder, anxiety disorder and medical/neurological primary diagnosis (e.g., fetal alcohol syndrome, prenatal substance abuse, fragile X syndrome) should be considered since they may be concurrent with or mistaken for speech, language, or learning disorders.

DSM-IV groups together a number of LLDs that share the following criteria:
- Performance is significantly below that expected for IQ or age.
- A discrete developmental disability in the absence of MR.
- Commonly presents as school refusal, emotional or behavioral problems.
- Fifty percent have co-morbid psychiatric disorder and/or other LLDs.
- Most show strong evidence of heritability.

Reading disorder (dyslexia)

Difficulty with reading, in most cases involving a deficit in phonological-processing skills. 4% of school-age children (range 2–10%). Male predominance. There is often a family history of dyslexia. Familial risk to first-degree relatives has been found to be between 35% and 45%, compared with the population risk of 3% to 10%. Mapped to genes and specific neurobiological profile, with associated interventions proposed by Shaywitz.[2]

20% have co-morbid ADHD or CD. Management includes 1:1 remedial teaching and parent involvement improves long-term outcome.

Disorder of written expression

Often coexists with dyslexia and manifests as difficulties with spelling, syntax, grammar, and composition. Occurs in 2–8% of school-age children with a 3:1 male predominance. Difficulties may first emerge with the shift from narrative to expository writing assignments.

Mathematics disorder

Female predominance and occurs in 1–6% of school-age children. Often associated with visuo-spatial deficits and attributed to right parietal dysfunction. Family members (e.g., parents and siblings) of children with mathematics disorder are 10 times more likely to be diagnosed with mathematics disorder than are members of the general population.

Communication disorders

Includes expressive and receptive language disorders, phonological disorder and stuttering.

Expressive language disorder

This is diagnosed when scores from standardized tests measure delays in expressive language, not due to sensory or motor deficit or environmental deprivation and in excess of delays expected based on scores of nonverbal intelligence and receptive language abilities. The difficulties with expressive language interfere with academic or occupational achievement. Approximately 3% to 5% of children have a developmental expressive language disorder.

Mixed receptive-expressive language disorder

This is diagnosed when scores from standardized tests measure delays in both receptive and expressive language, not due to sensory or motor deficit or environmental deprivation and in excess of delays expected based on scores of nonverbal intelligence abilities. The difficulties with receptive and expressive language interfere with academic or occupational achievement. Prevalence of either a developmental expressive or receptive language disorder ranges from 1% to 13% of the population.

Phonological disorder

This is defined as a failure to develop expected speech sounds appropriate for age and dialect that compromises academic/occupational achievement or social communication. The deficit is out of proportion to MR, sensory deficits or environmental deprivation, if present. Prevalence of phonological disorder ranges from 1% to more than 20%.

Stuttering

This is defined as a disturbance in the normal fluency or time pattern of speech. Persons who stutter usually struggle with the initial syllables of multisyllabic words. Onset is usually between the age of three and six years of age with a male predominance of 3:1. Rates of natural, unassisted recovery are about 75%. Majority of cases are developmental, but may be acquired (e.g., head injury). Etiology is thought to be genetic, due to incomplete cerebral dominance and/or hyperdopaminergic state. Management utilizes speech therapy, and sometimes medication, such as antipsychotics (e.g., risperidone) or SSRIs.

Recommended further reading

1 AACAP (1998). Practice parameters for the assessment and treatment of children and adolescents with language and learning disorders. *J Am Acad Child Adolesc Psychiatry* **37**(10 supp), 46s–62s.
2 Shaywitz, S.M. *Overcoming Dyslexia: A New and Complete Science-Based Program for Reading Problems at Any Level.* New York: Vintage Press, 2005. http://www.childrenofthecode.org/

Elimination disorders—enuresis

DSM-IV-TR diagnostic criteria for enuresis

- Repeated voiding of urine into bed or clothes (whether involuntary or intentional).
- The behavior is clinically significant as manifested by either a frequency of **twice a week** for at **least three consecutive** months or the presence of clinically significant distress or impairment in social, academic (occupational), or other important areas of functioning.
- Chronological age is at least **five years** (or equivalent developmental level).
- The behavior is not due exclusively to the direct physiological effect of a substance (e.g., a diuretic) or a general medical condition (e.g., diabetes, spina bifida, a seizure disorder).

Specify type: nocturnal only, diurnal only, nocturnal and diurnal.

Prevalence

Reported to be 5–15% of 5-year-olds, with 15% remission rate/year every year after, and 1–2% by teen/adult years. Episodes are usually involuntary, occur at night, and are more common in males than females. Enuresis can result in low self-esteem and often becomes a focus for family conflict.

Subtypes

Nocturnal only (most common), diurnal only, nocturnal and diurnal.

Etiology

Genetic: 75% have a family history of enuresis. Other: generalized developmental delay; incomplete potty training; psychosocial stressors (e.g., birth of a sibling, hospitalization, starting school, domestic conflict); co-morbid psychopathology (e.g., depression); organic causes.

Work-up

For nocturnal enuresis: use general medical evaluation (including personal and family history, physical, height/weight chart, urinalysis and abdominal exam) to rule out UTI, neurological problems, diabetes mellitus, seizure, and drug side-effects. Consider abdominal x-ray to rule out constipation. After age eight, and with any diurnal component, strongly consider urological referral.

Management

Behavioral modification is the first-line treatment and includes restricting fluids at night, scheduling toileting times prior to bed, behavioral management (star charts without or without other rewards), night-lifting, bell and pad technique, bladder training:

- Often helpful to implement bowel regimen (see encopresis section 📖 p. 724).

- Pharmacological intervention: use only if behavioral treatment fails
  - DDAVP (desmopressin), which is less anticholinergic than imipramine and does not exacerbate constipation.
  - Imipramine: A TCA. Works due to anticholinergic effect by increasing sphincter tone. 80% have some improvements but tolerance may develop after six weeks.
  - Other pharmacologic intervention available, but mostly utilized by pediatric urologists.

Clinical pearl

Remember to get an EKG because of potential cardiac implications of tricyclic antidepressants; also weigh benefits and risks because of risk of death with overdose and/or cardiac side-effects.

Encopresis

> **DSM-IV-TR diagnostic criteria for encopresis**
>
> - Repeated passage of feces into inappropriate places (e.g., clothing or floor) whether involuntary or intentional.
> - At least **one** such event **a month** for at least **three months**.
> - Chronological age is **at least four years** (or equivalent developmental level).
> - The behavior is not due exclusively to the direct physiological effects of a substance (e.g., laxatives) or a general medical condition except through a mechanism involving constipation.
>
> Code with or without constipation and overflow incontinence.

The DSM criteria are probably physiologically irrelevant. Episodes are almost always involuntary.

Prevalence
1–3% of children five year old and older. Most encopresis has resolved by adolescence. More common in males than females.

Subtypes
With or without constipation and overflow incontinence.

Etiology
May be caused or related to fecal withholding due to pain, power struggle, inattention to bowel needs, oppositionality, or physiological problem. Up to 95% involves some form of fecal constipation. Hirshprung's disease rarely cause of encopresis. Often related to ADHD.

Work-up
Medical history to rule out neurologic problems, drug side-effects, nutritional problems, and Hirschsprung's disease. History of frequency and form of stools is essential. Physical exam with complete abdominal exam, rectal exam, and abdominal X ray usually sufficient.

Management
Utilize fiber, water, and laxative to promote consistent soft stools. Can become increasingly aggressive with laxative use in order to promote *complete* bowel clean-out if initial conservative efforts are not effective. Educate parents and child in order to minimize embarrassment and family conflict. Consistent behavioral approach to toileting and soiling can be helpful, no matter what the cause. Parent should reward stool in the toilet, as opposed to clean underwear.

Disorders of eating, sleeping and thriving

Sleep problems

Complaints about difficulty initiating or maintaining sleep are common. Although organic pathology can be the cause of sleep problems at any age, frequent problems prior to age three are most likely due to immaturity and/or environment and can be corrected by working with parents on consistent interactional patterns around bedtime. After age three, psychiatric pathology can be considered, although environment is the most likely cause, with physiologic problems in a far second place. The clinician should have a low threshold for considering oppositionality or "bedtime resistance" for complaints between ages three and five. After five years of age, the clinician should consider all the above, but with increasing consideration of mental health concerns if the sleep problem is impairing and associated with other peer, school, or family difficulties. It is also important to consider formal sleep problems, such as sleep apnea, sleep walking, sleep terrors, nightmare disorder, and narcolepsy. Adolescents have an increased difficulty falling asleep due to a shift in their circadian rhythm, although they may present to the clinician with a parental complaint of oversleeping, since their overall need for sleep does not decrease.

Clinical pearl

Behavioral interventions around bedtime and sleep hygiene cure most sleep problems.

Make questions about sleep part of your routine exam. Be certain to include questions about napping, especially in adolescent patients (see Chapter 11 📖 p. 469).

Sleep disorders

Classified as for adult sleep disorders. The main syndromes that manifest in children and adolescents are: nightmare disorder; sleep terror disorder; and sleepwalking disorder. Management is the same as for adults. Refer to Chapter 11 for more details.

Motor skills disorder/developmental coordination disorder

There are a number of conditions affecting children where the primary problem involves an impairment of motor function. This may manifest as a delay in developmental milestones and includes impairments of coordination, fine motor skills, and gross movement. Gross motor impairments suggest genetic etiology while fine motor impairments suggest environmental causation. Treatment involves physiotherapy, occupational therapy, and educational assistance.

Failure to thrive

Evaluation for physiological or developmental problems is imperative. It is important to correct any nutritional deficiency as soon as possible in order to prevent negative impact on development.

Clinical pearl

Refeeding alone is not adequate, since failure to thrive is often related to either a primary or secondary failure of the feeding process.

Obesity

Severe overeating is a behavioral phenotype associated with some genetic and behavioral conditions. In addition, medications such as mood stabilizers and antipsychotics are associated with dyslipidemia and obesity. As such, weight parameters should be monitored in all children.

Feeding and eating disorders of infancy and early childhood[1]

Pica

This is a common condition where there is persistent (>1month) **eating of non-nutritive substances** at a developmentally inappropriate age (>1.5 yrs). Common substances are: dirt, clay, stones, hair, feces, plastic, paper, wood, string, etc. It is particularly common in individuals with developmental disabilities and may be dangerous or life threatening depending on the substance ingested. Consequences may include toxicity, infection, or GI ulceration/obstruction. Typically occurs during second and third years of life, although young pregnant women may exhibit pica during pregnancy. Hypothesized causes include: nutritional deficiencies; cultural factors (e.g., clay); psychosocial stress; malnutrition and hunger; brain disorders (e.g., hypothalamic problem).

Rumination

This is the voluntary or involuntary **regurgitation and re-chewing** of partially digested food. Occurs within a few minutes post-prandial and may last 1–2 hrs. Regurgitation appears effortless and is preceded by belching. Typical onset 3–6 months of age, may persist for several months and then spontaneously remit. Also occurs in older individuals with MR. May result in weight loss, halitosis, dental decay, aspiration, recurrent RTI, and sometimes asphyxiation and death (5–10% of cases). Causes include: MR; GI pathology; psychiatric disorders; psychosocial stress. Treatment includes physical examination and investigations; behavioral methods; nutritional advice.

Eating disorders: anorexia nervosa and bulimia nervosa

Occur mostly in females, with a typical onset around age 15–19 (although onset is by no means is limited to this age range). Treatment is challenging, and with very high relapse rates. Assessment, Diagnosis, and treatment is similar in adolescents and adults. (see 📖 *pp. 450–461*).

Recommended further reading

1 Ellis, C.R. and Schnoes, C.J. (2002). www.emedicine.com

Attachment disorders

Attachment

May be defined as the organization of behaviors in the young child that are designed to achieve physical proximity to a preferred caregiver at times when the child seeks comfort, support, nurturance, or protection. According to AACAP Practice Parameters, preferred attachment appears in the latter part of the first year of life as evidenced by the appearance of separation protest and stranger wariness. John Bowlby described the formation of healthy secure attachment from early infancy, as well as a normal pattern of separation anxiety commencing between 6 and 9 months, peaking between 12 and 18 months and decreasing during the third year. Its developmental course appears to be the same across cultures and is the same for infants who are in day care, raised in nuclear families, or reared in larger social groups.[1] Infants become attached to caregivers with whom they have had significant amounts of interaction and lack of attachment to a specific attachment figure is exceedingly rare in reasonably responsive caregiving environments; signs of reactive attachement disorder (RAD) are not typically reported in the absence of serious neglect.

Ethology and attachment

The history of attachment theory is closely allied to the development of ethology, the study of animal behavior in its natural environment. Konrad Lorenz (an Austrian doctor) and Nico Tinbergen (a Dutch biologist) are recognized as the fathers of ethology, and shared the Nobel Prize in 1973 for their contributions to the field. Some of their most important discoveries were the identification of imprinting, fixed action patterns (FAPs), and innate releasing mechanisms (IRMs)—all of which have informed the understanding of infant attachment behavior. Lorenz classically described imprinting in ducklings and Greylag goslings, the phenomenon where young animals form an immediate and irreversible social bond with the first moving object they encounter. The phenomena of FAPs and IRMs were first observed in the herring gull and the stickleback, and formed a basis for understanding the complex innate mechanisms that facilitate mother-infant bonding during the first weeks.

During the 1950s and 1960s, John Bowlby and Margaret Ainsworth used ethological principles to study the formation of healthy and abnormal attachment in children. Ainsworth developed the Strange Situation Procedure, an experiment that she used in several cultural settings to establish universal patterns of attachment. Healthy attachment was classically described as "secure," while "insecure" attachment encompassed "anxious," "resistant," and "avoidant" types. These latter concepts are recognized in contemporary nomenclature under the diagnoses "separation anxiety disorder" and "reactive attachment disorder". Bowlby also coined the term "critical period" to describe the stage during which the infant is most responsive to developing secure attachment.

Reactive attachment disorder of infancy and early childhood (RAD)

Prolonged hospitalizations of the child, extreme poverty, or parental inexperience may predispose to the development of pathologic care, but grossly pathological care does not always result in the development of RAD. Persistence of RAD is exceedingly rare in children adopted out of institutions into more normative care environments and there are no data compatible with the idea that there is a critical period for attachment formation.

Key features

Early onset of markedly disturbed and developmentally inappropriate social relatedness across contexts that begins before age five. RAD is the result of "pathogenic care", and is distinguishable from PDD (RAD is not diagnosed when PDD is present), and may manifest as either **inhibited** or **disinhibited** subtypes. Pathogenic care is evidenced by either persistent disregard of child's basic emotional needs or phsycial needs, or repeated changes of primary caregiver that prevent formation of stable attachements.

Epidemiology

Estimated prevalence is less than 1%. The prevalence is suggested to be from 30% to 40% in foster care.

Symptoms

Excessively inhibited, hypervigilant, or highly ambivalent and contradictory responses such as avoidance or resistance to comforting or frozen watch-fulness in inhibited type. Excessive familiarity with relative strangers or lack of selectivity in choice of attachment figures in disinhibited type. Older children may present with peer problems or superficial connection to others.

Differential

MR; PDD; ADHD, CD, ODD; LD; social phobia; PTSD.

Assessment

Detailed history and direct observation of the child in the context of his/her relationships with primary caregivers.

Management

Therapy that focuses on establishing an attachment relationship with the child and ameliorating disturbed attachment relationships with caregivers. Coercive treatments (e.g., holding therapy, rebirthing) are potentially dangerous and not recommended.

Recommended further reading

1 Haugaard J.J. and Hazan C. (2004). Recognizing and treating uncommon behavioral and emotional disorders in children and adolescents who have been severely maltreated: reactive attachment disorder. *Child maltreatment* **9**: 154–160.

Anxiety disorders—overview[1,2]

Anxiety and fear are an inherent part of the human condition and in times of danger are often adaptive. As a result of changing developmental and cognitive abilities during childhood, the content of normal fears and anxieties shifts from concerns about concrete external things to abstract internalized anxieties. Anxiety disorders are characterized by excessive anxiety or worry causing significant distress and/or impairment in functioning and their relative prevalence reflects this shift in content. Thus specific disorders appear more common during specific stages of development. Children may not be able to recognize that the fear is excessive or unreasonable.

Epidemiology

Anxiety disorders are among the most common psychiatric disorders in youth. Prevalence rates range from 5–15% with 8% requiring clinical treatment. Age of onset varies for each disorder but range from early childhood to 12 years. Separation anxiety disorder and specific phobia usually have onset in early childhood, generalized anxiety disorder (GAD) occurs across all age groups, while obsessive-compulsive disorder, social phobia, and panic disorder tend to occur in later childhood and adolescence. Co-morbidity is common and 60–70% have two anxiety disorders and 25–30% has three anxiety disorders. Anxiety disorders are very common with depressive and bipolar disorders, ADHD, CD, and substance abuse.

Etiological factors

Genetic vulnerability; temperament that exhibits "behavioral inhibition" (timidity, shyness, and emotional restraint with unfamiliar people or situations); anxious attachment; negative life events; dysregulation of 5-HT and NA systems; S allele in 5HTTLPR promoter gene; hypertrophy and hyper-responsiveness of the amygdale to emotional stimuli.

Organic causes of anxiety

Medical conditions such as hyperthyroidism; cardiac problems such as arrhythmias; respiratory and neurological diseases. Substances such as alcohol; caffeine; cocaine; amphetamines; cannabis; LSD; ecstasy; etc.

Assessment

- Physical examination and interview with child.
- Interview with parents including developmental and family history and collateral information from teachers if release of information can be obtained.
- Instruments: K-SADS; DISC; CBCL; The Screen for Child Anxiety Related Emotional Disorders (SCARED); The Revised Children's Manifest Anxiety Scale (RCMAS); The Multidimensional Anxiety Scale for Children (MASC); The Pediatric Anxiety Rating Scale (PARS); The State-Trait Anxiety Inventory for Children (STAI-C); The Social Phobia and Anxiety Inventory for Children (SPAI-C); The Social Anxiety Scale for Children-Revised (SASC-R); The Fear Survey Schedule for Children-Revised (FSSC-R); The Children's Yale-Brown Obsessive-Compulsive Scale (CY-BOCS).

Anxiety disorder treatment principles

- Cognitive behavior therapy (CBT) is supported by a number of controlled studies as the psychological treatment of choice for pediatric anxiety disorders. Focuses on relaxation training, exposure and response prevention, and cognitive restructuring.
- Psycho-education and parent training is very important, particularly for younger children.
- Psychodynamic therapies include group, family, and individual/play techniques.
- Pharmacological: SSRIs are first-line agents if CBT is not available or ineffective. There is no evidence to select a specific SSRI for a particular anxiety disorder, but available studies demonstrated efficacy of fluvoxamine in GAD, and social phobia (SP), sertraline for GAD, fluoxetine for GAD and SP. There are positive studies with fluoxetine, sertraline, fluvoxamine, citalopram, and paroxetine in childhood OCD. The effect size SSRIs in childhood anxiety disorders is bigger than in depressive disorders. Available data suggest that suicidal activation (🕮 *p. 756*) still needs to be considered in childhood anxiety disorders regardless of mood symptoms and the significance and safety/follow-up plan should be discussed with patients and families. Severity of anxiety symptoms and family history predicts less favorable outcome and one year of maintenance of the medication after stabilization is suggested. Combined CBT and pharmacotherapy is supported by some studies but can be reserved for slow or poor responders. There are some data supporting use of buspirone and benzodiazepines (alprazolam and clonazepam) in older children and adolescents with resistant symptoms. BDZs can be helpful with acute or short term management in some cases or in some children who are very sensitive to side-effects of SSRIs (weigh benefit of BDZs with risk of abuse and possible paradoxical activating response).

Recommended further reading

1 Labellarte, M.J., Ginsburg, G.S., Walkup, J.T., Riddle, M.A. (1999). The treatment of anxiety disorders in children and adolescents. *Biological Psychiatry* **46**, 1567–1578.
2 Dadds, M.R. and Barrett, P.M. (2001). Practitioner review: psychological management of anxiety disorders in childhood. *J Child Psychol Psychiat* **42**, 999–1011.
3 Myers, K. Winters, N.C. (June 2002). Ten-year review of rating scales. II: Scales for internalizing disorders. *Journal of the American Academy of Child & Adolescent Psychiatry* **41**(6):634–659.
4 Morris, T.L., March, J.S. (2004). *Anxiety Disorders in Children and Adolescents*, 2nd ed. The Gulford Press, New York, NY.

Generalized anxiety disorder (GAD)

Key features

Characterized by developmentally inappropriate and excessive worry (apprehensive expectation) and anxiety on most days about things and the child find it to difficult to control. Severe enough to cause distress and/or dysfunction. Children are often perfectionist and self-critical. Most common anxiety disorder of adolescence with approximately 4% prevalence in this group. More common in females during adolescence. Only 1/3 seek treatment.

Symptoms

In addition to excessive anxiety and difficulty controlling their worry for six months, presence of **one** of the following items in children is enough (three items are required in adults) to make the diagnosis of GAD: Restlessness, fatigue; poor concentration/mind going blank; irritability, sleep disturbances; muscle tension.

Other symptoms in children can be:

- Somatic symptoms (headache; stomach pains or "irritable bowel"; rapid heart beat; shortness of breath).
- Nail biting.
- Hair pulling.

Co-morbidity

Very high rates—up to 90%. Other anxiety disorders, depression, bipolar disorder, ADHD, conduct disorders, and substance abuse are most common.

Management

Psyhoeducation; CBT; SSRIs; BDZs (see end of chapter for overview).

Specific phobias[1]

Key features
Excessive fear of an object or situation with distress and phobic avoidance that lasts at least six months. In children, anxiety may be expressed by crying, tantrums, freezing, or clinging. There may be anticipatory anxiety and exposure can precipitate a panic attack. Children may not be able to recognize that the fear is excessive or unreasonable.

Causes
Familial pattern in some cases; paired conditioning and sensitization.

Epidemiology
Very common (10% in some studies) 2:1 female to male ratio.

Co-morbidity
Other anxiety disorders, depression; substance abuse.

Subtypes
Animal phobias; natural, environment phobias (especially 5–10 year-olds); blood/infection/injury phobias; situational phobias (e.g., elevators, closed spaces); other.

Management
Psycho-education; CBT is the mainstay, including relaxation training and graded exposure; SSRIs.

Recommended further reading
1 Velting, O.N. and Albano, A.M. (2001). Current trends in the understanding and treatment of social phobia in youth. *J Child Psychol Psychiat* **42**, 127–140.

Panic disorder with or without agoraphobia[1,2]

Key features

Recurrent, unexpected panic attacks are the hallmark of this disorder, together with a period of at least one month during which the child is concerned about having another attack and the possible consequences of an attack and exhibits significant behavioral changes related to the attacks. These latter features are referred to as anticipatory anxiety. The first attack must be unexpected. A panic attack is defined as "a discrete period of intense fear" or discomfort that has an abrupt onset, reaches a peak in 10 minutes, and it is accompanied by at least 4 of 13 somatic or cognitive symptoms. Panic attacks are more common, but panic disorder (PD) cannot be diagnosed if panic attacks are better accounted for by another anxiety disorder (e.g., occurring on exposure to a feared social/phobic situation).

Symptoms

Somatic symptoms include shortness of breath, accelerated heart rate, chest pain, choking sensations, dizziness, tingling or numbing sensations, hot/cold flashes, sweating, trembling and nausea and cognitive symptoms include fear of dying, going crazy and losing control. In young children somatic symptoms predominate. Agoraphobia may or may not coexist with the disorder, but is usually present and the essential feature is anxiety about being in a situation in which escape would be difficult or help unavailable should a panic attack occur.

Epidemiology

The prevalence of PD in community samples ranges between 0.5% and 5.0, and in pediatric psychiatric clinics from 0.2% to 10%. Panic attacks are reported to be equally prevalent in males and females. Clinical studies have shown that the most of the PD pediatric patients consulting the clinics are older adolescents, Caucasian, female, and middle class. Peak onset is 15–19 yrs.

Co-morbidity

Depression, bipolar disorder, substance abuse, and other anxiety disorders (especially social phobia) are most common.

Management

Exclude organic causes; psycho-education; CBT; SSRIs; BDZs (see end of chapter for details).

Recommended further reading

1 Larsen, L.H. (2002). www.eMedicine.com
2 Furukawa, T.A., Watanabe, N., Churchill, R. (2006). Psychotherapy plus antidepressant for panic disorder with or without agoraphobia: systematic review. *Br J Psychiatry* **188**: 305–312.

Social phobia (social anxiety disorder)

Key features

Social phobia (SP) is extremely common and often undiagnosed and is the third most common mental health disorder in America. It is characterized by marked fear of one or more social or performance-related situations where the child is exposed to scrutiny and in which embarrassment may occur. Exposure to social situations usually causes an anxiety reaction (may be a panic attack) that is distressing for at least six months and recognized as inappropriate. Thus situations are either avoided or endured with discomfort. This may lead to agoraphobia and in severe cases school refusal.

Children may not be able to recognize that the fear is excessive or unreasonable. There must be evidence of the capacity for age-appropriate social relationships with familiar people and anxiety must occur in peer settings, not just with interactions wit adults. In children anxiety may be expressed by crying, tantrums, freezing, or shrinking from social situations with unfamiliar people.

Epidemiology

SP is most common in adolescents with an estimated prevalence of 5–15% as opposed to only 1% in children. Selective Mutism (SM) is seen in less than 1% of children in community settings and may represent SP with early onset. SP is more common in girls and the average age of onset for both genders is 12 years. Family studies demonstrate a twofold increased risk for SP in the relatives of SP probands, while twin studies show a threefold increased risk in monozygotic twins.

Co-morbidity

High rates of other anxiety disorders (especially GAD, simple phobia, and panic disorder) in approximately 30–60% cases, with mood disorders (20%) and substance abuse also frequent co-morbidly.

Prognosis

Although the prognosis for treated SP is fair to good, co-morbid conditions may persist and hinder educational and social progress. Those who experience symptoms in two or more situations have a poorer outcome than those experiencing symptoms in a single situation only.

Management

High levels of clinician awareness in diagnosing SP; individual and family assessments; psycho-education; CBT; SSRIs.

Separation anxiety disorder

This represents increased and inappropriate anxiety for at least four weeks centered around separation from attachment figures or home, which is developmentally abnormal and results in impaired normal functioning. It starts before age 18 and occurs in about 3.5% of children and 0.8% of adolescents.

Causes

Genetic vulnerability; anxious, inconsistent, or overinvolved parenting; and regression during periods of stress, illness, or abandonment.

Symptoms

Anxiety about actual or anticipated separation from or danger to attachment figure; sleep disturbances and nightmares; somatization; and school refusal (especially in adolescents).

Co-morbidity

Depression; anxiety disorders (panic with agoraphobia in older children); ADHD; oppositional disorders; learning disorders; and developmental disorders.

Assessment

Full physical examination; attempt interview individually and with parents; parental interview including full developmental and family history; collateral from school if consent obtained.

Treatment

Family/group therapies; CBT and play therapies; bridging back to school; SSRIs.

Selective mutism

Key features

Selective mutism (SM) primarily affects children and often manifests at school when the child cannot speak when called upon by teachers. The child may designate a friend or family member to serve as an interpreter and whispers in that person's ear in order to communicate.

Epidemiology

SM is seen in less than 1% of children in community settings and may represent Specific Phobia (SP) with early onset. Slightly more common in females.

Co-morbidity

Social phobia and other anxiety disorders, communication disorder, and general medical condition that causes abnormalities of articulation.

Prognosis

Usually starts before age five but may not come to clinical attention before entry into school. It may persist for only few months or may continue for several years. Anxiety symptoms may become chronic in some cases co-morbid with social phobia.

Management

Psycho-education; CBT, together with cooperation with the family and the school personnel; SSRIs (if CBT is not available or not helpful).

Recommended further reading

1 Bergman, R.L. Piacentini, J., McCracken, J.T. (2002). Prevalence and description of selective mutism in a school-based sample. *Journal of the American Academy of Child & Adolescent Psychiatry.* **41**(8), 938–946.

Obsessive-compulsive disorder (OCD)

Description

OCD is a disabling neuropsychiatric condition characterized by obsessions (recurrent intrusive thoughts, ideas or images) and compulsions (repetitive ritualistic behaviors). These symptoms cause significant impairment in terms of time (>1hr/day), distress, and interference in functioning.

Clinical features

Clinical presentation

Common obsessions include contamination fears (dirt, germs, or illness), aggressive/harm obsessions (excessive worries about danger, catastrophic events, such as death or illness happening to self or loved ones), separation, hoarding and saving, symmetry/ordering and doing things "just right." Intrusive sexual thoughts and religious obsessions are more common in adolescence than in childhood. Common compulsions are washing, checking (e.g., locks), repetitive counting, arranging, touching, and hoarding.

Diagnosis

A clinical diagnosis should include the following: psychiatric interview with the child; interview with parents, including complete developmental and family history; symptom rating and monitoring of severity over time using the Children's Yale-Brown Obsessive-Compulsive Scale (CY-BOCS); review of systems, with special attention to neurological and infectious disease signs, symptoms, and history.

Differential diagnosis

Normal developmental rituals; Tourette's/tic disorders; Sydenham's chorea; pediatric autoimmune neuropsychriatic disorders associated with streptococcal infections [PANDAS]; OCD spectrum disorders (including trichotillomania, onychiophagia [nail biting], chronic skin picking, other impulse control disorders, body dysmorphic disorder); eating disorders; psychotic disorders; depressive and anxiety disorders; side-effects of stimulants; rarely, basal ganglia disease.

Co-morbidity

80% have at least one co-morbid psychiatric disorder. Common co-morbid conditions include the following: major depression and other mood disorders; other anxiety disorders; OCD spectrum disorders; tic disorders; disruptive behavioral disorders, particularly ADHD and oppositional defiant disorder; speech/developmental disabilities; eating disorders; pervasive developmental disorders.

Epidemiology

Prevalence rate in pediatric population is 2–4%. Studies suggest a bimodal distribution of incidence with one peak in childhood and another in adulthood. Mean age of pediatric onset OCD is 10.3 years. Mean age at assessment is 13.2 years. Boys tend to have earlier age of onset than girls. May occur in children as early as 3 years of age. Male/female ratio for cases with onset prior to 10 years is 7:1 and for onset after puberty is 1:1.5; average male-to-female ratio in pediatric OCD is 3:2. Mild subclinical obsessions and compulsions are common in the general population (4–19%). Approximately one-third to one-half of adult OCD cases have a childhood onset.

Etiology

Causes

The causes of OCD remain to be fully elucidated; however there are several hypotheses regarding its etiology and etiopathogenesis. Due to the effectiveness of serotonin reuptake inhibitors in treating OCD, serotonergic abnormalities are potentially involved in the development and expression of the disorder. OCD is associated with several basal ganglia illnesses, including tic disorders, Huntington's chorea, and Sydenham's chorea; basal ganglia abnormalities in OCD are also supported by neuro-imaging studies.

Genetics

OCD is highly familial. OCD and subclinial OC symptoms are present in 18–30% of first-degree relatives. Relative risk in family members of affected children is approximately 25% (double that found in relatives of adult-onset cases). Studies suggest that genetic and nongenetic factors are about equally important in risk for developing OCD.

Treatment

Psychotherapy

Cognitive behavior therapy (CBT), involving graded exposure to anxiety-provoking stimuli and ritualizing prevention (exposure and response prevention—ERP) is recommended as a first-line intervention. Family therapy and Behavioral family intervention (BFI) are important and effective approaches that target the affective and cognitive aspects of the parent-child relationship as well as the entanglement of the OCD in the family context.

Pharmacotherapy

First-line agents include selective serotonin reuptake inhibitors (SSRIs: fluoxetine, sertraline, fluvoxamine, paroxetine, citalopram, and escitalopram) and the TCA, clomipramine. Maintenance therapy for at least 1–2 years to avoid relapse. Relapses common and long-term treatment advised after two relapses. In adults, higher doses of SSRIs often appear to be required for positive results in OCD versus doses used for anxiety or depression.

Combination therapy

Expert consensus guidelines for children who have OCD recommend starting treatment with either CBT or with the combination of CBT and pharmacotherapy; this decision depends upon the severity of the OCD and any co-morbid conditions that may benefit from pharmacotherapy.

Prognosis

Pooled mean persistence rates are 41% for full OCD and 60% for full or subthreshold OCD. Earlier age of onset, longer duration of illness, and inpatient status predicted an increased persistence. Co-morbid psychiatric conditions as well as poor initial treatment response are poor prognostic factors. Co-morbid tic or mood disorders are associated with increased OCD severity.

Recommended further reading

1 Leonard, H.L., Ale, C.M., Freeman, J.B., Garcia, A.M., Ng, J.S. (2005). Obsessive-Compulsive Disorder. *Child and Adolescent Psychiatric Clinics of North America* **14**, 727–743.
2 Geller, D.A. (2006) Obsessive-Compulsive and spectrum disorders in children and adolescents. *Psychiatric Clinics of North America* **29**, 353–370.
3 American Psychiatric Association. *Diagnostic and Statistical Manual of Mental Disorders.* 4th ed., text revision (DSM-IV-TR). Washington (DC): American Psychiatric Association (2000).

Pediatric autoimmune neuropsychriatic disorders associated with streptococcal infections (PANDAS)[1,2]

Description

A subgroup of children with a pediatric onset of either OCD or a tic disorder who have an abrupt onset of symptoms following a group A β-hemolytic streptococcal infection.

Clinical features

- Presence of OCD and/or a tic disorder meeting DSM-IV criteria.
- Prepubertal symptom onset.
- Dramatic onset and acute exacerbations with an episodic course of symptom severity.
- Temporal association between symptom exacerbation and group A β-hemolytic streptococcal infection (GABHS).
- Associated neurological abnormalities (e.g., choreiform movements) present during symptom exacerbations.

Epidemiology

The average onset of symptoms is 6.3 ± 2.7 years of age for tics and 7.4 ± 2.7 years of age for OCD (in PANDAS). There is a male predominance of approximately 2.6:1.

Etiology

The causes and etiopathogenic mechanisms are unknown. Evidence for an autoimmune etiology, involving the presence of serum antibodies that cross-react with neurons of the caudate, putamen, and globus pallidus is supported by:

- Magnetic resonance imaging studies, revealing enlargements of the caudate, putamen, and globus pallidus, which point to potential regional inflammatory changes.
- Frequent presence of antineuronal antibodies among patients.

There is evidence for a genetic predisposition; the rates of tic disorders and OCD in first-degree relatives of children in the PANDAS subgroup are higher than those in the general population, and similar to those previously reported for tic disorders and OCD.

Assessment

The determination that a child fits the PANDAS profile is made through prospective evaluation and documentation of the presence of streptococcal infections in conjunction with at least two episodes of neuropsychiatric symptoms, as well as demonstrating a negative throat culture or stable titers during times of neuropsychiatric symptom remission.

Treatment

Antibiotic treatment of infection. Treatment of OCD symptoms with CBT and/or pharmacotherapy is recommended if symptoms are very severe and/or if they persist following treatment of infection. Penicillin prophylaxis may be considered for children who meet all criteria for PANDAS and who have an ongoing risk of streptococcal exposure. Children with PANDAS may benefit from immunomodulatory treatments.

Recommended further reading

1 Leonard, H.L., Ale, C.M., Freeman, J.B., Garcia, A.M., Ng, J.S. (2005). Obsessive-compulsive disorder. *Child and Adolescent Psychiatric Clinics of North America* **14**, 727–743.
2 Snider, L. and Swedo, S.E. PANDAS current status and directions for research. (2004). *Mol Psychiatry*, **9**, 900–907.

Tic disorders

A tic is an involuntary, rapid, recurrent, nonrhythmic movement and/or vocalization. The frequency of tics may vary from a few times per week to more than 100 times per minute. Tics vary in intensity and amplitude, typically diminish during sleep or activities that need concentration, and can be intensified by anxiety, stress, fatigue, and excitement. Any attempts to suppress tics will frequently leads to a commonly described feeling of discomfort that builds until the tics are performed. Tics are frequently preceded by strong emotions, premonitory urges, or bodily sensations. Tics are generally manifested as either motor or vocal and are further categorized as either simple or complex. **Simple motor** tics (e.g., eye blinking, nose wrinkling, shoulder shrugging) usually last less than several hundred milliseconds. **Complex motor** tics (e.g., jumping, touching, pressing, facial contortions) usually last seconds or longer. **Simple vocal** tics (e.g., throat clearing, grunting, sniffing) are meaningless sounds. **Complex vocal** tics involve speech and language and include the sudden and spontaneous expression of words; speech blocking; repetition of words; echolalia; coprolalia (expression of socially unacceptable words or phrases). Tic disorders are generally described as one of the following: Tourette's disorder; chronic motor or vocal tic disorder; transient tic disorder; tic disorder not otherwise specified (NOS).

Chronic motor or vocal tic disorder

- Single or multiple motor or vocal tics, but not both motor and vocal.
- The tics occur many times/day nearly every day or intermittently throughout a period of more than one year (without a tic-free period of more than three consecutive months).
- The onset is before age 18 years.
- Criteria have never been met for Tourette's disorder.

This is more common than Tourette's, with a better long-term outcome. There is considerable variation in the severity of tics. The first symptoms at an average age of 7.8 years. Tics are often transient, tend to improve after adolescence, but may persist into adult life. The symptoms of chronic motor tics start significantly later than the symptoms of Tourette's. Tic severity is correlated with early age of onset. Similar etiology and treatment as Tourette's disorder (see p. 748).

Transient tic disorder

- Single or multiple motor and/or vocal tics.
- The tics occur many times/day nearly every day for at least 4 weeks, but for no longer than 12 consecutive months.
- The onset is before age 18 years.
- Criteria have never been met for Tourette's disorder or chronic motor or vocal tic disorder.

This is the most common of all tic disorders. The prevalence is approximately up to 20% of children. Onset of tics is generally at 8.5 ± 3.0 years of age.

Tic disorder NOS

Disorders characterized by tics that do not meet criteria for a specific tic disorder.

Tourette's disorder[1,2]

> ### Clinical features
> - Characterized by *multiple* motor *and* one or more vocal tics.
> - The tics occur many times/day nearly every day or intermittently throughout a period of more than one year (without a tic-free period of more than three consecutive months).
> - The onset is before age 18 years.

Approximately one-half of cases begin with a single tic, usually eye blinking. On average, phonic/vocal tics begin many years after the onset of motor tics and usually are simple in character (see 📖 *p. 746*).

Diagnosis
Comprehensive clinical interview, including medical and family history. Supplementary assessment instruments, such as the Yale Global Tic Severity Scale (YGTSS) are useful in following the course of illness severity.

Differential diagnosis
Obsessive-compulsive disorder (OCD); obsessive-compulsive spectrum disorders (OCS).

Co-morbidity
The most frequent co-morbidities in patients with Tourette's are ADHD, OCD, and OCS. Other co-morbidities include learning disorders, mood disorders, anxiety disorders, and other impulse control disorders.

Epidemiology
The average age of onset of symptoms is 7 years but typically ranges from 3 to 8 years. Tic severity is usually greater around ages 7 to 12 years, with a steady decline until age 20 years. Prevalence is approximately 5–30/10,000. Tourette's affects about 1% of school-aged children, whereas the estimated prevalence rates for all tic disorders (Tourette's, chronic motor or vocal tic disorder, and transient tic disorder) range from 4% to 18%. Tourette's disorder is four times more frequent in males than in females. Younger age of onset of Tourette's is associated with more severe tics.

Etiology
The causes of Tourette's remain to be fully elucidated. Studies have recognized several risk factors, including pre- and perinatal stresses/insults (e.g., delivery complications, and fetal exposure to high levels of coffee, cigarettes, or alcohol), and various bacterial and viral infections. Abnormalities in the dopamine system and the basal ganglia have been implicated. Current evidence regarding co-morbidity and family and molecular genetic, neuroimaging, and treatment studies suggest that Tourette's, OCD, and chronic tic disorder arise from a common neurobiologic pathway. Volumetric MRI studies have shown larger dorsolateral prefrontal regions in children. Functional neuroimaging studies have found

that voluntary tic suppression involves deactivation of the putamen and globus pallidus, coupled with partial activation of prefrontal cortex and caudate nucleus.

Family studies report a history of tics in the range of 8–57% of parents of affected children. Studies report increased rates in monozygotic twins and in first-degree relatives and transmission within Tourette's families is consistent with autosomal dominant and common polygenic modes of inheritance. In children who are so predisposed, tics may first emerge upon treatment of ADHD with stimulants.

Treatment

Successful treatment does not necessarily mean the complete suppression of tics but, rather, a substantial reduction in their frequency and intensity.

Psychotherapy

Psycho-education and counseling for mild symptoms. The best-studied behavioral intervention for Tourette's is *habit reversal*, which consists of various techniques focused at increasing the awareness of tics and developing a competing response to replace the target tic when the patient is first aware that tics are about to occur. Other behavioral interventions, such as relaxation methods, may also be effective.

Pharmacotherapy

Effective treatments include the following: D_2 receptor antagonists (typical antipsychotics), including haloperidol and pimozide; atypical antipsychotics, including risperidone, ziprasidone, quetiapine and aripiprazole; alpha-2 adrenergic receptor agonists, including clonidine and guanfacine. Typical antipsychotics carry risk of extrapyramidal symptoms and tardive dyskinesia. Atypical antipsychotics also carry risk of weight gain and lipid abnormalities. Other medications that havesome data supporting their effect in reducing tics are tetrabenazine, pergolide, ropinirole, and clonazepam. For more severe and refractory cases, direct interventions in neural pathways may be effective (bilateral capsulotomy or deep brain stimulation).

Recommended further reading

1 Khalifa, N., Von Knorring, A. (2005). Tourette syndrome and other tic disorders in a total population of children: Clinical assessment and background. *Acta Pædiatrica* **94**, 1608–1614.

2 Shavitt, R.G., Hounie, A.G., Rosario Campos, M.C., Miguel, E.C. (2006). Tourette's syndrome. *Psychiatr Clin N Am* **29**, 471–486.

Post-traumatic stress disorder (PTSD)[1,2]

Key features

A syndrome characterized by a triad of symptoms: intrusive re-experiencing of a traumatic event, avoidance, and hyperarousal. Formally recognized in children since the 1980s. Symptoms variable in young children, but similar to adult pattern in older children.

Traumatic event

Diagnosis requires exposure to a trauma with response involving fear, helplessness, horror, or disorganized, agitated play (in young children).

Epidemiology

Prevalence varies according to age and severity of trauma, but develops in approximately 3–6% of children exposed to a trauma. Most exposed do not develop the disorder and those that are affected usually have a pre-existing vulnerability (i.e., "an unnatural response to an unnatural event").

Risk factors include family and personal history of anxiety disorder, previous traumata and relationship disruptions.

Clinical presentation in young children[3]

Although this information is still being investigated, it has been suggested that young children may have certain specific symptoms:

- Compulsive repetitive play representing part of the trauma and failing to relieve anxiety.
- Recurrent recollections of the event.
- Nightmares, night terrors, and difficulty going to sleep.
- Constriction of play.
- Social withdrawal.
- Restricted affect.
- Loss of acquired developmental skills, especially language regression and toilet training.
- Decreased concentration and attention.
- New aggression.
- New separation anxiety.

Depression is often co-morbid but it is not part of the core disorder. Adolescents are more likely to exhibit symptoms consistent with DSM-IV criteria.

Co-morbidity

Common in PTSD, with depressive disorders, anxiety disorders, and substance abuse frequent in adolescents. In young children, the development of behavioral disorders is common after a traumatic event.

Clinical assessment

- Direct interview with child (drawing/play methods useful in young children).
- Interview with parents including developmental and family history and account of the trauma.
- Instruments include K-SADS-PL and the Children's Post-Traumatic Stress Reaction Index can be helpful, but are not diagnostic.

Treatment of PTSD (see 📖 p. 434 for adult overview)

- Good evidence suggests use of CBT in several clinical trials. Additional focus on psycho-education and managing anxiety symptoms.
- Pharmacologic interventions that target specific symptoms may be beneficial. Some open trials suggest SSRIs are also useful.

Recommended further reading

1 Perrin, S., Smith, P., Yule, W. (2000). The assessment and treatment of post-traumatic stress Disorder in children and adolescents. *J Child Psychol Psychiat* **41**, 277–89.
2 Yule, W. (2001). Posttraumatic stress disorder in the general population and in children. *J Clin Psychiatry* **62** (suppl 17), 23–28.
3 Perrin, S. Smith, P. Yule, W. (2000). The assessment and treatment of post-traumatic stress Disorder in children and adolescents. *J Child Psychol Psychiat* **41**, 277–89.
4 Yule, W. (2001). Posttraumatic stress disorder in the general population and in children. *J Clin Psychiatry* **62** (suppl 17), 23–28
5 Scheeringa, M.S., and Gaensbauer, T.J. (2000). Post-traumatic stress disorder. In *Handbook of Infant Mental Health*. C.H. Zeanah (ed.). New York: The Guilford Press.

Depression in children and adolescents[1]

Unipolar depressive disorders are common, familial, and recurrent in young people, and usually persist into adulthood. Adolescent-onset depression confers greater risk for recurrence in adulthood than childhood-onset. Co-morbidity with these disorders is the rule rather than the exception (approx. 50–70%). Childhood and adolescent depression are commonly associated with poor psychosocial, family, and academic function. Risk of suicide requires early detection and treatment of depressive symptoms. 5–10% of youth do not fit criteria for major depressive disorder (MDD), but still have significant impairment and increased risk for suicide and later MDD.

Major depressive disorder (MDD)

Epidemiology

- Prepubescent: estimated prevalence is 2% with 1:1 gender ratio.
- Adolescent: estimated prevalence is 4–8% with a 1:2 male to female ratio.

Risk factors

Family history/parent with mood disorder; prior history of anxiety disorder, loss of a parent; abuse; negative life events; family conflict.

Etiology

Pre-existing cognitive distortions (e.g., pessimism) and bias toward threat and distress and away from reward, altered serotonergic and noradrenergic neurotransmission, interaction of life stress and "s" allele of 5HTTLPR promoter gene.

Clinical features

Childhood depression symptoms may include sad or depressed mood, anhedonia, change in appetite, sleep problems, anergia, amotivation, irritability, guilt, poor concentration, and morbid ideation or thoughts of suicide. Children and adolescents may present with psychomotor retardation but more often present with irritability and agitation. With a high level of co-morbidity, differential diagnosis is crucial and challenging. (See Chapter 7 ⬛ p. 271 for further details on MDD).

Co-morbidity

Treatment of co-morbid conditions is integral to the management of depression. Common co-morbid conditions include anxiety disorders, substance abuse, and dysthymia. It is also important to consider contribution of ADHD, eating disorders, medical conditions, and the contribution of a history of childhood abuse. Note: Children with bipolar disorder (BD) more often have a family history of bipolar disorder, and may have depressed phase symptoms of hyperphagia, hypersomnia, and psychosis.

Differential diagnosis

- Pre-existing anxiety disorder leading to depressive symptoms.
- ADHD leading to functional impairment and interpersonal difficulty.
- Substance use disorders and depressogenic substances/medications.

- Psychotic disorders with affective flattening, and medical conditions resulting in depressive symptoms.
- Undiagnosed medical conditions mimicking depressive symptoms (e.g., endocrine disorders, neurologic disorders, autoimmune disease, etc.)
- 10 to 20% with a MDE will later manifest bipolar diathesis.

Dysthymic disorder

Epidemiology

- 0.5–1.7% in children and 1.6–8% in adolescents.
- May be a precursor to MDD or co-morbid ("double depression").

Clinical features and course

- Pervasive and chronic low mood or irritability for at least one year.
- Fewer symptoms than MDD.
- Often there is a protracted course, which leads to double depression: MDD superimposed on top of a pre-existing dysthymic disorder.
- (See page 📖 p. 286 for further details on dysthymia).

Treatment for adolescents with depression study[2]

(TADS) is a randomized controlled trial that evaluates the effectiveness of fluoxetine, CBT, fluoxetine plus CBT, and placebo. Medications were administered double-blind; CBT and combined treatment were administered unblinded. Response: "much or very much improved": 71.0% for the combination of fluoxetine and CBT, 60.6% for fluoxetine alone, 43.2% for cognitive-behavioral psychotherapy alone, and 34.8% for placebo. Thus, the combination of fluoxetine and cognitive-behavioral psychotherapy appears to produce the greatest improvement in symptoms of major depression. Fluoxetine alone is effective, but not as effective as the combination of fluoxetine and CBT. Cognitive-behavioral psychotherapy alone is less effective than fluoxetine and not significantly more effective than placebo. Almost 30% of TADS participants had suicidal ideation at the start of the study; 2% had intense suicidal ideation. Suicidality decreases substantially over 12 weeks of treatment. Improvement in suicidal ideation is greatest for the combination of fluoxetine and CBT and least for fluoxetine alone. Importantly, fluoxetine does not appear to increase suicidal ideation. In contrast, harm-related behavioral events though uncommon were more common in patients receiving fluoxetine as follows: fluoxetine (11.9%), the combination of fluoxetine and CBT (8.4%), cognitive-behavioral psychotherapy (4.5%) and placebo (5.4%). Thus, consistent with its impact on suicidal ideation, cognitive-behavioral psychotherapy may protect against these events in patients taking fluoxetine.

Recommended further reading

1 Birmaher B., Brent, D.A. (2006). Work Group on Quality Issues. Practice parameters for the assessment and treatment of children and adolescents with depressive disorders. *J Am Acad Child Adolesc Psychiatry*, in press.
2 March, J. at www.aacap.org

Management of depression in youth

Assessment

- Thorough evaluation is needed for assessment of depressive symptoms and medical and psychiatric co-morbidity.
- Patient and parent should always be interviewed, with patient interviewed independently.
- Repeated suicide assessments should be part of every stage of assessment and treatment.
- Collateral information from teachers, primary care providers, social services, etc. should be obtained.
- Rating scales include Beck Depression Inventory and Child Depression Inventory. Scales are useful for symptom screening, assessing severity, or monitoring improvement (see Chapter 2 📖 p. 37).
- Laboratory/medical investigations may be necessary, especially if history warrants and/or patient has not responded to previous regimens of evidence based treatment. CBC with diff, platelets, lytes, BUN, Cr, glucose, thyroid panel, liver functions, vitamin levels such as B_{12} and folate, or other labs as indicated by patients' presentations.

Treatment

- Approach may vary by duration, severity, and co-morbidity.
- All treatment should include psycho-education, support, and involvement of family and school.
- Treatment should include acute, continuation, and maintenance phases.
- Psychotherapy is a reasonable initial treatment in mild to moderate depression. CBT and Interpersonal Therapy (IPT) are most extensively researched and data supports their efficacy (see 📖 Chapter 21).
- Pharmacotherapy
  - Fluoxetine is the only FDA approved medication for children at this time, and has the most evidence for efficacy. Starting dose: 5–10mg per day for one week, then increase to 20mg if tolerated. If needed, may slowly increase dose after 4–8 weeks. Higher doses may be used and may be helpful for those who are not having side-effects.
  - There is some, but less support for other SSRIs, more in adolescents than children (e.g., sertraline, citalopram, and for the SNRI venlafaxine). Open trials support the use of bupropion, but there have been no RCTs.
  - Tricyclic Antidepressants are not supported by trials and have been associated with cardiac toxicity.
  - Concern about increase in suicidality has led to extensive examination of antidepressants use, best evidence indicates 2 additional patients with spontaneously reported worsening or emergent suicidal events (ideation or attempt) for every 100 youths treated, with no completions.
  - For patients with a clear seasonal component, light therapy has been shown to be efficacious.

- Combination treatment should be considered in all cases, particularly chronic or refractory depression. There is evidence that mild to moderate depression may respond to psychotherapy alone.
- Diagnosis and treatment of parental depression will make treatment response in the child more likely.

Continuation and maintenance treatment

For a single, first episode, continuation treatment should be provided for 6–12 months after complete symptomatic remission. Recurrent depression likely requires longer treatment.

- Psychotherapy: monthly CBT has been shown to prevent relapse of depression.
- Pharmacotherapy: there is evidence that pharmacotherapy should be continued for at least six months after a single MDE and for at least 12 months for recurrent MDD after complete symptoms remission to decrease risk of recurrence.

FDA BLACK BOX WARNING: SSRIs and suicidality

Suicidality in children and adolescents—Antidepressants increased the risk of suicidal thinking and behavior (suicidality) in short-term studies in children and adolescents with MDD and other psychiatric disorders. Anyone considering the use of SSRIs or any other antidepressant in a child or adolescent must balance this risk with the clinical need. Patients who are started on therapy should be observed closely for clinical worsening, suicidality, or unusual changes in behavior. Families and caregivers should be advised of the need for close observation and communication with the prescriber. Prozac® is approved for use in pediatric patients with MDD and OCD. Pooled analyses of short-term (4–16 weeks) placebo-controlled trials of 9 antidepressant drugs (SSRIs and others) in children and adolescents with MDD, OCD, or other psychiatric disorders (a total of 24 trials involving over 4,400 patients) have revealed a greater risk of adverse events representing suicidal thinking or behavior (suicidality) during the first few months of treatment in those receiving antidepressants. The average risk of such events in patients receiving antidepressants was 4%, twice the placebo risk of 2%. No suicides occurred in these trials.

Recommended further reading

1 Bridge, J.A., Salary, C.R., Birmaher, B., Asare, A.G., Brent, D.A. (2005). The risks and benefits of antidepressant treatment for youth depression. *Annals of Medicine* **37**, 404–412.

Suicide and suicidal risk in young people

Epidemiology

Approximately 20% of adolescents have experienced suicidal ideation, about 6% have had suicidal ideation with intent and a plan, while 1–4% of males and 1.5–10% of females have attempted suicide. The rate of suicide in adolescents is around 8/100,000, with a 3–4 fold higher risk in males than females. The risk of suicide in individuals who attempt is 0.5 to 1% per year. Approximately 2,000 adolescents in the United States committing suicide each year. Eighty percent of attempters and 90% of completers have at least one Axis I disorder.

- Most adolescents who complete suicide use a firearm, and overdose is the most common method of attempt.

Risk factors for children and adolescents who attempt suicide

- Availability of lethal means.
- Personal history of suicide attempt.
- Life stressors (school, family discord, loss of relationship).
- Current depression, substance abuse, conduct disorder, borderline personality traits, especially in combination.
- Psychological characteristics (hopelessness, negative cognitions, impulsivity).
- Family history of psychopathology and/or suicidal behavior.
- History of sexual, physical, and/or emotional abuse.

Associated disorders: Most commonly major depression, with particularly high risk in bipolar disorder, mixed; substance use disorder, schizophrenia, anxiety disorders, cluster B symptomatology, and mood disorder co-morbid with substance abuse.

Assessment

- Ideation, plans, and intent.
- Reasons for living.
- Events that would increase risk of self-harm.
- Access to lethal means of self-harm.
- Current self-injurious behavior.
- Patient's ability to collaboratively develop and implement a plan for safety.

Management

- Treatment should be in the least restrictive safe environment
- Patient should be hospitalized if:
  - There is persistent wish to die and intent to act on suicidal ideation AND
  - He or she cannot guarantee safety.

- Treatment should establish safety plan, instill hope, determine appropriate level of care, and increase support.
- Outpatient care must involve a caregiver able to provide adequate supervision and support.
- A child presenting with suicidal ideation should not be assessed and discharged without plan for follow-up.
- Patients should be seen frequently and have 24 hour access to crisis response.

Psychotherapy

- There are no definitive studies in children at present, but CBT that addresses cognitions and chain analysis of the attempt and dialectical behavior therapy have been shown efficacious in adults.
- Other treatments for depression, such as standard CBT and IPT may help depressive symptoms, but haven't been shown to reduce risk for recurrent suicide attempt.
- Long-term contact and patient engagement in treatment reduce suicide risk.

Pharmacotherapy

- Any pharmacotherapy for a suicidal child or adolescent must be carefully monitored, and side-effects or new behaviors reported immediately.
- Treat underlying disorders and identify target symptoms.
- Lithium has been shown to decrease suicide rates in adults.
- Use of SSRIs:
  - Evidence that use of SSRIs to treat depression reduces risk of suicide completion.
  - FDA evidence of 1.78-fold increase in ideation with no increase in completions.
- As with all medications, carefully monitor for new suicidal ideation, agitation. Weigh risks with benefits: Many more depressed youth will respond to antidepressants than will experience a suicidal event.
- Patients should be seen for follow-up within one week of start of a new medication and with each increase (to monitor suicide risk).
- Refer to your institution for guidelines on monitoring antidepressant therapy in youth.

Prevention

- Asking children and adolescents about suicidal ideation does not increase their risk of attempt.
- Evidence shows that patients at greatest risk will reveal suicidal ideation and plan if asked directly.
- Screening for depression and other disorders that lead to suicide allows identification of those at risk.
- Psycho-education of parents, the public, and the media.
- Firearms must be secured in all homes with children, most urgently in homes of those youth with any suicidal risk.

A pathway to suicidal behavior

Predisposing factors   e.g., previous attempt, psychiatric disorder
↓
Precipitating factors   e.g., "domino effect"
                                       (suicide in community or in the media)
↓
Opportunity   e.g., access (to a gun), privacy
↓
Attempt

Gun control and adolescent suicide (a U.S. perspective)

Accessibility to firearms, particularly handguns, influences the rate of teen suicides. Firearms are the most common method of suicide by youth. The increase in the rate of youth suicide (and the number of deaths by suicide) over the past four decades is largely related to the use of firearms as a method. Handguns were used in nearly 70% of teen suicides in 1990, up 20% since 1970. The most common location for the occurrence of firearm suicides by youth is the home. A home with a handgun is almost ten times more likely to have a teen suicide than a home without. In fact, for youth under the age of 16 and in those with little evidence of psychopathology, a gun in the home is the single biggest risk factor for completed suicide. There is a positive association between the accessibility and availability of firearms in the home and the risk for youth suicide. The risk conferred by guns in the home is proportional to the accessibility (e.g., loaded and/or unsecured firearms) and the number of guns in the home. If a gun is used to attempt suicide, a fatal outcome will result 78% to 90% of the time. Public policy initiatives that restrict access to guns (especially handguns) are associated with a reduction of firearm suicide and suicide overall, especially among youth.

Youth Suicide by Firearms Task Force

Bipolar disorder in children and adolescents

Background

Mania has been observed in children in the 19th century by Esquirol and in the 20th century by Kraepelin, Kasanin, and Bleuler. Kraepelin believed that mania in children was rare, but noted that 0.5% of his manic patients had their first episode by 10 years of age. Historically, bipolar disorder (BD) has not been studied well in children, although much research activity is now underway.[1]

Epidemiology

Given the controversy in characterizing pediatric BD, there is no data on the prevalence of prepubertal BD. One published study (Lewinsohn) showed a lifetime BD prevalence of approximately 1% in youths 14–18 years old (predominantly BD type II and cyclothymia) with an additional 5.7% youths with subsyndromal BD symptoms. Retrospective reports of adults with BD show that 60% reported BD onset before 20 years of age and 10–20% reported BD onset before 10 years of age.[2] BD affects both sexes equally.[3] Ninety percent of BD youth have normal IQ.[3]

Clinical presentation

Although the presentation of BD in mid to late adolescence is considered similar to adult BD, the presentation of pediatric BD has been debated. Many children have less than the 4–7 days duration specified in the DSM-IV criteria for hypomania or mania respectively. The symptoms that most differentiate pediatric BD from other clinical conditions are *euphoria*, *grandiosity*, *increased energy*, and *increased sexuality*. Pediatric BD is characterized by a predominance of mixed episodes and/or rapid cycling, with many *more episodes* per year than adult BD, and fewer periods of remission, and a high rate of *co-morbid* ADHD and anxiety disorder. The National Institute of Mental Health Roundtable on pubertal BD in 2001 categorized pediatric BP phenotypes in terms of **"narrow"** (DSM-IV definitions of mania and hypomania) and **"broad"** (includes common clinical presentation of severe irritability, mood lability, temper outbursts, symptoms of depression, anxiety, hyperactivity, poor concentration, and impulsivity), although recent longitudinal and neurocognitive characterization of this latter group suggests that it is distinct from BD. Diagnosis of BD is complicated by the age-specific symptom presentation. For example, increased self-esteem and goal-directed activity may be consistent with child's normal development. Psychosis, most commonly auditory hallucinations, has been reported in 16–60% of youth with BD with the prevalence of psychosis lower in adolescent mania than adult mania.[2]

Pediatric BD is highly co-morbid with ADHD, oppositional defiant disorder, conduct disorder, anxiety disorders (particularly panic disorder), substance abuse, and PDD (particularly Asperger's disorder[2]). Adolescents with BD are at *increased risk of completed suicide*, particularly those in a mixed state.[3]

Biological features consistent with BD

Neuropsychology

Difficulties in attentional set shifting and visuospatial memory, misinterpretation of sad, happy, and fearful child faces (but not adult faces) as angry.[2]

Brain morphology

White matter hyperintensities in cortical and subcortical brain regions and smaller amygdalar size, smaller parietal and temporal lobe cortical gray matter, reduced gray matter volume in the dorsolateral prefrontal cortex (DLPFC), and decrease in hippocampal volume.[2]

Functional and metabolic brain imaging

With a Stroop test probe, left thalamus and putamen activation was increased. With a visuospatial working memory task, greater activation in the DLPFC, bilateral anterior cingulate, left thalamus, and right inferior frontal gyrus.[2]

BD is highly genetic as evident with the increase of BD spectrum in high-risk studies with offspring of BD parents and link between early age of onset and risk of BD among first-degree relatives of youth with BD. Molecular-genetics studies point to familial transmission in early onset BD; however, no reliable indicators of genetic risk have been found to date.[2]

Differential diagnosis

Pediatric BD could be differentiated from ADHD by the symptoms of grandiosity, elation, flight of ideas, hypersexuality, and a decreased sleep. In older adolescents, mood-incongruent delusions, hallucinations, and thought disorder may lead BD to be misdiagnosed as schizophrenia. Irritability and mood lability could be present in a PDD and substance abuse.[2] Evaluation should exclude non mood-related emotional and behavioral disturbances, developmental delays, child abuse, delirium, tumors, infections, metabolic disorders, and seizure disorders.

Management

Treatment requires the combination of a pharmacologic agent plus psychosocial interventions.[3] There have been few prospective studies on the efficacy and safety of psychotropic medications in the treatment of pediatric BD. Open trials have supported the use of lithium, mood stabilizers (valproate and carbamazepine) and second-generation antipsychotic (SGA) medications. The combination of SGA and mood stabilizers appears to be effective in acute treatment of pediatric BD and continued stabilization for a six-month period.[2] There are no proven psychotherapy treatment methods for pediatric BD. A few published preliminary studies focused on child and family focused cognitive behavior therapy, manual-based multifamily group treatment, and a manual-based family-focused therapy.[2] Psychosocial intervention may include psycho-education, relapse prevention, stress reduction, problem-solving skills, and family functioning.[3] It is vital to monitor sleep and to make sure that hyposomnia is addressed as this may head off an incipient manic episode.

Depression can be treated with maximizing neuroleptics and mood stabilizers; if depression persists, then antidepressants can be used cautiously, after mood stabilization. Sometimes, depressive symptoms can be relieved with reduction in levels of mood stabilizers.

Recommended further reading

1 Weller, E.B., Weller, R.A., Sanchez, L.E. Bipolar Disorder in Children and Adolescents In M. Lewis *Child and Adolescent Psychiatry: A Comprehensive Textbook*, 3rd ed. Philadelphia: Lippincott Williams and Williams, 2002.

2 Pavuluri, M.N., Birmaher, B., Naylor, M.W. (2005). Pediatric bipolar disorder: Review of the past 10 years. *J Am Acad Child Adolesc Psychiary* **44**, 846–871.

3 AACAP (1997). AACAP Official Action. Practice parameters for the assessment and treatment of children and adolescents with bipolar disorder. *J Am Acad Child Adolesc Psychiary* **36,** 138–157.

Schizophrenia in children and adolescents

Background

The presentation of schizophrenia is most common in late adolescence and early adulthood. However, rare cases of the disorder in childhood were identified by Kraepelin, DeSanctis, and Bleuler in the early 20th century.[1] Beginning with DSM-III, childhood-onset schizophrenia (onset of psychosis by age 12) was recognized as a disorder that is clinically and neurobiologically continuous with the adult-onset disorder.[1] (See psychosis chapter for more details [book] p. 258).

Epidemiology

Childhood schizophrenia is rare and probably less common than autism; however, major epidemiologic studies have yet to be conducted.[2] Reported sex ratios across studies have varied between a 2:1 male predominance to essentially equal sex ratios. Children with schizophrenia are generally in the low average to average intelligence range. There is some evidence that children with schizophrenia may be more common in both the low and high socioeconomic classes.[2]

Clinical presentation

The premorbid course of childhood schizophrenia includes impairments in language, motor, and social development. Auditory hallucinations are the most frequently reported symptom. Other symptoms may include delusions and thought disorders. The diagnosis of childhood schizophrenia is made when the DSM-IV symptoms are present for the required duration in a child by age 12 and other disorders have been ruled out.

Biological features

Consistent with childhood schizophenia are as follows[3]:

Neuropsychology

Poor neuropsychological functioning in attention, working memory, and executive function.

Brain morphology

Increase in lateral ventricular volume with decreased cerebellar volume and midsagittal thalamic area.

Functional and metabolic brain imaging

Frontal hypometabolism, decreases in the ratio of N-Acetylaspartate (NAA) to creatine in the frontal cortex and hippocampus.

Smooth pursuit eye movements: abnormalities in ratio of eye speed to target speed, increased global level of aberrant eye tracking, and increased anticipatory saccades. Many of these features are more common in the asymptomatic offspring of schizophrenic parents.

The genetic nature of schizophrenia is seen in the increase of schizophrenia and schizophrenia spectrum disorders in offspring studies and adoption studies. Recent studies suggest a significant elevation of schizophrenia spectrum disorders in relatives of childhood-onset subjects versus adult-onset and control subjects. There may be a greater rate of cytogenic abnormalities.[3]

Obstetric complications

Although a meta-analysis demonstrated increased in adult schizophrenia, obstetric complications are not, as previously hypothesized, associated in childhood-onset schizophrenia.[3]

Differential diagnosis

Psychotic illnesses are rare in young children and present a particular challenge in both diagnosis and management. Very young children under six years have preoperational cognitions and thus "reality testing" is blurred by a range of normal fantasy material. Imagined friends, transient hallucinations under stress, and loose associations may all occur as part of the normal spectrum of childhood experience.

Differential diagnosis includes mood disorders (such as psychotic symptoms associated with depression or bipolar disorder), PDD, post-traumatic stress disorder/dissociative disorders, OCD, nonpsychotic emotional and behavioral disturbances, organic conditions (e.g., TLE, thyroid disease, brain tumor, SLE, and substance misuse disorders). Evaluation must include developmental delays, child abuse or neglect, language disorders, and cultural beliefs. Organic conditions such as substance use or acute intoxication, delirium, tumors, infections, metabolic disorders, or seizure disorders should be evaluated.[3]

Management

Treatment requires the combination of a pharmacologic agent plus psychosocial interventions.[3] First-line pharmacologic agents for the treatment of the psychotic symptoms associated with schizophrenia include traditional neuroleptic or the Second-Generation (SGA) medications. The SGA medications are often preferred because they are effective in positive symptoms and may be more effective in negative symptoms. In addition, SGA agents have a more favorable risk profile (compared to typical antipsychotics, such as Haldol®) in terms of extrapyramidal and tardive dyskinesia side-effects. Adjunctive agents (for example: antidepressants, antiparkinsonian agents, benzodiazepines, and mood stabilizers) are commonly used to address co-morbid conditions (such as depression and substance abuse), associated symptoms (such as agitation, dysphoria, or mood instability), or mediation side-effects. Psychosocial interventions recommended include psycho-educational therapy for the patient and the family. Therapies for the patient include education about the illness and treatment, social skills training, relapse prevention, life skills training, and problem solving strategies. Therapies for the family include education about the illness and treatment and coping strategies. Co-morbid depression is common and should be managed with psychotherapy and SSRIs. Patients with schizophrenia, particularly those with prior high functioning subchronic course are at high risk for suicide and should be managed/monitored accordingly.

Recommended further reading

1 Nicholson, R., Rapoport, J.L. (1999). Childhood-onset schizophrenia: Rare but worth studying. *Biol Psychiatry* **46**,.1418–1428.
2 Volkmar, F.R., Tsatsanis, K.D. Childhood Schizophrenia In M. Lewis, Child and Adolescent Psychiatry: A Comprehensive Textbook, 3rd ed. Philadelphia: Lippincott Williams and Williams, 2002.
3 AACAP (2000). AACAP Official Action. Summary of the Practice Parameters for the Assessment and Treatment of Children and Adolescents With Schizophrenia. *J Am Acad Child Adolesc Psychiary* **39**, 1580–1582.

Substance abuse in children and adolescents[1]

Substance use disorders (SUDs) are increasingly common in young people. Assessment is multi-faceted and includes:

- Use, assessed for DSM criteria of abuse or dependence.
- Child or adolescent's attitudes of the substance of abuse and patterns of use.
- Impairment in social and academic function.
- Interference in child or adolescent's development.
- Extent of parental knowledge of use and consequences of use.
- Presence of co-occurring disorders.

Risk factors

Individual, including biogenetic risk (attention deficit disorder, especially in combination with conduct disorder; sensation seeking; in girls; early onset of puberty).

- Parent and family risk factors (parental substance abuse, family discord, abuse, parental criminality, low parental monitoring and supervision).
- Peer-related risk factors (peer antisocial behavior and substance use).
- Co-morbid psychiatric disorders (especially anxiety and depression).
- Increased risk after onset of adolescence.

Co-morbidity

Youths with SUDs often experience aggressive and suicidal behaviors, disruptive behavior disorders (ODD, CD, ADHD), mood disorders, anxiety disorders, and bulimia nervosa (often these conditions precede SUD, but sometimes mood disorders are secondary to substance use and its consequences).

Management

- Treatment in the least restrictive, effective environment.
- Explanation and maintenance of appropriate confidentiality.
- Abstinence is the ultimate goal of treatment, interim goals include improvement in function and reduction of use.
- Treatment should include family involvement.
- Interim goals Include Improvement in function and reduction of use, established with techniques of motivational interviewing (MI), identification of triggers for craving and use, alteration of routines and peer group, ongoing participation in support groups.
- Identify and treat co-occurring disorders.
- Use of urine drug screening at assessment and for monitoring.

Pharmacotherapy management

- Assessment of risk of abuse of medication.
- Assessment of dangers of simultaneous use of medication and substance (some evidence that treatment of underlying depression with SSRIs, bipolar disorder with lithium, and of ADHD with stimulants can reduce risk for substance use).

- Treatment of any withdrawal symptoms.
- Substitution therapies (e.g., methadone) are rarely used in children and adolescents.

Therapeutic management

Therapies are not well studied in children, but include:
- CBT (use feelings and behaviors and relapse prevention), see 📖 *p. 1016*.
- Family therapy.
- Self-help groups (AA, NA).
- MI and motivational enhancement therapies.
- Parent management training, see 📖 *p. 1029*.

Children at risk for noncompliance with treatment often have younger age of onset, more extensive use, polysubstance use, deviant behavior, less school and social involvement, and/or limited family support.

Characteristics of successful treatment include longer duration, sufficient intensity, appropriate follow-up, family involvement, cultural sensitivity, involvement of social-services agencies, development of a drug-free lifestyle, and involvement in self-help groups.

Recommended further reading

1 Bukstein, O.G., Bernet, W., Arnold, V., *et al.* (2005). Work Group on Quality Issues. Practice parameters for the assessment and treatment of children and adolescents with substance use disorders. *J Am Acad Child Adolesc Psychiatry* **44**(6), 609–621.
2 Working Group on Quality Issues. (2005). Practice parameters for the assessment and treatment of children and adolescents with substance use disorders. *J Am Acad Child Adolesc Psychiatry* **44**(6), 609–621.

Child abuse—general issues

In recent decades there has been growing awareness that the abuse of children can take many forms. All forms of child abuse involve the elements of power imbalance, exploitation, and the absence of true consent. Federal legislation provides a foundation for states by identifying a minimum set of acts or behaviors that define child abuse and neglect. The Federal Child Abuse Prevention and Treatment Act (CAPTA) (42 U.S.C.A. §5106g), as amended by the Keeping Children and Families Safe Act of 2003, defines child abuse and neglect as, at minimum:

- Any recent act or failure to act on the part of a parent or caretaker which results in death, serious physical or emotional harm, sexual abuse or exploitation.
- An act or failure to act which presents an imminent risk of serious harm.[1]

Categories of abuse

Emotional abuse

Failure to provide for the child's basic emotional needs such as to have a severe effect on the behavior and development of the child. This may include persistent coldness, hostility, or rejection by the caregiver and can be seen as the "willful destruction or significant impairment of a child's confidence." Other abuse types often result in emotional abuse.

Physical abuse

Where there is physical injury to the child and it is known, admitted, or reasonably suspected that the injury was inflicted by another person; or where a guardian knowingly fails to prevent injury or acted without due regard for the safety of the child; or where the nature of the injury is inconsistent with the account of how it occurred. (Includes Munchausen syndrome by proxy 📖 p. 776).

Physical neglect

Persistent or severe exposure of a child to danger or the persistent failure to fulfill the child's basic needs (food, sleep, diaper changing, clothing, warmth, shelter, or medical needs) that is likely to result in serious impairment of the child's health and development. This may also occur when an adult guardian persistently pursues or allows a child to follow a lifestyle inappropriate to the child's developmental needs or which jeopardizes his/her health. Leaving a child unattended or inadequately supervised may also qualify as physical neglect.

Failure to thrive

Failure to meet expected weight and growth norms or developmental milestones, which does not have a basis in a hereditary or medical condition.

Sexual abuse

Any child below the age of consent will be deemed to have been sexually abused when any person, by design or by neglect, causes that child to be involved in any activity that might reasonably be expected to lead to the sexual arousal or gratification of that or any other person, including organized networks. This definition holds regardless of whether there has been genital contact and whether or not the child is said to have initiated the behavior.

Abuse by young people or children

This involves activities between children/young people of a sexual or physical nature where one or more of the following characteristics is present: lack of true consent; inequalities in power (such as age, developmental stage, or size); actual or threatened coercion. A distinction must be made between behavior normally expected between young people/children and behavior that is clearly of an abusive nature.

Recommended further reading

1 http://www.childwelfare.gov/

Child abuse—assessment, management, and psychiatric outcome

The management of child abuse involves many professionals including police, social workers, educationalists, and health workers. Thus a multidisciplinary approach is required in order to fully assess the extent or risk of abuse and to provide the appropriate interventions. Working with child abuse is stressful and may invoke strong feelings and opinions, and supervision of the clinician is recommended.

Principles of assessment and management of child abuse

- Early detection in children at high-risk or presenting with alerting signs.
- A multidisciplinary approach is essential with early consultation across disciplines.
- Maintain confidentiality where necessary and possible, yet be aware of mandated reporting responsibilities.
- Assessment should be measured, sympathetic and above all child-centered.
- Attempt to engage and involve parents/care providers at all stages and keep them informed in all but the most exceptional circumstances.
- Evaluate the child's physical, emotional, cognitive, and sexual development, as well as the child's position in the family.
- Evaluate the family in terms of: degree of social isolation and support, levels of stress, emotional maturity of the parents, parental relationship, role of nonabusing parent, and family dynamics.
- Consider extra-familial factors such as: deficiencies in support services, failure of interprofessional communication, sociopolitical environment.
- Important to clarify the family's perception of the problem and to gain their cooperation with changes/interventions required.
- Remove/hospitalize child if there is an immediate risk of, or ongoing, abuse.
- Consider whether siblings are at risk.
- Involve social services early. Report to authorities and specified agencies as mandated by regulations.
- Balance the benefits/costs of nonintervention versus that of intervention.
- Above all, put the needs of the child first.

Psychiatric outcome of chronic abuse

Children who are abused have an extremely high rate of psychiatric disorders, both during the abuse and later on. CBT has been shown to reduce risk for PTSD and depression in sexually abused children; parental treatment has been shown to improve outcome in children by increasing parental monitoring of child behavior and support to the child around the issue of abuse and its disclosure.

Some of the most common disorders potentially associated with previous abuse
- PTSD.
- Dissociative disorders.
- Conversion disorders.
- Borderline personality disorder.
- Depression.
- Paraphilias.

Refer to 📖 *p. 846 for further details.*

Child abuse—alerting signs

The following are signs that may alert one to abuse, but it is important to remember that other causes may exist, and also that these behaviors should be viewed within the context of other information at one's disposal. The parent may also have unusual behavior (e.g., unusually demanding, uncaring, or dismissive of the child). There may also be obvious parent-child interactional problems (e.g., they don't look at each other or have an overly negative relationship).

Signs of possible emotional abuse
- Low self-esteem, continual self-deprecation.
- Sudden speech disorder.
- Significant decline in concentration.
- Socio-emotional immaturity.
- Rocking, head-banging, or other neurotic behavior.
- Self-mutilation.
- Compulsive stealing.
- Extremes of passivity or aggression.
- Running away.
- Indiscriminate friendliness.

Signs of possible physical abuse
- Unexplained injuries or burns, especially if recurrent.
- Improbable excuses given for injuries.
- Refusal to discuss injuries.
- Untreated injuries or delay in reporting them.
- Excessive physical punishment.
- Limbs kept covered in hot weather; avoidance of swimming, physical education classes, etc.
- Fear of returning home.
- Aggression toward others.
- Running away.

(Note: "Injuries" may occur for other reasons such as: genuine accidents; hematological disorders; natural skin pigmentation; skin conditions such as impetigo or nevi; rare bone diseases; swelling of eye due to tumor; undiagnosed birth injury such as fractured clavicle.)

Signs of possible physical neglect
- Constant hunger.
- Poor personal hygiene.
- Constant tiredness.
- Poor state of clothing.
- Frequent lateness or nonattendance at school.
- Untreated medical problems.
- Low self-esteem.
- Poor peer relationships.
- Stealing.

Signs of possible failure to thrive

- Significant lack of growth.
- Weight loss.
- Hair loss.
- Poor skin or muscle tone.
- Circulatory disorders.
- Loss of previously attained developmental milestones.

Physical/medical

- Bruises, scratches, or other marks to the thighs or genital area.
- Itch, soreness, discharge, unexplained bleeding from the rectum, vagina, or penis
- Pain on passing urine or recurrent urinary tract infection.
- Recurrent vaginal infection.
- Venereal disease.
- Stained underwear.
- Unusual genital odor.
- Soiling or wetting in children who have been trained.
- Discomfort/difficulty walking or sitting.
- Pregnancy, particularly when reluctance to name father.

Signs of possible sexual abuse

Behavioral

- Lack of trust in adults or overfamiliarity with adults.
- Fear of a particular individual.
- Social isolation, withdrawal, and introversion.
- Sleep disturbances (nightmares, irrational fears, bed wetting, fear of sleeping alone, needing a nightlight).
- Running away from home.
- Girls taking over the mothering role.
- Reluctance or refusal to participate in physical activities or to change clothes for activities.
- Low self-esteem.
- Drug, alcohol, or solvent abuse.
- Display of sexual knowledge beyond child's years.
- Unusual interest in genitals of adults, children, or animals.
- Expressing affection in inappropriate ways.
- Fears of bathrooms, showers, or closed doors
- Abnormal sexualized drawing and precocious sexual behavior.
- Fear of medical examinations.
- Developmental regression.
- Poor peer relations.
- Over-sexualized behavior.
- Eating disorders.
- Compulsive masturbation.
- Stealing.
- Psychosomatic complaints.
- Sexual promiscuity.

Munchausen syndrome by proxy[1]

Munchausen syndrome by proxy (MBP) is a factitious disorder that involves an adult perpetrator and a child victim. It can easily be confused with the adult factitious disorder "Munchausen syndrome," which is when the adult intentionally feigns symptoms to assume the sick role themselves (see 📖 p. 972). In MBP, the adult intentionally exaggerates the situation to place the sick role on the child, and experiences the gain "by proxy." There are an estimated 600 cases per year, though most go undetected due to the often savvy deception of the ill adult, and the general desire of clinicians to believe parental reports. MBP frequently shows up in pop culture TV and literary references.

General facts about MBP

- This is a form of abuse that can result in harm or death to the child.
- The perpetrator is usually the child's mother (93–98% are females, usually the mother or female caregiver).
- The perpetrator appears to be using the child's induced illness to meet her own psychological needs (e.g., desire to be in control, the center of attention, or receive attention from doctors and other professionals).
- External gains (e.g., money, legal advantages) are not the primary motivation, but may be present.
- The Pediatric Condition Falsification (PCF) can be covert and elaborate, and is only limited by the creativity of the perpetrator.
- The result is over- or undertreatment of the condition.
- The PCF can range from exaggerating actual symptoms to deliberately creating symptoms by various methods.
- Family, physicians, and other caregivers can be easily drawn into what is often a convincing deception.
- The child (or family) may be aware of the PCF, yet not report the abuse.
- Examples of PCF reports include allergies, neurological or gastrological conditions, or poisoning.
- Even convicted perpetrators can go on to abuse again, even under the closest of surveillance.
- Children tend to do well when separated from the perpetrator, despite objections that the parent must remain present for the child to be well.

What to look for

No one symptom is pathognomonic. Look for a trail of medical and social clues that do not otherwise add up:

- Child was doing well in the past and now is not.
- Parental subjective reported symptoms do not match objective findings.
- Child gets better when the parent is not around the child.
- Child gets worse when the parent is around the child.
- Unexplained findings on toxicology reports.
- Observation confirms the PCF.

- History of death or unexplained illness in a sibling of the child (previous abuse makes current abuse more likely).
- "Doctor shopping" in order to subject the child to repeated procedures.
- The caregiver perpetrator often has personality disorder traits.

Differential diagnoses

- Anxious or easily frightened caregivers mothers who overly seek doctors' attention and exaggerate symptoms to avoid being dismissed.
- Parents (some with dependence issues) who allow a child to feign symptoms to keep them home from school.
- Parents who exaggerate an illness to gain advantage in a legal custody battle.
- Other physical, sexual abuse, or neglect (e.g., failure to thrive) that is disguised by falsely reporting medical symptoms.
- Many children who experience MBP had an initial illness that was over- or undertreated. The treatments or tests may have potential sequelae.
- Actual complicated medical illnesses that is difficult to diagnose.

What to do when you suspect MBP

- Familiarize yourself with the literature to look for all possible presentations.
- Gather all medical records for the child. Speak to the providers directly. There may be multiple providers from various clinics, hospitals, and emergency rooms. Bring in other family members and providers to gather all of the information.
- Consult specialists (pediatricians, psychiatrists, MBP specialists) to help with diagnosis. Obtain supervision for yourself.
- Corroborate all parental reports.
- If MBP is suspected, it is a form of abuse and needs reported according to your local rules and regulations.
- May need to, if legally cleared, monitor and document parental behavior by video surveillance.

Recommended further reading

1 Ayoub, C., *et al.* (May 2002). Position paper: Definitional issues in Munchausen by proxy. Child Maltreatment. **7**(2), 105–111.

Prescribing in children and adolescents

This section will review selected psychopharmacologic agents used in the treatment of children and adolescents. Other references review pharmacokinetic and pharmacodynamic properties of these medications in detail and should be reviewed prior to prescribing psychotropic medication to a pediatric population.

Many medications currently utilized in clinical practice are "off label"—they have FDA approval but not indication for specific pediatric illnesses. When using psychotropic medications, one should follow the most recent evidence in the scientific literature and also review the manufacturer's label or reprint in the Physicians" Desk Reference. One must also provide informed consent to family members regarding the current knowledge of safety and efficacy both from short and long term trials. As such, **risks, benefits, alternatives**, and **consent** must be thoroughly reviewed and documented for the patient and *all* legal guardians before prescribing medication, and a review of this information should be repeated routinely throughout treatment and with each dosage adjustment. There are subtle nuances to prescribing medication for children and adolescents, and information changes as time and evidence progresses. As such, review of the recent literature as well as supervision and consultation with an expert in child and adolescent psychopharmacology should be sought prior to prescription or administration of these medications in the youth population. In addition, a physical examination from the primary care physician is typically recommended due to the baseline evaluation outlined for many of the medications.

Psychopharmacotherapy is one adjunct in the treatment of mental illness in children and adolescents. Medications should be used cautiously but judiciously in conjunction with psychological, social and educational interventions. Check with your institution for options, guidelines, and protocols on the administration and implementation of psychiatric treatment in the pediatric population.

Stimulants

Stimulant class issues

Stimulants are among the most effective psychotropic medications in clinical use today. In general there is a 70% response rate when a single stimulant is used, i.e., methamphetamine (MPH) or dextroamphetamine (DEX) alone.[1] Nearly 90% will respond if both stimulants are tried.[2]

Short-term trials have reported improvements in interrupting, fidgeting, on-task behavior, compliance, sustained attention and social interactions.

Mode of action

An indirect sympathomimetic that increases release of dopamine and norepinephrine in the brain.

Indications

ADHD and narcolepsy.

Absolute and relative contraindications

Structural cardiac defects, psychosis, bipolar disorder without a concomitant mood stabilizing medication, tic disorders, substance abuse (especially if considering a short-acting stimulant).

Clinical effects

Increased concentration and attention and decreased impulsivity; may also improve aggression and explosivity in children with these co-morbid symptoms.

Principles of prescribing[2]

- Start low and titrate systematically, as often as weekly.
- Document an accurate diagnosis and psychotropic trials.
- Monitor response with parent and teacher rating scales to assure adequate response of symptoms throughout the day.
- Check heights, weight, BP, and pulse regularly.
- Observe for rebound effects such as mood changes, or disruptive symptoms as medication wears off (worse with shorter-acting stimulants).
- Address insomnia by educating about sleep hygiene and behavioral strategies. Sometimes, late-day stimulants may reduce rather than increase insomnia. If all else fails, may use low doses of melatonin, or antihistamines to help with sleep latency.
- The current standard of care is to provide stimulant treatment year-round and on weekends, in order to target multiple domains of impairment both within and outside of school.
- The second-line treatment after a child has failed a stimulant is generally another stimulant from the alternative group (amphetamine or methylphenidate), before trying a nonstimulant medication.[2]
- Special prescribing and dosing considerations may be required for co-morbid medical problems.
- Sometimes one must exceed the labeled maximum recommended doses of a stimulant in patients with only a partial response who are otherwise tolerating the medication.

Note: the consensus from practice is that doses may go higher than the PDR recommendations on rare occasions

Stimulant contraindications
- Previous sensitivity to stimulant medication.
- Glaucoma.
- Symptomatic cardiovascular disease: Structural, Arrhythmias.
- Hyperthyroidism.
- Hypertension.
- Family history of sudden death.

FDA package inserts also warn against use with concomitant motor tics, marked anxiety and that MPH can lower the seizure threshold (recent clinical literature reveals tics may not be worsened by stimulants and that stimulants can be utilized in children with well controlled seizures). Caution in use with history of drug dependence.

Stimulant baseline and monitoring information
- Document an accurate diagnosis and psychotropic trials.
- Obtain baseline BP, Pulse, HGT, WGT. Baseline EKG may be warrranted.
- Yearly physical exam, more frequently if needed.

Common side-effects of stimulants
Most common
- Headache, stomachache/nausea, delayed sleep onset, appetite suppression.
- Studies have shown that consistently medicated children have a temporary slowing in growth rate (on average, a 2cm or less change in growth in height, 2.7kg less change in growth in weight over three years).

Less common
- Psychosis, mood lability, aggression, seizures, tics.

Special considerations for prescribing in children
The typical prescribing practice is to use the medications only if needed, chose the medication with best risk to benefit profile, obtain full consent/assent after detailed disclosure of all options and risks, start at the lowest dose, and increase only if needed after adequate number of days on that dose. Circumstances may suggest increased doses or shortening titrations (severity of illness, previous tolerance of higher starting dose). However, to minimize side-effects and complications, the most prudent course remains starting low and titrating slowly.

Many of these drugs and doses are not FDA approved in children, and there have specific regulations about monitoring potential side-effects. Check with the standard of practice and recognized guidelines before using any drugs in children.

Recommended further reading

1 Spencer, *et al.* (1996). Pharmacotherapy of attention-deficit hyperactivity disorder across the life cycle. *J Am Acad Child Adolesc Psychiatry* **35**: 409–32.
2 Elia, *et al.* (1991). Methylphenidate and dextroamphetamine treatments of hyperactivity: are there true nonresponders? *Psychiatry Res* **36**(2): 141–55.

Stimulant medications for ADHD— quick guide

	General Duration (hrs)	Available doses (mg)	Starting dose (mg)	Max. dose (mg/d)
Short-acting				
Methylphenidate (Ritalin®)	3–5	5, 10, 20	5mg bid	60
Methylphenidate (Methylin®)	3–5	5, 10, 20 tab 2.5, 5, 10 chew 5/5mL, 10/5mL sol.	2.5–5mg bid	60
Dextroamphetamine (Dexedrine®)	4–5	5, 10	2.5–5mg bid	40
Dexmethylphenidate (Focalin®)	4–5	2.5, 5, 10	2.5mg bid	30
Intermediate-acting				
Methylphenidate Sustained-Release (Ritalin SR®)	4–5	20	20mg/d	60
Mixed amhetamine salts (Adderal®l)	4–6	5, 7.5, 10, 12.5, 15, 20, 30	2.5–5mg bid	40
Dextroamphetamine capsules (Dexedrine Span®)	8	5, 10, 15	2.5–5mg bid	40
Methylphenidate Extended-Release (Metadate ER®)	8	10, 20	10mg	60
Methylphenidate Long-acting (Ritalin LA®)	8	10, 20, 30, 40	20mg qam	60
Long-acting				
Oros Methylphenidate (Concerta®)	12	18, 27, 36, 54	18mg qam	54–72
Methylphenidate Controlled-Delivery (Metadate CD®)	10–12	10, 20, 30, 40, 50, 60	20mg qam	60
Mixed Amphetamine Salts Extended-Release (Adderall XR®)	12	5, 10, 15, 20, 25, 30	10mg qam	40
Dextromethylphenidate Long-Acting form (Focalin XR®)	8–12	5, 10, 15, 20	10mg qam	20
Daytrana (Methylph-enidate transdermal®)	9–14	10, 15, 20, 30 per 9 hour patch	10mg/ patch	30mg/ patch
Pemoline (Cylert®)	12–14	Not used	—	112.5

FDA age approval for ADHD medications

Trade Name	Generic Name	Approved Age
Adderall®	amphetamine	3 and older
Concerta®	methylphenidate (long acting)	6 and older
Cylert®	pemoline	6 and older. Not used in U.S.
Daytrana®	methylphenidate transdermal	6 and older
Dexedrine®	dextroamphetamine	3 and older
Dextrostat®	dextroamphetamine	3 and older
Focalin®	dexmethylphenidate	6 and older
Metadate ER®	methylphenidate (extended release)	6 and older
Metadate CD®	methylphenidate (extended release)	6 and older
Ritalin®	methylphenidate	6 and older
Ritalin SR®	methylphenidate (extended release)	6 and older
Ritalin LA®	methylphenidate (long acting)	6 and older

Short-acting stimulants

Methylphenidate "MPH" (Ritalin®)

(5, 10, 20mg tablets)
- Starting dose 5mg qam and lunchtime.
- Titrate to minimal effective dose by 5–10mg per dose per week, using 2–3 times daily dosing.
- *Duration 2–3 hours*.

Methylin
Another MPH formulation. (5, 10, 20mg tabs; 2.5, 5, 10mg chewables; 5/5mL, 10/5mL solution). Start at 0.3mg/kg/d divided bid or 2.5–5mg bid. Increase by 0.1mg.kg.dose or 5–10mg/day every 7 days.
- An alternate approach is to use a fixed-titration trial in which a full set of different doses is switched on a weekly basis and physician and parents determine, which was most efficacious with the least side-effects.
- PDR recommends a *maximum* daily dose of 2mg/kg/day up to 60mg/d.
- Children weighing less than 25kg should not receive single doses greater than 15mg.
- The consensus from practice is that doses may go higher the PDR recommendations on rare occasions (25mg per dose of MPH).
- *Duration 3–5 hours*.

Per dose, requiring 2–3 times daily dosing. Take last dose before 6 p.m.

Dextroamphetamine (Dexedrine®)

(5, 10mg tabs)
- Starting dose 5mg daily, increase by 5mg daily (by 10mg in teenage children) every 7 days if needed, to max of 60mg per day. Give in divided doses over 4–6 hour intervals. Longer lasting Dexedrine Span® (about 8 hours) is available.
- *Duration 4–5 hours*.

Dexmethylphenidate (Focalin®)

(2.5, 5, and 10mg tabs)
- Initial starting dose at 5mg daily (2.5mg bid).
- Titrate in 2.5 to 5mg increments to a max 20mg daily (10mg bid).
- Conversion from MPH: start Focalin at 50% of current MPH dose.
- *Duration 4–5 hours*.

Space doses at least 4 hours apart.

Intermediate-acting stimulants

Methylphenidate SR (Ritalin SR®)

(20mg tabs)
- Initially titrate with short acting Ritalin until 20mg reached. This can then be converted to the 8-hour sustained release (SR) preparation. Max total dose 60mg/day, or 2mg/kg/day in younger children.
- *Duration 4–8 hours.*

Space bid doses 8 hours apart.

Amphetamine/dextroamphetamine, "AMP/DEX" (Adderall®)

(5, 7.5, 10, 12.5, 15, 20, 30mg tabs)
- Starting dose 2.5mg in younger children, start 5mg (in a.m. or bid) in older children.
- Dose in 4–6-hour intervals.
- Titrate to a minimal effective dose by 2.5–5mg per dose per week in divided doses. An alternate approach is to use a fixed-titration trial in which a full set of different doses is switched on a weekly basis and MD and parents determine which was most efficacious with the least side-effects. PDR recommends a *maximum* daily dose of 40mg per day and that children weighing less than 25kg should not receive single doses more than 10mg
- *Duration 4–6 hours.*

The consensus from practice is that does may go higher than the PDR recommendations on rare occasions.

Methylphenidate (Metadate ER®)

10 and 20mg tabs
- Start at 10mg, titrate by 10mg every 7 days as needed to recommended max total dose of 60mg/ day.
- Do not crush, cut or chew.
- *Duration 4–8 hours.*

May need bid with 8 hour spacing.

Methylphenidate ER (Methylin ER®)

10 and 20mg tabs
- Start at 10mg, titrate by 10mg every 7 days as needed to recommended max total dose of 60mg/ day.
- Do not crush, cut or chew.
- *Duration about 4–8 hours.*

May need bid with 8 hour spacing.

Methylphenidate LA (Ritalin LA®)

10, 20, 30, 40mg capsule
- May be administered by swallowing as whole capsules or by sprinkling on applesauce.
- Initial starting dose is 20mg daily with weekly 10mg increments to a maximum dose of 60mg daily.
- *Duration is 8–12 hours.*

Methylphenidate ER (Concerta®)

18, 27, 36, 54mg caps.
- Must be swallowed whole (do not crush, cut, or chew).
- PDR recommendations:
  - Stimulant naive patients start at a dose of 18mg qam.
  - Dose conversions from short-acting methylphenidate.
  - 5mg bid or tid 18mg qam.
  - 10mg bid or tid 36mg qam.
  - 15mg bid or tid 54mg qam.
- Initial conversion dose should not exceed 54mg qam.
- After conversion, dose may be titrated by 18mg/day to maximum dose of 54mg/ day in children in divided doses (72mg/day in teens and adults).
- *Duration 8–12 hours.*

Methylphenidate (Metadate CD®)

10, 20, 30, 40, 50, 60mg caps.
- May be swallowed whole or broken apart and sprinkled on applesauce
- Initial starting dose of 20mg qam; Dosage may be adjusted in weekly 10–20mg increments to a maximum of 60mg/day.
- Do not crush, cut or chew
- *Duration is 8–12 hours.*

AMP/DEX (Adderall XR®)

5, 10, 15, 20, 25, 30mg caps.
- May be swallowed whole or broken apart and sprinkled on applesauce.
- Can switch from total daily dose of short-acting Adderall to 1 dose of XR.
- PDR recommendations:
  - Children 6 years of age or older initial starting dose of 10mg qam.
  - Titrate by 5–10mg on a weekly basis.
  - Maximum dose of 30mg/day (60mg/day in adults).
- Amphetamines are not recommended for children under the age of 3 and have not been studied in children under the age of 6.

Dexmethylphenidate (Focalin XR®)

5, 10, 15 and 20mg caps.
- May be swallowed whole or broken apart and sprinkled on applesauce.
- Initial starting dose at 5mg daily.
- Titrate in 5mg increments to a maximum dose of 20mg daily.
- *Duration is 8–12 hours.*

Methylphenidate PATCH (Daytrana®)

10, 15, 20, 30mg/9 hour patch.
- Start 10mg patch. Increase to next size patch every 7 days to optimal response (max 30). Placed on hip, rotate sites. Can have site irritation.
- Do not alter patch in any way.
- *Duration.*
Until removed (~9hrs), but may continue 5 hours after removal.

Methylphenidate PATCH dosing information

Dose Delivered (mg) over 9 hrs	Dosage Rate (mg/hr)	Patch Size (cm^2)	Methylphenidate Content/patch (mg)
10	1.1	12.5	27.5
15	1.6	18.75	41.3
20	2.2	25	55
30	3.3	37.5	82.5

Lisdexamfetamine dimesylate (Vyvanse®)

An amphetamine derivative prodrug, new to the market in 2007.
- 30, 50, 70mg capsules.
- Start 30mg once daily in a.m.
- If needed, titrate in 20mg increments at weekly intervals.
- Maximum dose is 70mg/day.
- Can take capsule whole or dissolved in water (take immediately if dissolved).

Nonstimulant medications for ADHD

Nonstimulants may be appropriate when patients have failed or not tolerated stimulants, or have certain co-morbid disorders such as tics, depression, anxiety, or substance abuse (given nonstimulants lack of abuse potential). Special prescribing and dosing considerations may be required for co-morbid medical problems.

Atomoxetine (Strattera®)

The only currently available nonstimulant labeled for the treatment of ADHD, both in children and adults. It works as a selective norepinephrine reuptake inhibitor. Potential side-effects include sedation, nausea, mild increases in blood pressure, headaches, and *rare* case reports of *hepatoxicity* or increased suicidal behaviors. Metabolized by the cytochrome 2D6 enzyme system, it has potential interactions with other drugs (e.g., fluoxetine, paroxetine). Clinicians prescribing atomoxetine should monitor blood pressures, pulses, mood and suicidal thoughts or behaviors, especially early in treatment, and advise of potential hepatoxicity (e.g., jaundice, malaise, nausea, elevations in liver function tests).

Bupropion (Wellbutrin®)

A noradrenergic and dopaminergic reuptake inhibitor, shown in randomized controlled trials in both children and adults to have efficacy in ADHD. It may be particularly helpful for youths with co-morbid depression. Potential side-effects reported include appetite suppression, insomnia, rashes, agitation, and *rare* cases of *seizures* (especially at higher doses, or in patients with previous seizures or eating disorders).

Tricyclic antidepressants[1]

Including imipramine, desipramine, and nortriptyline, have strong evidence for their efficacy in pediatric ADHD, however, use is typically limited to patients for whom stimulants are ineffective or contraindicated. All have anticholinergic side-effects, as well as potential orthostatic hypotension, tachycardia, and conduction delays, and are *potentially fatal in overdoses*. Children prescribed tricyclics should have baseline and repeated electrocardiograms, and checks of blood pressure and pulse to rule out signs of cardiovascular toxicity.

Alpha-2 adrenergic receptor agonists[2]

Including clonidine and guanfacine, have some evidence of efficacy in randomized controlled trials of ADHD. They are more effective for hyperactive/impulsive symptoms than inattentive symptoms. They may also be useful for treating co-morbid tic disorders and insomnia. Common side-effects are sedation, dizziness, low blood pressure, and rebound hypertension if doses are missed. There are case reports of rare *unexplained deaths* in children prescribed clonidine, *especially in combination with methylphenidate*. Close monitoring of electrocardiograms, blood pressures, pulses and tolerability is recommended prescribing alpha-agonists.

ADHD medication	Available Doses (mg)	Starting Dose	Maximum Dose
Atomoxetine (Strattera®)	10, 18, 25, 40, 60	0.5mg/kg/d	1.4mg/kg/d
Bupropion Wellbutrin® Wellbutrin SR® Wellbutrin XL®	75, 100 100, 150, 200 150, 300	1.5mg/kg/d	6.5mg/kg/d*
Imipramine (Tofranil®)	25, 50	1mg/kg/d	5mg/kg/d
Desipramine (Norpramine®)	25, 50	1mg/kg/d	5mg/kg/d
Nortiptyline (Pamelor®)	10, 25, 50	0.5mg/kg/d	2.5mg/kg/d
Clonidine (Catapress®)	0.1, 0.2	0.05mg bid	0.1mg qid
Guanfacine (Tenex®)	1.0	0.5mg bid	1.5mg tid

* Maximum single dose should not exceed 150mg for bupropion and 200mg for bupropion SR.

Recommended further reading

1 Popper, C.W.: Antidepressants in the treatment of attention-deficit/hyperactivity disorder. Journal of Clinical Psychiatry 1997; **58** Suppl, 14:14–29; discussion 30–1.
2 Connor, D.F, Fletcher, K.E., Swanson, J.M. (1999). A meta-analysis of clonidine for symptoms of attention-deficit hyperactivity disorder. Journal of the American Academy of Child & Adolescent Psychiatry **38**(12), 1551–1559.

Lithium use in children and adolescents[1,2,3]

Lithium is the best-studied mood stabilizer for children and adolescents who have bipolar disorder. At the time of this edition's release, it is the only medication approved by the U.S. Food and Drug Administration for the treatment of acute mania and bipolar disorder in adolescents (ages 12–18). Approximately 40–50% of children and adolescents who have bipolar disorder respond acutely to lithium therapy. Lithium is used to stabilize the extremes of mood fluctuations in bipolar children and to prevent recurrence of mood cycling. It is particularly useful to treat the manic symptoms of bipolar disorder and has also been beneficial in treating symptoms of depression that have not responded to typical antidepressants.

Precautions for lithium

- Lithium should not be administered to children with significant kidney problems.
- Lithium may be administered with caution to children with cardiac, thyroid, seizure, severe dehydration and sodium depletion problems.
- Lithium may cause cardiac defects (**Epstein's anomaly**) in the fetus if taken during the first three months of pregnancy and can be excreted in the breast milk of nursing mothers.
- Changes in the amount of **salt and water** in the body can affect blood levels of lithium. Decreases in overall body water may result from not drinking enough fluids, perspiring excessively (whether with exercise or during a febrile illness), excessive vomiting and diarrhea. This can lead to dehydration. Dehydration can increase the blood level of lithium. Abrupt decreases in the amount of salt in diet may lead to high lithium blood levels and too much salt in diet can lead to low blood levels of lithium. It is, therefore, important that the child drinks enough water and maintains average ordinary table salt intake, especially on hot, humid days.
- Be cautious giving other prescriptions or over-the-counter medications. Using lithium with nonsteroidal anti-inflammatory medications may increase blood lithium levels. To prevent interactions with lithium, always check with the patient's other providers and pharmacists to see if the child is taking other prescribed medications. Special prescribing and dosing considerations may be required for co-morbid medical problems.

Common side-effects of lithium

Includes fine tremor, increased thirst, increased urination, inability to concentrate urine, fatigue, weight gain, headache, gastrointestinal complaints (including nausea and diarrhea). These side-effects usually subside with continued treatment or a temporary reduction or cessation of dosage. Gradual increases in lithium dosage may be helpful in controlling gastrointestinal symptoms. Over time, many patients develop hypothyroidism. Rarer, but more serious is the impact on the kidney, including a decrease in GFR and proteinuria.

Baseline monitoring and laboratory work-up for lithium

The dosage of lithium will depend on the child's clinical response, lithium blood levels and the presence of any side-effects. Lithium is usually administered to obtain blood levels between **0.8 to 1.2mEq/L.**

- A complete blood count with differential (CBC with diff).
- Serum electrolytes (sodium, potassium, chloride).
- Pregnancy test for females.
- Kidney function tests (blood urea nitrogen or BUN and creatinine and possibly a twenty four hour urine collection for analysis of the volume and concentration of urine along with the presence or absence of protein in the urine).
- Thyroid function test.
- Cardiovascular function test—electrocardiogram (EKG).

Lithium blood levels will be monitored routinely during the initial phase of treatment as the medication dosage is adjusted. Once symptom improvement is noted, maintenance monitoring of lithium blood levels and electrolytes, kidney functioning and thyroid functioning will continue at a less frequent schedule.

Dosages and preparations of lithium

Lithium carbonate (immediate-release)
- Brand name: Eskalith®.
- Preparations: capsules 150 (generic) and 300mg.
- Starting dosage: 25mg/kg/d (2–3 daily doses).
- Target dosage: 30mg/kg/d (2–3 daily doses).
- Dosage range: 300–1800mg/day given 2–3 times/day.

Lithium carbonate controlled release (CR)
- Brand name: Eskalith CR®.
- Preparation: capsules 450mg.
- Starting dosage: 25mg/kg/d (2–3 daily doses).
- Target dosage: 30mg/kg/d (2–3 daily doses).
- Dosage range: 300–1800mg/day given 2 times a day.

Lithium carbonate slow release (SR)
- Brand name: Lithobid®.
- Preparation: capsules 300mg.
- Starting dosage: 25mg/kg/d (2–3 daily doses).
- Target dosage: 30mg/kg/d (2–3 daily doses).
- Dosage: 300–1800mg/day given 2 times a day.

Lithium citrate
- Brand name: Cibalith-S®.
- Preparation: syrup (8mEq/5cc).
- Starting dosage: 25mg/kg/d (2–3 daily doses).
- Target dosage: 30mg/kg/d (2–3 daily doses).
- Dosage: 300–1800mg/day given 2–3 times a day.

Lithium blood levels will be monitored routinely during the initial phase of treatment as the medication dosage is adjusted. Once symptom improvement is noted, maintenance monitoring of lithium blood levels, electrolytes, kidney functioning and thyroid functioning will continue at a less frequent schedule.

Recommended further reading

1 Kowatch, R.A., et al. (2000). Effect size of lithium, divalproex sodium, and carbamazepine in children and adolescents with bipolar disorder. *J Am Acad Child Adolesc psychiatry* **39**(6): 713–20.

2 Youngerman, J., Canino, I.A. (1978). Lithium carbonate use in children and adolescents. A survey of the literature. *Arch Gen Psychiatry* **35**(2): 216–24.

3 Smarty, S., Findling, R.L. (2007). Psychopharmacology of pediatric bipolar disorder. A review Psychopharmacology **191**(1): 39–54.

Anticonvulsants use in youth

Precautions for anticonvulsants

- Anticonvulsants should only be prescribed by physicians who are thoroughly familiar with potential risks, interactions, and proper monitoring of drug group.
- Should be administered with great caution in children with medical illnesses (especially liver and kidney disease).
- Can cause SERIOUS birth defects during pregnancy (esp. the first trimester).
- Drugs (especially carbamazepine) may interact with other medications.

Common side-effects of anticonvulsants

Nausea, vomiting, diarrhea, drowsiness, dizziness, cognitive problems, increase or decrease in appetite, weight gain.

Side-effects of specific anticonvulsants

Divalproex sodium (Depakote®)
- Elevation of liver function enzymes.
- Pancreatic inflammation.
- Decreased platelet levels.
- Hand tremor.
- Hair thinning.
- Polycystic ovarian disease.

Carbamazepine (Carbatrol®, Tegretol®, Equetro®)
- Decreased WBC.
- Decreases RBC and platelets.
- Agranulocytosis/aplastic anemia.
- Rash.
- Elevation of liver function enzymes.
- Hand tremor.
- Poor coordination/clumsy.

Oxcarbazepine (Trileptal®)
- Hyponatremia (rare).

Lamotrigine (Lamictal®)
- Skin rash, possibly rare and serious Steven-Johnson's syndrome.
- Can interact with other medication (esp. Depakote).

Topiramate (Topamax®)
- Increase risk of kidney stones, glaucoma, hyperthermia.
- Difficulty with memory, dizziness, poor sleep, weight loss.
- Laboratory tests for specific anticonvulsants.

Divalproex sodium (Depakote®)
- Baseline CBC with differential and platelets and LFTs.
- VPA blood level 8—12 hours after last dose after 5 days at steady state.
- Therapeutic trough levels roughly between 60 and 120mcg/mL.

Carbamazepine (Carbatrol®, Tegretol®, Equetro®)

- Baseline and periodic CBC with differential and platelets, LFT.
- Baseline EKG for children with cardiac history.
- Blood level 8–12 hours after last dose after 5 days at steady state.
- *Metabolic autoinduction* is likely to occur so blood levels may drop even when on a steady dose and compliant with regimen. This may require change in dosage.
- Therapeutic levels between 4 and 12mcg/mL.

Oxcarbazepine, lamotrigine, topiramate

- No baseline lab tests required.
- Consider creatinine, sodium levels. See 📖 *p. 798* for details.

Dosages and preparations for anticonvulsants

The typical prescribing practice is to use the lowest effective dose of medication with the best risk to benefit profile after explaining all options and obtaining full consent. To minimize side-effects and complications, the most prudent course remains starting low and titrating slowly. Special prescribing and dosing considerations may be required for co-morbid medical problems. Check the updated standard of practice and recognized guidelines before using any drugs in children. Doses are provided in ranges: refer to your institution standards for titration schedule, maintenance dosing, and max dosing.

Divalproex sodium (Depakote®)

- Tablets 125mg, 250, 500mg; Sprinkle capsules 125mg.
- Dosage 250–1500mg given bid.
- Peds dosing: 10–15mg/kg/day- increase by 5–10mg/kg q 7 days to max 60mg/kg/day divided qd-tid dosing.
- Dose to reach therapeutic blood level between 60–120 microgram/ml.

Divalproex sodium extended release (Depakote ER®)

- 250 and 500mg tablets; 500–1500mg once daily.
- Peds dosing: 10–15mg/kg/day: increase by 5–10mg/kg q 7 days to max 60mg/kg/day.
- Dose to reach therapeutic blood level between 60–120 microgram/ml.

Carbamazepine (Tegretol®)

- Chewable tablets 100mg; Liquid 100mg/tsp (5cc).
- Dosage 200–1600mg, given 2–3 times per day to obtain blood level 4–12 micrograms/ml.
- Peds dosing: varies by age range with max as low as 1000mg/d.

Carbamazepine (Carbatrol®)

- 200 and 300mg; dosage same as for Tegretol®

Carbamazepine XR (Tegretol XR®)

- 100, 200 and 400mg tablets.
- Dosage 400–1600mg, given 2–3 times per day.
- Peds dosing: varies by age range with max as low as 1000mg/d.

Carbamazepine ER (Equetro®)

- 100, 200, 300mg capsules: do not crush or chew beads.
- Dosage 400–1600mg bid in adults. Peds dosing is not available.
- Therapeutic levels 4–12microgram/mL.

Oxcarbazepine (Trileptal®)
- 150, 300, and 600mg tablets; syrup: 300mg/5cc.
- Dosage 300–2400mg, divided 2–3 times per day.
- Peds dosing: varies by age.

Lamotrigine (Lamictal®)
- 25, 100, 150, and 200mg tablets; 2, 5 and 25mg chewable tablets.
- Dosage 25–400mg divided into 2 dosages per day.
- *This drug requires very special dosing regimen to limit severe side-effects, esp. with valproate. Refer to manufacturer for full details before starting this medication!

Topiramate (Topamax®)
- 25, 50, 100, 200mg tablets; 15 and 25mg capsules.
- Dosage 200–400mg given twice a day.

Atypical antipsychotics

The atypical antipsychotics have established efficacy in the treatment of schizophrenia and bipolar disorder in adults. To date, none of these agents are labeled for treatment in children (except Risperdal® which received approval in the use of autism in late 2006). Although none are labeled by the FDA, many are used for the treatment of various conditions in pediatric populations. While there are current research projects studying these medications in this population, much remains unknown about the efficacy and long-term safety of this class of medications in the pediatric population.

Common side-effects
- Weight changes, diabetes and hyperlipidemia.
- Sedation.
- Cardiovascular.
  - QTc prolongation in all (especially ziprasidone)—caution in combination with other drugs.
- Orthostatic hypotension, tachycardia.
- Pericarditis.
- Agranulocytosis and neutropenia (clozapine).
- Prolactin level.
  - Risperidone > olanzapine > ziprasidone.
  - Clozapine, quetiapine and aripiprazole do not appear to increase prolactin in adults.
- Seizures (clozapine).
- Tardive dyskinesia, EPS, and withdrawal dyskinesia.
  - Significantly lower risk than with traditional antipsychotics.
- Neuroleptic malignant syndrome (rare).
- Liver dysfunction (rare).
- Cataracts.

Baseline history and laboratory work-up for atypical antipsychotics

(See 📖 chapter 6 for more details.)
Document family history of diabetes, hyperlipidemia, seizures, cardiac abnormalities and previous response or adverse event associated with atypical neuroleptics. For all atypical antipsychotics, the following monitoring should be completed at baseline and as directed thereafter:
- EKG: if positive family history of syncope, sudden death, arrhythmias.
- Complete at baseline and routinely throughout course of treatment (recommend following the consensus statement from the ADA and APA[1]).
- Vital signs.
- HGT, WGT, waist circumference, and BMI.
- Fasting blood glucose.
- Lipid profile.
- AIMS—scale to measure movement disorders. See 📖 *p. 213.*

Recommend further reading

1 Summary of the Practice Parameters for the Assessment and Treatment of Children and Adolescents with Schizophrenia. (2000). *J Am Acad Child Adolesc Psychiatry* **39**(12): 1580–82.

Dosages and preparations of antipsychotics

The typical prescribing practice is to use the lowest effective dose of medication with the best risk to benefit profile after explaining all options and obtaining full consent. To minimize side-effects and complications, the most prudent course remains starting low and titrating slowly. Special prescribing and dosing considerations may be required for co-morbid medical problems. **Most of these drugs and doses are not FDA approved in children.** Check the updated standard of practice and recognized guidelines before using any drugs in children. See chapter 6 for more details.

Risperdone (Risperdal®)

- 0.25, 0.5, 1, 2, 3, 4mg tablets.
- 1mg/ml liquid.
- M-tab 0.5, 1, 2, 3 and 4mg (disintegrating tablet).
- Intramuscular extended release 25, 37.5, 50mg.
- Dosage 0.5–6mg daily given in 1–2 doses.

Olanzapine (Zyprexa®)

- 2.5, 5, 7.5, 10, 15, and 20mg tablets.
- Zydis® (disintegrating tablet) 5, 10, 15 and 20mg.
- Intramuscular 10mg.
- Dosage 2.5–20mg given once daily.

Quetiapine (Seroquel®)

- 25, 50, 100, 200, 300, and 400mg tablets.
- Dosage 25–800mg given in divided doses daily.
- Consider ophthalmologic examination for cataracts.

Ziprasidone (Geodon®)

- 20, 40, 60, and 80mg tablets.
- Dosage 20–160mg daily given in divided doses.
- Specific monitoring: EKG at baseline and with subsequent dose titration to evaluate QTc.

Aripiprazole (Abilify®)

- 2, 5, 10, 15, 20, and 30mg tablets.
- 10, 15, 20, and 30mg oral disintegrating tablets.
- 1mg/ml oral solution.
- Dosage 10–30mg once daily.

Paliperidone (Invega Extended-Release Tablets®)

- New in 2007. Active ingredient of risperidone.
- 3, 6, 9mg.
- Dose: 3–12mg, once daily.
- Manufacturer's recommended starting dose in adults is 6mg.
- Causes modest increase in QT interval.

Clozapine (Clozaril®)

- 12.5, 25, 50, 100, and 200mg tablets.
- 25 and 100mg oral disintegrating tablets.
- Dosage 25–900mg given 2–3 times daily.
- Specific Monitoring:
  - CBC at baseline, then every 2 weeks for 6 months.
  - Consider EEG.

*There is restricted access to this drug due to monitoring requirements. Contact Novartis Pharmaceuticals for more information (see 📖 *p. 248* psychosis for more details).

Antidepressants commonly used in child and adolescent psychiatry

Antidepressants such as SSRIs are commonly used in the pediatric population for anxiety and depressive disorders. Research into the efficacy and usage of these medications in the pediatric population is not as well studied as in the adult population, and our understanding of their use continually advances. Currently, many of these medications are used off-label. To date, only fluoxetine (Prozac®) is FDA approved for pediatric depression, and only fluoxetine (Prozac®), sertraline (Zoloft®), fluvoxamine (Luvox®), and clomipramine (Anafranil®) are FDA approved for pediatric obsessive-compulsive disorder. As such, careful monitoring of efficacy, safety, and potential side-effects is essential. Special prescribing and dosing considerations may be required for co-morbid medical problems.

Precautions

- FDA black box warning (risk of suicidal thoughts and behaviors).
- Serotonin syndrome, withdrawal syndrome with abrupt discontinuation.
- Increased disinhibition agitation, mixed mania, hostility, induced mania.
- Screen thoroughly for bipolar disorder, special caution in this population (see mood disorders 📖 p. 346).

FDA BLACK BOX WARNING: SSRIs and suicidality

Suicidality in children and adolescents. Antidepressants increased the risk of suicidal thinking and behavior (suicidality) in short-term studies in children and adolescents with MDD and other psychiatric disorders. Anyone considering the use of SSRIs or any other antidepressant in a child or adolescent must balance this risk with the clinical need. Patients who are started on therapy should be observed closely for clinical worsening, suicidality, or unusual changes in behavior. Families and caregivers should be advised of the need for close observation and communication with the prescriber. Pooled analyses of short-term (4 to 16 weeks) placebo-controlled trials of 9 antidepressant drugs (SSRIs and others) in children and adolescents with MDD, OCD, or other psychiatric disorders (a total of 24 trials involving over 4,400 patients) have revealed a greater risk of adverse events representing suicidal thinking or behavior (suicidality) during the first few months of treatment in those receiving antidepressants. The average risk of such events in patients receiving antidepressants was 4%, twice the placebo risk of 2%. No suicides occurred in these trials.

Monitoring as a result of the Black Box warning

"All pediatric patients being treated with antidepressants for any indication should be observed closely for clinical worsening, suicidality, and unusual changes in behavior, especially during the initial few months of a course of drug therapy, or at times of dose changes, either increases or decreases.

Such observation would generally include at least weekly face-to-face contact with patients or their family members or caregivers during the first 4 weeks of treatment, then every other week visits for the next 4 weeks, then at 12 weeks, and as clinically indicated beyond 12 weeks. Additional contact by telephone may be appropriate between face-to-face visits."

Common side-effects of antidepressants

- Nausea, vomiting, diarrhea, constipation, heartburn, loss of appetite
- Headache, change in weight, decreased sex drive, anxiety, alteration in sleep pattern, vivid dreams. Bruising and increased clotting time is significant if patient is going to have surgery or has a preexisting clotting disorder.

Specific side-effects of antidepressants

Fluoxetine (Prozac®)

- Weight loss, headache, vomiting, insomnia, diarrhea and tremor.

Citalopram (Celexa®)

- Nausea, rhinitis, abdominal pain, diarrhea, insomnia, headache, fatigue.

Sertraline (Zoloft®)

- Nausea, vomiting, diarrhea, anorexia, agitation, insomnia.

Venlafaxine (Effexor®)

- Nausea, alteration in appetite, abdominal pain, vomiting, insomnia.
- Should be used with caution in children with high blood pressure, tachycardia, arrythmias.

Escitalopram (Lexapro®)

- Headache, abdominal pain.

Nafazadone (Remeron®)

- Somnolence, weight gain, dry mouth, agranulocystosis, neutropenia, and hypotension, cases of hepatic failure.

Trazodone (Desyrel®)

- Orthostatic hypotension, dizziness and priapism in males.

Monitoring and laboratory work-up

When starting an antidepressant, as always, review the risks, benefits, side-effects, and black box warnings. Once trial is initiated, patient should have weekly contact with clinician to assess safety and side-effects for the first 4 weeks, then every two weeks for the next month then at 12 weeks. Observe closely for any change in behavior, suicidality, or clinical worsening. For venlafaxine, obtain baseline EKG, BP, and pulse, and monitor with every dose change.

Dosages and preparations of antidepressants

The typical prescribing practice is to use the medications only if needed and chose the medication with best risk to benefit profile after explaining all options and obtaining full consent. To minimize side-effects and complications, the most prudent course remains starting low and titrating slowly. Special prescribing and dosing considerations may be required for co-morbid medical problems. Most of these drugs and doses are not FDA approved in children. Check the updated standard of practice and recognized guidelines before using any drugs in children.

Fluoxetine (Prozac®, Prozac Weekly®, Sarafem®)

- 10, 20, and 40mg capsules; 10mg tablet; 20mg/5mL liquid.
- Prozac dosage: 10–80mg once a day.
- "Prozac Weekly" dosage: 90mg once a week.

Sertraline (Zoloft®)

- 25, 50, 100mg tablets; 20mg/ml liquid.
- Dosage: 25–300mg once daily.

Citalopram (Celexa®)

- 10, 20, and 40mg tablets; 10mg/5ml liquid.
- Dosage: 10–60mg daily.

Escitalopram (Lexapro®)

- 5, 10 and 20mg tablets; 5mg/5ml liquid.
- Dosage: 10–40mg daily.

Fluvoxamine (Luvox®)

- Sometimes used in OCD, not much in MDD.
- 25, 50 and 100mg tablets.
- Dosage: 25–300mg daily.

Venlafaxine (Effexor®)

- Short acting dose.
- 25, 37.5, 50, 75, and 100mg tablets.
- Dosage: 25–375mg daily, divided bid or tid.
- Minimize single dose size.

Venlafaxine XR (Effexor XR®)

- 37.5, 75, 150mg capsules.
- Dosage: 75–300mg once or twice daily.
- FDA max is 225mg/day. Minimize size of single doses.

Buproprion (Wellbutrin®)

- Short-acting dose.
- 75 and 100mg tablets.
- Dosage: 75–300mg given once or twice daily.

Buproprion SR (Wellbutrin SR®)—12 hour

- 100, 150, 200mg tablets.
- Dosage: 100–400mg once or twice daily.

Buproprion XL (Wellbutrin XL®)—24 hour

- 150 and 300mg tablets.
- Dosage: 150–450mg daily.

Trazodone (Desyrel®)

- 50,100,150,300 mg tablets.
- Younger children: 1.5 to max 6mg/kg/day divided tid.
- Older children: 50mg bid/tid to max 6mg/kg/day or 400mg/day, in divided doses.

Paroxetine (Paxil®/Paxil CR®), duloxetine (Cymbalta®)

- Not typically used to treat children at this time.

Forensic psychiatry—civil law

Forensic introduction

Since the beginning of recorded history, man has struggled to understand the relationship between human behavior and culpability. One needs to look no further than ancient Greek literature and the Oedipus cycle to observe the agonizing scrutiny given to man's behavior and moral responsibility. Shakespeare's themes often delved into "madness and mayhem," guilt and retribution. Roman law makes mention of excusing "children because of their innocence and the insane because of the nature of their misfortune." This idea of responsibility more recently has extended to damages caused either by intention or by negligence (Tort actions).

In earlier times judgments were executed by kings and rulers who were advised by priests and prophets. In modern history the king/ruler has been replaced by judge and jury and the priest/prophet by the expert witness. The professional expertise requested by the court has involved any field that is beyond the understanding of a layman. Other than the pathologist, the expert most frequently called in to court is the psychiatrist. Although forensic psychiatry has evolved into a subspecialty with approved training programs and board certification, the treating clinician is frequently called into the judicial setting. The following chapters are designed to provide reference for those who are court ordered to provide assessments or subpoenaed to testify before the court.

There are many other forensic legal issues that often engulf the treating psychiatrist. These involve the body of legislation and judicial decisions that affect the practice of psychiatry. No other specialty so often involves holding and/or treating a patient who does not consent to such treatment. Historically, medicine and psychiatry subscribed to a paternalistic approach to the patient. Recently, this emphasis has shifted and the treating clinician is responsible for understanding the full extent and limitations of his/her responsibilities.

Finally, the following information may prove satisfying to those who hold a fascination with the field of forensic psychiatry.

Civil forensic psychiatry

- I. Forensic Psychiatry [CMG].
  - Definition.
  - Roles and Responsibilities.
  - Ethical Considerations.
- II. Forensic Report [AS].
- III. Forensic Witness [AS].
- IV. Theoretical Basis of Patient's Rights [CMG].
  - Bill of Rights.
- V. Civil Commitment [SHB].
  - Voluntary.
  - Involuntary.
  - Outpatient.
- VI. Consent.
  - Informed Consent [RP].
  - Right to Treatment [CMG].
  - Right to Refuse Treatment [CMG].
  - EMTALA [CMG].
- VII. Substitute Decision Making [RP].
  - Competence.
  - Guardianship.
  - Power of Attorney.
  - Advanced Directives for Psychiatric Treatment.
- VIII. Confidentiality [RP].
  - HIPAA.
  - Duty to Warn/Protect.
  - Drug and Alcohol Records.
  - Subpoenas.
- IX. Malpractice [CMG].
- X. Juvenile Issues [SHB].
  - Juvenile Rights.
  - Juvenile Court.
  - Child Custody.
  - Child Abuse and Termination of Parental rights.
- XI. Special issues [MS].
  - Driving Privileges.
  - Impaired Practitioner.
  - Gun Ownership.
  - Fitness to Return to Duty.

Forensic psychiatry

Definition

Forensic psychiatry is a subspecialty of psychiatry dealing with the interface between psychiatry and the law. As a subspecialty of psychiatry it concerns the psychiatric issues involved in legal matters as well as the legal issues that arise in the practice of clinical psychiatry. This specialty is practiced in correctional facilities, in psychiatric hospitals, in courtrooms and in consultation to groups and individuals. The accrediting body for forensic psychiatrists in the United States and Canada is the American Board of Psychiatry and Neurology, and postgraduate training programs are supervised by the Accreditation Council for Graduate Medical Education (ACGME). The primary organization for forensic psychiatrists in the United States and Canada is the American Academy of Psychiatry and the Law (AAPL). Forensic psychiatry encompasses both criminal and civil issues and the following topics among others:

- Psychiatric disability.
- Civil Competencies.
- Parental Fitness/ Child custody.
- Conservators and guardianships.
- Criminal Competencies.

- Testimonial capacity.
- Insanity defense.
- Diminished capacity.
- Psychiatric malpractice.

Roles and responsibilities

The responsibilities of the forensic psychiatrist consist of providing evaluations and consultations regarding legal and psychiatric matters in accordance with APA and AAPL ethical guidelines. This includes evaluations, opinions, and testimony relating to diverse subjects including civil and criminal matters. Typically forensic psychiatrists are asked to answer specific questions posed by referral sources such as the courts, attorneys, government agencies, civil institutions and others.

Ethical considerations

"Forensic psychiatry is a subspecialty of psychiatry in which scientific and clinical expertise is applied to legal issues in legal contexts embracing civil, criminal, and correctional or legislative matters: forensic psychiatry should be practiced in accordance with guidelines and ethical principles enunciated by the profession of psychiatry" (American Academy of Psychiatry and the Law, adopted 5/20/85).

The ethical considerations at the core of forensic psychiatry relate to the following topics: confidentiality, consent, honesty, "striving for objectivity" and the qualifications of practitioners. Confidentiality is limited in forensic evaluations and must be *explicitly explained* to the evaluee prior to initiation of any evaluation. A typical statement found in a forensic report might read as follows, "The nature and purpose of the interview and the limits of confidentiality were discussed in detail and the patient's consent was obtained prior to initiation of the interview." In other words, it was explained to the evaluee that the examiner is employed by the court (or other agency) and any information proffered during the examination will be transmitted to the courts. Of note it is considered a requirement of truly objective forensic evaluations to interject at appropriate intervals, a reminder of the evaluee's right to avoid self-incrimination under the Fifth Amendment. For example, when an evaluee, begins to disclose information that might incriminate him/her, he/she should be reminded by the evaluating forensic psychiatrist of the limitations of confidentiality. The tendency for an evaluee to treat the evaluating forensic psychiatrist as a clinician and, therefore, to disregard the limits of confidentiality is referred to as "**slippage**." Consent to evaluation must be obtained from the evaluee or substitute decision maker with knowledge of these constraints.

Every effort must be made by the forensic evaluator to achieve as great a degree of objectivity as possible. Finally, forensic evaluations and consultation should be practiced only within the individual practitioner's sphere of training and expertise.

The World Psychiatric Association asserts that, "Under no circumstances should psychiatrists participate in legally authorized **executions** nor participate in assessments of competency to be executed." The American Psychiatric Association is similarly opposed on moral grounds to the death penalty; however, currently the APA does not specifically restrict evaluations for competency to be executed. Within the American Academy of Psychiatry and the Law discussion continues regarding not only the legitimacy of the death penalty itself but the role of the forensic psychiatrist in treating inmates to regain competency for execution.

> "**Dual agency**" is the term used when a forensic psychiatrist acts in more than one capacity with regard to a specific client. The forensic psychiatrist is obligated to remain as impartial as possible; acting as both the treating physician and the forensic expert, for example, constitutes a conflict of interest which should be avoided.

Forensic ethics

There are several core issues at the heart of forensic ethics above and beyond those expected of other physicians; these are in part dictated by the forensic psychiatrist's unique role. Among these are the following:

- Confidentiality—the limitations of confidentiality inherent in forensic evaluations.
- Consent—obtaining consent for evaluations with limited confidentiality as well as from collateral sources.
- Honesty—toward evaluees regarding the nature of the process and the ability of evaluations to help, harm, or have no effect on the evaluee's case and about the limits of one's expertise or knowledge.
- "Striving for objectivity"—because no individual can be completely objective, the stated goal in forensic psychiatry is to strive for the greatest degree of objectivity possible and to complete only work for which one has adequate qualifications such as forensic training and certification.

Please see the relevant sections of the text for further information on these ethical principles in context.

The forensic report

The forensic report is the distilled product of a forensic evaluation, which may be comprised of one or multiple interviews with an evaluee, collateral sources, record review (medical, psychiatric, and legal), and testing data, either neuropsychological or biological. The purpose of the report is to answer the psychiatric-legal question posed. It differs from a clinical psychiatric report, which addresses diagnostic issues and therapeutic goals. The forensic report is the most important format for the psychiatric opinion offered. On many occasions this report is the only input the forensic psychiatrist will have with the court. It can have irreversible consequences. An ideal forensic report should therefore be thorough, clear, concise, easily understood, and as objective as possible.

To better understand the making of a report, consider the following psychiatric legal scenario: A young male with a long history of bipolar disorder robs a convenience store. He is later apprehended. The arresting officer finds the defendant extremely talkative, proclaiming, "I started all the religions in the world. The chief administrative judge follows my secret cult."

- *The psychiatric-legal* question: is this defendant competent to stand trial?
- *The legal criteria/standard*: "**Dusky Standard.**" Specifically, does the defendant understand the charges against him and can he assist his attorney in his own defense? Additional elements to consider in this case are the defendant's ability to understand the judicial procedure, to act appropriately in a court of law, and to utilize the available information to assist his/her attorney, while suffering from a manic episode with delusions of grandeur.
- *Psychiatric data*: obtained from a detailed interview of the defendant, including a cognitive assessment, reality testing, and capacity to comprehend legal concepts, as well as collateral information.
- *Opinion*: the answer to the legal question posed by the court and the reasoning behind the conclusion.

There are two schools of report writing:
  - American Board of Forensic Psychiatry Format (ABFP).
  - Legal Format.

They differ in the format in which the above information is organized and presented but consider the following categories essential to any forensic report:
  - Identifying Information.
  - Source of referral.
  - A bibliography of all sources of information including medical records, interviews etc.
  - Statement regarding the limits of confidentiality.
  - The psychiatric-legal question and the appropriate criteria.
  - The psychiatric data.
  - The expert opinion.
  - Rationale behind the opinion.

The legal format resembles a brief and need not include a diagnosis or a formal mental status. It presents the opinion of the author and supports that opinion with the facts and observations documented. The ABFP format more closely resembles a traditional psychiatric evaluation.

Psychiatrists are divided over answering the ultimate question. It is generally preferable to give opinions on whether the evaluee meets the standards of the legal definition rather than to answer the ultimate question, which is the domain of the fact finder.

The expert witness

The psychiatric expert witness plays multiple roles in the courtroom. The expert witness gives evidence as close to objective as possible with regard to his or her opinion on the psychiatric issues in question. The forensic expert can serve as educator to the court, shedding light on key psychiatric issues in simple language that promotes an understanding of the psychiatric legal question before the court. Expert witness testimony can be instrumental in criminal and civil cases. For the most part, however, the adversarial system in American courts is mirrored in the recruitment of expert witnesses by both sides.

Types of witnesses

It is essential to differentiate an expert witness from a witness of fact. The treating psychiatrist is often called as a witness of fact whereas a forensic psychiatrist is hired to objectively render an opinion on a specific legal question.
- For example, an inpatient psychiatrist who was treating the patient at the time of a suicide can be subpoenaed to court to testify as a witness of fact.

An expert witness in such a scenario would be an independent psychiatrist retained by an attorney on either side of the dispute to provide expert opinion regarding the psychiatric legal questions. Some questions put to the expert might include the following: whether the event was foreseeable; whether the treatment met the standard of care; or whether appropriate precautions were taken to prevent suicide. Similarly, the treating psychiatrist may be subpoenaed to provide information regarding a patient who is subsequently involved in litigation or charged with a crime. Again an independent evaluator might be called as an expert witness to provide an opinion regarding the psychiatric legal questions.

Depositions

Another form of input to a psychiatric-legal situation in court is via deposition. This occurs during the discovery phase of the proceedings. The format is a structured question-answer session conducted under oath with opposing counsel present as well as a court reporter. No judge is present and objections are noted, but no rulings are made. Often video/audio recordings are made. Material from the deposition may or may not be presented at the trial. Another situation in which depositions are utilized arises when the expert is either not required or cannot be present in court to testify. In civil cases, the questions to be covered are often presented to both sides as part of the discovery process to prevent any unnecessary surprises and to facilitate potential settlement without the expense and time necessary for a trial.

Proceedings in court

Direct examination

Testimony begins under oath with the attorney who retained the expert asking questions that include his/her training and qualifications and that proceed to his/her findings and opinions. If a report has been completed, it is often presented as evidence at this time. The attorney will often follow the report closely in his/her questioning. The opinion is expressed within "reasonable medical certainty," the definition of which varies depending on the source. However, it is often understood as "more likely than not."

Tests for admissibility
The tests for admissibility of evidence/testimony, include the **Frye Test** and the **Daubert Test**. The Frye test calls for a theory to be generally accepted in the scientific community. The Daubert test requires four criteria be met:
- That the theory has or can be tested.
- That the theory has been peer reviewed.
- That the potential rate of error is known.
- That the theory is generally accepted.

The federal rules of evidence use the Daubert test. In many states the Daubert test has superseded the Frye test.

The hypothetical question
This is used to give a basis for the expert's opinion. All the facts assumed in the question are in evidence. An expert may testify on a hypothetical question without having examined the evaluee. The hypothetical question is used less often with the modern rules of evidence.

Hearsay rules
Provide that the expert base his/her opinions solely on his/her examination and the facts in evidence. More modern rules allow exceptions for psychiatric testimony because it is customary to consider the information given by collaterals when forming an opinion.

Cross examination
The opposing counsel has the opportunity to clarify, challenge, and discredit the testimony of the expert. The judicial system allows the credibility of the witness and his/her work to be challenged at this point. A competent expert witness stays calm and answers questions to the best of his/her ability. He/she may refuse to answer a question when (s)he thinks the question violates privilege, but may be required to answer if the judge allows the question. The witness may ask the judge for clarification on a question. Staying neutral and not advocating for a cause are important when maintaining credibility.

Redirect examination
The retaining attorney has the opportunity to re-examine the expert to clarify his/her position and repair any damage to his/her credibility. Questions are limited to those used in cross-examination. No new questions can be introduced at this time.

Re-cross-examination
The opposing attorney can ask questions about issues generated in the redirect exam.

Challenges on the stand

Underprepared expert

Lack of readiness will put a witness in an embarrassing position. The expert is allowed to carry all his/her documentation and his/her report to the stand and should feel free to consult them before responding to a question. An astutely written report with a carefully prepared index can avoid the spectacle of looking hassled while searching for information.

Neutrality

Although bias is often almost impossible to avoid, the expert is urged to be objective. When the expert gives the appearance of an advocate for a cause his/her credibility is damaged. It is important to keep in mind that an expert is paid for his/her time not his/her opinion.

Adversarial judicial system

The judicial system promotes advocacy ethics. That is the attorney is expected to present the best defense for his/her client's position. This is different from an ethical witness who is expected to be objective and to honestly report the facts on which he or she based a carefully rendered opinion.

Preparation for testimony

Pretrial conference

The forensic report is "discoverable." Opposing counsel has the right to view the report before testimony. It is recommended to meet with the attorney before Court to review the direct examination and to discuss and plan for the cross-examination.

An ethical witness will not change his/her opinion at the request of the attorney, but the best presentation of the expert's findings and opinion along with preparation for probable questions and strategy by opposing counsel is permissible and advisable.

Presentation

It should be remembered that juries are, in most cases, comprised of lay persons with varying degrees of familiarity with the expert's field. Speaking as plainly as possible, while not giving the appearance of condescension, is helpful in assisting juries to understand unfamiliar concepts. Confidence and modesty are important when communicating with the jury or the judge. Dressing professionally, staying focused on the issues, speaking clearly, and providing short confident answers have all been shown to impress jurors and judges favorably. Treating the cross-examination by an overly zealous attorney as an opportunity to educate the jury is more helpful than engaging in a duel.

- Experience: In today's world of seemingly universal media coverage, testimony is bound to provoke anxiety. The experience becomes easier with experience and solid preparation. Participating in mock trials and seeking mentorship have proven helpful.

Theoretical basis of patient's rights

In the United States the structure and function of the U.S. government are based on the U.S. Constitution. The Bill of Rights was added as an addendum to the Constitution in order to provide additional protection against infringement of individual rights and the rights of the individual states to self-determination by the powers granted to the federal government in the Constitution. The Bill of Rights comprises ten individual amendments outlining specific rights of individuals.

To appeal a ruling by a lower court to the United States Supreme Court (USSC), one must demonstrate that there has been a violation of a constitutional right since verdicts rendered in lower level courts are considered to have been tried "in fact" and a determination made. That is to say that when a case has been tried, the truth has been determined "in fact" and that fact is reflected in the verdict. Therefore, appeals to higher courts must demonstrate a violation of law to be granted further consideration. An understanding of the relevant amendments is helpful for the practicing forensic psychiatrist. Not all of the amendments are as relevant today. The first ten Amendments are described opposite.

Amendment I

Grants the right to freedom of speech, religion and the press, peaceable assembly and to petition the government regarding grievances.

Amendment II

The right of individuals to bear arms and to form a militia.

Amendment III

Protection from quartering troops. (The obligation of the populace to give lodging to troops.)

Amendment IV

Protection against unreasonable search and seizure without probable cause and specifics regarding the nature of the evidence sought.

Amendment V

The right to due process of law (federal), to avoid self-incrimination and to avoid being tried more than once for the same offense (known as double jeopardy). The 5th Amendment also protects against eminent domain seizure without appropriate compensation.

Amendment VI

The right to a speedy trial, an impartial jury, to confront witnesses and to legal representation or to represent oneself in civil cases.

Amendment VII

The right to trial in civil cases and protection from judical verdicts contrary to those of the jury.

Amendment VIII

Protection against cruel and unusual punishment and excessive bail.

Amendment IX

Protection against infringement on the individual's rights by the rights outlined in the Constitution.

Amendment X

Reserves powers not granted to the Federal government or specifically denied to the individual states for the States and the people. Although this is clearly a truism, it was intended as a reassurance to the people and the States that the Federal government would not enact laws and enforce them upon the States without regard to the constitution and the Bill of Rights.

Further amendments to the Constitution have, of course, been made over time, most notably the 13th (abolishing slavery) and the 14th (guaranteeing equal rights under the law and the right to due process). The 14th Amendment has been interpreted to afford both substantive due process (in broad general principle) and procedural due process (in actual practice in courts and legal proceedings) of law to all citizens of the United States in state proceedings. The Supreme Court has also held that the 14th Amendment extends or "incorporates" many of the earlier amendments and applies them specifically to the states as well as the federal government, superseding any contrary state law.

Civil commitment

Components in deciding civil commitment statute
- Mental illness.
- Dangerousness.
- Treatability.

Civil commitment statute components
- Mental illness threshold.
- Danger to others.
- Danger to self (including self-mutilation without suicidality in some states).
- Gravely disabling (explicitly stated in three-fourths of states).
- Least restrictive alternative (required in two-thirds of states).

Types of civil commitments
- Voluntary hospitalization.
- Involuntary hospitalization.
- Involuntary outpatient treatment.

Voluntary hospitalization
A voluntary patient, as an individual, retains the right to decide to accept or to reject treatment, including medications and ECT, and retains the (modified) right to leave the hospital.

Essentially two types of voluntary admissions exist:

Informal admission
- Patient must be discharged immediately upon his/her request.
- No statutory period during which he/she can be held in the hospital following a request for discharge.
- Patient may leave the institution, often in the midst of treatment and against the advice of physicians who may not prevent it, assuming involuntary commitment is not justified.

Formal admission
- Includes a mandatory period (3–5 days), defined by statute, during which the hospital has the discretion to hold the patient against his/her wishes should they(s)he attempt to leave.
- Most states require patients to give informed consent for voluntary hospitalization and written notice of a desire to leave against medical advice (AMA).
- In the case of seriously mentally ill patients, where continued hospitalization is necessary to protect the patient or others, this provides time for the patient's family or the institution to seek an involuntary commitment from the court.

Intents of voluntary hospitalization
- To promote patient autonomy.
- To promote a collaborative relationship between physician and patient.

- To remove some of the stigma associated with admission for treatment of a mental disorder.
- To eliminate the coercive element associated with involuntary hospitalization.

Involuntary hospitalization
Legal bases
- Parens patriae: The state takes responsibility for those unable to care for themselves.
- Police power: The state has authority to prevent harm to the community, including harm to mentally ill persons themselves.

Two means
Emergency certification
- Effected in most instances by a licensed physician or other qualified individual such as a clinical psychologist or psychiatric nurse.
- It does not need to be reviewed by the court prior to the patient's admission.
- It is essentially a holding order prior to commitment.
- It is intended to provide a means for a time-limited admission without delay in the urgent situations presenting themselves most typically in hospital emergency rooms.
- In some states, involuntary commitments are granted by administrators or delegates on behalf of the county or state based on information presented at the time of application for immediate commitment.
- In most states, provision of emergency certification or immediate commitment is coupled with a provision for a probable-cause hearing by the court shortly after admission in order to review the necessity for hospitalization.

Filing of a petition for commitment with the court of proper jurisdiction
- This is preceded by or leads to an examination of the patient by one or more psychiatrists or other qualified individuals.
- The court then decides, on the basis of the written reports and oral testimony, whether the individual meets the commitment criteria outlined in the state statutes.

Intents of involuntary hospitalization
- Commitments are time limited and there is usually a statutory requirement that commitment status be reviewed on a periodic basis.
- In addition, an individual can always request a review of their status through a **habeas corpus** petition (Latin for "present the body," is the name of a legal action or writ by means of which detainees can seek relief from unlawful imprisonment).
- These are generally longer than emergency certifications.
- They provide due process protections through various procedural safeguards.

Due process safeguards for civil commitment
- Right to a hearing (although not necessarily a trial by jury).
- Exclusion of hearsay evidence.
- Right to remain silent and a warning of this right and its meaning.
- Standard of proof: the patient must be proved to require hospitalization by clear and convincing evidence; to be both mentally ill and represent a danger (to themselves or others). This is the minimum standard for commitments however states are permitted to maintain higher (but not lower standards).
- Requires notice of the allegations to the patient.
- Right to representation by an attorney.

Involuntary civil commitment to outpatient treatment
The scope and enforcement of outpatient commitment statues vary considerably from one jurisdiction to another.

Current APA task force report recommendations
- Outpatient commitment should not be limited to patients who meet criteria for involuntary hospitalization, but extended to prevent relapse or deterioration in those whose relapse would predictably lead to severe deterioration and/or danger.
- Predictions about relapse, deterioration, and/or future dangerousness should be based on documented episodes in the recent past.
- Outpatient commitment should be limited to those incompetent to make treatment decisions, but should be available to assist patients who, as a result of their mental illnesses, are unlikely to seek or comply with needed treatment.
- Outpatient commitment statutes must provide adequate resources for treatment.
- Statutes should authorize initial commitments of 180 days, with provisions for extensions based on specific criteria.
- A thorough medical examination should be required.
- Outpatient clinicians should be involved in the development of the treatment plan.
- Patients should be consulted about their treatment preferences and be given copies of their treatment plans so that they will be aware of the conditions with which they will be expected to comply.
- The statues should contain specific provisions to be followed in the event of noncompliance, including a court hearing if the noncompliance is substantial and further efforts to motivate compliance would likely fail.
- No recommendation is made about forced medication; but if it is authorized, it must be based on incompetence to make treatment decisions.

Consent

Informed consent

Informed consent is the process by which patients make decisions about their heath care options. It involves education and evaluation of the patient's understanding of the relevant issues. The process can occur in a single interaction between treatment provider and patient; often, however, several meetings between the treatment provider and the patient may be required in order to obtain adequate consent from the patient.

The process involves educating and evaluating the patient's understanding of the nature of his/her condition, potential risks and benefits of the proposed treatment, the course of the disease if left untreated and alternative treatments. The information provided should conform to the standard of what a "reasonable person" would want to know regarding these issues. Additionally, the patient must be able to communicate a choice and the rationale for his/her decision. In the absence of an adequate demonstration of all the factors above, a patient cannot be considered to have truly given informed consent.

For children and adolescents not considered emancipated minors, the treatment provider should obtain informed consent from the parents or guardians. Similarly, for patients who have been provided a legal guardian for medical decisions by the court, the medical provider should obtain informed consent from the guardian.

In the emergency setting, patients are presumed to be competent to provide informed consent unless they are acutely incapacitated and are unable to communicate their understanding and choice. In any emergency situation in which there is no adequate decision-maker or advance directives the patient should be treated to alleviate the immediate danger and the issues of informed consent revisited at a later date.

Disclaimer

These are general principles for the practitioner to follow when obtaining informed consent. There are, however, exceptions to these principles and appropriate consultation should be sought to resolved potential conflicts.

Significant problems can occur in the psychiatric population with respect to decision-making capacity leading to questions about the ability to give informed consent. Delusional, demented, delirious, manic, and extremely depressed patients, among others, may have limited capacity, either cognitively or affectively, to make decisions regarding their care and give truly informed consent.

Clinical vignette

A 42-year-old outpatient with depression states "Doctor, I will accept whatever treatment you recommend because I trust your judgment. I don't want to hear about the alternatives." There is no reason for the doctor to believe that the patient lacks decision-making capacity. Should the doctor proceed to treat the patient?

Answer

Yes. This scenario is referred to as a therapeutic waiver and is relatively rare today. The physician can proceed to treat the patient but must document the patient's refusal to be educated about the alternative treatments. The physician should also consider making future attempts to educate the patient.

Right to treatment

In 1929, G.A. Smoot proposed that "along with the power to control and restraint of the non compos goes the duty to care and provide for them." This is summed up as the "**quid pro quo**" theory of commitment, i.e., "this for that," meaning that patients are deprived of their liberty and are therefore due something in return, namely treatment for medical issues.

In 1960, Morton Birnbaum proposed that the court recognize a constitutionally protected right to treatment for the institutionalized mentally ill. He theorized that this was based on the 14th Amendment right to substantive due process in that those confined to inpatient facilities cannot be deprived of freedom and remain untreated while having committed no crime.

In *Rouse v. Cameron* (1966), Mr. Rouse was found not guilty of possession of a dangerous weapon by reason of insanity. The maximum sentence had he been tried was one year for this offense; however, he was involuntarily committed for an indefinite period. A district court refused relief in habeas corpus appeal based on his contention that he had received no psychiatric treatment at Saint Elizabeth's Hospital in Washington D.C. Judge David Bazelon in the D.C. Circuit Court of Appeals ruled that Mr. Rouse had a right to treatment under a D.C. statute that mandated treatment for the mentally ill who were involuntarily committed stating "the hospital need not show that the treatment will cure or improve him but only that there is a bona fide effort to do so."

In *Donaldson v. O'Connor* (and *O'Connor v. Donaldson,* the subsequent appeal), the most compelling series of landmark cases regarding the right to treatment, Kenneth Donaldson was committed to the Florida State Hospital at Chattahoochee and diagnosed with paranoid schizophrenia. Mr. Donaldson was at no time found to be dangerous to himself or others; many groups of family, friends, and other groups offered repeatedly to help care for him in the community, and yet he was denied release. As a Christian Scientist, Donaldson refused medication and ECT. During his 14½ years in Chattahoochee, his freedoms, including grounds privileges and OT, were restricted yet further as a matter of policy for treatment refusal.

The final USSC decision ruled that there is no constitutional basis for confining persons making the following holding "a state cannot constitutionally confine without more, a non-dangerous individual who is capable of surviving safely in freedom by himself or with the help of willing and responsible friends and family members."

Mr. Donaldson, upon his release, subsequently published a book about his experiences entitled *Insanity Inside Out.*

Right to refuse treatment

Patients have always had a right to refuse medication, except during emergencies. However under older, more "paternalistic" standards, the doctor would decide the appropriate course of treatment. Commitment was based on the need for treatment, so the right to refuse treatment as such was essentially nonexistent. It made little sense to admit a patient for treatment and then allow him to refuse that treatment.

At the heart of the discussion lies a fundamental question of patients' rights under the constitution versus their need for treatment. Constitutional arguments for right to refuse treatment include: the right to free speech (1st Amendment), the right to be free from cruel and unusual punishment (8th Amendment), the right to due process (14th Amendment), the right to privacy (penumbra of 1st, 4th, 5th, and 9th Amendments), and the "rights-driven model"—concerned with the individual's autonomy.

Of note, 1–15% of involuntary patients refuse medication at one time or another. In cases reviewed by courts, refusals are overridden 90% of the time, whereas in internal (psychiatric) reviews refusals are only overridden 65–80% of the time.

In the 1970s, there was a shift toward dangerousness as the criterion for commitment and, therefore, the question of the competent patient's right to refuse treatment arose.

In *Wyatt v. Stickney*, patients were entitled to the least restrictive treatment setting, freedom from unnecessary or excessive medication, the right to be excluded from experimental research without consent and the right to refuse ECT or lobotomy without consent and consultation with counsel.

In *Kaimowitz v. Michigan Department of Mental Health* (1973), John Doe was illegally detained for the purpose of experimental psychosurgery and held as a criminal sexual psychopath without trial. The Court ruled it was impossible to obtain true informed consent from an involuntary patient. Under Nuremburg standards; this required free will while involuntarily committed subjects were felt to be inherently coerced.

The 1st Amendment protects freedom to generate new ideas, which psychosurgery obviously limits. Rules governing treatment refusal may vary according to state law, treatment setting and jurisdiction. As a result of this decision experimentation on prisoners virtually came to a complete stop and very strict standards are currently in place to protect prisoners' rights.

An apt quote from Justice Benjamin Cardozo states that "every human being of adult years and sound mind has a right to decide what shall be done with his own body" (*Schoendorff v. Society of New York Hospital* 105 NE 92, 93 [1914]).

Concerns have always existed regarding the patient's rights versus the quality of patient care. Models for addressing patient refusal have developed over time with the two most noteworthy being the Rennie and Rogers models. In *Rennie v. Klein* (1979), a district court mandated written consent forms, patient advocates to serve as informal counsel and informal review by independent psychiatrists before medications could be forced on patients. Forced medications were permitted in emergencies.

The background to this (treatment-driven model or second-doctor decision maker) was a class action suit in New Jersey State Hospitals in the context of understaffing, polypharmacy, and no warning to patients of long-term side-effects.

In *Rogers v. Commissioner* it was ruled that "neither competent nor incompetent patients may be forcibly medicated or secluded except where there is a substantial likelihood, or a result, of extreme violence, personal injury, or attempted suicide" (rights-driven model). This was modified slightly by the court's citing a previous case (the case of Richard Roe III) that a judge, using substituted judgment, could authorize antipsychotic medication for an outpatient who refuses treatment.

However, in dicta (non-binding opinion), the USSC stated: "For purposes of this discussion, involuntarily committed mental patients do retain liberty interests protected directly by the constitution and these interests are implicated by the involuntary administration of antipsychotic drugs."

The Massachusetts Supreme Court Decision in Rogers amounted to a decision that a committed mental patient is competent until adjudicated incompetent by a judge and that a judge may then use a "substituted judgment standard" to decide what the patient would have wanted had (s)he been competent rather than what might be considered objectively to be in his/her best interests.

Washington v. Harper: the USSC held that the administrative scheme to override treatment refusals without a judicial hearing was constitutionally adequate to meet both substantive and procedural due process. The liberty interest of the prisoner can, therefore, be overcome by an administrative appeals process with a lay representative.

In *Riggins v. Nevada*, the court required that the state demonstrate that the antipsychotic Mellaril was required during Riggins' trial to render him competent with the assertion that this violated his 14th Amendment rights. The court did not address the right to refuse this treatment if this refusal would render him incompetent.

Finally in *Sell v. U.S.* (2003), the issue was the right to restore competence after a serious but nonviolent offense. The standard established was that incompetence to consent or danger should be used to override refusal. Failing these methods, involuntary treatment can be used if the following can be demonstrated: medically appropriate treatment is being provided, this treatment is unlikely to undermine the fairness of the trial, this is the least intrusive alternative available, and the treatment must advance governmental trial-related interests.

Rogers and Rennie offer two different approaches. Rogers is a rights-driven model relying on state statutes and common law principles. Rennie is a treatment-driven model. More recently decisions have favored the treatment-driven approach of Rennie and the case of *Youngberg v. Romeo* encouraged deference to professional judgment.

The right to refuse treatment and treatment over objection follow a variety of standards from state to state.

For example some states merely require a qualified second opinion to treat over refusal whereas others require the clinician to present before an administrative board.

For more information on the standards in a specific state, check with the State Mental Health Code, an attorney specializing in mental health law, and/or a forensic psychiatrist licensed in the state.

Emergency Medical Treatment and Active Labor Act (EMTALA)

The Emergency Medical Treatment and Active Labor Act (EMTALA) is a statute that governs when and how a patient may be refused treatment or transferred from one hospital to another and under what medical conditions. EMTALA was passed as part of the Consolidated Omnibus Budget Reconciliation Act of 1986 (COBRA), which includes a host of related statutes not relevant to this discussion.

The Emergency Medical Treatment and Active Labor Act applies to "partipating hospitals" that have entered into "provider agreements" under which they will accept payment from the Department of Health and Human Services or Centers for Medicare and Medicaid Services. This includes virtually all hospitals in the United States (excepting military facilities). EMTALA provisions apply to all patients, not just Medicare patients.

The avowed purpose of the statute is to prevent hospitals from rejecting patients, refusing to treat them, or transferring them to "charity hospitals" or "county hospitals" because they are unable to pay or are covered under the Medicare or Medicaid programs.

The Emergency Medical Treatment and Active Labor Act is primarily, but not exclusively, a nondiscrimination statute. It provides that no patient who presents with an emergency medical condition but is unable to pay may be treated differently from patients who are covered by health insurance.

Physicians may also be held liable for decisions they make that are covered under EMTALA. In the event that a decision by one of its employees or staff physicians makes a facility liable under EMTALA, hospitals may seek to assert a claim for reimbursement from the involved physician. Some physicians and staff have been held partially liable for decisions made to refuse care to individual patients.

An Emergency Medical Condition is defined under EMTALA as, "A medical condition manifesting itself by acute symptoms of sufficient severity (including severe pain) such that the absence of immediate medical attention could reasonably be expected to result in placing the health of the individual or, with respect to a pregnant woman, the health of the woman or her unborn child in serious jeopardy, serious impairment in bodily functions, or in a pregnant woman who is having contractions there is inadequate time to effect a safe transfer to another hospital before delivery, or the transfer may pose a threat to the health or safety of the woman or her unborn child." For any person found to be suffering from an emergency medical condition, the hospital is obligated to either provide them with treatment until they are stable or to transfer them to another hospital according to the statute's directives.

Substitute decision-making

Competence

Competence is a legal term, not a medical term, and can only be determined by a court of law. The equivalent medical term generally used is "decision-making capacity." Competence refers to the ability to make a decision and is task-specific; that is a person may be competent to make medical decisions but not competent to make a will. Types of competencies include testamentary capacity (ability to make a will), capacity to make medical decisions, capacity to manage finances, capacity to marry, capacity to enter into a contract, and parental fitness. Competence includes the ability to understand the relevant information, the ability to appreciate the situation and its consequences, the ability to manipulate the information rationally and relevantly and the ability to communicate a choice. An individual is presumed to be competent unless demonstrated to be incompetent in a court of law. The burden of proof lies with the party alleging incompetence to demonstrate to the court that the person is incompetent. The standard of proof is clear and convincing evidence.

Physicians are often called upon to determine a patient's decision-making capacity, particularly to make medical decisions. In hospitals, primary teams will often consult psychiatrists to make assessments regarding a patient's competence. The psychiatrist should inform the primary team that he/she can only make a decision as to the patient's decision-making capacity. The information that the patient must understand, appreciate, and manipulate rationally is the same information required for informed consent. Furthermore, consideration should be given to the potential for undue influence from family, caretakers, or staff on the patient's decision. The patient may agree with a doctor's decision to proceed with treatment, but this does not mean that the patient has the capacity to make that decision. For example, if a patient desires a voluntary admission for inpatient psychiatric treatment, but is grossly disorganized, hallucinating and incoherent (see *Zinermon v. Burch* for further details), an involuntary admission may be more appropriate.

Guardianship

Following a petition of the court and a finding of incompetence, the court will appoint a guardian for the incompetent person who is then referred to as a "ward." The guardian may be of the person, of the estate, or both. A court may appoint a guardian for a specific purpose (limited guardian) or for general purposes (plenary guardian). The exact type of guardianship is determined by the specific incapacity of the individual. Should an individual deemed by the court to be incompetent present for voluntary admission, he/she cannot sign voluntary admission papers. The guardian must be involved in making medical decisions for the patient including admission to the hospital. Some states allow a guardian to sign admission papers for a medical inpatient admission, yet do not permit a guardian to sign a voluntary admission for inpatient psychiatric treatment. Without advanced directives, an involuntary admission would have to be initiated.

Mental health advance directives

If a patient is competent and is not currently an involuntary psychiatric inpatient, the patient may choose to execute an advance directive. This practice has traditionally been applied to medical treatment. More recently, this has been extended in many jurisdictions to include psychiatric care. A mental health advance directive is a document that details the person's preferences for treatment in case he/she should become incompetent and unable to express his/her preferences regarding treatment. These are often quite specific and can designate a preferred inpatient facility for treatment as well as specific medications to be tried and/or avoided. Consent for ECT and participation in research can also be addressed. It should be noted that no physician can be forced to provide treatment that he or she considers inconsistent with professional standards to meet the terms of an advance directive. This document should be reviewed periodically with the patient as treatment protocol and/or the patient's preferences may change. Furthermore, there may arise scenarios that had not been envisioned by the treatment provider or the patient when the advance directives were originally executed.

Power of attorney

Alternatively, an individual may designate another to make decisions for the individual when he or she no is no longer competent to make these decisions. The person designated under the Power of Attorney will then make medical decisions and/or financial decisions for the individual. When the Power of Attorney extends to medical decisions, informed consent for all treatment must be obtained from the designated decision maker.

Often a patient may have both executed an advanced directive document and appointed a power of attorney. Specific exceptions exist in certain jurisdictions to the above information.

Clinical vignette

Mary is an 82-year-old female with a court-appointed "guardian of person" in Pennsylvania. Mary is depressed and suicidal and ECT is determined by the treatment team and the guardian to be the best treatment. Can the guardian consent to ECT?

Answer

No. Pennsylvania law specifically prohibits a guardian from consenting to ECT, unless the authority to consent for ECT is specifically written into the Order of Court appointing the guardian. Therefore, the guardian and treatment team will be required to appear before the court to obtain a specific Order of Court authorizing the guardian to consent for ECT. A similar process to obtain an Order of Court authorizing ECT is necessary for patients who do not have a court-appointed guardian. Please note: these laws can vary from state to state.

Confidentiality

Introduction

Confidentiality is the term used to describe the patient's expectation of privacy of his/her records, and privilege is the term used to describe the clinician's obligation to withhold confidential information. This is comparable to the attorney-client or priest-confessor privilege.

In the treatment setting, confidentiality traditionally has required that information shared between the treatment provider and patient remain confidential unless the patient gives explicit permission to the provider to disclose information to a third party. Confidentiality is one of the most important factors in the development of a therapeutic relationship between treatment provider and patient. Today, information may have to be shared with third party payers, government agencies who are engaged in determining payments for temporary and permanent disability, as well as other agents or third parties.

An important first step in protecting confidentiality is to discuss with the patient what information is confidential and what information is not confidential and to whom information will be disclosed and for what purpose. It is also important to discuss with the patient exceptions to the normal rules of confidentiality.

HIPAA

Patients have the right to have their medical information held confidential. Laws governing confidentiality vary from state to state. Originally passed to promote greater control over electronic record keeping, but extended to encompass a host of other confidentiality issues, the Health Insurance Portability and Accountability Act (HIPAA) is the federal law governing confidentiality. HIPAA supersedes corresponding state laws unless the state laws are more restrictive. In the latter case, the state laws should be followed.

In general, while the hospital/provider owns the medical record, the patient can determine to which parties the medical record can be released. This includes other treatment providers.

- For example, a psychiatrist cannot release information in the patient's medical record to the patient's primary care physician unless the patient signs an authorization to release the information. However, in order to ensure treatment continuity, information relevant to the care of the patient can be communicated to members of the current treatment team. Relevant information may also be provided to third party payers in order to secure payment.

HIPAA confidentiality requirements extend to family, friends and relatives. In fact, it contravenes guidelines to even affirm that a patient is receiving care in an institution without the consent of the patient. Furthermore confidentiality requirements extend even if the patient is not currently receiving treatment. Lawyers and police officers wishing to obtain information about whether a patient is currently receiving treatment should be referred to the legal department of the facility for further information. However, to receive collateral, freely offered and unsolicited information from third parties, the treatment provider does not need to obtain explicit consent from the patient. Such collateral information may provide valuable information for the care of the patient. In cases in which the patient has either a parent or legal guardian involved in treatment, treatment providers must exercise judgment about discussing with these parties information the patient has specifically requested be confidential. Confidentiality regarding treatment of children and adolescents is generally regarded to hold true (including such information as drug use and sexual activity) with the exception of information that might be potentially life threatening (such as an admission of a suicide plan).

Emergency situations constitute an exception to the typical rules of confidentiality. For example, for a patient in the emergency room, the treatment team may contact outside providers or other third parties known to the patient in order to obtain critical information necessary for treatment without express written consent, although this is usually attempted.

Duty to warn/to protect

Another exception to the general expectation of privacy/confidentiality is based on a ruling from the landmark **Tarasoff** case. In the Tarasoff case, the treatment provider was determined to have a duty to protect third parties from potential harm by a patient. For example, if a patient discloses to a therapist that he or she intends to kill or seriously harm an identifiable person and this constitutes a realistic threat (not a threat by a homeless man in Cleveland to kill Tony Blair), then the therapist has a duty to warn and/or protect the targeted person. The specific requirements regarding the duty to warn and/or protect vary with the individual circumstances, but may include the therapist directly contacting the targeted person as well as law enforcement to inform them about the threat.

Drug and alcohol records

Drug and alcohol records also receive special protection that is reported under the Code of Federal Regulation (CFR, Title 42, Chapter 1, Part 2). The purpose of these protections is to restrict the disclosure and use of the records of patients in any federally assisted drug and alcohol program (CFR, Title 42, Chapter 1, Part 2, section 2.3). Disclosure of these records must comply with the federal regulations. It is important to note that under the code for drug and alcohol records that fall under the regulations, these records may "not otherwise be disclosed or used in any civil, criminal, administrative, or legislative proceedings conducted by any Federal, State, or local authority" (CFR, Title 42, Chapter 1, Part 2, Section 2.13).

- For example, these records may not be disclosed to law enforcement or other officials or even an individual who has obtained a subpoena (CFR, Title 42, Chapter 1, Part 2, Section 2.13).

Subpoenas

Subpoenas

A subpoena is a command requiring an individual to do something. It is issued by a court at the request of a party or a party's attorney. For example *appearance subpoena* requires the personal appearance of a person at a certain place and time to provide testimony. A subpoena *duces tecum* requires the appearance of the individual along with documents or papers relevant to the legal controversy. The receipt of a subpoena by a clinician should immediately trigger consultation with an administrator and/or attorney for advice regarding an appropriate response. Some court rules require notice to opposing counsel of the intent to serve subpoenas on any witnesses. A reasonable amount of advance notice should be provided to individuals who are served with subpoenas, especially professionals. However, a properly served subpoena should not be ignored or disregarded. This may lead to sanctions by the court, up to and including imprisonment. In some states a subpoena alone is insufficient for the production of documents or testimony regarding a person's mental health treatment. In addition to the subpoena, the patient's written consent must be obtained. If the consent is not readily obtainable, the court may issue an order requiring the individual to testify regarding the confidential mental health treatment information.

Clinical vignette

The wife of a patient calls the inpatient ward asking whether the patient is on the inpatient ward. What should the treatment provider do?

Answer

The treatment provider should neither acknowledge nor deny the presence of the patient on the ward. Instead, the provider should state that they can't confirm the patient's presence on the ward but if such a person is on the ward, a message may be passed along to them.

Clinical vignette

George M is a 32-year-old outpatient who carries a diagnosis of sedative/hypnotic dependence. Dr. S is concerned about Mr. M obtaining sedative/hypnotics from multiple providers without telling Dr. S. How should Dr. S proceed to contact the other providers?

Answer

Dr. S should discuss with Mr. M his diagnosis and the concerns that Dr. S has that Mr. M is obtaining medications from multiple providers. Dr. S should clarify with Mr. M what medications Mr. M is currently obtaining from other providers and for what purpose. Dr. S should then discuss with Mr. M contacting the other providers and what information is to be released and for what purpose. If Mr. M consents, then the other providers may be contacted, using whatever means of written consent is approved by Dr. S's teaching facility.

Recommended further reading

1 Health Insurance Portability and Accountability Act (HIPPA) of 1996, 29. U.S.C.A. 1181, et seq. *Tarasoff v. Regents of the University of California.* Cal. 1976.
2 CFR, Title 42, Chapter 1, Part 2, Section 2.13. http://www.access.gpo.gov/nara/cfr/waisidx_02/42cfr2_02.html

Malpractice

Malpractice is pursued as a civil suit or **"tort."** It alleges that a wrong has been committed and the tort attempts to "make whole" again the plaintiff who has been wronged through the mechanism of financial remuneration. It is not a criminal proceeding and the standards of evidence are substantially different. Malpractice is considered an unintentional tort as opposed to an intentional tort, which would constitute purposefully causing harm.

In general, psychiatric malpractice is relatively uncommon compared to other specialties. The leading causes of suits against psychiatrists for malpractice are incorrect treatment, suicide, drug reaction, incorrect diagnosis, improper supervision, unnecessary commitment and sexual misconduct. Studies demonstrate that in general the best protection against lawsuits is a good working relationship with one's patients. Patients who are satisfied with their physician and their care are less likely to sue.

In order to prove malpractice it must be demonstrable that four key elements exist, easily remembered as "the four Ds":

- **Duty**—the clinician has established a demonstrable relationship with the plaintiff and therefore, has a duty toward them; (i.e., a treatment relationship is established). In the absence of a relationship of this type no malpractice is possible. As an example, someone stops you on the street and asks whether one type of antidepressant is better than another. You give your opinion, noting it to be "just my opinion." The individual subsequently gets this medication from his PCP; his/her depression fails to improve (a depression of which you were unaware); she or he subsequently commits suicide. In this case there is no doctor-patient relationship and, therefore, no duty on your part. The circumstances are certainly unfortunate but individual clinicians are not held responsible for all the misfortunes that befall individual patients, only those for which they are directly responsible.
- **Dereliction of duty**—the clinician has somehow varied from the accepted standard of care through gross negligence, willful misconduct, or other means. In some cases, these can be interpreted as intentional torts such as intentional infliction of emotional injury, battery and etc. These are usually cases in which the clinician has strayed extremely far beyond the usual treatment relationship; for example, having sex with a client or using illicit drugs with them. Simply prescribing for a patient a medication which is considered reasonable by most practitioners as treatment for the patient's condition, but which later is demonstrated to have a previously unknown side-effect, is not the responsibility of the clinician acting in good faith according to reasonable standards.

- **Damages**—must be demonstrated by the plaintiff, which would entitle the plaintiff to be reimbursed by a tort action, the financial component intended to substitute for the physical, emotional, or other damages she or he may have suffered. There must be a demonstrable damage for malpractice to be affirmed. The patient must be able to show that she or he has suffered from some condition directly caused by the clinicians mistreatment, such as chronic depression treated only with psychoanalytic psychotherapy without mention of medication, which could potentially lead to substantial improvement.
- **Direct causation**—the damages caused are a direct result of the clinician's action or lack thereof. The plaintiff is able to demonstrate damage, be it physical or psychic, as a direct result of the clinician's actions. The standard used in malpractice cases is "the preponderance of the evidence," generally interpreted as roughly 51% or essentially just enough evidence to convince that it is more likely true than not.

Malpractice suits in psychiatry (as in all other specialties) must demonstrate that all four elements are present in order to present a reasonable malpractice case. In the past, the "reasonable practitioner" standard was used in judging malpractice; that is to say, did the physician adhere to the standard of care for his/her specialty? Recently many states have begun to move toward a **"reasonably prudent practitioner"** standard, which holds the physician to a higher level and may allow a finding of malpractice even if the physician demonstrates that she or he adhered to the standard of care.

Physician's **protection against malpractice** suits comes in several forms. A good and open relationship with one's patients, frequent discussions of the risks and benefits of particular treatments and reasonable alternatives, documentation of the decision-making process, all limit the risk of litigation against the clinician. Likewise, adherence to best practice guidelines lessen the likelihood of malpractice suits. Furthermore, these practices can provide powerful evidence that a practitioner has carefully thought through a problem, discussed the risk-benefit ratio of treatment with his/her patient and acted in good faith by making the best decision she or he could with the information available.

Juvenile rights

Definitions

- Minor: a person who has not yet reached the age of majority (18 in most states).
- Emancipated minor: common law doctrine that severs the mutual rights and obligations of the parent-child relationship. This terminates a parent's duty to support and control the minor. This does not affect the minor's protection under the law. Emancipated minors include those who live outside the family home and are employed or self-supporting, married, or emancipated by a court of law.
- Mature minor: an individual who, though not fully emancipated, is potentially competent to make certain decisions.
- Age of consent: is the age at which a minor can consent to sexual intercourse (16 in most states).

Juvenile's rights

- Medical care: when a child needs medical care, it is the responsibility of the parent or guardian to provide informed consent prior to treatment.
- Mental health care: more than 50% of states have laws that provide that minors have a right to access information and treatment regarding substance abuse without parental consent. Some states have enacted statutes addressing the ability of minors to consent to both inpatient and outpatient mental health treatment.
- Reproductive rights: most states have laws that permit minors to seek counseling and treatment for venereal disease without notification of their parents or guardians.

Juvenile court

Definitions
- Juvenile: Person who has not reached the age at which one is treated as an adult by the criminal justice system. Majority of states consider this age to be 18.
- Delinquent: Youth who committed an act that would be a crime if committed by an adult.
- Status offender: Youth who committed an act prohibited by the law that would not be a crime if committed by an adult. Examples: truancy, curfew violation.
- Guardian ad litem: A person appointed by the court to protect the interests of the juvenile. Focus is on child's "best interests," not necessarily what the child wants.

Epidemiology (data from 2002)
There were 1.6 million delinquent cases handled by courts with juvenile jurisdiction.
- Gender: 74% delinquents were males and 26% were females.
- Age: 57% of all the delinquency cases processed by the juvenile courts involved youths age 15 or younger.
- Race: 78% of the juvenile population were Caucasian and 16% were African American.
- Violent crimes: Of all the arrests 55% were Caucasian, 43% African American, 1% Native American and 1% Asian youth.

Juvenile justice system structure and process
- Taken into custody: The juvenile equivalent of adult arrest is being "taken into custody."
- Referral: Referred to juvenile court.
- Court intake: Mostly the responsibility of the probation department and/or prosecutor's office. Two options: dismiss case or handle case informally.
- Detention: Courts may hold juvenile in detention centers if the court believes it is in the best interest of the community or the child. In all states a detention hearing must occur within a specified period.
- Prosecutorial direct file: The prosecutor may be required to file a case in criminal court based on a state statute or may have the discretion to file from a predetermined list of charges in either juvenile or adult court.
- Delinquent petition: Also known as petitioning. If the case is handled by juvenile court a delinquent petition is filed which states the allegations and requests the juvenile court to adjudicate the youth delinquent.
- Waiver petition: Filed when the prosecutor or intake officer believes that a case under jurisdiction of the juvenile court would be more appropriately handled in criminal court.
- Adjudication hearing: Equivalent to a trial where witnesses are called and facts of the case are presented. Rather than being found "guilty" youth are "adjudicated delinquents."
- Disposition hearing: Equivalent to adult criminal court sentencing hearing.
- Juvenile aftercare: Similar to adult parole.

Special evaluations in juvenile court

- Juvenile's waiver of Miranda rights: The right to avoid self-incrimination (5th Amendment) and the right to advice of counsel during police questioning (14th Amendment).
- Competency to stand trial evaluations: Standards and procedures are the same as in adult court. Should be requested in the following cases:
  - Age 12 or younger.
  - Diagnosis or treatment for a mental illness or mental retardation.
  - "Borderline" level of intellectual functioning, or record of "learning disability."
  - Observations by others at pretrial events suggesting deficits in memory, attention, or reality testing.
- Insanity defense in juvenile court: Rare. If applicable, focus is on rehabilitation and not punishment.
- Juvenile waivers to adult court: Focus is on punishment rather than rehabilitation; "do the crime, do the time."

A juvenile offender who has committed a serious offense may be waived from juvenile court to adult court. Sometimes this is a discretionary waiver, when the prosecutor files a motion to have the young offender tried as an adult. After a hearing, where evidence is presented for and against a waiver, the judge decides whether the offender should be tried as a juvenile or as an adult. Sometimes, this is a mandatory waiver, in which the law requires the young offender to be tried as an adult. Many states have passed laws allowing prosecutors to file adult charges against juveniles for certain serious offenses, without having to apply for a waiver.

Generally, a court with criminal jurisdiction over a case excluded by statute from juvenile jurisdiction may waive it and transfer the child to juvenile court if such a transfer is "in the interests of the child or society." This is known as the **reverse waiver**. However, the court may not transfer a case of any child who (1) has previously been convicted of an excluded offense; (2) has previously been waived/transferred once to juvenile court and adjudicated delinquent; or (3) is accused of first degree murder and was at least 16 at the time of commission of the act.

Following a plea or a trial in a case in which pretrial transfer was either denied following a hearing or prohibited solely because the child was 16 and charged with first degree murder, the court may nevertheless order the case transferred to juvenile court for disposition purposes, as long as the juvenile has not pled or been found guilty of any excluded offense. In either situation, the law specifies various factors that must be considered in making the transfer determination, which are identical to those considered in discretionary waiver hearings.

Once a child has been convicted of a felony as an adult, all subsequent felony charges against the same child must be heard in adult criminal court, unless a reverse waiver has been granted. A juvenile tried in adult court has all the rights granted to an adult defendant, including the right to a jury trial.

Child custody

Child custody and guardianship are legal terms, used to describe the legal and practical relationship between a parent and his or her child, such as the right of the parent to make decisions for the child, and the parent's duty to care for the child.

Statistics

In the United States in 2005, there were 7.5 new marriages per 1,000 people, and 3.6 divorces per 1,000, a ratio that has remained fairly constant since the 1960s. The claim that "half of all marriages end in divorce" became widely accepted in the United States in the 1970s, on the basis of this statistic, and has remained conventional wisdom. Divorce affects about one million children each year, and approximately 10% of divorces involve custody litigation.

The main causes for divorce in 2003/2004 were:
- Extra-marital affairs—27%.
- Family strain—18%.
- Emotional/physical abuse—17%.
- Midlife crises—13%.
- Addictions, e.g., alcoholism and gambling—6%.
- Workaholism—6%.

Evaluation

Most divorces involving children do not result in custody hearings. More often than not, the parties agree on custody/visitation schedules; however, when the issue of suitability of one parent/guardian is raised, a custody hearing is held. This often involves an independent evaluation by a forensic psychiatric /psychological professional.

Evaluators

Treating clinicians are advocates or agents for children and ideally are partners with parents or guardians in the therapeutic alliance. In contrast, the forensic evaluator, while guided by the child's best interests, has no duty to the child or his/her parents. The forensic evaluator reports to the court or attorney involved rather than to the parties being evaluated. Thus, the aim of the forensic evaluation is not to relieve suffering or treat, but to provide objective information and informed opinions to help the court render a custody decision. Forensic evaluators must be mindful of this role and convey this in full to all parties before beginning the evaluation, similar to any forensic evaluation.

Sources of requests for evaluations include parents, attorneys, judges, court clerks, or family relations officers. Child custody hearings are heard in Family Court.

Three major questions

According to the APA (1982) three major questions that should be addressed in the evaluation include:
- What is the quality of the reciprocal attachment between parent and child?
- What are the child's needs and the adults' parenting capacities?
- What are the relevant family dynamics at play?

Interviews are conducted with each parent individually, each child alone, and the child with each parent individually. The interviews may also include the parents together without the child, the child together with both parents, or the child with his or her siblings.

Determination of with whom the child resides is based on the "best interests of the child" standard.

Family law proceedings that involve issues of residence and contact often generate the most acrimonious disputes. Although many parents cooperate when it comes to sharing their children, not all do. For those that engage in litigation, there seem to be few limits. Court filings quickly fill with mutual accusations by one parent against the other, sometimes including allegations of sexual, physical, and emotional abuse, "brain-washing," parental alienation syndrome, sabotage, and manipulation. It is these infrequent superheated custody battles that make headlines and can distort the public's perceptions about the prevalence of such disputes and the adequacy of the court's response.

Child custody—types of custody

Dealing with child custody and visitation is one of the most difficult aspects of divorce, particularly if one parent wants sole custody of the child. There are two types of custody:

Physical custody

Physical custody means that a parent has the right to have a child live with him or her. Some states will award joint physical custody to both parents when the child spends significant amounts of time with both parents. Joint physical custody works best if parents live relatively near each other, because it lessens the stress on children and allows them to maintain a somewhat normal routine.

When the child lives primarily with one parent and has visitation with the other, generally the parent with whom the child primarily lives will have sole physical custody, with visitation awarded to the other parent.

Legal custody

Legal custody of a child means having the right and the obligation to make decisions about a child's upbringing. A parent with legal custody can make decisions about schooling, religion, and medical care, for example. In many states, courts regularly award joint legal custody, which means that the decision making is shared by both parents.

If parents share joint legal custody and one parent excludes the other parent from the decision-making process, the excluded parent can ask the judge to enforce the custody agreement, which will involve another hearing. No fines or jail time is involved, but this leads to further expense, embarrassment, and friction, which may be harmful to the child.

Sole custody

One parent can have either sole legal custody or sole physical custody of a child. Courts generally do not hesitate to award sole physical custody to one parent if the other parent is deemed unfit—for example, because of alcohol or drug dependency, a new partner who is unfit, or charges of child abuse or neglect.

However, in most states, courts are moving away from awarding sole custody to one parent and toward enlarging the role a divorced father plays in his children's lives.

- For example, even when courts do award sole physical custody, the parties often still share joint legal custody, and the noncustodial parent enjoys a generous visitation schedule. In such a situation, the parents make joint decisions about the child's upbringing, but one parent is deemed the primary physical caretaker, while the other parent has visitation rights.

Unless one parent causes direct harm to the children, it is not advisable to seek sole custody. Even in light of allegations of harm, courts may allow supervised visitation, while still ordering joint legal custody.

Joint custody

Parents who do not live together have joint custody (also called shared custody) when they share the decision-making responsibilities for and/or physical control and custody of their children. Joint custody can exist if the parents are divorced, separated, or no longer cohabiting, or even if they never lived together. Joint custody may be:

- Joint legal custody.
- Joint physical custody (where the children spend a significant portion of time with each parent).
- Joint legal and physical custody.

It is common for couples who share physical custody to also share legal custody, but not necessarily vice-versa.

Joint custody arrangements

When parents share joint custody, they most often develop a schedule that accommodates their work requirements and housing arrangements and the children's needs. If the parents cannot agree on a schedule, the court will impose an arrangement. A common pattern is for children to split weeks between each parent's house or apartment. Other joint physical custody arrangements include:

- Alternating months, years, or six-month periods.
- Spending weekends and holidays with one parent, while spending weekdays with the other.

There is another joint custody arrangement in which the children remain in the family home and the parents take turns moving in and out, spending their out-time in separate housing of their own. This is called "bird's nest custody."

Pros and cons of joint custody

Joint custody has the advantage of assuring the children continuing contact and involvement with both parents. It also alleviates some of the burdens of parenting for each parent.

There are, of course, disadvantages:

- Children must be shuttled back and forth.
- Parental noncooperation or ill will can have serious negative effects on children.
- Maintaining two homes for the children can be expensive.

It is advised that parents who have joint custody maintain detailed and organized financial records of expenses should future claims of financial responsibility arise.

Child abuse

As of 1966, all 50 states had laws making the reporting of child maltreatment mandatory. The Adoption Assistance and Child Welfare Act (AACWA) is a federal statute passed in 1980, which requires states to make reasonable efforts to prevent removal of maltreated children from parental custody.

Definitions
- Child neglect and abuse: The physical or mental injury, sexual abuse, negligent treatment or maltreatment of a child under the age of 18 by a person who is responsible for the child's welfare under circumstances that indicate that the child's health and welfare is harmed or threatened thereby.
- Sexual abuse: The employment, use, persuasion, inducement, enticement, or coercion of any child to engage in (or assist any other person to engage in) any sexually explicit conduct or simulation of such conduct for the purpose of producing any visual depiction of such conduct, or the rape, molestation, prostitution, or other forms of sexual exploitation of children, or incest with children.

Four major types of child maltreatment
- Physical abuse: A nonaccidental injury, or an injury that is not compatible with the history of the injury or the child's level of development.
- Sexual abuse: The use of a child as an object of gratification for adult sexual needs or desires.
- Emotional abuse: When a person conveys to a child that she or he is worthless, flawed, unloved, unwanted, or endangered.
- Child neglect: Failure to provide for a child's emotional or physical needs. There are four forms of child neglect:
  - Physical neglect.
  - Educational neglect.
  - Emotional neglect.
  - Child endangerment.

Epidemiology
According to the 2004 National Child Abuse and Neglect Reporting System there were an estimated 3.5 million children that were the subjects of a Child Protective Services investigation or assessment. Of these, 66% were transferred for further investigation, and 34% were screened out for no further investigation. About 25.7% of those evaluated resulted in a finding that the child maltreatment was substantiated or indicated. The most common form of reported abuse was neglect (60%), physical abuse (18%), sexual abuse (10%) and psychological abuse (7%).

Perpetrators of child abuse
- 84% are parents or a parent acting with another person.
- 58% are female and 42% are males.
- Females are more likely offenders when the victim is young (under the age of three).
- Males are more likely offenders when the victim is older.

Clinical markers of abuse (Mudd and Findlay, 2004)
- Long delay before parents seek help.
- History provided does not fit injuries observed.
- Child has history of repeated physical injuries.
- Time frame does not fit injuries.
- History does not fit developmental skills of child.
- Different histories given to different health care professionals.
- Injuries blamed on siblings or others.
- Child accuses caretaker of abuse.

Child abuse and termination of parental rights

National Clearinghouse on Child Abuse and Neglect Information, July 2001:
- Ends the legal parent-child relationship.
- The standard of proof is "clear and convincing evidence."
- Once terminated, the child is legally free to be placed for adoption with the objective of securing a more stable, permanent family environment that can meet the child's long-term parenting needs.

Most common statutory grounds for involuntary termination of parental rights include
- Severe or chronic abuse or neglect.
- Abuse or neglect of other children in the household.
- Abandonment.
- Long-term mental illness or deficiency of the parent(s).
- Long-term alcohol or drug-induced incapacity of the parent(s).
- Failure to support or maintain contact with the child.

The Adoption and Safe Families Act (ASFA)
Was passed in 1997 to address problems from the Adoption Assistance and Child Welfare Act (AACWA) of 1980.
- ASFA requires that a permanency plan be made within 12 months of a child's entry into foster care and also sets rules regarding the termination of parental rights.
- AFSA requires state agencies to seek termination of the parent-child relationship when:
  - A child has been in foster care for 15 of the most recent 22 months.
  - A court has determined: (1) A child to be an abandoned infant; or (2) The parent has committed murder of another child of his/her own; committed voluntary manslaughter of another child of his/her own; aided or abetted, attempted, conspired, or solicited to commit such a murder or such a voluntary manslaughter, or committed a felony assault that has resulted in a serious bodily injury to the child or to another child of the parent.
  - The above factors become grounds for terminating parental rights when reasonable efforts by the state to prevent out-of-home placement or to achieve reunification of the family after placement have failed to ameliorate the conditions and/or parental behaviors that led to state interventions.

In parental rights termination, the focus is on parenting capacity, not on the best placement for the child.

Clinical criteria for termination of parental rights
(Rosner 2nd Edition)
- Evaluation should include examination of the child individually with both biological parents and foster parents. All should be informed of the limitations of confidentiality.
- A review of all records from the child's school, medical records, psychiatric treatment, child protective services, or agency records should be carried out to obtain history and collateral information.

- A thorough evaluation of the child's stated parental preference must be explored in the context of a child psychiatric evaluation.
- The child's perception of the parent's abuse, neglect, and unavailability should be assessed.
- Evaluation of the child's development, including medical examinations, developmental milestones, and psychological testing should be completed.
- Parental attitudes, knowledge of parenting skills, the parents own development and emotional maturity should also be assessed.
- Determination of how parents coped with stressors/demands during their child's development.
- Evaluation of the parent's perspective about his/her own difficulties and alleged reasons for termination of parental rights.
- Psychiatric mental status examination of involved parents to assess for possible psychopathology.
- Assessment of child-parent interaction in an unstructured play setting is useful in detecting covert hostility, anger, and detachment.

Special issues

Driving privileges

Essence

Presence of a mental disorder per se does not imply impaired driving capacity. However, patients with mental disorders may experience symptoms that can interfere with their ability to operate motor vehicles safely. According to the AMA physician handbook[1] "clear evidence of substantial driving impairment implies a strong threat to patient and public safety." Many states have laws or rules that either require or allow physicians to report potentially dangerous patients.

Background

The law in most states allows a breach of confidentiality under various circumstances, such as reporting to the state police or DMV when a medical or psychological condition is likely to impair the patient's ability to safely operate a motor vehicle. The agency will determine whether to pursue further investigation. Accurate assessment of the impact of symptoms on functional abilities is difficult. Psychiatrists have no special expertise in assessing the ability of their patients to drive.[2]

Epidemiology

Deaths and injuries from motor vehicle accidents are the leading cause of death in persons aged 2 through 33 years, and a leading cause of injury-related deaths among 65 to 74-year-olds and older age group.[3] Although seniors do not drive as often as younger counterparts, they account for a disproportionate number of accidents.

Legal

Mental disorder, whether organic or otherwise, as per DSM-IV, with symptoms of:
- Attention deficits (e.g., preoccupation, hallucinations, delusions).
- Suicidal ideation.
- Excessive aggressiveness, presenting as clear and present danger.
- Substance abuse precludes driving privileges and may warrant a special driving examination (DMV) to determine driving competency.

Clinical

Age per se is not a critical factor in losing the capacity to drive safely; rather it is the loss of health through Illness which becomes increasingly common with advancing age. It is important to advise patients about the potential impact of their illness (e.g., hallucinations, mania) and treatments (effects of psychotropic medications on alertness and coordination, potentiation by ETOH) on driving ability as well as the importance of discussing with their treating physician(s) the desirability of choosing medications.

---

1 American Medical Association: Physician's Guide to Assessing and Counseling Older Drivers (2003). Chicago, IL. (Web-based version at www.ama-assn.org/ama1/pub/upload/mm/433/chapter8.pdf/. Last accessed March 2006).
2 American Psychiatric Association POSITION STATEMENT. The Role of the Psychiatrist in Assessing Driving Ability (1993). APA Document Reference No. 930004. The American Psychiatric Association, Washington, D.C.
3 Metzner, J.L. (2004). Commentary: Driving and Psychiatric Illness. *J Am Acad Psychiatry Law* **32**, 80–82.

Assessment

Cognition, vision, and motor function deficits interact cumulatively. Assess information processing ability (attention, concentration, memory); sustained attention; visual spatial functioning; impulse control; judgment and problem solving (U.S. Department of Transportation, Federal Highway Administration, May 1991, Publication no. FHWA-MC-91-006.). In addition to MSE, obtain collateral information regarding ADLs and family concerns. Moderate dementia usually precludes driving safely; moderate cognitive impairment is less clear but should prompt regular follow up if evidence of driving impairment is absent as patients and families often overestimate the patient's driving abilities. Acute mental illness (mania, psychosis) precludes safe driving, but chronic, treated mental illness may not interfere with driving.

Pitfalls

Issues include dual agency, confidentiality, and expertise. Driving cessation is often a life-changing decision that should be based on clear predictable evidence of dangerousness to self or others.

Impaired physician[4]

Definition

Physician who is unable to fulfill professional responsibilities secondary to a psychiatric illness, a physical illness, or condition of abuse of alcohol or other drugs. The APA definition of impairment is inability to practice medicine with reasonable skill and safety.

Epidemiology

Lifetime prevalence of impairment is between 8 and 15%; ETOH 2.3–3.2%; other substances 0.9–2%; psychiatric conditions 0.9–1.3%; no increase compared to general population.

Etiology

Acute (respiratory, cardiac), chronic (thyroid, diabetes mellitus), or progressive degenerative (multiple sclerosis) illness, normal aging, psychiatric disorders including mood, anxiety, adjustment, personality disorders, substance abuse, cognitive impairment, behavioral problems (boundary violations, disruptive behaviors, dishonesty).

Signs

Boundary issues (taking advantage of patients for monetary or personal gain, prescribing to family and friends, inappropriate socializing, confidentiality breaches); disruptive behaviors (inappropriate anger, resentment, words or actions towards others; inappropriate/inadequate responses to patient or staff needs).

Symptoms

Poor personal hygiene, multiple physical complaints, personality/behavior changes, inappropriate tremor/sweating, slow or rapid speech, mood swings, bizarre acts and behaviors, disorganized office or clinic schedules, irrational altercations with patients/staff, frequent absences, decreased work tolerance, frequent lateness, deteriorating performance, inappropriate orders, medical records in disarray, unavailability on call, subject of hospital gossip or rumors.

4 Booker, T., Bush, M.D. *The Physician Who Becomes Impaired.* Division of General Internal Medicine. Beth Israel Deaconess Medical Center, available www.bidmc.harvard.edu

Treatment

Appropriate treatment of mental and/or physical illness, drug or alcohol dependence, on an inpatient or outpatient basis (40% of physicians do not have a PCP). Hospital diversion programs, FFD (fitness for duty) exam, state licensing authority action, revocation of license or practice privileges, remediation.

Conclusion

All physicians are susceptible. Prevention and early interventions are key. Most states have a board or agency that accepts reports/referrals for intervention and rehabilitation of impaired physicians.

Gun ownership

Key features

Most violent acts are committed by people who are not mentally ill and who have no history of mental illness. A significant correlation does exist between mental illness and self-directed violence (suicide).

Epidemiology

Firearms-related injuries are the second leading cause of injury mortality (57% suicide, 39.5 % homicide or "legal intervention", 2.7% unintentional). Firearms-related violence is considerably higher in the U.S. than in other developed, industrialized nations.[5]

Assessment

Inquire about firearm ownership whenever clinically appropriate or necessary as judged by the psychiatrist.[6] Risk factors for violent acts include substance abuse, family violence and child abuse, discrimination, economic hardship, unemployment, and the availability of weapons. For persons with mental illness, the risk increases disproportionately with substance abuse (up to five times), a history of violent acts, and the lack of treatment and social supports are also risk factors.

Legal

State jurisdictions differ in the degree to which they regulate firearms possession and use. Involuntary mental health commitment precludes the right to own firearms in some states.

Conclusion

Inquire about firearm availability. Educate patients and families about risks of gun ownership and proper safety precautions (safe storage, ammunition stored separately).

Fitness for duty[7]

Key features

Mental illness is a major cause of disability in the workplace and may preclude an employee from performing his or her job safely and effectively. The key to determining an individual's level of function or impairment is assessment of

---

5 Krug, E.G., Dahlberg, L.L., Mercy, J.A., Zwi, A.B., Lozano, R. World report on violence and health. Geneva: World Health Organization (2002).

6 American Psychiatric Association. Doctors Against Handgun Violence ENDORSEMENT. APA Document Reference No. 200107.

7 American Medical Association. A physician's guide to return to work/edited by James B. Talmage, J. Mark Melhorn, AMA press 2005.

actual symptoms and their relationship to specific job responsibilities rather than application of diagnostic labels.

Background

A psychiatric fitness for duty examination is an objective assessment of the mental health of an employee in relation to his/her specific job requirements (includes examination, report of diagnostic findings and treatment options, and opinion about fitness for duty).[8] Questions usually comprise 1) presence and nature of a psychiatric problem, 2) ability of the examinee to perform the job in a safe and effective manner. Several levels of formality: pre-employment screening or physical examination, return-to-work-letter, evaluation and treatment-plan implementation, impairment rating, Social Security Disability evaluation, independent medical evaluation.

Referral

Usually employer mandated rather than voluntary; prompted by marked negative change in job performance (pattern of interpersonal conflicts, insubordination, excessive use of sick leave, intoxication while on duty, pattern of poor judgment, sexual inappropriateness, bizarre or threatening behavior, high rate of errors); boundary violations, unethical or illegal behavior, maladaptive personality traits, poor motivation to return to work, diagnostic uncertainty, multiple co-morbidities, presence of psychosis, violence, anger or lethality issues, secondary gain or malingering.

Examination

Specific psychiatric evaluation (including collateral information, job performance data, PMH), thorough history including prior periods of disability, treatment etc; relevant areas of history reviewed in detail, addiction evaluation, expanded MSE if evidence for possible cognitive deficits: concentration, memory function (remember instructions etc). Psychological and/or neuropsychological testing, laboratory studies (UDS, other substance abuse tests) or other examinations and tests, as indicated. Physical examination if indicated to document neuropsychiatric impairments (apraxia, aphasia etc).

Assessment

Remain objective (distinguish among what is known, observed, stated, or perceived). Gather job responsibilities and performance; obtain job description; awareness of essential job functions is necessary to determine whether an employee can perform his or her job adequately. Symptoms rather than diagnoses determine one's functioning; delineate nature and extent of psychiatric impairments, and separate those pertinent to the claim.

Include:

- DSM-IV-TR diagnoses,
- whether the illness interferes with safe and effective work at the specific job (assess fitness for duty and employability by comparing the patients work capacity to workplace demands),
- areas of impairment (including insight and judgment),
- conditions for an employee to work safely (be specific and thorough),

8 Anfang, S.A., Faulkner, L.R., Fromson, J.A., Gendel, M.H. (2005). The American Psychiatric Association's Resource Document on Guidelines for Psychiatric Fitness for Duty Evaluations of Physicians. *J Am Acad Psychiatry Law* **33**(1), 85–88.

- recommendations for treatment especially if not currently adequate,
- If there is no impairment, clearly explain, without simply stating, "no impairment present."

Practical considerations

Clarify specific assessment question. Explain limits of confidentiality (state purpose, process of evaluation, who will receive report, limited scope of doctor-patient relationship), obtain release of information (document if refused sometimes mandated). Do not confuse or equate impairment with disability. Distinguish ongoing psychosocial stressors (anxiety over possible relapse, marital problems at home), socially unacceptable disabilities in disguise (substance abuse crisis behind complaints of a low back pain), vocational dissatisfaction, employer relations issues (desire to punish the boss), legal issues (causality dispute or desire for cash compensation). May omit sensitive personal information if not relevant. Store and dispose of confidential health information appropriately.

Forensic psychiatry—criminal law

The criminal justice system— structure and sequence

Court structure

State and federal courts

The American court system is comprised of the 50 separate state court systems and the United States or federal court system. Trial courts focus on ascertaining facts through the testimony of witnesses and the examination of physical evidence, while appellate courts review the application of law to facts already ascertained by trial courts.

Most cases involving civil or criminal law are initially filed in state or local trial courts. These cases can then, in most states, be appealed at the State Intermediate Court of Appeals. The final court of appeal for most state cases is the State Supreme Court of Appeals.

United States or federal district courts handle cases involving federal statutes, the U.S. Constitution, or civil cases between individuals from different states where the amount of money at stake is greater than $75,000. Cases from U.S. district courts can be appealed to the U.S. Circuit Courts of Appeal, and final recourse can be had at the U.S. Supreme Court.

Civil division

Civil cases involve disputes between citizens. A civil wrong is called a **tort**. Tort law is an effort to restore the rights of the injured party, usually by means of financial compensation. Intentional torts are done with the prior knowledge that damage may result. Examples in psychiatry include false imprisonment or sex with patients. Unintentional torts are also called **negligence**, which in the medical field is called **malpractice**. Negligence occurs when there is a breach of duty that directly results in actual damages to the affected party.

Family division

In many states, a family court division exists. In some states, the jurisdiction of the family division is further subdivided into orphan's or probate court. The following general matters may fall within the family court division, although there are marked variations between states:

- Delinquency: violation of criminal law by minors, status offenses (minors accused of age-based offenses, e.g., truancy, running away from home, underage drinking). Juveniles may be tried in the criminal court as adults by the process of judicial waiver, often based on seriousness of the offense or repeat offending.
- Child protective proceedings: child abuse and neglect.
- Adoption.
- Divorce: including issues of child custody, visitation, and child support.
- Probate: process of legally establishing the validity of a will.
- Involuntary mental health commitments.
- Guardianship: assignment by the court of a competent adult to care for minor children or incompetent adults.

Criminal division

Criminal cases involve disputes between citizens and the state. Depending on the state, criminal cases are usually heard in state district courts or state circuit courts, the latter usually having jurisdiction for the more serious criminal infractions. Crimes are usually divided between felonies and misdemeanors, the latter usually carrying penalties of up to two years incarceration in local jails while the former usually result in incarceration in the state prison system. Additionally, there are summary offenses or citations that carry short sentences usually of no more than 90 days.

Sequence of events in the criminal justice system

- Crime→investigation→arrest→charges filed.
- Initial appearance→preliminary hearing→bail hearing→grand jury or information→arraignment→trial→sentencing.

Notes/definitions

- The function of the **preliminary hearing** is to discover whether there is probable cause that the accused committed a known crime within the jurisdiction of the court. That is to say, at the preliminary hearing it is determined if there is sufficient evidence to hold the case for court. In some jurisdictions, this function is served by a grand jury.
- At **arraignment**, the accused is informed of the charges, advised of the rights of criminal defendants and asked to enter a plea.
- **Bail** is money given to the court to assure a defendant's appearance at court. If he appears, the money is returned. Bail amounts are set high when an individual is deemed a danger to the community or a flight risk. If the individual does not appear at court, the money is forfeited.
- **Sentencing** choices that may be available include incarceration, probation (allowing the offender to remain at liberty but subject to certain conditions and restrictions such as supervision by the probation office, drug testing and/or treatment, or mental health treatment), fines (money paid to the state), or restitution (money paid to the victim).
- **Parole** is the conditional release of a prisoner before the prisoner's full sentence has been served.

The criminal justice system—trial

Trial

A trial is defined as the examination of evidence and applicable law by a competent tribunal to determine the issue of the specified charges or claims.

- **Burden of proof** is defined as the obligation to prove allegations that are presented in a legal action. In criminal cases, there is a legal burden, or burden of persuasion, which is the obligation that remains on a single party for the duration of the claim. The presumption of innocence creates a legal burden for the prosecution to prove all elements of the offense and disprove the defense.

- The **standard of proof** is the level of proof required in a legal action to convince the court that a given claim is true. In the United States, the legal context determines the standard of proof that is applied. Probable cause is a relatively low standard of proof used to determine whether a search is warranted and used by a grand jury to issue an indictment. The standard of proof known as "preponderance of the evidence" or "balance of probabilities" is met when evidence argues that a given proposition is more likely to be true than not true, effectively meaning that there is a greater than 50% probability of its veracity. This standard of proof is used in civil actions. "**Clear and convincing evidence**" is an intermediate standard of proof used in some civil procedures in which the party with the burden of proof must convince the trier that a claim is substantially more likely than not to be true, sometimes thought to correspond to a probability of approximately 75%. This is often the standard used when the deprivation of rights is at issue (excluding criminal cases), such as in cases involving civil incompetence or involuntary commitment. In most criminal cases, the standard of proof is "beyond a reasonable doubt." This is generally interpreted as meaning that the evidence would not allow for a reasonable person to have a doubt such as would cause him or her to hesitate in the most important of his or her affairs.

- In a trial, the judge or jury are the "fact finders" who determine whether certain facts have been proven to the determined standard.

- Witnesses are individuals who present to the court and swear an oath to give truthful evidence in a legal action.
  - **Witnesses of fact** are those who have first-hand knowledge about a crime or event through their observations.
  - An **expert witness** is one who by virtue of education, profession, publication, or experience is believed to have special knowledge of a subject beyond that of the average person, such that others may rely upon his opinion. Psychiatrists may be called to this role by parties in a civil or criminal action. The qualifications of an expert witness are frequently called into question in a legal action. The validity of scientific expert witness testimony is most frequently evaluated by the **Frye test** or the **Daubert test**. The Frye test calls for a theory to be generally accepted in the scientific community. The Daubert test requires four things to be shown: (1) that the theory has or can be tested, (2) that the theory has been peer-reviewed,

(3) that the potential rate of error is known, and (4) that the theory is generally accepted. The Federal Rules of Evidence use the Daubert test.

Sentence

- When an offender is found guilty, the judge issues the sentence. The sentence generally involves a period of imprisonment, a fine, and/or other punishments against a defendant convicted of a crime. The ability for a judge to use discretion in setting a sentence varies. Under mandatory sentencing policies, the law limits judicial discretion such that a defendant convicted of a certain crime must be punished with at least a minimum number of years in prison. The Federal Sentencing Guidelines are rules that set out a uniform sentencing policy for convicted defendants in the United States Federal Court System. The guidelines are discretionary, meaning that judges consider them but are not required to adhere to their standards in making decisions. Common considerations in determining sentences are deterrence of the individual from future crimes, protection of the community, incapacitation of the offender for further criminality, rehabilitation of the offender, restoration to the victim for damages suffered, and societal retribution inflicted upon the offender. There are several basic theories of sentencing in criminal jurisprudence:
  - **Restorative justice** focuses on crime as an act against another individual or community rather than against the state. The victim plays a major role in the process and receives some type of restitution from the offender.
  - **Retributive justice** is a theory in which punishments are seen as restoring an imbalance in the social order created by the criminal.
  - **Transformative justice** seeks to treat an offense as a relational and educational opportunity for victims, to offenders, and other members of the affected community and look at the root causes and comprehensive outcomes of crime.

Appeal

- An appeal is the act of challenging a judgment to a higher judicial authority. The appellate court is typically deferential to a lower court's findings of fact and usually focuses of on the application of law to those facts.

Crime

Property crime

Property crime includes burglary, larceny, motor vehicle theft, and arson.
- **Burglary** is the unlawful entry of a structure to commit a felony or theft.
- **Larceny** is the unlawful taking, carrying, leading, or riding away of property from the possession of another.
- Motor vehicle theft consists of the theft or attempted theft of a motor vehicle.
- Arson is the willful or malicious burning or attempt to burn, with or without intent to defraud, of a building, vehicle, or personal property of another.

Crimes against person

Violent crimes other than homicide

May vary by state. For example, as defined by the Pennsylvania Crimes Code:
- **Kidnapping**—the unlawful removal of a person by force, threat, or deception (or without consent by a guardian in persons under age 14) by a substantial distance or confinement of a person for a substantial period of time, with intent to hold the person for ransom or reward or as a shield or hostage, to facilitate commission of a felony, to inflict bodily injury on or to terrorize the victim or another, or to interfere with the performance of public officials.
- **Aggravated assault**—attempting to, knowingly, or recklessly causing serious bodily injury to another, under circumstances demonstrating extreme indifference to the value of human life.
- **Simple assault**—attempting to, knowingly, or recklessly causing bodily harm to another.
- **Recklessly endangering** another person—recklessly engaging in conduct which could or does place another person in danger of serious bodily injury or death.
- **Terroristic threats**—with intent to terrorize another, communicating a threat to commit a crime of violence, cause evacuation of a place of assembly, or otherwise cause serious public inconvenience.
- **Stalking**—engaging in conduct toward another person which demonstrates intent to instill fear of bodily injury or to cause substantial emotional distress.
- **Harassment**—with intent to harass, annoy, or alarm another, a person threatens, attempts to, or proceeds to strike, shove, or kick another person; follows the person; attempts to engage in acts with the person that serve no legitimate purpose; or communicates in a lewd or threatening manner either to or about the person.

Homicide

Homicide is the killing of one person by another. **First-degree** murder requires premeditation and malice aforethought such that the actor possesses *mens rea*, (literally "guilty mind", and describes the criminal intent of the person). Murder in the **second degree** is defined as an unpremeditated homicide committed during the perpetration of another felony. In some states, murder in the **third degree** is defined as homicide with *mens rea* but without premeditation. **Voluntary manslaughter** results when an actor inflicts injury willingly upon another without the intention of killing the victim, but death results. In other states, voluntary manslaughter is committed when an actor kills a victim under serious provocation or under the unreasonable belief that the killing is justified. **Involuntary manslaughter** is committed when an actor causes the death of another person while doing an unlawful or lawful act in a reckless or grossly negligent manner. Justifiable homicide is an intentional killing that is exculpated due to special circumstances, some of which include prevention of serious crime, self-defense, and the actions of a public servant in the execution of his or her duty.

Sexual offenses and sex offenders

Please refer to the next section of this chapter.

Juvenile crimes

Considerations

Persons under 18 years of age are generally charged as juveniles and, as such, are under the jurisdiction of the juvenile court system.

The differences in the procedural safeguards and placements are described under another section.

Sentencing cannot extend past the defendant's 21st birthday.

It should be noted here that, in most jurisdictions, juveniles charged with serious crimes who are 14 years of age and older are automatically waived to adult court, where they are tried as adults. They can then be transferred back to juvenile court if so determined by a hearing. This is discussed further in another section. (See Juvenile court 📖 *pp. 840–51*).

Types of offenders

- A delinquent is an offender who committed an act that would be considered a crime if committed by an adult.
- A status offender is an offender who committed an act that is prohibited by law because of the age and/or status of the offender, such as, truancy, violation of curfew, running away, or underage drinking.

Sexual offenses and sex offenders

Terminology

- **Paraphilia**—recurrent, intense sexually arousing fantasies, sexual urges, or behaviors, involving nonhuman objects, the suffering or humiliation of oneself or one's partner, children, or other nonconsenting persons, occurring over a period of at least six months.
- **Pedophilia**—paraphilia consisting of recurrent, intense, sexually arousing fantasies, sexual urges, or behaviors involving sexual activity with a prepubescent child or children (generally age 13 or younger). The individual needs to be at least 16 years of age and at least 5 years older than the child/children involved in the fantasy/action.
- **Sex offender**—a person who has been convicted of a sex offense, as defined by state or federal law. There is great variation between states; however, the **Wetterling Act** mandated sex offender registration with law enforcement for a period of ten years or life. Subsequently **Megan's Law** has mandated community notification by web site, and registration periods may be for 10 to 25 years to life. The federal government mandates that states maintain web sites and provides assistance to those states unable to do so; however, the details of each state's site and regulations vary tremendously. States vary about how much information is made available, e.g., home and work address, telephone numbers and specific details of offenses. The duration of notification on web sites varies by state but is becoming longer in general, particularly with newer federal legislation superseding state law. Many states also require minors convicted of sexual offenses to register for varying periods.
- **Sexually Violent Predator** (SVP)—an individual who has been convicted of committing a sexually violent act and has been determined by experts appointed by the state to pose a substantial risk of committing further sexually violent offenses. The individual must also suffer from a mental illness or abnormality that increases the likelihood of recidivism and sexually violent re-offending. The standards for the necessary psychiatric component are extremely variable across states but may include paraphilias (such as pedophilia), other Axis I disorders and even Axis II disorders such as antisocial personality disorder. States differ in their inclusion criteria for what constitutes a sexually violent act, but examples include rape, forcible sodomy, sexual penetration with an object, and aggravated sexual battery. Many states have provisions that enable an individual designated as a SVP to be civilly committed following release from incarceration. These commitments are often indefinite in term and may require only minimal review of the offender's treatment or progress toward potential release (see Sexual offenders, 📖 p. 885).

Many objections have been raised to these commitments under the color of constitutional protections; however, the U.S. Supreme Court has repeatedly ruled that since these are civil and not criminal matters, and that issues such as **double jeopardy** (the right not to be tried twice for the same offense), **ex post facto** (arbitrarily extending the length of a sentence after it has been set), **substantive due process** (the right to fair treatment under the law), and **equal protection** (under the 5th, 7th, 9th and 14th Amendments; see Bill of Rights for further details) do not apply.

Epidemiology of sexual offense

- As of 2003, there were approximately 455,000 convicted, registered sex offenders.
- Nearly 60% of sex offenders are under conditional supervision in the community.
- Most individuals with paraphilic disorders report age of onset between ages 10 and 20.
- Median age of victims of imprisoned sexual offenders is less than 13 years old.
- Approximately 96% of sexual assaults are committed by men. The majority of sexual offenses committed by women tend to be against children.
- Most sex offenders (80–95%) assault people they know.
- Approximately one-third of sex offenders report assaulting both males and females.
- Some sex offenders have committed many assaults before they are caught. Some also report they have committed multiple types of sexual offenses (such as exhibitionism, voyeurism, public masturbation, possession of child pornography and child molestation), involving both family and nonfamily members, male and female victims, and victims of different ages.
- Many sex offenders have a record of nonsexual crimes as well. This is most true of rapists who often have multiple violent and criminal offenses of a nonsexual nature.
- Individuals who perpetrate sexual offenses display high rates of mental illness overall, including substance abuse, personality disorders, and other psychiatric co-morbidity.
- Some studies have shown that fewer than 30% of sex crimes are reported to law enforcement.

Rape

- Anger, power, and control are believed by many to be the primary motivators for rape, rather than sexual gratification.
- Although the median age of rape victims in the United States is 22 years old, approximately 30% are under age 11 at the time of the assault.
- Offenders often have committed relationships.
- By the time they enter treatment, it is estimated that the typical rapist has assaulted seven victims on average.

Sexual offenses against children

- 80% of child sex offenders are male.
- Female child sex offenders often have a higher level of psychopathology than do male sexual offenders and are at times involved through association with a male sex-offender partner or significant other.
- Those who offend against children often victimize adults as well, and vice-versa.

- A majority of child molesters are heterosexual and may also have sexual relations with appropriate adult partners.
- 90% of child victims know their offender, with almost half of the offenders related to the victim. Young victims who know, or who are related to their perpetrator are the least likely to report the crime to the authorities.
- 55% to 75% of child victims are female.
- Female children are more commonly victims of "hands-off" offenses (such as exhibitionism, voyeurism, and public masturbation) whereas male victims suffer more commonly from "hands-on" offenses.

Recidivism

- Sexual offenders released from prison are rearrested four times more frequently than nonsexual offenders, though the majority of these rearrests are for nonsexual offenses.
- A significant portion of sex offenders who commit another sexual offense do so within a year of their release from prison.
- Exhibitionists have the highest rates of recidivism and the greatest number of victims, often in the hundreds before arrest.
- The likelihood of re-offending increases significantly with greater numbers of prior offenses.
- Antisocial orientation or lifestyle, deviant sexual preferences, and a history of treatment drop-out have also been associated with higher rates of recidivism for sexual offenses.
- Sex offender treatment programs, cognitive behavior therapy, and pharmacotherapy (predominantly selective serotonin reuptake inhibitors [SSRIs] and antiandrogen therapy) have all been demonstrated to modestly reduce the risk of sexually re-offending.

Assessment tools

- Psychological testing—Abel, Becker, Kaplan Cognition Scale, Bumby Cognitive Distortions Scale, Attitudes Toward Women Scale, Burt Rape Myth Acceptance Scale, Clarke Sexual History Questionnaire, Hare Sex Knowledge and Attitude Test, Multiphasic Sex Inventory, Hare Psychopathy Check List.
- Psychophysiologic assessment—penile plethysmography (PPG), polygraphy.
- Risk of recidivism assessment instruments—There are many tools for assessing the likelihood of recidivism including the Abel Assessment for Sexual Interest (AASI-2), the Rapid Risk Assessment for Sexual Offender Recidivism (RRASOR), Sexual Violence Risk-20 (SVR-20), STATIC-99. Refer to p. 883 for additional information about these instruments.

Mental illness and criminal behavior

- Most crimes are not perpetrated by persons with mental illness.
- Most persons with mental illness do not commit criminal acts.
- The rate of criminality is slightly higher among individuals with mental illness than among the general population.
- Individuals with substance use disorders, psychotic disorders, traumatic brain injury, impulse control disorders, paraphilias, and personality disorders are found in a higher percentage in the prison population than they are in the population-at-large.
- Female prisoners are more likely to have mental illness than are male prisoners.
- Among those individuals who commit criminal acts, substance use disorders (particularly alcohol abuse or dependence) are the most prevalent psychiatric diagnoses.
- In individuals with mental illness, the presence of a co-morbid substance use disorder greatly increases the likelihood of the commission of a criminal act; likewise, a high percentage of offenders incarcerated in prison who are diagnosed with a mental illness also have a co-morbid substance use disorder.
- As a group, persons with schizophrenia commit homicide at a higher frequency than do individuals without schizophrenia; however, only about 5% of violent crimes are committed by individuals with a psychotic disorder, and most individuals with schizophrenia do not commit violent acts. Acute symptomatology (particularly command auditory hallucinations) accounts for a substantial portion of the increased relative risk.
- Persons with Axis II diagnoses commit more criminal offenses, as a group, than do individuals without personality disorders. Diagnoses of antisocial, borderline, narcissistic, and paranoid personal disorder are the most common Axis II diagnoses found in the prison population.
- Among incarcerated individuals, female prisoners are more likely to have a mental illness than are male prisoners.
- The patterns of criminal behavior (e.g., nature of the offense, motivation for the crime, and characteristics of the victim) for persons with and without mental illness are fairly parallel.
- Dynamic factors (including presence or absence of social support, housing stability, employment, medication compliance, and recent substance use) are strongly correlated with the perpetration of criminal acts by those both with and without mental illness.

Risk assessment for violence

Psychiatrists are frequently asked to perform violence risk assessments in the following circumstances: planning for discharge from inpatient facilities, testifying at civil commitment hearings, determining risk to potential victims who may be targeted by patients, and forcing treatment over refusal.

The assessment of a patients, dangerousness or risk for violence to others can be performed in a purely clinical manner or in combination with actuarial instruments. **Actuarial methods** refer to techniques that utilize mathematics to combine information.

The factors that have predictive value with respect to future violence can be divided into static and dynamic factors. **Static factors** include base rates of violence in the population of which the patient is a part: male gender, younger age, lower socioeconomic status, lower educational achievement, past history of violence, presence of a mental disorder, psychopathy (traits of both antisocial personality disorder and narcissistic personality disorder, usually assessed by Hare psychopathy checklist), poor employment adjustment, history of juvenile delinquency, criminal history, dysfunctional upbringing (physical abuse or a parent who was a substance abuser or a criminal).

Dynamic risk factors include:
- Severity of current psychiatric symptoms.
- Anger.
- Current substance abuse.
- Presence of violent fantasies with a specific target.

With regard to psychiatric illness, severity of present symptoms is more predictive and significant than simple presence or absence of a diagnosis. Most dangerous are symptoms characterized as threat/control/override; these include persecutory delusions or delusions involving thought insertion and/or mind and behavior control. Presence of hallucinations, per se, is not predictive of violence, but **command hallucinations with violent content** may be, especially when accompanied by delusional ideation.

In juveniles, specific violence risk factors include poor school performance, unstructured free time, lack of supervision, poor reputation within their neighborhood, and gang affiliation.

Violence risk can be communicated as a listing of factors that place a patient at risk for violent behavior, with specification of static and dynamic factors. Results of actuarial instruments, if used, should also be included. Specific recommendations that target modifiable factors are most helpful.

Dispositions for mentally ill offenders

With the national trend toward de-institutionalization, more mentally ill offenders enter the criminal justice system each year. The interventions made within and outside of the criminal justice system and the community reintegration opportunities offered to this population vary greatly and affect rates of recidivism and subsequent incarceration.

Diversion

This is the process by which a mentally ill offender is "diverted" from the criminal justice system and into the mental health system prior to adjudication. This can occur before or during formal arraignment, or at the preliminary hearing when evidence is examined for bringing a case to trial. Often, in lieu of a formal trial, an inmate will be offered the option of mental health or drug court as a more appropriate venue for hearing his/her case, with an emphasis on treatment, rather than punishment by incarceration. Both mental health and drug courts emphasize strong working relationships with case mangers, parole or probation officers and other forensic services and community supports.

Mental health courts

Mental Health Courts attempt to address the problem of repeat offenses in the **seriously and persistently mentally ill** (SPMI) population. The concept behind the Mental Health Court is that those suffering from an SPMI with a history of minor offenses would be better served in the community, receiving treatment that would likely decrease their re-offense rate, as the primary issue is felt to be their mental illness. Criteria for identifying individuals referred to mental health courts vary not only between states but even within states, at the county level. Individuals with histories of questionable mental illness, severe personality issues, more serious arrest records and more serious charges (particularly violent or sexual offenses) are less likely to be selected for mental health court. Mental health courts generally use probationary periods as a means of guaranteeing adherence to a treatment regimen, and utilize various levels of housing dependent on the individual's level of function. Examples include long-term structured residencies, group homes, and other supportive living arrangements. Treatment is mandated and failure to meet criteria including medication management, house rules, group attendance, and drug or alcohol use is considered a violation that may lead to a move to a more restrictive setting or, at worst, incarceration.

Drug and alcohol courts

Drug and alcohol courts work on a similar model to mental health courts, usually with a continuum of care allowing a gradual step-down toward societal reintegration. Criteria for selection in drug courts generally favor the nonviolent, nonsexual offenders with a long history of severe substance abuse/dependence and concomitant minor (often property) crimes. These are often referred to as drug or alcohol related crimes and involve possessing illegal substances, being intoxicated under conditions in which such behavior is prohibited, or engaging in illegal nonviolent activities to procure substances. Parole and probation are again used as tools to encourage compliance with treatment for drug and alcohol or often dual diagnosis issues. Offenders generally progress from inpatient programs such as therapeutic community model housing to three-quarter and halfway houses, to partial programs, to intensive out-patient programs and eventually outpatient treatment. Electronic moni-toring is often used if the offender is residing in unsupervised housing in the community while attending various levels of outpatient programs. A strong emphasis is placed on sobriety, involvement in treatment and support programs such as AA and NA; failure to meaningfully participate may lead to parole or probation violations, a move to a more restrictive setting or, at worst, incarceration.

Transfers

For those offenders within the correctional system suffering from a serious mental illness (for example an offender who is found to be delusional, hallucinating, and disorganized, and considered incompetent to stand trial), transfer to a more intensive level of care may be appropriate. This may include private hospitals, state forensic units, or "competency restoration units." Standards vary significantly from state to state, but for involuntary commitments in order to regain competency, the offender is still entitled to a hearing, an opportunity to hear the "evidence" of mental illness, legal representation and an opportunity to present evidence. A judge then makes a determination based on the evidence presented to whether the offender meets the minimum criteria ("clear and convincing evidence") for commit-ment.

For offenders who are tried and found not guilty by reason of insanity (NGRI), a reasonable relationship must exist between the sentence they would likely have served if convicted and the time in a mental institution. If the offender is still found to be mentally ill and dangerous, he/she can be transferred from a forensic to the civil treatment unit, by way of civil commitment, with the same burdens of due process.

For some defendants who are found to be incompetent to stand trial and who are transferred for treatment, it becomes apparent that compe-tency is unlikely to be regained (due to severe and treatment resistant mental illness, mental retardation or organic brain injury among others) and transfer to a civil treatment facility is possible if the same criteria described above are met. In these cases, charges are often dismissed by a judgment of **"nolle prosequi"** (meaning "we shall no longer prosecute," made by a prosecutor after charges but before verdict, essentially dropping the case) with the understanding that the patient will receive the appropriate level of care for his illness. In cases where the prosecution is not prepared to noll pross, the defendant can be released on bond and be similarly treated in the civil arena. The rationale is that awaiting a trial that is not likely to occur due to the defendant's incapacity is a significant waste of the court's time and resources.

For additional information on transfers, please refer to "Transfers between correctional and mental health systems", 📖 *p. 884.*

Criminal competencies

The forensic psychiatrist is often asked to render an opinion regarding a criminal defendant's capacity to make certain decisions regarding specific issues as these relate to the defendant's case. The definition of competency, a legal acknowledgement of an individual's capacity to accomplish a task, varies with regard to what function the defendant is being assessed for, and a defendant may well be competent for one purpose but not for another.

In the United States, the concept of **criminal competency** is related to the 6th Amendment, the right to a fair trial, and the 14th Amendment, relating to due process. The defendant must be competent to proceed with trial, to maintain the integrity of the process in an adversarial system, to maintain fairness, and to maintain the retributive value of the proceeding, that is the defendant must understand why he or she is being tried and/or punished. There are a number of criminal competencies relating to the series of events that occur in the criminal justice process.

Competence to waive Miranda warnings and to make a statement

After arrest, the defendant is presented with his or her Miranda rights. These include the right to remain silent, the information that the arrestee's statements can be used against him or her in court, and the right to an attorney (including the right to an attorney for indigent individuals). The defendant may waive these rights if he or she rationally and voluntarily makes a decision to do so, with the understanding of what rights are being waived. In the case of *Colorado v Connelly* (1986), the U.S. Supreme Court held that the confession to a murder given by a man acting upon command auditory hallucinations was acceptable because there was no coercive police activity. An evaluation of competency to waive Miranda warnings should include a determination that the Miranda warning was provided and that a signed waiver or related document was obtained. Recordings or transcripts of the arrest and interrogation can assist in demonstrating the mental status of the defendant at the time that the waiver was made and also suggest the presence or absence of coercion. Educational, past medical, and past psychiatric records should be reviewed to further demonstrate the defendant's previous cognitive status. This may clarify the defendant's ability to remain silent, as well as his or her ability to understand what choices existed. Reading ability is particularly important to assess in cases involving defendants who sign documents that were not read aloud to them. Malingering must always be considered, given that the retraction of a confession is a significant secondary gain.

Competence to stand trial

In order to proceed with a criminal trial, the defendant must be competent to stand trial.

The standard for this was defined by the U.S. Supreme Court in 1960, in the case of **Dusky v USA**. The court held that a defendant must be able to understand the charges held against him or her and be able to cooperate with his or her attorney in his or her own defense. This implies a rational understanding of the procedure rather than the ability to simply recount the facts. The defendant must be able to understand the charges and their relation to him or her, the available legal defenses, the likely outcomes, the roles of the various courtroom personnel, the role of his or her own counsel, and to possess the ability to interact appropriately and effectively with counsel. Finally, the defendant must be able to behave in an appropriate manner in the courtroom. The criteria stipulate that the defendant must lack the ability, not the willingness, to participate in the trial; furthermore, the defendant's knowledge of the legal situation and the proceedings must be "reasonable," and not necessarily complete.

Competence to stand trial is first and foremost a function of the defendant's current mental status. By federal standards, incompetence requires that a "present mental disease or defect renders the defendant unable to understand the nature and consequences of the proceedings against him or to assist in his own defense." A defendant is therefore presumed to be competent; thus, the burden of proof lies with the defendant. The standard for proving incompetence is by preponderance of the evidence.

Competence to plea and waive the right to trial and/or attorney

When a defendant goes to trial, he or she may enter into a plea bargain. This involves the agreement on the defendant's part to plead guilty to a crime, in return for either a decrease in the severity of the charge or a guarantee that the sentence will be less severe than the maximum allowed by law. In the 1992 case of *Godinez v Moran,* the U.S. Supreme Court ruled that a defendant who is found competent to stand trial is also competent to "knowingly and voluntarily" waive any of his constitutional rights, including the right to a jury trial and the right to counsel. This ruling superseded a previous ruling which held a higher standard for waiving constitutional rights than for standing trial.

Competence to be executed

In the 1986 case of **Ford v Wainright**, the U.S. Supreme Court found that a defendant must be competent to undergo capital punishment. The court stated that the defendant must know that he or she is in fact being executed, as well as the reason for the execution. The court held that the reasons for not executing an incompetent defendant include the lack of retributive value, the lack of deterrence, and that "it simply offends humanity."

Criminal responsibility

For an act to be considered a crime, two factors are necessary: the actus reus, or criminal act, and the mens rea, or criminal intent. In a criminal trial, a defendant may attempt to be exculpated of criminal responsibility by attempting to use the insanity defense or to have the charge and sentence mitigated by making an argument for diminished capacity.

Not guilty by reason of insanity (NGRI)

The notion that an insane individual may be exempt from sanctions for what would otherwise be a criminal offense has a long history in Western and Middle-Eastern law. The persistent legal question has been how to define insanity in legal terms. In the United States, the most commonly used legal standard of insanity for determining criminal responsibility is the **M'Naghten test**. This standard states that for an individual to be acquitted on the basis of insanity "it must be clearly proven that at the time of committing of the act, the party accused was laboring under such defect of reason, from disease of the mind, as not to know the nature or quality of the act he was doing, or if he did know it, that he did not know he was doing what was wrong." The M'Naghten test is fundamentally based on a defendant's cognition at the time of an act. It has been criticized because it does not take into account a defendant's ability to control his or her impulses or conform his or her behavior to the requirements of the law.

In response to this critique, the American Law Institute (ALI) promulgated another standard for insanity that included both cognitive and volitional arms, stating that a person is not responsible for criminal conduct "if at the time of such conduct as a result of mental disease or mental defect he lacks substantial capacity either to appreciate the criminality of his conduct or to conform his conduct to the requirements of law." Recently, however, most states and the federal government have abolished the volitional component and retained only the cognitive component. In most jurisdictions, the burden of proving insanity rests on the defense by a standard of clear and convincing evidence.

Statistics of the NGRI defense

- Defendants in less than 1% of all felonies raise the NGRI defense.
- Three-quarters of these do not succeed in receiving an NGRI verdict.
- Almost 70% of cases that do result in a successful NGRI verdict are pled before a judge rather than a jury.
- There is minimal literature on recidivism rates of NGRI acquittees, but the available resources reveal a rate varying from almost 3% in Oregon to 65% in Connecticut.
- An NGRI acquittee is more likely to be a young female of lower socio-economic status with less education.
- On average, an NGRI acquitee is detained for as much time, or longer, than a defendant found guilty of a similar defense.

Guilty but mentally ill (GBMI)

Other states, approximately 20 in all, have adopted yet another verdict, guilty but mentally ill (GBMI), in recognition of the fact that some defendants suffer mental illness at the time of the crime, but do not meet the standards for legal insanity. The state of Pennsylvania, for example, uses the ALI definition of insanity as the criterion for mental illness in the GBMI defense, while preserving the M'Naghten rule as the criterion for the NGRI defense. The practical difference between NGRI and GBMI is that, in receiving the former verdict, the defendant is absolved of criminal responsibility and is remanded for psychiatric treatment, whereas with the latter the defendant is sentenced as if he or she had been found guilty. A determination is then made about the need for treatment for the mental illness. When the defendant completes the course of treatment for the illness in a psychiatric facility, he or she is then required to serve the rest of his sentence. This is in contrast to an insanity defense acquitee, who would be eligible for release when deemed no longer dangerous. The GBMI verdict has been criticized on the grounds that it may mislead jurors that a defendant receiving this sentence, may receive a lesser sentence, or that some other allowance may be made for the presence of the mental illness.

Diminished capacity

The diminished capacity defense is an affirmative defense that argues that an actor's ability to form **mens rea** was compromised at the time of the act. This argument requires a distinction between crimes of general intent and crimes of specific intent. General intent is the intent to commit a particular act. Specific intent constitutes one of the elements of certain offenses as defined by law and requires **mens rea** (meaning "guilty mind," criminal intent of the person). Specific intent adds another layer of culpability to general intent, e.g., "premeditated" murder. Diminished capacity can be introduced as an affirmative defense in crimes that reqiure specific intent. In jurisdictions in which this defense is accepted, it can lead to a reduction in the charge and mitigation of the sentence (e.g., manslaughter as opposed to first degree murder).

Death penalty issues

Currently in the United States, 38 states and the federal government have capital statutes. In 2005, 60 people were executed, all by lethal injection, and at the end of the year 2004, 3,314 prisoners were being held around the country under sentence of death. Psychiatrists can be involved in the process of capital punishment in several ways: evaluations and testimony with regard to aggravating and mitigating factors in the crime, that will bear on whether the sentence of death is or is not imposed; assessments for competency to be executed; the treatment of offenders and who are under sentence of death.

There is no clear consensus among forensic psychiatrists on ethical issues in most death penalty matters. The ethical guidelines of the American Medical Association proscribe professional participation in an execution; however, this has typically been narrowly defined as direct administration of the lethal agent. Among the published opinions of the American Psychiatric Association's (APA) Ethics Committee on the Principles of Medical Ethics, it is stated that it is ethical to provide a competency evaluation prior to an execution, if the prisoner is informed of the nature and purpose of the evaluation, the limits of confidentiality, and has legal representation. The APA's position is that it is *not ethical to treat an individual who is incompetent to be executed with the aim of restoring said individual to competency.* However, psychiatric treatment is at times provided to individuals on death row who are incompetent to be executed, with the justification that the treatment is medically necessary and alleviates suffering, although the treatment may indeed restore such individuals' competency to be executed.

In the case of **Atkins v. Virginia** (2002), the U.S. Supreme Court ruled that execution of a **mentally retarded** individual violated the 8th Amendment's prohibition against cruel and unusual punishment. In **Roper v. Simmons** (2005), the Supreme Court held that the 8th and 14th Amendments forbid the imposition the death penalty on juveniles who were under the age of 18 at the time of their crime was committed.

Mitigators and aggravators

When deciding between capital punishment and a lesser sentence, state law often asks juries or judges to consider the aggravating or mitigating circumstances of a case. **Aggravating factors** are relevant circumstances supported by evidence that make a harsher penalty appropriate. Although aggravators differ between states, examples include the commission of the capital crime during the commission of another felony, the youth of the victim, payment received or expected for the capital crime, the use of torture during the commission of a capital crime, and the continuing high risk for dangerousness despite incarceration.

Mitigating factors are circumstances that would predispose to the imposition of a lesser sentence. These also vary by jurisdiction, but may include the commission of the capital offense while the actor was under the influence of extreme mental or emotional disorder, the participation or consent of the victim to the homicidal act, the commission of the act under circumstances which the defendant reasonably believed to be a justification or extenuation, duress or domination of the actor by another individual that led to the commission of the capital offense, and a substantial defect in the capacity of the actor to appreciate the criminality of the capital offense or to conform his or her conduct to the requirements of the law due to a mental disorder or intoxication. A forensic psychiatrist may be called upon to testify to the defendant's state of mind at the time of the offense and the presence of mental disorder or intoxication at the time of the act. This testimony may be used as evidence for or against the existence of mitigating factors during the sentencing.

Correctional psychiatry

The United States has the highest number of incarcerated individuals of any nation worldwide. On average, over two million inmates reside in the correctional system in the United States at any given time. More than half are inmates of state and federal prisons. In addition to directly preventing individual crime by removing the inmate from society and serving as a deterrent to others, the intended purposes of incarceration have encompassed both rehabilitation and retribution.

Mental illness in the correctional system

According to the last Bureau of Justice statistics report, in 1999:

- Over a quarter million mentally ill persons were in a prison or jail. This constitutes 16% of the incarcerated population.
- Mentally ill inmates were more likely to have committed a violent offense than an offense against property.
- Six in ten mentally ill offenders were under the influence of alcohol or drugs at the time of their offense.
- Six in ten mentally ill state inmates reported receiving mental treatment since their admission to prison.
- Over three-quarters of mentally ill inmates had been sentenced to time in jail, prison, or probation at least once prior to their current sentence.

Treatment in the correctional setting

All levels of correctional facilities, from lockups to federal prisons, have significant populations suffering from mental illness. Jails and lockups incarcerate offenders who may require acute psychiatric and substance abuse treatment and are often understaffed and underfunded to recognize those requiring treatment. These inmates require early identification and prompt treatment. Poor funding and understaffing often result in inadequate recognition and response. State and federal prisons house inmates for a longer duration, providing opportunities for greater recognition of mental illness and more extensive long-term interventions. These include psychopharmacology, psychotherapy, drug and alcohol rehabilitation, and sex offender treatment programs. These opportunities, however, are often missed due to time, staffing, and cost constraints within the correctional system, leaving many inmates untreated or undertreated for much of their sentences.

Screening evaluations are used in the great majority of larger institutions to facilitate referral for mental health treatment. Screening practices vary widely depending on the location and the institution and screening tools are many and varied in their complexity and utility.

The 8th Amendment, which prohibits cruel and unusual punishment, has been interpreted to require adequate treatment for both physical and mental illness. That is to say, all post-adjudication offenders are entitled to treatment within correctional facilities and to reasonable provisions for care post-release.

There is a high incidence of substance abuse and drug-seeking behavior in the incarcerated population, complicating the treatment process.

Inmates may wish to pass their sentences in an overmedicated state to ease the monotony and stress of extended incarceration. Furthermore, black market trading in prescription medications exists: illicit alcohol and illegal drugs and medications may be traded or sold by inmates within institutions. This consideration should be borne in mind by the prescribing physician.

Within institutions, inmates with severe psychiatric illness, developmental disabilities, and brain injuries, among others, are often separated from the general population, to minimize the risk of exploitation and victimization. Inmates treated in mental health units who are deemed capable of being safely maintained in the general population, are often gradually reintroduced to avoid incident. Institutional mental health units may be further subdivided into acute, subacute, and dual-diagnosis units. Mental health treatment options vary significantly by county, state, and institution. Mental health units are generally staffed by psychiatrists and nurses, and sometimes by therapists and psychologists and other support staff trained in correctional issues.

Inmates with severe illness requiring further evaluation or hospitalization may be transferred to forensic psychiatric facilities, such as state hospitals for inpatient treatment, or to mental health units within the Department of Corrections that have been licensed as inpatient treatment facilities. Inmates are protected by the same constitutional rights to refuse treatment as are noninmates, and involuntary commitment procedures must include a hearing presenting the inmates the right to confront the allegations facing them, the opportunity to present arguments and evidence on their own behalf, and the right to representation. The burden of proof required to obtain an involuntary commitment varies between states, but the minimum standard is "clear and convincing evidence" of illness requiring transfer to a treatment facility, with the burden of proof on the party seeking the commitment.

Special considerations

- **Suicide prevention**: lock-ups and jails are increasingly housing seriously mentally ill offenders. These offenders often have co-morbid substance abuse problems and are subjected to the same overcrowding and cramped conditions as other inmates in U.S. correctional facilities. These conditions add to the stress of incarceration. Shame and guilt associated with arrest, along with an insufficient or inaccurate understanding by the offender of his or her legal situation, may compound this stress. This can place offenders, both mentally ill and otherwise, at high risk for suicide. The rate of suicide is highest in lock-ups followed by jails, then prisons. The first eight hours of incarceration are often the most critical period for potential suicide prevention. Perhaps somewhat counter-intuitively, the typical suicide involves a young, intoxicated offender, with minimal legal history and minor charges. Suicide is a notoriously difficult event for even experienced practitioners to predict; therefore, caution should be exercised in making judgments regarding safety in a population already under severe psychosocial stressors.

- **Dual agency**: in general, dual agency is strongly discouraged. However, in the correctional setting, practical considerations sometimes require the clinician to perform court ordered evaluations and treatment on the same offenders, constituting dual agency including, for example, parole evaluations. When this occurs, a careful and thorough discussion with the inmate regarding the limits of confidentiality is of the utmost importance. The American Psychiatric Association Task Force (2000) Guidelines state, "It is the responsibility of the psychiatrist to set forth clearly to the inmate any such limitation on confidentiality as part of the informed consent process."
- **Duty to the individual** versus **duty to the institution**: the goals for treatment often require a consideration of both the safety of the individual and the security of the institution as a whole, with its many inmates and staff. Confidentiality is generally assumed not to extend to situations involving an immediate danger to the patient or others, a clear and present danger of escape or riot, or situations requiring urgent transfer to a special unit or another institution.

Malingering

- DSM-IV-TR definition: the intentional production of false or grossly exaggerated physical or psychological symptoms, motivated by external incentives.
- Motivation for malingering includes avoidance of punishment or an undesired activity, procurement of benefits or medications, or retaliation against a perceived injustice.
- Can vary from full fabrication of symptomatology (pure malingering) to conscious exaggeration of actual symptoms (partial malingering).
- Some individuals may downplay or deny symptomatology for secondary gain, which has been termed dissimulation.
- Factors associated with malingering include history of legal problems, substance dependence, antisocial personality disorder, homelessness, and being single.
- Thorough knowledge of symptoms as they present in a "genuine" illness goes a long way in helping to diagnose malingering.
- Factors that increase suspicion for malingering include:
  - "Symptom display" in excess of what is typical for a given disorder (e.g., a patient feigning cognitive deficits who is unable to add 1+1, or a patient feigning schizophrenia who endorses seeing large monsters or experiencing constant hallucinations).
  - Display of illness only in selective settings or at certain times, particularly when the patient knows that he/she is being observed.
  - Symptoms relayed in an overly zealous or scripted manner; conversely, answers provided in an evasive, fairly vague manner.
  - Positive endorsement of virtually all symptoms inquired about, particularly ones that are uncharacteristic for a given disorder.
  - Discrepancy between what is reported, observed, learned from testing, and what is known about the typical presentation for a disorder (e.g., in psychosis, the presence of isolated hallucinations (particularly visual) or command hallucinations that are always obeyed; in severe depression, absence of psychomotor retardation or other neurovegetative symptoms).
  - Inconsistency in history provided or patient presentation over time.
  - Contradictory collateral information.
  - Prior history of malingering.
  - Patient refusal to comply with testing or to accept that no diagnosis is present.
  - Patient insistence on receiving only a certain medication or class of medications.
  - Atypical treatment response (overly rapid improvement, absence of improvement, unusual side-effects).
- If malingering is suspected, consider possible reasons for secondary gain, seek collateral information, evaluate over several sessions, and consider ordering psychological or physiological testing. May also choose to obtain a second opinion.

- Psychological testing that can be employed in the detection of malingering includes the **Minnesota Multiphasic Personality Inventory-2** (MMPI-2), **Miller Forensic Assessment of Symptoms Test** (M-FAST), and **Structured Inventory of Malingered Symptomatology** (SIMS).
- Keep in mind that a patient can malinger certain symptoms but still suffer from psychiatric illness.
- If it is determined that a patient is malingering, one may still be able to intervene therapeutically after considering the underlying reason for the malingering (e.g., for a patient who is feigning suicidality out of fear that he will be attacked by his cell mate, attempt to arrange for a transfer to another cell).

Assessment tools

General diagnostic instruments

- Millon clinical multiaxial inventory-III (MCMI-III)—a self-administered questionnaire consisting of 175 true-false items, focusing predominantly on personality pathology.
- Minnesota multiphasic personality inventory-2 (MMPI-2)—a self-administered questionnaire consisting of 567 true-false items that is designed to assist in the diagnosis of psychopathology and the elucidation of patterns of personality; widely researched and highly utilized, requires between 60–90 minutes to complete.
- Schedule of affective disorders and schizophrenia (SADS)—a semistructured interview with emphasis on both current and lifetime mood and psychotic disorders.
- Structured Clinical Interview for Diagnosis (SCID)—a structured interview that examines both current and lifetime diagnoses; widely utilized both clinically and in research studies. The SCID-I is utilized to assess for DSM-IV Axis I diagnoses, whereas the SCID-II is used to detect Axis II pathology.

Screening instruments for malingering

- Miller forensic assessment of symptoms test (M-FAST)—a 25-item screening instrument designed to provide an estimate of the likelihood that a subject is feigning psychiatric illness.
- Structured inventory of malingered symptomatology (SIMS)—a 75-item screening instrument developed to assist in the detection of malingered psychopathology and neuropsychological symptoms.

Competency assessment instruments

- Competency screening test (CST)—a 22-item sentence-completion inventory designed to assess the defendant's knowledge of and attitudes about the components of the trial and its various participants.
- Georgia competency court test (GCCT)—a structured interview involving the completion of 21 questions, ascertaining a subject's knowledge of the basic elements of a courtroom and the roles of the primary participants involved in a trial.
- MacArthur competence assessment tool–criminal adjudication (MacCat-CA)—a 22-item structured interview designed to assist in the pretrial assessment of competency to stand trial for persons over the age of 18. Utilizes vignettes and objectively scored questions to assess a subject's capacity to understand, reason about, and appreciate the various elements involved in a trial, including his/her role in the process.
- McGarry's competency assessment instrument—a 13-item instrument scored on a 5-point scale using a semistructured interview. Some of the items include quality of relating to the attorney, appraising legal strategy, and self-defeating versus self-serving goals.

Instruments for use with sexual offenders

- Abel assessment for sexual interest-2 (AASI-2)— an assessment instrument designed to evaluate sexual interest and to obtain information regarding involvement in abusive or problematic sexual behaviours, for use with adult or adolescent sexual abusers. Includes self-report elements and objective measurements of sexual preference. Sometimes utilized with convicted sex offenders to monitor response to treatment and continued pedophilic preferences.
- Sexual violence rating scale (SVR-20)—a 20-item tool designed to assess the risk of sexual recidivism for previously convicted sexual offenders by examining risk factors.
- STATIC-99—a 10-item actuarial scale designed to estimate the long-term probability of sexual and violent recidivism among adult males convicted of a prior sexual offense.
- Penile plethysmography (PPG)—measures penile tumescence when presented with various visual stimuli.

Other focused assessment tools

- Hare psychopathy checklist revised (PCL-R)—a 20-item clinical rating scale utilized to assess for psychopathy; the inventory is scored following the administration of a semistructured interview and the review of collateral information.
- Polygraph examination—a method utilized to detect lies, involving the interview of a subject by a trained examiner and the subsequent analysis of recorded physiological measurements (heart rate, respiratory rate, blood pressure, and skin conductivity) obtained during the interview. Defendants in the United States can refuse examination and the results are often inadmissible in court (jurisdiction-dependent). Accuracy rates vary widely across different studies.
- Rorschach psychodiagnostic (Inkblot) test—a projective assessment tool involving a subject's interpretation of a set of 10 inkblots, designed to reveal underlying thought process, psychodynamic processes, and personality characteristics. There are multiple scoring systems, although the Exner System is among the most popular and widely studied.

Transfers between correctional and mental health systems

Pretrial

Jails and lockups house a large number of psychiatrically unstable inmates. Inmates are at a high risk for emergencies, including suicide, particularly in the initial days of incarceration. Jails are ill equipped to manage these situations and transfer for inpatient treatment may be required. An acute emergency may warrant an immediate transfer to a local hospital. Inmates so transferred remain under arrest and are accompanied by correctional officers. For less emergent situations, inmates are transferred to inpatient forensic units in various state or city hospitals. These hospitalizations serve to treat psychiatric illness and also to restore competence in inmates found incompetent to stand trial. Involuntary admission to an inpatient treatment setting requires the same due process as an involuntary admission in the community. (See Civil commitments and Right to refuse treatment, 📖 p. 820).

Sentenced prisoners

Psychiatric illness is more prevalent in correctional institutions than in the general population. Deinstitutionalization, among other factors, has led to growing numbers of the mentally ill in correctional rather than hospital facilities. These patients, now inmates, require treatment for their illness while incarcerated. This treatment may include hospitalization when their needs are not met within the correctional system. Again, in an emergency situation, this may require transfer to a local hospital accompanied by a correctional officer. Recently, this more often involves a transfer to a mental health unit licensed as an inpatient treatment facility and contained in one of the state prisons. The same procedural safeguards are required for involuntary admissions as those required in the community setting.

NGRI acquittees

Disposition of acquitees is a hotly debated issue. Cases of NGRI acquittees reoffending provoke public outcry. While John Hinckley continues to spend his life at St Elizabeth Hospital, public policy regarding disposition of the NGRI acquitees remains vague and varies depending on jurisdiction. To hold an individual against his or her will in a treatment setting for a period of time exceeding what would have been his or her sentence had he or she been convicted raises issues regarding the violation of civil liberties. Trends in accepting NGRI acquittees in society have swung both ways over the last few decades.

Disposition

Most NGRI acquittees are transferred to state hospitals for treatment of their psychiatric illness. The Supreme Court has held, however, that an insanity acquitee cannot be held in a mental health facility unless it is proven that he or she is both mentally ill and dangerous. Although some states in the United States have moved toward encouraging shorter hospital stays, followed by conditional release into the community, other states have moved in the opposite direction and abolished the NGRI defense altogether. Of the states that continue to have the defense, lengths of hospitalizations tend to be comparable to the criminal sentence for the crimes for which these persons were initially charged.

There is also some correlation between the seriousness of the original offense and length of hospital stay. A long criminal history starting at a young age and psychopathy are factors that tend to prolong stays in forensic state hospitals.

Conditional release

Some jurisdictions employ a conditional release. When NGRI acquittees are no longer a threat to themselves or society, they are released into the community. There are curtailments to their freedom, including following a closely scrutinized treatment plan. The treatment plan is under the jurisdiction of an agency or the court system. Any violation could lead to a rehospitalization. Although the rates of rehospitalizations have increased concomitant, there has been a concomitant decrease in criminal recidivism.

Sexual offenders

The history of legislation relating to sexual offenders is one of public outcry following discovery of a horrendous crime and a legislative backlash against sexual offenders. "Sexual psychopath" legislation has now become "SVP" (sexually violent predator) legislation, with many states legislating involuntary commitment to inpatient facilities for treatment following completion of a criminal sentence. The criteria required for the SVP label is as follows: a history of a sexually based violent offense, an assessment that the offender is likely to re-offend, and a psychiatric condition that could predispose the offender to re-offending. The definition of the psychiatric condition has been extended in some states to the point of including "any condition congenital or acquired" that might affect the "cognitive or affective" state of the offender in such a way as to predispose him or her to re-offend. Definitions include Axis I and II disorders and in some cases are so broad as to exclude virtually no condition. The involuntary treatment is accomplished through the civil commitment process and, therefore, the Supreme Court has repeatedly ruled that criminal protections such as double jeopardy, ex post facto, and substantive due process do not apply.

This is a complex issue involving overlapping legislation on the state and national level, with rapid and frequent changes. The interested reader is referred to more comprehensive sources for more information.

Recommended further reading

1 Rosner, Richard (ed.) (2003). *Principles and Practice of Forensic Psychiatry*. London: Arnold press, 2nd edn.
2 Simon, Robert I. and Liza H. Gold (eds.) (2004). *The American Psychiatric Publishing Textbook of forensic Psychiatry*. Washington, DC: American Psychiatric Publishing.

Intellectual and developmental disabilities

Introduction

More than any other specialty in psychiatry, mental retardation (MR), also referred to as intellectual disability (ID) and developmental disorders presents a multifaceted, complex discipline, encompassing everything from molecular genetic diagnostic techniques to provision of adequate social supports. Confronted by multiple physical, psychiatric, social, occupational, communication, and educational problems (to name but a few), it is prudent to collaborate in a team model. However, MR can be one of the most rewarding specialties: dealing with children, adolescents, adults, the elderly, families, and other caregivers; utilizing a multidisciplinary approach through collaboration with other health care professionals, psychologists, teachers, and community services; significantly impacting upon the quality of life of both patients and their family/caregivers.

There are great variations in the range and quality of services for the MR population in different geographical areas (meaning that "local knowledge" is essential). With the closure of large institutions, there are more individuals with MR living in the community. This means that the provision of assessment and treatment services is a collaborative effort of primary medical care, mental retardation case management, educational or vocational services, mental healthcare, family or caregivers, and the individual with MR.

The role of the psychiatrist in working with individuals with MR includes:

- Establishing the reason for developmental delay in infants and young children, working with primary medical care (📖 see *p. 898*).
- Establishing the nature and extent of the MR and developmental disorders and the clarification of special educational needs for children of school age, working with special educators.
- Assessing longer-term social care needs particularly in advance of transitional stages, working with the multidisciplinary team (e.g., adolescence, later life—📖 see *p. 900*).
- Assessing behavioral problems or possible psychiatric problems in children or adults.
- Ensuring physical problems, sensory impairments, or other disabilities are not overlooked and facilitating access to general medical services and other specialist assessments.

A structured approach is essential because of the complexity of needs in many people with MR (📖 see *p. 894*). The ultimate aim of the process of assessment is to determine need and to inform what types of intervention and/or treatment may be effective (and to the benefit) of the person concerned (i.e., social, educational, psychological, medical, or psychiatric). The process should be open and transparent, with clear communication between the clinical team, the person with the problem (when possible), and family/caregivers. All too often problems arise when expectations are unrealistic, or where there are misunderstandings about the actual role of particular members of the clinical team. The clinician may act as a focal point in the collation and dissemination of information, and providing treatment recommendations.

Historical perspective

In 1968, ICD-8 (WHO) classified "mental retardation" according to severity of intellectual impairment (by IQ assessment) and social factors. The 1970s/1980s saw major policy changes, emphasizing integration with mainstream resources and education, away from institutions and to the community. Many people with MR moved from hospitals and institutions to group homes in the community.

Understanding of the etiology of MR expanded from the 1950s onwards, for example, the discovery of the genetic basis of Down syndrome in 1959. By the 1970s most standard textbooks recognized multiple etiologies (genetic and environmental), separating pre-, peri-, and postnatal causes. Chromosomal karyotyping, identifying metabolic abnormalities, and isolating infectious agents, allowed for laboratory diagnoses, rather than reliance on clinical observation.

Pharmacological treatments of epilepsy, behavioral disturbance, movement disorders, and psychiatric co-morbidity; dietary treatments of metabolic disturbances; behavioral and cognitive approaches; improved assessment/management of social/occupational functioning, communication problems, and educational needs have improved the services and quality of life for individuals with MR and their families. Problems still exist (e.g., inadequacy of funding for community care/resources, unequal distribution of specialist services), but the outlook for people with MR in this, the 21st century, is more promising than it was at the turn of the last.

Classification[1]

The internationally agreed upon term is mental retardation (used in both ICD-10 and DSM-IV-TR). The DSM-IV-TR diagnosis of mental retardation requires significantly sub-average intellectual functioning (IQ approximately 70 or below) on an individually administered IQ test, deficits in adaptive functioning and onset prior to age 18 years.

Both ICD-10 and DSM-IV-TR also agree on the use of the terms mild, moderate, severe, and profound to describe the degree of mental retardation, with arbitrary "cut-offs" varying only slightly:

IQ range for categories	DSM-IV-TR	ICD-10
Mild	50–55 to 70	50–69
Moderate	35–40 to 50–55	35–49
Severe	20–25 to 35–40	20–34
Profound	Below 20–25	Below 20

DSM-IV-TR diagnostic criteria for mental retardation

- Significantly subaverage intellectual functioning: an IQ of approximately 70 or below on an individually administered IQ test (for infants, a clinical judgment of significantly sub-average intellectual functioning).
- Concurrent deficits or impairments in present adaptive functioning (i.e., the person's effectiveness in meeting the standards expected for his or her age by his or her cultural group) in at least two of the following areas: communication, self-care, home living, social/interpersonal skills, use of community resources, self-direction, functional academic skills, work, leisure, health and safety.
- The onset is before age 18 years.
- Code based on degree of severity reflecting level of intellectual impairment:
  - mild mental retardation: IQ level 50–55 to approximately 70.
  - moderate mental retardation: IQ level 35–40 to approximately 50–55.
  - severe mental retardation: IQ level 20–25 to approximately 35–40.
  - profound mental retardation: IQ level below 20 or 25.
  - mental retardation, severity unspecified: when there is a strong presumption of mental retardation but the person's intelligence is not testable by standard tests.

DSM-IV-TR additional features

- Onset before age 18.
- Deficits/impairments in present adaptive functioning in at least two areas:
  - Communication.
  - Self-care.
  - Home living.
  - Social/interpersonal skills.
  - Use of community resources.
  - self-direction.
  - functional academic skills.
  - Work.
  - Leisure.
  - Health.
  - Safety.

ICD-10 guidelines

Mild

- Delay in acquiring speech, but eventual ability to use everyday speech.
- Generally able to independently self-care.
- Main problems in academic settings (e.g., reading, writing).
- Potentially capable of working.
- Variable degree of emotional and social immaturity.
- Problems more like the normal population.

Minority with clear organic etiology, variable associated problems (autism, developmental disorders, epilepsy, attentional and conduct disorders, neurological and physical disabilities).

Moderate

- Delay in acquiring speech, with ultimate deficits in use of language and comprehension, as well as reading and writing. May be capable of simple supervised work.

Severe

- Similar to moderate, but with lower levels of achievement of visuospatial, language, or social skills. May have motor impairment and associated deficits.

Profound

- Comprehension and use of language very limited.
- Basic adaptive and functional skills limited at best.
- Organic etiology clear in many cases.
- Severe neurological and physical disabilities affecting mobility common.
- Associated problems (pervasive developmental disorders, epilepsy, visual and hearing impairment) more common.

American Association of Intellectual and Developmental Disabilities-AAIDD

(Previously known as the American Association on Mental Retardation).

DSM-IV-TR and ICD-10 use comparable diagnostic codes but vary in their definitions of MR. AAMR utilizes a different approach in providing an extended definition that focuses on the individual's needs and what can be done to improve functioning.

Recommended further reading

1 Schalock, R.L. et al. Users Guide: Mental Retardation Definition, Classification, and Systems of Supports, 10th ed. AAIDD. 2007.

Impairments, disabilities, and handicaps

Mental retardation is being rethought to be named as ID. In fact, they both describe a constellation of impairments with associated disability and handicap, the etiology of which may be known (e.g., Down syndrome) or unknown (e.g., childhood disintegrative disorder). The WHO[1] has proposed a system of classification, which helps define needs and direct interventions/treatments, without making specific etiological assumptions.

Impairment

- Any loss or abnormality of psychological, physiological, or anatomical structure or function.
- A deviation from the norm.
- Characterized by losses or abnormalities that may be temporary or permanent, that have affected the acquisition of skills and learning ability.
- Includes the existence or occurrence of an anomaly, defect, or loss in a limb, organ, tissue, or other structure of the body, or a defect in a functional system or mechanism of the body, including the systems of mental functioning.
- Is not contingent upon etiology.
- Have implications for treatment and prognosis and, in many instances, genetic counseling.

Disability

- Any restriction or lack (resulting from impairment) of ability to perform an activity in the manner or within the range considered normal for a human being.
- Concerned with compound or integrated activities expected of the person or of the body as a whole (e.g., tasks, skills, and behaviors).
- Includes excesses or deficiencies of customarily expected activities and behavior, which may be temporary or permanent, reversible or irreversible, and progressive or regressive.
- The process through which a functional limitation expresses itself as a reality in everyday life.

Handicap

- A disadvantage for a given individual, resulting from impairment or disability that limits or prevents the fulfillment of a role that is normal for that individual.
- Places value on this departure from a structural, functional, or performance norm by the individual or his/her peers in their cultural context.

---

1 World Health Organization (1980). *International Classification of Impairments, Disabilities, and Handicaps* (10th rev.). Geneva: World Health Organization, 1980.

- Is relative to other people and represents discordance between the individual's performance or status and the expectations of their social/cultural group.
- A social phenomenon, representing the social and environmental consequences for the individual stemming from his/her impairment or disability.

The process of assessment— a structured approach

When a person with MR presents to services because of a particular problem (e.g., "challenging behavior," see 🕮 *p. 932*), the task for the clinician is to determine the underlying cause, which will include predisposing, precipitating, and perpetuating factors. Causation may in fact be multifactorial, and because of this a structured approach is best. Some aspects of assessment may be well documented (e.g., the etiology of the MR), particularly when the patient is an adult. Any "diagnostic formulation" should always take note of previous assessments and highlight what further assessments may be helpful.

- Intellectual impairment: assessed using standardized tests (e.g., Wechsler scales, Kaufman scales, Stanford Binet).
- Severity of MR ICD-10 or DSM-IV criteria (🕮 see *p. 890*).
- Disabilities: assessments of functioning (e.g., Vineland Adaptive Behavior Scales, American Adaptive behavior Scales, Scales of Independent Behavior).
- Handicap: assessment of quality of life and life experiences (e.g., Life Experiences Checklist).
- Etiology of MR: see Assessing causation 🕮 *p. 898*.

Other aspects of assessment will include:

- Full physical examination; as this may identify undiagnosed problems, which the patient may be unable to communicate.
- Mental state examination; see Psychiatric co-morbidity in the MR population 🕮 *p. 926*, which may go unrecognized and untreated. This includes temperament, usual behavior patterns, current medication.
- Communication difficulties; which may include formal speech and language assessment.
- Environmental and social factors; which may be contributing to the problem.

Current support network

Assessment will involve not only talking to the patient, but also gathering information from previous documentation (including current treatments/previous diagnoses), family/caregivers, other support services, and teachers. The aim is to view the current problem in the light of past experiences, known problems, and current situational factors. A longitudinal approach is advised (i.e., does the current presentation reflect a recurrent problem, is it part of progressive functional decline, or does it represent a new, unidentified problem/unmet need?). It is useful to document the current supports received by the patient, and any important contacts for future reference.

Needs assessment

Should it be the case that the person's needs have changed, then there may be a statutory responsibility to complete a formal "needs assessment," taking into account the wishes of the person (if they have capacity to make the kinds of decisions required) and others involved in care provision. This includes social care, educational, and health care needs.

Etiology

A specific cause for MR can be identified in about 80% of severe and 50% of mild cases. About 50–70% of cases will be due to a prenatal factor, 10–20% perinatal, and 5–10% postnatal. The identification of etiological factors is important because it allows for discussion of the risk of recurrence in future pregnancies. A known cause can allow for discussion of likely disabilities, possible cognitive impairments, and prognosis. This can be useful for planning supports/services, access to education, and optimizing environmental factors (see Needs and priorities, 📖 p. 903).

Modern classifications of etiological factors are often based on timing of the event.

Genetic causes
- Autosomal chromosome disorders (e.g., Down syndrome, 📖 p. 904).
- Sex chromosome disorders (📖 see p. 914).
- Deletions and duplications (📖 see p. 906).
- Autosomal dominant (📖 p. 910) and recessive (📖 p. 912) conditions.
- X-linked recessive and dominant (📖 p. 916) conditions.
- Presumed polygenic conditions (e.g., neural tube defects, pervasive developmental disorders).
- Mitochondrial disorders, maternally inherited (e.g., myoclonic epilepsy with ragged red fibers-MERRF).

CNS malformations of unknown etiology
About 60% of all CNS malformations do not have a known genetic or exogenous cause. The types of malformation seen indicate the timing of the causative event, but not its nature.

External prenatal factors
(See nongenetic causes of MR, 📖 p. 920) particularly in the early stages (during blastogenesis or organogenesis). Infection; exposure to medication, alcohol, drugs, and toxins; maternal illness (diabetes, hypothyroidism, hypertension, malnutrition), and gestational disorders.

Perinatal factors
Occurring around the time of delivery. Neonatal septicemia; pneumonia; meningitis/encephalitis; other congenital infections; problems at delivery (asphyxia, intracranial hemorrhage, birth injury); other newborn complications (respiratory distress, hyperbilirubinaemia, hypoglycemia).

Postnatal factors
Occurring in the first years of life. CNS infections, vascular accidents, tumors; causes of hypoxic brain injury (e.g., submersion); head injury (e.g., accidents, child abuse); exposure to toxic agents (e.g., lead poisoning); psychosocial environment (e.g., poverty, psychotic illness).

Other disorders of unknown etiology
For example, cerebral palsies, epilepsy, autistism spectrum disorders, childhood disintegrative disorders (📖 see Chapter 16).

Types of malformation and the timing of the causative event

Timing (in gestation)	CNS event	Malformation
3–7 weeks	Dorsal induction	Anencephaly, encephalocele, meningomyelocele, other neural tube closure defects
5–6 weeks	Ventral induction	Prosencephalies and other faciotelencephalic defects
2–4 months	Neuronal proliferation	Microcephaly or macrocephaly
3–5 months	Neuronal migration	Gyrus anomalies and heterotopias
6 months (to 1st year of life)	Neuronal organization	Myelination, disturbed connectivity (dendrite/synapse formation), disturbed proliferation of oligodendrocytes and myelin sheets

Assessment of causation

This requires comprehensive history taking from the parents (examination of prenatal records), and a careful physical examination of the child.

Factors in the history

- Family history: parents: ages; consanguinity; medical history; any previous pregnancies (including abortions, stillbirths). Wider family: any history of MR; specific cognitive impairments; congenital abnormalities; neurological or psychiatric disorders.
- Gestational history: general health and nutrition; maternal infections; exposure to medication, drug and alcohol use, toxins, radiation; chronic medical conditions; history of pre-eclampsia, abnormal intrauterine growth, or fetal movements.
- Birth of child: gestational age; multiple pregnancies (birth order); duration of labor; mode of delivery; any complications; any placental abnormalities. Examination of birth records (Apgar scores, weight, length, head circumference).
- Neonatal history: need for special care (respiratory distress, infections, hypoglycemia, hyperbilirubinemia), baby checks (physical examination, Guthrie test).
- Childhood history: weight gain, growth pattern, feeding pattern, sleeping pattern, early developmental milestones. History of childhood illnesses (especially CNS infections or seizures, metabolic/endocrine disorders) and accidents. General systemic inquiry.

Physical examination

- Look for evidence of any dysmorphic features and note whether these are seen in close relatives (e.g., skin—pigmentation, dermatoglyphics; facial features; musculoskeletal abnormalities).
- Full physical examination of all systems including neurological examination for localizing signs.
- If suggested by the history/examination, ophthalmological and audiological examinations should be arranged.

Investigations

- Standard routine tests will include CBC, lytes, urine screen, LFTs, TFTs, glucose, infection screening (blood and urine), and serology (ToRCH—toxoplasmosis, rubella, cytomegalovirus, herpes simplex virus; HIV).
- Where dysmorphic features are evident, or physical signs indicate, arrange X rays of skull, vertebrae, chest, abdomen, hands, feet, and long bones; cardiac/abdominal ultrasound.
- If metabolic disorder is suspected (e.g., progressive course) arrange screening tests of blood and urine.

Benefits of genetic evaluation

For the individual patient
- Identification of appropriate medical and nonmedical therapies.
- Presymptomatic screening for associated complications/functional disabilities.
- Educational planning.
- Elimination of unnecessary testing and evaluations.

For parents
- Anticipatory guidance.
- Education and advocacy.
- Referral to appropriate medical and social service agencies.
- Referral to support groups.
- Reproductive counseling, carrier testing, prenatal diagnosis.
- Family networking.

Critical periods of changing needs in MR—adolescence

This may be a difficult transitional period; issues that may require attention include:

Engaging with adult services

Loss of the additional support provided by supported mainstream, or special schools, may lead to problems if there is not a smooth transition to adult services. Where appropriate (or available) this may include moving to social educational/day centers or school-to-work programs. Some countries have specific legislation to ensure that needs are identified early (e.g., "transitional planning" from the age of 14 under the U.K. Education Act 1993, U.S. Department of Education Individuals with Disabilities Education Improvement Act (IDEIA, 2004)).

Social/economic independence

• Employment/meaningful work activities: depending on the level of the skill and the abilities of the individual, this may be in a self-contained highly supervised workshop, or supported employment opportunities that often include the support of a "job coach" to assist in the transition. Despite changing attitudes, there are considerable barriers to finding work in the open job market, although for some this may be worth pursuing.
• Living arrangements: loss of additional social supports may actually increase the burden of care shouldered by the family. For some, the wish for independence or the lack of family support may be best met with a variety of community and supported living arrangements where support may be tailored to individual needs. Community living for individuals with MR range from small two and three bed group homes with 24 hours 7 day's week supervision, to living in a home with minimal supervision, to living independently, or living with a foster or host family.

Health and mental health needs

Finding consistent medical, mental health and clinical staff to work with individuals and families with MR continues to be a life long challenge. Often, coordinated care is limited and fragmented. MR is a lifespan problem and very few practitioners specialize in this area or understand the issues that a person with MR has across childhood, adolescence, adult, and aging.

Sexual relationships

Societal views may find it difficult to accept the fact that people with MR have normal sexual desires, which can be more of a problem for families/care givers than the individuals themselves. Nonetheless, issues raised by appropriate sexual relationships will include consideration of contraception, understanding of the responsibilities of parenthood, issues of commitment and marriage. Many people, particularly with mild MR, are capable of being successful parents and provide a stable environment for children with appropriate support.

Critical periods of changing needs in MR—Later adulthood

Changing health needs

With increasing age, health needs may be unrecognized or there may be failure to access services. Despite issues of capacity and consent to medical treatment, everyone has a right to best practice, state of the art, high standard of medical care, and no individual regardless of disabilities should be neglected.

Changing mental health needs

These may relate to changing symptomatology over time, altered tolerance of medication, and additional specific age-related cognitive impairment (e.g., due to chronic intractable epilepsy, early onset Alzheimer's disease in Down syndrome).

Aging caregivers

The ability of caregivers to continue to provide the same level of care for their children ought to be considered before a crisis is reached. This requires an ongoing assessment and life planning of supports. Increasing reliance on caregivers may also lead to social isolation, and it is prudent to raise the issue of planning for the future at an early stage. Family planning should include; pre-arranged living wills, inheritances, and family trusts. Issues of bereavement may complicate support arrangements due to the consequent life changes (e.g., may need to move out of the family home and entail learning to be with new caregivers and people who will have problems of their own). There may be cultural differences in preferences and expectations, and these should be sympathetically addressed.

Family issues

Parents of a child with MR

Having a child with MR is a major, often unexpected and potentially overwhelming experience for families. Individual responses vary, but with the variety of supports and resources available, the majority of parents adapt well to the situation and show remarkable resilience and resourcefulness. Depression and guilt are quite common responses in parents and should not be overlooked. Important positive factors include: having a good relationship with their partner and the support of relatives, friends, and support services including "respite" care. Needs and priorities will vary over time and should be identified early and addressed collaboratively with the involvement of parents and other caregivers in any key decisions.

Prenatal screening issues

Prenatal diagnostic screening can place parents in the unexpected position of having to make difficult choices even before the birth of their child. Advice and counseling are a necessary and important part of the screening process, and should not be ignored even when testing is regarded as "routine." The mistaken assumption that screening "guarantees" a healthy child may lead to even greater feelings of disappointment and anger, magnified further by anxious times after the birth, with a baby in a special care unit. Although some conditions can be diagnosed at birth, often parents only realize there is a problem when their child fails to reach developmental milestones, or develops seizures after an apparently "normal" infancy. Often the response is one of bereavement or guilt, and parents may need support to "work through" their feelings.

The importance of diagnosis

While challenging in some cases, clear diagnosis is ideal for multiple reasons. Some MR etiologies may have potential health risks that should be closely monitored. The psychological and social expectations for a certain diagnosis may guide the treatment plan. Clear diagnosis may allow access to specific supports including parent groups and education regarding what the future may hold (i.e., usual course, associated problems, and prognosis over time). For inherited conditions, the issue of further genetic counseling/testing of family members needs to be addressed. Provision of clear information allows individuals to make informed decisions about being tested and to weigh the risks of having other affected children.

The effect on other family members

Although it was previously thought that having a child with MR impacted adversely on other unaffected siblings (often leading to the removal of the child from the family), there is little evidence that this is the case and worries about long-term damage appear unfounded. In fact, brothers and sisters of individuals with MR appear to be drawn to the caring professions and many end up working as doctors, nurses, teachers, or providing support for children with special needs. Grandparents and other family members may be a useful supportive resource for parents.

The pros and cons of external support

For caregivers, informal support may actually be more valuable than formal (professional) support. Frequent appointments or regular home visits may be more disruptive than helpful for some families. Developmental delay brings with it associated problems (e.g., longer time until the child can walk, achieve continence, acquire language/communication skills, and establish a normal sleep pattern). The social, financial, and psychological impact on caregivers should be acknowledged and appropriate help and support provided. For infants and children, schooling may be both a benefit (in terms of learning social skills, support/respite for parents, and close contact with teachers/other parents) and a burden (particularly if the necessary academic support and services are not locally available). Transitional periods (e.g., adolescence/early adulthood) are accompanied by parental anxieties as well as changes in how needs are met. Advance planning will go some way to alleviate increased caregivers stress. Caregivers may also be concerned about what will happen to their child when they are no longer able to care for them and the open discussion of these issues, with provisional planning, may help avert crises.

Needs and priorities

- Early, accurate diagnosis.
- Early Intervention (early intervention shows improved prognosis).
- Informative genetic advice to parents and other family members.
- Access to high-quality primary (and secondary) health care.
- Advice and access to appropriate help and support (practical help, financial assistance, social and educational needs).
- Help and advice with any communication problems (communication aids, learning of sign language).
- Consideration of the needs of caregivers (education, support groups, respite care).
- Well-coordinated care using a team approach.
- Provision of specialist and domiciliary help with specific behavioral problems.
- "Safety net" of open access to increased support when necessary including a crisis intervention plan.
- Acknowledgment that individual needs will vary and change over time.

Genetics of mental retardation

Chromosome abnormalities are the most common known cause of MR, occurring in 4–28% of all cases.

Down syndrome

Down syndrome (DS) is the most common genetic cause of MR with an incidence of 1 in 600 to 800 births. The first descriptions of the trisomy 21 phenotype were by Jean-Etienne-Dominique Esquirol (1838), Edouard Seguin (1846) and later by John L. H. Down in 1862. It took more than a century for Jerome Lejeune to discover the extra-chromosomal origin of Down syndrome.

Etiology

95% caused by the *nondisjunction of human chromosome 21* during meiosis (mother producing a diploid gamete) or nondisjunction during a first or second mitotic event (extra chromosome can be of either paternal or maternal origin), 5% caused by Robertsonian translocations (fusion 14/21 or 13, 15, 22). Mosaicism (mixture of normal and trisomic lines) occurs in 2–5% resulting in IQ in the 70s and less pronounced dysmorphic features. Nondisjunction increases with increasing age, thus increased maternal age is a risk factor for the disease (age-adjusted incidence/1000 births 0.5 at age 25, 0.7 at age 30, 5 at age 35, 25 at age 40 and 34.6 at age 45). Elevated transcript levels of the more than 350 genes on the chromosome have been detected and the variability in transcript level likely accounts for the phenotypic divergence in individuals with trisomy 21.

Clinical features

DS individuals have characteristic facial dysmorphology of a flat facial profile; underdeveloped nasal bridge, close set eyes with epicantal folds, upslanting palpebral fissures, Brushfield's spots (gray or very light yellow spots of the iris), small low-set ears, high-arched palate, protruding tongue, instability of atlanto-axial joint, and narrowed hypopharynx (leading to sleep apnea). Individuals have a small and hypocellular brain (reduced 10–20%) and are invariably cognitively impaired, with most in mild to moderate MR range (35<IQ<70). Individuals have an increased risk of seizure disorder (5–10%). Brains of individuals with DS show histopathology of Alzheimer's disease presenting by the fourth decade. A greater incidence of eye defects including strabismus (20%), blocked tear ducts, nystagmus, late-life cataracts and keratoconus are seen. Developmental delay, especially in the area of speech, with slow growth and short stature is typical. Hypotonia occurs frequently in newborns. Most individuals have short broad hands with atypical dermatoglyphic features (single transverse palmar creases). Syndactyly (webbed fingers) and clinodactyly (in-curving fifth fingers) are often present. There is an increased incidence (40%–50%) of congenital heart disease (ASD, VSD, MVD and PDA), childhood onset leukemia, esophageal atresia, umbilical and inguinal hernias, Hirschsprung disease, thyroid dysfunction, diabetes, and immune dysfunction (elevated IgG, IgM, decreased T cells). Males have delayed puberty and problems with spermatogenesis (unless mosaic). Females have normal onset of menstruation and are fertile, but have problems with ovulation and undergo early menopause. Medical complications result in decreased life expectancy.

Psychiatric co-morbidity in DS

Approximately 18% of children and 30% of adults with DS have associated psychiatric co-morbidity, usually depression ~10%. Less commonly bipolar disorder, obsessive-compulsive disorder (OCD), Tourette's disorder or schizophrenia are seen. There is an increased risk of autism (1–11% in various survey studies of DS).

Deletion and duplication disorders

ά-thalassemia

An x-linked mental retardation syndrome (cryptic deletion on 16 pter-p13.3 in the ATRX gene), characterized by severe MR in males, dysmorphic facies including epicanthic folds, nasal bridge, midface hypoplasia, a full and everted lower lip, giving the mouth a "carp-like" appearance, widely spaced frontal incisors, microcephaly, hemoglobin H inclusions, cryptorchism and genital abnormalities, mild foot deformity, skeletal abnormalities and scoliosis. Similar phenotype is seen in the X-linked form.

Crit du chat

Partial monosomy; karyotype 5p-(varies from deletion of a small band at 5p15.2 to the entire arm of 5p); de novo mutations (90%), or inherited as balanced parental translocation (paternal 5–6:1). Occurs in 1:20,000–50,000 births.

Clinical features include "cat-like" cry (possibly due to abnormal laryngeal development), low birth weight, feeding difficulties, hypotonia, microcephaly, rounded face, hypertelorism, micrognathia, dental malocclusion, epicanthic folds, low-set ears, hypotonia, speech delay, severe/profound MR and self-aggressive behavior.

Prader-willi syndrome (PWS)

Caused by paternal microdeletion in PWACR 15q11-q13 (70%, M:F 1:1) or maternal uniparental disomy (25%, M:F 4:3) or methylation defect (5%) with a prevalence range from 1:10,000–1:20,000.

Clinical features hypotonia, poor cry, poor sucking reflex with difficulty feeding, FTT, somnolence, developmental delay in the first year of life with a transition to uncontrollable hyperphagia leading to morbid obesity and possible death without monitoring. Typical abnormal facies include narrow bi-temporal diameter, triangular shaped mouth, almond shaped eyes, strabismus, thin upper lip and cleft palate. Other abnormalities include musculoskeletal anomalies (incurved feet, clubfoot, congenital hip dislocation, abnormalities of the knee and ankle, scoliosis), heart disease, GI problems (obstruction, duodenal ulcer, rectal prolapse, gall stones), respiratory disease (asthma, cor pulmonale), renal calculi, hearing deficits, endocrine dysfunction (diabetes, hypothalamic dysfunction with short stature, and hypogonadism) and low normal intelligence to moderate MR. There can also be severe behavioral disturbances which may even resemble conduct disorder (see 📖 p. 708).

Angelman syndrome

Four known genetic mechanisms can lead to Angelman syndrome (AS):
- Molecular deletions involving the Prader-willi/Angelman critical region (PWACR 80%).
- Paternal uniparental disomy (2%).
- Imprinting defects.
- Mutations in the ubiquitin-protein ligase E3A gene (UBE3A).

Patients present with normal prenatal and birth history, normal head circumference and absence of major birth defect. Feeding difficulties may be present in the neonate and infant. Delayed, but forward progression of development (no loss of skills) is evident by 6–12 months and can be associated with truncal hypotonus and unsteady gait. Patients have normal metabolic, hematologic, and chemical laboratory profiles and structurally normal brain using MRI or CT (mild cortical atrophy or dysmyelination).

Consistently seen clinical features (100%)

Severe developmental delay, movement or balance disorder, ataxic gait, and/or tremulous limbs; apparent happy demeanor with frequent laughter/smiling; excitable personality, hand-flapping, hyperactivity, speech impairment, from nonverbal to minimal use of words (receptive speech better than expressive).

Frequently seen features (more than 80%)

Delayed, disproportionate growth in head circumference, usually microcephalic by age two years. Microcephaly is more pronounced in those with 15q11.2–q13 deletions, seizures (86%; onset usually <3 years of age) severity usually decreases with but is lifelong, abnormal EEG, with a characteristic pattern, as mentioned earlier. EEG abnormalities can occur in the first two years of life and can precede clinical features and are often not correlated to clinical seizure events.

Associated features of AS (20%–80%)

Flat occiput, occipital groove, protruding tongue, tongue thrusting, suck/swallowing disorders, feeding problems and/or truncal hypotonia during infancy prognathia (projecting jaw), wide mouth, wide-spaced teeth, frequent drooling, excessive chewing/mouthing behaviors, strabismus, hypo-pigmented skin, light hair, and eye color compared to family (seen only in deletion cases), hyperactive lower extremity deep tendon reflexes, uplifted flexed arm position especially during ambulation, wide-based gait with pronated or valgus-positioned ankles, increased sensitivity to heat, abnormal sleep-wake cycles and diminished need for sleep, attraction to/fascination with water; fascination with crinkly items such as certain papers and plastics, abnormal food-related behaviors, obesity (in the older child), scoliosis, constipation.

Di George syndrome

Most frequent interstitial deletion (22q11.2) found in man with a prevalence of 1:5000 live births. Velo-cardoi-facial syndrome is an associated phenotype related to this deletion.

Clinical features include dysmorphic facial features (microcephaly, cleft palate/submucous cleft, small mouth, long face, prominent tubular nose, hypoplasia of adenoids—nasal speech, bulbous nasal tip, narrow palpebral fissure, minor ear abnormalities, small optic discs/tortuous retinal vessel/cataracts); congenital heart defects (75%: fallot tetralogy, VSD, interrupted aortic arch, pulmonary atresia, truncus artereiosus), hypocalcemia (60% seizures, short stature, hearing problems, renal problems, inguinal/umbilical hernia); hypospadias (10% males), MR (mild 2/3, moderate 1/3) and increased risks for psychiatric disorders, attention-deficit hyperactivity disorder (ADHD; 35–55%), autism spectrum (14%), schizophrenia (25% adults).

Miller-Dieker syndrome

(Type I lissencephaly) is a neuronal migration disorder, caused by microdeletions along the short arm of chromosome 17 (17p13.3) with a complete spectrum of cortical malformations which includes lissencephaly, associated pachygyria, and ventriculomegaly. Lissencephaly and congenital brian abnormalities are also associated with X chromosome mutations.

Clinical features: craniofacial dysmorphism (includes tall prominent forehead), bitemporal narrowing, widely spaced eyes, upward slanting palpebral fissures, short nose with upturned nares, flared thin alae (the flaring part of the nose), protuberant upper lip, thin down-facing vermillion border, flattened midface, micrognathia and flattened ear helices.

Rubenstein-Taybi syndrome (RTS)

Spontaneous mutations involving the specific locus 16p13.3 including balanced translocations, inversions, or microdeletions cause disruption of the human c-AMP regulated enhancer binding (CREB) protein. Incidence is 1:125,000 (M:F = 1:1).

Clinical features: obligatory features of RTS are mental retardation with dysgenesis of the corpus callosum, characteristic facies, and broad, short, terminal phalanges of the thumbs and halluces (great toes). The characteristic facial features include a microcephaly, downward slanting palpebral fissures, and partial ptosis, strabismus, glaucoma, iris coloboma. Low-set ears, a beaked nose, small pouting mouth, maxillary hypoplasia, abnormally set teeth, and a high arched palate. Other abnormalities include: cardiac anomalies (including pulmonary stenosis with hypertension, mitral-valve regurgitation, patent ductus arteriosus); GU anomalies (including hypoplastic kidneys, cryptorchidism, shawl scrotum); GI problems (megacolon constipation); collapsible larynx (leading to sleep apnea) and epilepsy in 25%. Behavioral problems include sleep difficulties, stereotypies and self-injurious behaviors.

Smith-Magenis syndrome

An interstitial microdeletion of the retinoic acid-induced gene 1 (RAI 1) at chromosome 17p 11.2. Incidence is 1:25,000–50,000.

Clinical features: exemplified by multiple congenital anomalies and moderate mental retardation, abnormalities of sleep/wake circadian rhythm (75%) and other psychopathologies. Distinct craniofacial dysmorphic phenotype includes: brachycephaly, prominent forehead, flattened midface, strabismus, myopia, broad nasal bridge, atypical ears, prognathism (projected jaw), and down-turned mouth with cupid's bow. Otolaryngologic abnormalities in 94%; eye abnormalities in 85%; rapid eye movement; hearing impairment in 68% (65% conductive and 35% sensorineural); cardiac abnormalities in 37%; scoliosis in 65%; brain abnormalities such as ventriculomegaly in 52%; renal anomalies in 35%; low thyroxine levels in 29%; low immunoglobulin levels in 23%; forearm abnormalities in 16%; and other minor abnormalities such as seizures and genital abnormalities. Other abnormalities include a hoarse, deep voice; a short stature; broad hands with brachydactyly; and self-injurious behaviors such as head banging, wrist-biting, onychotillomania, and polyembolokoilamania, self-hugging (auto amplexation/embracing), stereotypy; signs of peripheral neuropathy (decreased deep tendon reflexes, decreased sensitivity to pain, bony markers of pes cavus or planus); delayed speech and motor development.

Williams syndrome

Williams syndrome is caused by a submicroscopic deletion of 1.55 Mb in the chromosome band 7q11.23, which includes 26–28 genes (possible candidate genes include those for cytoskeletal proteins LIMK-1 and 2, CLIP and elastin). Incidence is 1:7500. Patients have cardiovascular problems, particular elfin-like facial features and several typical behavioral and neurological abnormalities.

Clinical features facial abnormalities include a broad forehead, wide mouth, full cheeks and lips, oval ears and dental abnormalities; hypercalcemia; hyperacusis, growth failure, supravalvular aortic stenosis (SVAS) with sudden death occurring in 1:1000 affected, genitourinary abnormalities, asymmetrical kidneys, nephrocalcinosis, bladder diverticuli, urethral stenosis, pulmonary artery stenosis, delayed and impaired mental development with mean IQ varying from 40 to 79, a poor visual–motor integration, attention deficits and hyperactivity. Language skills are relatively spared, particularly remarkable social use of language. Behaviorally patients are socially disinhibited and are excessively friendly and may have exceptional musical abilities.

Wolf-Hirschorn syndrome

A subtelomeric deletion of the short arm of chromosome 4 (4p16.3) that includes the WHSC1 gene and genes on the telomeric side of WHSCI. The majority of cases (87%) comprise de novo deletions of preferential paternal origin. Incidence is one per 50,000 births with a female predilection of 2:1.

Clinical features: include typical Greek warrior helmet appearance of the nose, pre- and post-natal growth delay, congenital hypotonia, mental retardation and seizures. Craniofacial defects: microcephaly, broad forehead, prominent glabella, hypertelorism, high arched eyebrows, short philtrum, micrognathia, hypotonia, growth retardation, dysgenic corpus callosum and severe mental retardation. Many survive into adulthood.

Langer-Giedion syndrome

Or type II trichrhinophalangeal syndrome is caused by a deletion of long arm of chromosome 8 in the region q24.11–q24.13.

Clinical features include hearing loss, submucous cleft palate, skin and joint laxity, melanocytic nevi, myopia, growth delay, mental deficiency, epilepsy, psychological disturbances, sarcomatous changes in exostoses uretrohydronephrosis, hematometra, endocrine problems like diabetes mellitus and hypothyroidism, epiphyseal dysplasia, avascular necrosis of femoral head and decreased reproductive fitness.

Autosomal dominant disorders

This group of disorders includes the phakomatoses- congenital neurocutaneous disorders.

Neurofibromatosis

Neurofibromatosis NF1 (chromosome 17q11.2, incidence 1 in 3000 to 4000) and NF2 (chromosome 22q12.2, 1:40,000 incidence) are dominantly transmitted, with half of cases arising from new mutations.

Clinical features predominant phenotypic characteristic of NF1 is the development of benign neurofibromas and schwannomas that arise in the myelin nerve sheaths of peripheral or cranial nerves. Other clinical manifestations include malignant tumors (gliomas, meningiomas, ependymomas or malignant peripheral nerve sheath tumors), skin discoloration, and skeletal dysplasia. Leads to varying levels of mild cognitive impairment in 40–65% of patients.

Von Hippel-Lindau

A hereditary tumor syndrome associated with inactivation tumor suppressor gene, pVHL (3p25–26). Incidence of 1:36,000 live births.

Clinical features brain and spinal cord hemangioblastoma, retinal hemangioblastoma, pheochromocytoma, renal cell carcinoma, renal cysts, and pancreatic cystadenoma and mental retardation.

Sturge-Weber syndrome (SWS)

Is a congenital neurocutaneous syndrome with a facial capillary malformation (port-wine stain), abnormal blood vessels of the brain (leptomeningeal angioma), and abnormal blood vessels in the eye predisposing to glaucoma. Prevalence estimated at 1:50,000 live births (M:F 1:1). Etiology of SWS remains unclear. Familial cases are rare, and the lack of clinical similarity in monozygotic twins has pointed to somatic mutation as a possible means of disease transmission.

Clinical features: frequently develop seizures, headaches, and migraines, stroke-like episodes with hemiparesis, focal neurologic impairments, visual problems, and cognitive deficits. Mental retardation rates of 50 to 60% have been reported.

Tuberous sclerosis (TSC)

A multisystem genetic disorder caused by mutations in the tumor suppressor genes, TSC1 (9q34, harmartin, 40% cases) or TSC2 (16p13, tuberin). Incidence is 1:7000–10,000.

Clinical features: characterized by abnormal growths in a wide range of organs including the skin (adenoma sebaceum, ash leaf spots (96%), shagreen patches, depigmented nevi, café-au-lait spots, fibromas of nails, pitted tooth enamel), heart (rhadomyoma, harmartoma), kidneys (Wilm's tumor, renal cysts) and central nervous system (cortical tubers, subependymal nodules, subependymal giant cell astrocytomas). Epilepsy is a major manifestation; mental retardation, specific learning disabilities, autism spectrum disorders and ADHD also occur.

Autosomal recessive disorders

Phenylketonuria

An autosomal recessive mutation of phenylalanine hydroxylase gene on chromosome 12 q22–24.1 with a prevalence of 1:15,000. The enzyme converts phenylalanine to tyrosine. The disorder is diagnosed postnatally using the *Guthrie test* and is preventable by adhering to a strict diet low in phenylalanine as soon as the diagnosis is made.

Clinical features fair hair/skin, blue eyes (lack of pigment due to tyrosine deficiency), neurologic signs (stooped posture, broad-based gait, hyperreflexia, tremor, stereotypies). Behavioral problems include hyperactivity, temper tantrums, perseveration, echolalia. Prognosis is lower than average IQ even with treatment.

Sanfilippo syndrome

Mucopolysaccharide (MPS III) is a group of four MPS disorders that are caused by the deficiency of enzymes involved in the breakdown of the GAG heparan sulphate. Heparan-N-sulphatase (17q25.3, most severe and most common), α-N-acetylglucosaminidase (17q21.1), acetyl-CoA N-acetyl transferase (variably mapped to chromosome 14,21 and to a 8.3 cM (16 Mbp) span in the pericentromeric region of chromosome 8).

N-acetylglucosamine-6-sulphatase (12q14.9) are deficient in subtypes A, B, C and D, respectively. The clinical phenotypes are similar in all subtypes. Prevalence is 1:25,000–325,000.

Clinical features: severe MR, claw hand, dwarfism, hypertrichosis, hearing loss, hepatotsplenomegaly, biconvex lumbar vertebrae, and joint stiffness. Behavioral problems include restlessness, sleep problems, and oppositional behaviors. There is a poor prognosis with many dying between ages 10–20 years of respiratory tract infections.

Hurler syndrome

Mucopolysaccharidosis type IH (MPS IH) is a lysosomal storage disease resulting from mutation of alpha-L-iduronidase (4p16.3) with an incidence of 1:76,000–144,000.

Clinical features: progressive MR (eventually severe to profound), skeletal anomalies (short stature, kyphosis, flexion deformities, claw hand, long head, characteristic facies), hearing loss, hepatosplenomegaly, umbilical/inguinal hernia, corneal opacity, gingival and tongue hypertrophy, respiratory and cardiac valvular problems. Death is often caused by cardiac or respiratory failure and usually occurs before the second decade of life.

Laurence-Moon syndrome

Associated with multiple loci (11q13, 11q21, 15q22, 3p13) aka Laurence-Moon-Biedl (incorporating Bardet-Biedl syndrome which shares clinical features, but additionally there is central obesity and polydactyly) syndrome is an autosomal recessive disorder characterized by retinitis pigmentosa, hypogenitalism, mental retardation, and renal abnormalities. Prevalence is 1;125,000–160,000.

Clinical features: mild to moderate MR, short stature, spastic paraparesis, hypogenitalism (most males infertile), night blindness (due to red cone dystrophy), NIDDM, renal problems (diabetes insipidus, renal failure).

Joubert syndrome

Is an autosomal recessive disorder presenting with hypotonia, ataxia, developmental delay, breathing abnormalities in the neonatal period, and oculomotor apraxia. Three causative loci have been mapped JBTS1/CORS1 at 9q34.3, JBTS2/CORS2 at 11 centromere, and JBTS3/CORS3/AHI at 6q23.

Clinical features: severe MR, hyperapnea ("panting like a dog"), cerebellar dysgenesis, hypotonia, ataxia, tongue protrusion, facial spasm, abnormal eye movements, cystic kidneys, syndactyly/polydactyly. Behavioral problems include self-injurious behavior.

Sex chromosome disorders

Turner syndrome (TS)

Occurs in phenotypic females missing all or part of one sex chromosome, with the most common karyotypes as follows: 45, X; 45, X/46XX or XY mosaics; 46, XiXq; 46, XdelXp; 46, XrX; and many of these latter groups have a 45, X cell line as well. It is the most common genetic disorder of females, estimated to occur in approximately 1/2000–5000 live female births.

Clinical features: the most constant features of TS remain short stature and early ovarian failure. While a small number patients, with ring or marker chromosomes interrupting the x-inactivation center may have mental retardation, the majority of girls and women with TS have normal intelligence. Congenital cardiovascular defects are found in approximately 50% of girls with TS, but clinically severe defects requiring surgical correction affect only 10–15%. The increased risk for aortic dissection is probably the most serious medical problem facing girls and women with TS.

Trisomy X 47,XXX

These are relatively common, occurring in 0.1% of live-born female infants.

Clinical features: most have a normal phenotype with only a few congenital malformations reported in the literature. 70% have a learning disorder. 33% show some mental or behavioral problems usually of minor significance. There may be an increased incidence of schizophrenia. Female infants with 47, XXX have also been reported to experience delayed menarche, reduced fertility (children have normal karyotypes), and premature ovarian failure.

Klinefelter's syndrome (KS)

Is the most common sex chromosome disorder, occurring in 1:400–1: 1100 male births and in 1:300 spontaneous abortions (50% are due to paternal and 50% maternal nondisjunction).

Clinical features: during childhood, these individuals often appear normal with an asthenic body type (taller ~4cm, slim and long-limbed). By puberty, hypogonadism becomes evident with small testes and underdeveloped secondary sexual characteristics, low levels of testosterone and elevated levels of gonadotropin. KS patients are almost always infertile. The median IQ in KS is ~90 (10–15 points lower than 46, XY karyotype). They display behavioral problems that include immaturity, insecurity, shyness, poor judgment, and inappropriate assertive activity.

XYY male

Sex chromosome trisomy; karyotype 47, XYY; 1:1000 male births.

Clinical features: controversial suggestion of higher incidence in prison populations, as with Klinefelter's the IQ may be 10–15 points lower than average, behavioral problems commonly seen. The commonest indication for a 47, XYY male to be karyotyped will be developmental delay and/or behavior problems.

X-linked disorders

Fragile X syndrome (Martin-Bell syndrome)

The most common inherited cause of MR results from an expanded CCG triplet repeat sequence in the untranslated region (UTR) of the FMR1 (FRAGILE X MENTAL RETARDATION 1, FRAXA, Xq27.3) gene in its most severe form and by CCG repeat expansion in the UTR of two other genes, FMR2 (FRAXE, Xq28) and FMR3 (FRAXE, Xq28) in its milder form. Premutated alleles exhibit an expansion in the CGG trinucleotide sequence from 50–200 repeats (normal 6–54 repeats, mean = 30). Penetrance is low, but greater in males than females (due to the "protective" effects of the second normal X chromosome in females). FAS affected males have repeats between 230–1000+. Transmitting males and obligate females have repeats between 43–200. The prevalence of FRAXA (FMR1) mutation is 1:4000 in males and 1:8000 females. The prevalence of FRAXE (FMR2 and 3) mutation is 1:50,000 males.

Clinical features: FRAXA features are variable, subtle, and often cannot be detected before adulthood. May include: large testicles and ears, smooth skin, hyper-extensible fingers, flat feet, mitral valve prolapse, inguinal and hiatus hernia, facial features (long, narrow face with under-development of the mid-face, macrocephaly), epilepsy (~25%), variable MR (borderline to profound), behavioral features appear to be similar to those seen in ADHD (80% of males with fragile X syndrome and in 35% of females with the full mutation) and autism (30%), hand flapping/waving, repetitive mannerisms, shyness, gaze avoidance, poor peer relationships, communication difficulties (e.g., delayed language development, conversational rigidity, perseveration, echolalia, paliphrasia (involuntary repetition or words), cluttering and overdetailed/circumstantial speech, psychiatric problems (e.g., mood and personality disorders). Brain imaging: reduced posterior cerebellar vermis, enlarged hippocampus and caudate nuclei, enlarged ventricles.

Fragile X-associated tremor/ataxia syndrome (FXTAS)

FXTAS is a neurological syndrome that has been shown to develop in males and occasionally females with premutation alleles with aging. While the patients do not have Fragile X syndrome, they can develop distinctive symptoms. The disorder consists of tremor, ataxia, peripheral neuropathy, and cognitive deficits. Significant brain atrophy and white-matter disease is usually seen. FXTAS is thought to be related to CGG sequence in the FMR1 gene that is repeated only about 55–200 times (a premutation expansion). Common features of the affected individuals of the family include slow psychomotor development with delayed speech, reading and writing, cognitive and behavioral troubles, and chronic anxiety. Other neurological and psychiatric symptoms have been seen in individuals with this mutation including psychosis, infantile spasms and seizures.

Hunter syndrome

Also known as mucopolysaccharidosis type II, Hunter syndrome is an X-linked recessive lysosomal storage disease caused by deficiency of iduronate-2-sulfatase. The disorder maps to Xq27–28 and has an incidence of 1:132,000–280,000 (more common in male Ashkenazi Jews 1:34,000). 20% have complete depletion of iduronate sulphatase and 2 subtypes are recognized. Type A (more common) has progressive MR and physical disability with death before age 15 years. Type B is a milder form with minimal intellectual impairment and better prognosis.

Clinical features: psychomotor retardation, facial dysmorphism ("gargoylism"), dysostosis multiplex with arthrogryposis of fingers and toes, gibbus, claw hand, pes cavus, cervical cord depression, eye defects (retinitis pigmentosa, papilledma, hypertrichosis), umbilical/inguinal hernia, hepatosplenomegaly, cardiomyopathy, chronic diarrhea, and hearing impairment.

Lesch–Nyhan disease

This is caused by X-linked recessive mutation in the gene for the hypoxanthine-guanine phosphoribosyltransferase (HPRT, Xq26–27) enzyme. Males are generally affected. Recent experience indicates that the complete disease does occur rarely in females as a consequence of nonrandom inactivation of the paternal or maternal X chromosome carrying the normal HPRT gene. The prevalence of HPRT deficiency in the population is not accurately known, although an estimate of the minimum frequency of the disorder in Canada is 1:380,000 births.

Clinical features: characterized by hyperuricemia, hyperuricosuria, and severe neurologic dysfunction (including choreoathetosis, spasticity, transient hemiparesis), microcephaly, mental retardation (usually severe), epilepsy (50%) and self-mutilating behaviors (biting of lips, inside of mouth, fingers). Management: Even treating hyperuricemia does not appear to reduce behavioral problems. SSRIs are used for the self-mutilating behavior and teeth are generally removed.

Oculocerebrorenal syndrome of Lowe

This is caused by a mutation of the OCRL-1 gene, an enzymatic protein with phosphatase activity and a small G protein ATPase located on Xq26.1. Occurrence in females has been described associated with balanced X: autosome translocations involving the Xq26 locus, explained by the inactivation of the normal X chromosome by the translocation.

Clinical features: patients have moderate to severe MR (up to 25% have normal IQ), short stature, hypotonia, epilepsy (30%), eye abnormalities (congenital cataracts), renal tubular acidosis and abnormalities of the musculoskeletal system. Behavioral problems include temper tantrums, hand-waving movements, self-injurious behavior (especially in early adolescence).

Menkes disease

A rare X-linked recessive disorder related to the loss of a copper-transporting adenosine triphosphatase (ATP7A, Xq12–q13) involved in the export of dietary copper from the gastrointestinal tract and its transport into organelles.

Clinical features include progressive cerebral degeneration with psychomotor deterioration and seizures, connective tissue alteration with hypopigmentation of skin and hair, and recurrent episodes of hypothermia with failure to thrive. Neuropathology studies show neuronal degeneration in cerebral and cerebellar cortices and in the basal ganglia. Early treatment with copper may be of some benefit.

Norrie disease

A rare X-inked recessive condition caused by mutation in the Norrie Disease Protein (NDP) gene, located on chromosome Xp11.1.

Clinical features include congenital blindness in males due to degenerative and proliferative processes in the neuroretina. 50% of patients have various degrees of mental retardation and psychotic features and 33% develop progressive sensorineural deafness, usually in the second decade.

Pelizaeus–Merzbacher disease (PMD)

An X-linked myelination disorder, caused by defect or altered dosage of the proteolipid protein gene (PLP1), a major structural component of myelin in the CNS. PLP1 gene duplications account for 50%–75% of cases and point variations for 15%–20% of cases; deletions and insertions occur infrequently. PMD is typically found in males. In females heterozygous for a PLP1 gene mutation, oligodendrocytes expressing the mutated X chromosome probably undergo apoptosis and are gradually replaced by oligodendrocytes expressing the normal X chromosome.

Clinical features: vary considerably, although commonly nystagmus, ataxia, spasticity and mental retardation.

X-linked hydrocephalus

This is the second most common cause of hydrocephalus after neural tube defects with an incidence of approximately 1:30,000 male births. It is caused by mutations in L1CAM gene on Xq 28.

Clinical features: There is a broad spectrum of clinical and neurological abnormalities but the main clinical features of this spectrum are corpus callosum hypoplasia, mental retardation (ranging from mild to profound), Adducted thumbs, Spastic paraplegia and Hydrocephalus (CRASH syndrome). Severely affected patients with massive hydrocephalus have pre- or perinatal death and mildly affected patients may have mild MR as the only abnormality.

Aicardi syndrome

Rare X-linked disorder (200–500 reported cases) mostly female, but three known males with a confirmed diagnosis have a 47, XXY karyotype.

Clinical features: include a triad of infantile spasms, agenesis of the corpus callosum, and distinctive chorioretinal lacunae. Polymicrogyria or pachygyria, periventricular and intracortical gray matter heterotopia, choroid plexus cysts and papillomas, ventriculomegaly and intracerebral cysts are frequently present. Most patients with Aicardi syndrome have severe developmental delay, but a few cases have only mild learning disabilities. Consistent facial features include microcephaly, a prominent premaxilla, low-set ears, upturned nasal tip, decreased angle of the nasal bridge, and sparse lateral eyebrows. Often there is hypotonia, epilepsy, scoliosis, vertebral and rib defects. Behaviorally patients present with lack of communication, fatigue/sleep problems, aggression (25%), and self-injurious behaviors.

Rett syndrome (see 📖 p. 716 for more details)

Predominantly affects girls, incidence 1:10,000–15,000. Significant loss of intellectual function is associated with this clinical disorder.

Clinical features: A severe clinical phenotype, which is an important cause of severe mental retardation. The syndrome is characterized by progressive loss of intellectual functioning, fine and gross motor skills, deceleration of head growth, and development of stereotypic hand movements at 6–18 months after birth. Initial stages resemble autism.

Etiology: Most cases associated with mutations in the MeCP2 gene located in the chromosome Xq28 region, which is important for gene regulation in the nervous system.

Prognosis; associated with progressive loss of function. Treatment is symptomatic.

Nongenetic causes of MR

Congenital hypothyroidism

A treatable cause of mental and growth retardation due to loss of thyroid function; incidence 1:3500–4000, but now screened for in neonatal period and treated early with thyroxine. If untreated, leads to typical clinical picture of lethargy, difficulty feeding, extremity edema, constipation, macroglossia, and umbilical hernia.

Fetal alcohol syndrome (FAS)

One of the major causes of MR, incidence of 0.2–3 per 1000 live births, 10–20% of cases of mild MR may be caused by maternal alcohol use. Important factors include: the quantity and timing of drinking, bingeing, other drug use (including smoking), genetic variation, and low socio-economic status. May be due to the effects of alcohol on NMDA receptors, which may alter cell proliferation. While FAS represents the most extreme end of a clinical spectrum, fetal alcohol exposure also has adverse effects on development including learning abilities and behavior.

Clinical features:

- Perinatal problems: irritability, hypotonia, tremors.
- Facial features: microcephaly, small eye fissures, epicanthic folds, short palpebral fissures, low nasal bridge with short or upturned nose, midface hypoplasia, underdeveloped philtrum, thin upper lip.
- Growth deficits: small overall length, joint deformities,
- CNS features: high incidence of mild MR, associated behavioral problems (hyperactivity, sleep problems), optic nerve hypoplasia (poor visual acuity), hearing loss, receptive and expressive language deficits,
- Other physical abnormalities: ASD, VSD, limb anomalies (inability to completely extend elbows, clinodactyly).

Other toxins

For example, maternal exposure to phenytoin, cocaine, coumarin anticoagulants (e.g., warfarin), infant hyperbilirubinemia or child exposure to lead.

Infective agents

ToRCH (toxoplasmosis, rubella, cytomegalovirus, herpes), syphilis (treponema pallidum), HIV, and other viral and bacteria causes of meningitis and encephalitis.

Hypoxic ischemic damage

Refers to cerebrovascular physiologic factors associated with asphyxia and cell damage and death in the central nervous system, which may occur in the ante-, peri-, or postnatal period. Associated risk factors include intrauterine growth retardation, multiple gestation, prematurity, or birth trauma. Type and extent of damage mediated by this mechanism vary depending on the infant's gestational age and other clinical factors.

Developmental abnormalities

- Disorders of head growth and shape—microcephaly and macrocephaly, craniosynostosis syndromes.
- Brain developmental disorders—Arnold-Chiari Malformation, abnormalities of the corpus callosum, hydrocephalus, holoprosencephalies, disorders of neuronal migration (lissencephaly, schizencephaly, heterotopias, pachygyria, polymicrogyria).

MR disorders of unknown etiology

Childhood disintegrative disorder

Clinical features: Rare disorder affecting more males than females, characterized by normal development until the age of ~4 years of age, followed by profound regression with disintegration of behavior, loss of acquired language and other skills, impaired social relationships, and sterotypies. The developmental regression is at an older age than "typical" children with autism. There is an increased risk of seizures. Must be differentiated from Landau Kleffner syndrome and electrical status epilepticus in slow wave sleep (ESES).

Etiology: Unknown, but may follow minor illness or viral encephalitis.

Prognosis: Poor, with the development of severe MR. For more details, 📖 see p. 716.

Cornelia de Lange syndrome (Brachmann-de Lange syndrome)

A largely sporadic disorder with presumed genetic disorder with an incidence of 1 in 10,000–30,000.

Clinical features: Hypertrichosis (hirsutism, synophrys [eyebrows that meet midline], long eyelashes), facial features (depressed nasal bridge, eye abnormalities, prominent philtrum, thin lips, down-turned mouth, anteverted nostrils, widely-spaced teeth, high arched palate, low-set ears, short neck), limb deformities (missing digits, dysplasia, especially in upper extremities), crytorchidism/hypoplastic genitals in males, congenital heart defects, low-pitched cry. Associated with GI problems, visual and hearing impairment, and learning and behavior problems. Usually IQ is below 60 (range 30–85).

Etiology: In a subset of patients, there is a heterozygous mutation in the gene named NIPBL located on 5p13.1 for which the exact function in humans is not clear. Many cases are sporadic.

Prognosis: Poor, with development of severe MR. Sleep disturbance, self-injurious behavior, mood disorders, and autistic like features are common.

Epilepsy and MR

Epilepsy can present a diagnostic and management challenge when it occurs in people with MR. It may begin at any age, presentations may change over time, and multiple forms may occur in the same individual. The prevalence of epilepsy in the MR population is ~40% in the MR population as a whole, and is higher in severe MR (30–50%).

Common pitfalls

Epilepsy may be misdiagnosed in patients with MR, particularly when there is a history of sudden unexpected aggression, self-mutilating behaviors, or other stereotypic movements. These may include staring spells, rapid eye blinking, exaggerated startle response, or unexpected intermittent lethargy. For patients who have been prescribed anticonvulsants for events not considered to be true seizures, a careful withdrawal of medication under close medical supervision may be an option.

Nonepileptic seizures can also occur in patients with or without epilepsy.

Certain epilepsy-related behaviors may be confused with psychiatric symptoms, e.g., hallucinations in somatosensory partial seizures, psychosis-like episodes during complex partial seizures in the frontal or temporal lobe, or postictal confusion or psychosis.

Diagnosis of epilepsy and MR

History and examination: It may be difficult to obtain accurate information, may need to rely on others for information (home video may be useful). Try to exclude other differential diagnoses (e.g., occult infection causing pain, migraine, effects of prescribed or illicit medications, movement disorder). Conduct a MSE, focusing on observed behaviors, identifications of any stressors (especially if anxiety provoking).

Investigations: baseline laboratory tests—basic metabolic profile, routine urinalysis, liver function tests, fasting glucose, lumbar puncture, toxicology screen. Consider neuroimaging studies, especially when the examination is abnormal: EEG (in complex cases video EEG may be particularly useful), PET or SPECT (to detect areas of hypometabolism).

Co-occurrence

Epilepsy is commonly associated with numerous causes of MR, e.g., Trisomy 21 (5–10%), Fragile X (10–25%), Angelman syndrome (90%), Rett syndrome (80%). This may be due to shared etiologies such as alterations in neuronal development and function, or co-existing brain lesions (migration disorders, neoplasm, vascular malformation).

Frequent seizures may lead to (or worsen) permanent loss of intellectual functioning (e.g., progressive partial epilepsies such as Rasmussen's syndrome, progressive myoclonic epilepsy, neuronal ceroid lipofuscinosis, mitochondrial encephalopathy with ragged red fibers—MERRF) emphasizing the need for accurate early diagnosis and institution of effective treatment to prevent often irreversible progression.

Epilepsy syndromes in infancy and childhood

Infancy: Early epileptic encephalopathy due to congenital or acquired abnormal cortical development; early myoclonic epileptic encephalopathy (metabolic disorders); infantile spasms/West syndrome (associated with tuberous sclerosis complex, ToRCH infections, congenital brain malformations); severe encephalopathic epilepsy in early infancy (EEG with high voltage bursts and intermixed flat suppressions).

Childhood: Lennox-Gastaut syndrome (mixed seizure disorder with abnormal interictal EEG, diffuse cognitive dysfunction); progressive myoclonic epilepsies (Unverrich-Lundborg, Baltic or Lafora disease); epilepsy with myoclonic-astatic seizures (Doose syndrome).

Treatment

This is typically the responsibility of a trained neurologist—collaboration with other specialists is vital.

Choice of treatment will depend on a number of factors:
- Accurate classification of the type of seizures/epilepsy syndrome,
- Possible antiepilepsy drug effects and interactions,
- Minimizing side-effects (especially cognitive impairment) and optimization of seizure control.
- After reasonable trials of at least two antiepilepsy medications, the patient should be considered for surgical evaluation as the potential for subsequent clinically significant medication response diminishes significantly.

Points to note
- Behavioral problems may be associated with antiepileptic drugs, and may be more common in patients with MR or brain injury (e.g., barbiturates, benzodiazepines, gabapentin, vigabatrin, levatiracetam).
- Communication difficulties may make assessment of side-effects more challenging.
- For intractable epilepsy, the benefits of surgery must be weighed against the possible risks of impairment as a direct result of the intervention (e.g., possible hemiparesis, memory deficit, language impairment).

Prognosis

There is wide variation in outcome; however, up to 70% of patients with MR can achieve good control of their epilepsy without major side-effects.

Psychiatric co-morbidity in the MR population[1,2,3]

Although originally thought to be mutually exclusive, it is now clear that psychiatric disorders do occur more frequently in the MR population than in the general population. Confusion of primary and secondary diagnoses may lead to underrecognition, particularly in individuals with one diagnosis that "overshadows" the other, as in the case of autistim spectrum disorders and mood disturbance. Certain genetic syndromes have unique susceptibilities to certain disorders. There is a lack of longitudinal studies making prediction of outcome difficult. Furthermore, typical diagnostic instruments and criteria are often difficult to apply to the MR population and may need to be modified.

Schizophrenia

Appears to be slightly greater in the MR population with few differences in symptomatology, except in severe MR cases where there may be unexplained aggression, bizarre behaviors, mood lability, or increased mannerisms and steotypies. Etiology: Common brain mechanisms with possible genetic influences may have a role in an increased risk.

Bipolar affective disorder

Prevalence may be greater than in the general population, with difficulty in making the diagnosis in severe MR. Symptom "equivalents" may include hyperactivity, wandering, mutism, temper tantrums.

Depressive disorder

Appears to be greater than in the general population. Biological features tend to be more marked, with diurnal variations. Irritability may be more prominent than feelings of sadness. Suicidal thoughts and acts may occur in borderline–moderate MR, but are less frequent in severe MR. Interpretation of suicidal acts however, could be difficult to distinguish from self-injurious behaviors. Other causes of mood disturbance (e.g., perimenstrual disorders) should also be considered.

Anxiety disorders

May be difficult to differentiate from depression, except where there are situational features.

OCD

Reported to be more prevalent in MR. Differential diagnosis: ritualistic behaviors, tic disorders, behavioral manifestations of autistim spectrum disorder. It may be difficult to elicit the true OCD from behavioral or motoric mannerisms associated with MR (i.e., the compulsive behaviors may not be linked to any obsessive thoughts as in typical OCD).

ADHD

Often prominent in children with MR (up to 20%). Stimulants may be helpful in mild MR with clear target symptoms, but efficacy in more severe MR is unclear.

Personality disorder

Unclear whether personality disorder is more common in this population due to the possibility of population sampling bias.

Recommended further reading

1 Deb, S., Thomas, M., Bright, C. (2001). Mental disorder in adults with intellectual disability.
2 The rate of behavior disorders among a community-based population between 16–64 years. Journal of Intellectual Disability Research 45(6), 506–514.
3 Whitaker, S. and Read, S. (2006). The prevalence of psychiatric disorders among people with intellectual disabilities: an analysis of the literature. Journal of Applied Research in Intellectual Disabilities.

Overview of management approaches—considerations and choices

Cautionary notes

- Attributing "treatment success" to a particular intervention may miss the "real" reason for improvement e.g., return of familiar caregiver, more structured environment (if admitted to specialist center), or treatment effects on "undiagnosed" primary condition (e.g., anticonvulsant used for aggressive behavior may actually be treating underlying epilepsy).
- Many conditions may run relapsing-remitting courses, leading to erroneous conclusions about effectiveness of an intervention, which only become clear when symptoms return despite treatment.
- Improvement (or worsening) of symptoms may reflect normal maturational processes or, conversely, further pathological degeneration.
- Because of the wide variation in etiology (genetic, environmental, psychological, social) and the complexity (and variable degree) of cognitive impairments, most trials of treatment are by nature empirical. Most management plans will inevitably be individually tailored and the current "evidence base" for many treatment modalities is limited.
- Issues of consent to treatment should be seriously considered in a population who may have varying degrees of *capacity* (see Ethics and the law section, 📖 Chapter 17).

A therapeutic environment

Provision of care and support should always be within an appropriate setting. Support may be: general (care provided by usual caregivers, schools, community teams) and/or specific (addressing particular needs e.g., special education, parental support groups, physical or psychiatric problems, maladaptive behaviors). Although, in general, every effort will be made to sustain a "normal" environment (i.e., remaining at home, integration into "mainstream" schools, use of local community resources), often more specialized environments are necessary.

Factors influencing management choices

- The nature of the problem (i.e., biological, psychological, social).
- The degree and etiology of the MR.
- Co-morbid physical conditions (which may restrict choice of medication).
- Situational factors (i.e., practicalities of instituting various treatment options, supports, ability to monitor progress).

Admission to specialist environments

Sometimes disabilities or problems may be too severe or too complex to manage with standard community resources:

- The degree of MR or the specific cognitive impairments require well-structured, predictable environments that cannot be provided elsewhere.
- The degree of physical impairment requires more intensive specialist nursing, or a safer environment where medical care is close at hand (e.g., severe treatment-resistant epilepsy).
- The severity of behavioral problems prohibits management at home (e.g., abnormally aggressive or disinhibited behavior that constitutes a serious risk of harm to themselves or others).
- The person requires treatment for a co-morbid psychiatric disorder, which has failed to respond to initial treatment.

Other reasons

- Respite placements to allow individuals and their families some relief from the intensity of long-term care.
- Assessment of complex problems—to disentangle environmental from illness factors, or where treatment requires close monitoring.
- "Crisis" admissions due to an acute breakdown of usual supports.

"Behavioral phenotypes"[1]

Many genetic causes of MR are associated with characteristic patterns of behavior. Recognizing these "behavioral repertoires" may help in diagnosis and management, and forms the basis for ongoing research into the genetic basis of some behavioral problems. Examples include: Down syndrome (oppositional, conduct, and ADHD); fragile X syndrome (autism, ADHD, stereotypies e.g., hand flapping); Lesch-Nyhan syndrome (self-mutilation); Prader-Willi syndrome (OCD, multiple impulsive behavior disorder e.g., hyperphagia, aggression, skin picking); Smith-Magenis syndrome (severe ADHD, stereotypies—"self-hugging," severe self-injurious behaviors, insomnia); Williams syndrome ("pseudomature" language ability in some; initially affectionate and engaging; later anxious, hyperactive, and uncooperative): Velocardioiofacial syndrome (ADHD symptoms, expressive language deficits, psychosis in adolescence).

1 Einfeld, S. L. (2004). Behavior phenotypes of genetic disorders. *Current Opinion in Psychiatry* **17**, 343–348.

Overview of management approaches—treatment methods

Behavioral treatments

May be used to help teach basic skills (e.g., feeding, dressing, toileting), establish normal behavior patterns (e.g., sleep), or more complex skills (e.g., social skills, relaxation techniques, assertiveness training). Behavioral techniques may also be used to alter maladaptive patterns of behavior (e.g., inappropriate sexual behavior, phobias).

Cognitive therapies and CBT

For borderline, mild, or moderate MR, cognitive approaches may be adapted to the level of intellectual impairment. These may be effective in the teaching of problem-solving skills, the management of anxiety disorders and depression, dealing with issues of self-esteem, anger management, and treatment of offending behaviors (e.g., sex offenders).

Psychodynamic therapies

May be helpful in addressing issues of emotional development, relationships, adjustment to life events (e.g., losses, disabilities, and bereavement). The range of approaches varies from basic supportive psychotherapy, to more complex group and family therapies.

Pharmacological treatments

Cautions

- Co-morbid physical disorders (e.g., epilepsy, constipation, cerebral palsy) increase the need to closely monitor adverse effects.
- Atypical responses such as increased (or reduced) sensitivity, and "paradoxical" reactions are more common, hence low doses and gradual increases in medication are advisable.
- The evidence base for many drug treatments is lacking and many claims for efficacy are at best based on small, open, uncontrolled trials.

Antipsychotics

For the treatment of co-morbid psychiatric disorders (e.g., schizophrenia and related psychosis) and acute behavioral disturbance. May also be effective in managing autistim spectrum disorders, self-injury, social withdrawal, ADHD, and tic disorders.

Antidepressants

Effective for the treatment of depression, OCD, and other anxiety disorders. They have also been used in the management of violence, self-injury, "nonspecific" distress, and other compulsive behaviors.

Anticonvulsants

There is some evidence for the use of anticonvulsants in the treatment of episodic dyscontrol (e.g., carbamazepine), but this may be due to better control of underlying epilepsy.

Lithium

Aside from the treatment of bipolar affective disorder and augmentation of antidepressant therapy, lithium may have some utility in reducing aggressive outbursts.

Beta-Blockers

May be useful in conditions of heightened autonomic arousal (e.g., anxiety disorders), which may be at the root of aggressive behavioral disturbance.

Stimulants

(e.g., methylphenidate) For the treatment of ADHD (see child and adolescent psychiatry 📖 *p. 702*).

Behavioral disorders and "challenging" behavior

Behavioral disorders are frequently encountered among individuals with mental retardation, ranging from minor antisocial behaviors to seriously aggressive outbursts. Depending on the sampling procedures, prevalence estimates of aggression have range between 2% to 20% of the MR population[1]: Aggression is found higher in males, is more frequent in higher functioning individuals and higher rates in the 20 to 30 year range.[2,3] While most aggression involve punches, kicks, and slaps, weapons are involved with 17–29% of MR individuals who present with aggressive behavior[1], Survey research on staff supporting individuals with MR indicate that 40 to 50% living in institutions have shown one or more forms of challenging behavior during their stay, and 9% rates reported for those living in the community group homes.

Studies of behavioral disorders in the MR population identify six relatively consistent groupings of the types of pathological behaviors1 that may create a significant burden for parents/caregivers.

Aggression

- Aggressive or unusual behaviors: Shouting, screaming, general noisiness; anal poking/fecal smearing (may reflect constipation); pica (consumption of nonfood items) self-induced vomiting/choking; stealing.
- Aggressive outbursts: Against persons or property.
- Severe physical violence: Rare.
- Self-injurious behavior: Skin picking, eye gouging, head banging, face beating (prevalence 10% to 15% overall, more common in severe/profound MR).
- Social withdrawal.
- Stereotypic behaviors (some of which may be self-injurious).
- Hyperactive disruptive behaviors.
- Repetitive communication disturbance (perseveration and echolalia).
- Anxiety fearfulness (fight or flight scenario).

When these behaviors are particularly severe, they are often termed "challenging."

Recommended further reading

1 Alen, D. (2000). Recent research on physical aggression in persons with intellectual disability: An overview. *Journal of Intellectual and Developmental Disability.* **25**, 41–57.

2 Smith, S., Branford, D., Collacott, R. A., Cooper, S. A., & McGrother, C. (1996). Prevalence and cluster typology of maladaptive behaviours in a geographically defined population of adults with learning disabilities. *British Journal of Psychiatry.* **169**, 219–227.

3 Einfeld SL., & Aman M. (1995). Issues in the taxonomy of psychopathology in mental retardation. *J Autism Dev Disord.* **25**, 143–67.

Assessment of behavioral problems should cover a number of interrelated domains:

- **Cognitive functioning** and adaptive behavior as multidimensional constructs; severity of intellectual impairment, language/communication ability, memory (visual/verbal), performance of specific tasks; executive functions (e.g., complex motor and abstract verbal tasks), problem solving and social competency.
- **Temperament**: behavioral flexibility, particularly high emotionality, high activity, poor sociability.
- **Physical problems** such as epilepsy, cerebral palsy, cardiac problems, GI problems, endocrine problems, visual/hearing and other sensory impairments.
- **Medication**: particularly psychotropic drugs may produce or mask cognitive, behavioral, or emotional problems. Sometimes a slow systematic reduction and a medication-free time period may be helpful to assess how medication contributes to the presentation.
- **Psychological factors**: primary reinforcers e.g., food, drink, pain (often undetected and difficult to measure in the severe MR group). Secondary reinforcers e.g., praise, environment, restrictive interventions (withholding reinforcement or attention/response cost, taking a preferred item away).
- **Communication difficulties**: frustration with typical forms of communication—verbal/nonverbal (sign language and gestures) and augmentative communication devices (pictures, electronics).
- **Adverse experiences**: common to the general population, and also particular to the MR population, e.g., delay in developmental milestones, experiences within institutions, social rejection, trauma/victimized (neglect, and emotional, physical, or sexual abuse).
- **Environmental factors**: living conditions, stability and continuity of day-to-day activities (most common factors: multiple short-term residential placements; young, inexperienced and multiple changes in care staff). The quality of the care environment may be directly responsible for behavioral problems and assessment should include factors such as: social relationships, specific environmental stressors, consistency of care, and lack of stimulation and meaningful activities.
- **Co-morbidity**: persons with MR are three to four times more likely to have a psychiatric disorder compared to the general population. Psychiatric disorders may complicate the presentation of behavioral problems e.g., ADHD; conduct disorder; oppositional defiant disorder; tic disorders; anxiety disorders—fears/phobias, separation anxiety, post-traumatic stress disorder (PTSD), OCD; depressive disorder; bipolar disorder; pervasive developmental disorders.

Prevalence rates of Dual Disabilities estimated that 20%–40% of people with MR have a diagnosable psychiatric disorder (John Jacobson, National Association of Dual Disabilities). Accurate diagnosis and appropriate treatment may significantly improve behavioral problems and quality of life.

Behavioral disorders—assessment and principles of management

At all stages in assessment and management, it will be essential to involve parents, care givers, and other allied professionals (e.g., teachers) both as sources of information and in implementing any proposed interventions.

Assessment

Include comprehensive analysis of the person's life experiences, current situations (school, home, work, leisure), personality and health condition.

A comprehensive evaluation including following is also necessary:
- Exclusion of psychiatric disorder.
- Exclusion of bio-medical/physical disorder (and assessment of general state of health).
- Trauma assessment.
- Assessment of sensory and physical impairments (vision, hearing, etc.).
- Assessment of communication difficulties (including formal speech and language assessment).
- Assessment of specific cognitive impairments (including formal psychological/neuropsychological testing).
- Identification of environmental and social factors.
- Use of functional behavioral analysis, behavioral diaries (by care givers/staff). ABCs—antecedents, behaviors, and consequences.

Positive approaches
(Positive behavior support)

Following assessment, specific factors should be addressed—psychiatric/physical causes, reduction of stimuli/reinforcers, modification/removal of environmental factors, social issues.

Positive behavioral approaches may involve:
- Environmental adaptations: Prevention strategies e.g., sensory or relaxation rooms. Areas of the residence/program with low stimulation and sensory activities.
- Communication adaptations: Making accommodations for impairments of hearing, vision, and language (including use of pictures, schedules, sign language, augmentative communication and electronic speech devices).
- Educational interventions both for families/caregivers (to improve understanding) and for patients (to ensure educational needs are individualized and being appropriately met in the least restrictive setting).
- Social interventions/Social skills training to address unmet needs at home, work, and community, with family/caregivers, or to widen access to other services or facilities (to provide opportunities for social interaction through social-skills groups, and improve support networks).
- Behavioral interventions/behavioral supports: Applied behavior analysis (ABA) and social skills training using differential reinforcement procedures (DRO), self-assessment/self monitoring, token reinforcement

(including response cost/withholding reinforcement and level systems), coping and problem solving, use of replacement/alternative behaviors through functional equivalence training and functional alternative techniques for response to attention-seeking behaviors, stereotypies, and aggressive/disruptive responding (these are interventions which are usually limited to specialists in MR treatment).

- Cognitive approaches: Cognitive behavior therapy (CBT), dialectical behavior therapy (DBT) and psychotherapy for individuals with moderate to borderline learning disabilities. At an appropriate level for degree of cognitive impairment and language abilities and insight, interventions may range from simple imitation to relaxation/breathing techniques to counseling on specific issues relating to contracts for safety for dangerous behavior.

- Sensory integration interventions: Using auditory, visual, tactile, vestibular, and deep pressure for relaxation and the de-escalation of challenging behavior.

- Pharmacotherapy: Including specific co-morbid conditions (e.g., ADHD—stimulants/non-stimulant; OCD—SSRIs; antidepressant treatment; tic disorders—antipsychotics; epilepsy—anticonvulsants). Sometimes a trial of antipsychotic treatment may be useful for serious aggression, hyperactivity, or stereotypies (often depot formulation; caution in epilepsy; increased risk of EPS symptoms). Other options for aggression, agitation, or self-injurious behaviors (mainly empirical evidence): anticonvulsants, lithium, beta blockers, and buspirone. For self-injurious behaviors alone there are a few studies that show some evidence for opiate antagonists (e.g., naltrexone). Refer to the Child and Adolescent chapter for more on pharmacotherapy in this population.

- Physical interventions (i.e., physical/mechanical restraint): From splints and headgear to isolation/seclusion (to protect individuals and others from injury/damage to property) have been deemed as nontherapeutic by most professional groups, including the National Association for Dual Disabilities (NADD), AAIDD/AAMR, National Alliance on Mentall illness (NAMI), serving individuals with learning disabilities. Position statements expressed that restraint and/or isolation should not be used as a behavioral modification intervention. If these restrictive interventions are required, restraints/isolation interventions should only be used for safety purposes, as a last resort, when all lesser restrictive interventions have failed and for the least amount of time necessary.

Any restrictive intervention should be closely monitored to ensure compliance, acceptability, and therapeutic response. Every restraint/seclusion episode should be followed by a patient and staff debriefing. In the case of medication, side-effects should be minimized and if treatment is deemed ineffective, drugs should be carefully withdrawn and monitored with a side-effects profile (to avoid secondary problems). Check with your organization to learn the specific rule and regulations related to the use of seclusion and/or restraints.

Behavior support plans[1]

Introduction

Individuals with MR may have behaviors that respond to a well-thought-out behavioral plan. Effective behavior support should result in changes in problem behaviors and life style options of a patient or student in a classroom. The behavior support plan represents the culmination of the assessment process, and is typically completed by individuals with previous training in creating a behavioral support plan. This plan is the team's action plan, outlining the specific steps to be used to promote the individual's success and participation in daily activities and routines. In order to be most effective, behavior support plans should be both carefully developed and clearly written using plain language, incorporate the values of the family and support team, identify any prerequisite resources and training needs for implementation, and include individual components that are both easy to use and easy to remember.

Purpose

The purposes of a behavior support plan are to:
• Provide a clear description of the problem being addressed.
• Define the changes in the physical setting, staff behavior, and physiological support that will occur in an effort to change the magnitude of the problem.
• Provide a process by which the effectiveness of these changes will be monitored and assessed.

In addition, support plans should be based on functional assessments, gathering information through indirect procedures (such as interviews, rating scales and direct observations in natural settings) that result in understanding of the basic assumptions, predictors, and functions surrounding the behaviors.

Page 938 provides an outline of a suggested behavior support plan format. Under the specific categories are general suggestions to consider when formulating a behavior support plan. In addition, a behavior plan has been devised to serve as a general example. Remember, when devising your own behavior plan, target behaviors and behavior interventions must be tailored to meet the needs of the specific individual and all of their unique needs within their environment.

Recommended further reading

1 Kerr, M.M., & Nelson, M.C., *Strategies for Addressing Behavior Problems in the Classroom*. 5th ed., Upper Saddle River, New Jersey: Pearson Merrill Prentice Hall: 2006. http://prenhall.com/kerr

General example of a behavior plan

Behaviors/symptoms

List behaviors or symptoms that will be addressed:
- Verbal/physical aggression.
- Poor anger management.
- Noncompliant for demands.

Etiology/functions of challenging behaviors

Attempt to identify the cause/reason/etiology of the behavior being exhibited.
- Behaviors appear to be related to poor impulse control, cognitive distortions about others' intentions, limited intellectual functioning, attempts at situational control and difficulties with managing feelings.
- Patient has difficulty following directions, controlling anger and self-calming, once situations begin to escalate.
- Patient exhibits poor impulse control, escape and avoidant behaviors for demand related situations and attention seeking behaviors when denied requests.

Replacement behaviors

Once etiology is established, identify alternative or replacement behaviors that the patient will learn to do instead of the problem behavior.
- Teach anger-management skills, positive attention-seeking skills, and teach the patient to respect the space of others.

Diagnosis

List the disability (medical or mental health diagnosis).
- PTSD.
- Depressive disorder, NOS.
- Borderline intellectual functioning.
- Impulse control disorder.
- History of sexual abuse/educational problems.

Interventions

List the interventions that will be implemented. Tailor interventions as needed to specific needs of the patient. Basic examples:
- Reinforcement of all positive social interactions.
- Provide high degree of structure with clear expectations/low stimulating environment. Aim for predictable consistency.
- Encourage group participation. Small groups as opposed to large groups.
- Limit items and make activities short.
- Provide cues about upcoming difficult transitions or tasks where extra control will be needed.
- Give short detailed bits of information when presenting a task.
- Present information in linear sequential manner.
- Begin patient on token economy point card system.
- Intensive problem-solving training through the use of worksheets.

- Assist patient in recognizing triggers for frustration and teach new ways to control them. Utilize preference of relaxation techniques (deep breathing, writing in journal).

Data collection

List any type of data to be collected to assist in determining efficacy of plan.
- Frequency counts.
- Patient report.
- Clinical notes.
- Direct observation.

Preferred reinforcers

List patient's preferred reinforcers, e.g.:
- Music.
- Writing in journal/reading.
- Movies.
- Computer games.

Consult-liaison psychiatry

Introduction

Consult-liaison (CL) psychiatry is concerned with the diagnosis and management of psychiatric and psychological illness in general medical populations. It is unique among the psychiatric subspecialties in that it concerns itself not with a particular subset of disorders, or treatment of patients of a particular age range, but patients within a particular clinical setting. The development of a distinct subspecialty of CL psychiatry is in some ways a result of the separation of psychiatric specialists from their medical and surgical colleagues and practices.

The subspecialty is a relatively recent innovation and dates in its current form since the 1960s. Motivations to its development were the low rate of outside referral in proportion to prevalence of the disorders in the population under review and increasing medical specialization leading to lack of confidence and competence with psychiatric/psychological problems. The role that these problems play in the course and outcome of physical illness is well documented and increasingly appreciated across medical practice. Treatment research that has better defined successful interventions, as well as the decrease in stigma associated with emotional disorders has generated more activity in this field.

The role of the CL psychiatrist will be defined, more than the other subspecialties, by custom and practice in the hospital concerned. The consultation aspect of the job covers episodic referrals made for advice on diagnosis, prognosis, need for further investigations, or management. It may include patients where the request is to consider taking over care. The liaison aspect refers to a closer relationship with a unit, with involvement in unit planning, staff support, policy development, and training as well as involvement in individual clinical cases. The balance between the liaison and consultation aspects of the job will depend on the specialty concerned, and the hospital type.

In many hospitals, specialists in this field are often identified under a broader division of behavioral health, and the model is one of both general CL work across medical specialties and behavioral health personnel imbedded within specialties. CL psychiatrists often further focus on medical subspecialties such as hematology/oncology, obstetrics and gynecology, transplantation, or neurological illnesses.

The main workload will in general include:
- Diagnosis of new psychiatric illness in general patients.
- Management of pre-existing psychiatric illness in general patients.
- Somatic presentation of psychiatric illnesses.
- Psychiatric and emotional complications of physical illness.
- Management of medically unexplained symptoms.
- Management of behavioral disturbance.
- Assessment and management of altered mental status.
- Assessment following attempted suicide and deliberate self-harm.
- Assessment of alcohol and drug abuse.
- Problems related to childbirth and the puerperium.
- Issues related to capacity and legal powers.

Working in the general hospital

CL psychiatry is unusual in that you will work as a psychiatrist based in a general hospital. This can bring its own difficulties and challenges as well as rewards. General hospital physicians in the various specialties will have their own ideas about psychiatry, as well as about the indicated treatment in any given case (which may differ from your own). Nonetheless it is well to remember that you have a range of skills and knowledge that will be useful and are not often known by your medical colleagues. You should rely on these and your own judgment, backed up by senior colleagues, in difficult situations. Always remember that you are a physician first and foremost. Don't assume that the primary medical team has done all that is indicated or necessary to assure medical stability or clarity in a given patient.

When you come to work in a general hospital you may feel initially overwhelmed. There are many new disorders, altered presentations of familiar disorders, a new tempo of working, and patients suffering from complicated medical conditions (e.g., ICU patients), which may go beyond your medical training. CL psychiatry takes a variety of types of referrals and they will vary by the type of hospital, the population served, and the specialty mix within the hospital. The person receiving the referral should take details of the patient, his/her inpatient primary treatment team and contact persons, and the nature of the problem, including its urgency. It is important to clarify what questions the treatment team want addressed. It is also important to clarify that the patient and parents (with pediatric patients) understand that a psychiatric referral has been made and all agree to this.

Where the situation is not an emergency, it can be useful to review any psychiatric or departmental records for previous contacts, prior to assessing the patient. On arrival to the unit, review the medical record of this and previous admissions and speak to a senior member of the treatment team. Clarify the patient's diagnosis and any investigations or treatments planned. Discuss the patient with the nursing staff—they often have useful information regarding the patient's symptoms around the clock and their mood day to day. Arrange a private room for the interview if at all possible.

Introduce yourself to the patient as a psychiatrist or behavioral health specialist. Explain your role, which may be misunderstood by the patient, who may feel you are there to "see if I'm crazy." Addressing up front the patient's anxieties or misconceptions about the involvement of psychiatry in their care will contribute to a more productive and valid assessment overall. Stating that the medical team is concerned about some of the patient's symptoms and they want a specialist in these symptoms to give them some advice is often an acceptable phrasing for patients.

A written document should be placed in the medical chart as soon as possible after the completion of the consult. If this is not possible, a brief "holding" note can address any critical issues, pending completion of the full consult. It is important to discuss your findings with the medical team face to face.

If a definitive psychiatric diagnosis is possible, write this clearly in the notes, along with a provisional management plan and any treatment recommendations. Clarify if further psychiatric review is planned, and note which symptoms should result in more urgent concern. Thoroughly sign out all patients to the covering evening/ weekend psychiatrist.

Evaluation of decision-making capacity

One of the more difficult and complex psychiatric consultations occurs when the medical team inquires whether a patient is "competent" to make medical decisions. Although competency is a broad legal issue, which can only be decided in the United States by the court system, CL psychiatrists can help guide the team in determining whether the patient has the capacity to make individual decisions. A psychiatric capacity evaluation usually involves several steps:

- Determining the specific decision being asked of the patient.
- Examining whether the patient has the ability to give informed consent.
- Evaluating whether any psychiatric condition is interfering with the patient's judgment or ability to appreciate the medical decision.
- Working within a multidisciplinary team to determine the final decision.

Step 1: identify the question

Although medical teams have a legitimate interest in knowing whether a patient is competent to make decisions or requires a surrogate decision-maker, a blanket recommendation is frequently impossible because of the differing capacity requirements for simple versus complex decisions. For example, if a diabetic patient is asked to provide blood to check their glucose level, the extremely low risk to benefit ratio would require only limited understanding and ability to manipulate information. It is probably sufficient that they know that they have diabetes and understand that if they don't monitor and control their glucose, it could hurt them. In contrast, for a terminal cancer patient to participate in a phase I chemotherapy trial with very limited benefit and considerable side-effects, they would need to demonstrate a thorough appreciation of the issues involved.

Step 2: examine the patient's ability to give informed consent

Once a particular question has been identified (e.g., whether a patient can refuse an amputation in the setting of osteomyelitis and early gangrene), it is necessary to explore whether the patient has the ability to understand and provide informed consent. This evaluation can be done by any medical professional, and in many cases is most appropriately evaluated by the physicians who best understand the risks and benefits of what they are offering. As part of our evaluation, we need to confirm that they have an appreciation of:

- The nature of their illness or condition.
- The procedure, medication, or other treatment being offered to them.
- The most important risks and potential benefits associated with that treatment.
- Any alternative treatment options, as well as the consequence of avoiding any action.

Many times the patient conveys a limited understanding of these issues. This may reflect underlying cognitive deficits or medical problems; however, it is also possible that many of these areas have not yet been discussed with the patient. In that case, it is often prudent to ask the medical team to discuss these issues in your presence, while you examine the patient's ability to process and retain this information.

Step 3: evaluate the presence of psychiatric illness and determine whether it is influencing the patient's decision

Even if the patient's decision reflects a fair grasp of the elements of consent, it is necessary to determine whether their judgment is being influenced by mental illness.

- For example, if the patient with gangrene understands the nature of their infection and the risks of surgery versus delaying treatment, we would not support their making a decision to avoid surgery if the decision was based on auditory hallucinations telling them that they don't deserve to live. Therefore, a comprehensive psychiatric assessment, including an evaluation of how they have made their decision, is essential.

The psychiatric evaluation for a capacity assessment needs to be comprehensive, particularly focusing on cognitive functions, reasoning and judgment; however, it is otherwise similar to any thorough psychiatric examination. The primary difference lies in the additional examination of how the patient has made similar choices in the past and what role psychiatric symptoms are playing in their current decision.

Although it is common for psychiatric symptoms to be present, one of the biggest challenges in a capacity assessment is determining whether these symptoms alter the patient's judgment to the extent that they are unable to determine their treatment. For example:

- Depression is frequently seen in people with chronic illnesses. Does this mean that a terminal patient can never refuse treatment because their decision might be influenced by depression?
- Psychosis may alter the patient's reality testing; however, most psychotic individuals retain their ability to make medical decisions if their psychosis does not alter their reasoning in that area.
- Cognitive impairment is frequently variable, based on diagnosis, time of day, when medications were given and other factors. Is a patient able to make decisions if they can only describe them adequately at certain times?

Step 4: gather additional information

Frequently patients' decision-making capacity may not be clear-cut, and we are left with the task of developing a consensus. Other individuals who may guide your recommendation include:

- The patient's family, particularly the likely surrogate decision-maker. If they agree with the patient, then the issue of the patient's capacity is less critical to the outcome.
- A medical ethics/legal consultant. These individuals (often part of the hospital system) can help the team understand whether the patient is making a decision that is consistent with their prior decisions and expressed wishes, as well as whether forcing treatment would be ethically/legally reasonable.
- Social worker, physical and occupational therapists. They can be of great assistance in identifying the patient's surrogate decision maker and examining whether the patient is able to function independently.

Final consultation report

Once all these steps are completed, we can advise the medical team on the patient's capacity to make the identified decision. Although these psychiatric consultations can be difficult and time-consuming, they can also be highly rewarding, because the outcome almost always has an immediate and profound impact on the patient's life and health.

Evaluation of medically ill patients— depression and psychosis

Assessing medical patients for psychiatric disease can be a difficult task since the symptoms of psychiatric disorders may overlap with those of many medical conditions. Also, it can be difficult to determine whether patients have a treatable psychiatric syndrome, versus typical emotional reaction in the context of their medical burden, and/or a mood disorder secondary to drugs, alcohol, medical conditions, or medications. Yet, it is often the job of the Consult-Liaison (CL) psychiatry team to discriminate the subtle distinctions among the potential etiologies. There are clinical pearls that may be helpful when evaluating patients for depression, anxiety, and psychosis. Lastly, there are also characteristic psychiatric syndromes produced in the context of medical burden that will be discussed later in the chapter. Detailed information on diagnosis and treatment of individual conditions is discussed throughout other chapters in this handbook.

Depression

When assessing patients' depressive symptoms, it may be hard to tease apart whether disturbances in energy, sleep, appetite, and concentration are related to the medical condition itself or whether they are symptoms of depression. Since several of these symptoms may be caused by medical illness, the presenting symptoms may mimic major depressive disorder (MDD). On the other hand, if you exclude all overlapping symptoms and attribute them to the medical condition, it may be difficult to reach the diagnosis of MDD even when it is present. In cases such as these, which are many in the consult-liaison world, there are clinical pearls of depression that may be most useful to ask about.

Clinical pearls: is it depression or a medical cause?

All these factors weighed together can give you a better picture of the etiology of the depressed mood as well as the severity.

- Hopelessness: It can be helpful to know how patients view their situation. Do they have plans for the future? What do they think the future looks like for them? Do they think things will ever improve? Depressed people will tend to have a pessimistic view of the future.
- Anhedonia: Is the patient still doing things they enjoy doing (if they are physically able to)? If not, do they still wish they could do those things or have they lost interest for these things?
- Tearfulness: Are they crying a lot? Are they tearful most of the day? This is more consistent with depression.
- Consistency of the feelings: Are they depressed most of the day or are there periods of the day when their mood lifts? Depressed individuals usually have consistent episodes of decreased mood that last for weeks.
- Lack of reactivity: Are they flat in affect? Emotionless? These are more indicative of a clinical depression.
- Social isolation: Do they look forward to visitors/family? Are they uninterested in having visitors? One caveat to watch out for is for

patients who want visitors but are afraid to look weak or in the "sick role," i.e., depressed individuals may have decreased interest in spending time with family, and may not be happy even after visitors arrive.

- Collateral information: obtaining information from close family or friends can be crucial in the assessment of medical patients as they often add insight into the severity, duration, and temporal relationship of the symptom course.

The clinical picture taken together with DSM-IV-TR criteria will paint the picture of whether patients have clinical depression versus another etiology. If they are severely disabled, unable to participate in care, hopeless or suicidal it may be prudent to treat symptoms of major depression regardless of actual etiology. On the other hand, if the clinical picture looks less severe it may be reasonable according to one's clinical judgment to watch the depression for a few weeks to see if it improves on its own with correction of the underlying medical condition. If the medical condition is not expected to resolve in the near future, it may be helpful to treat the depression to improve mood and functioning level (see the depression chapter 📖 Chapter 7).

Psychosis

Psychotic symptoms can be characteristic of many disorders, namely withdrawal syndromes, delirium, dementia, and primary psychotic disorders. There are some helpful hints to consider when assessing psychosis and its underlying cause so as to differentiate primary psychotic disorders (i.e., due to psychiatric illness) from other syndromes with a secondary psychosis (i.e., due to a medical condition or substance use diagnosis).

Clinical pearls: is it psychotic disorder or a medical cause?
- Visual hallucinations: Visual hallucinations are more likely to be related to delirium, where as auditory hallucinations are more characteristic of a primary psychotic disorder.
- Daily fluctuations: A waxing and waning picture with alterations in attention and alertness are more likely something suggesting delirium as opposed to a primary psychotic disorder.
- Timeline: How long has the psychosis been occurring? Is this new? Was there a gradual decline? A primary psychotic disorder typically has an obvious prodrome and/or emotional stressor and typically occurs in younger patients with a family history of psychosis. Some forms of dementia can also present with psychotic features, and typically occur in older patients or patients with family history of dementia. When assessing for dementia, it is helpful to gain information from collateral sources about any cognitive or executive decline from baseline and how long the decline has been occurring. 📖 see *pp. 152–68* for more details on dementia.
- Vital signs: Withdrawal syndromes also can present with psychotic symptoms. It is helpful to look for any autonomic instability, vital sign changes, sweating, and tremor, which may suggest an underlying withdrawal from alcohol or other sedatives. Such changes would be less likely in a primary psychotic disorder (see 📖 *pp. 615–85*).

Evaluation of medically ill patients—anxiety

Anxiety

Anxiety is a common phenomenon in medically ill patients, yet the diagnosis and treatment may be difficult for a few reasons. First, many times medical patients don't meet full criteria for a DSM-IV-TR diagnosis of an anxiety disorder. However, despite not meeting criteria for a DSM-IV-TR diagnosis, medical patients often have realistic worries over health, finances, work and family all related to their medical illness and the losses it produces. It is important to assess the worry and anxiety and make a decision based on symptom severity and impairment whether treatment would help the anxiety. Another reason why diagnosis of anxiety may be difficult in medical patients is because it is difficult to assess whether symptoms of anxiety like shortness of breath, heart palpitations, dizziness, insomnia, diaphoresis, and restlessness are part of a medical illness or related to an anxiety disorder. In these situations there are some important aspects to consider in your assessment of anxiety.

Clinical pearls: is it anxiety or medical cause?

- Medical work-up: Assess for medical causes for symptoms first. Has the patient had a complete medical evaluation for the physical complaints? If the medical tests have come back normal (e.g., EKG, lab work, TSH, chest x-ray, PFTs), then diagnosis of anxiety disorder should be a diagnosis of exclusion.
- Substance abuse/ingestion: patients should have a urine drug screen (UDS)/urine toxicology to rule out substance intoxication or withdrawal as a cause for the physical complaints, agitation, subjective feelings of restlessness, and anxiety. If an overdose is suspected, levels of acetaminophen, aspirin, tricyclic antidepressants, and an ethanol level should also be checked. If clinically indicated, some institutions also have a more comprehensive serum drug screen to rule out other drugs of abuse. Find out what your institution screens for and always think about those substances that may not show up on your institution's drug screen (i.e., they may not pick up all metabolites of benzodiazepines or opiates, or may include drugs known to have local emphasis). Monitor for any possible withdrawal from drugs, especially alcohol or benzodiazepines which many be contributing to the subjective feelings of anxiety. Refer to the substance use chapter for details on the treatment of substance withdrawal (see 📖 pp.615–85).
- Past psychiatric history: does the patient have an underlying anxiety disorder that is being made worse by a new medical stressor?
- Characteristic symptoms associated with specific medical illnesses: patients with pulmonary disease, COPD, asthma, lung transplant patients and airway assisted patients on weaning trials can all have anxiety surrounding feelings of shortness of breath. Sometimes these findings can be mistaken for anxiety or panic disorder, and vice versa. Do the subjective match the objective findings? Assess mental processes surrounding these feelings. Does the patient feel like or fear

they are going to die? Have a sense of doom? Fear they are going crazy? It is helpful to know exactly what the patient is experiencing when they have the sensation of feeling short of breath. If they are having an anxiety/panic type reaction to the experience it may be an anxiety syndrome. However, there is often an overlap between true respiratory symptoms and anxiety, and treating both problems may be necessary.

Assessment of suicide attempt[1,2]

Assessment of suicidal ideation and self-harm are reviewed elsewhere (📖 see p. 60 "Asking about thoughts of self-harm" and 📖 p. 1100).

Psychiatric assessment of patients who have attempted suicide is mandatory once their medical condition allows. The involvement of mental health professionals in the assessment of patients following attempts relates to the following observations:

- In this population of patients, roughly 1% will die by completed suicide in the 24 months after the initial attempt, with the risk highest in the weeks following the original act. This represents a mortality by suicide 50–100 times that of the general population. The *two weeks* following discharge from inpatient psychiatry (and before community follow-up) is considered to be a *high risk* time for suicide attempt in psychiatric patients.
- The rates of completed suicide are significantly raised in all psychiatric disorders except intellectual disability/ mental retardation and dementia. Studies examining completed suicides in patients with mental illness show inadequate doses of therapeutic drug treatment, increased drop-out rate from follow-up, and increased presence of untreated co-morbidity.
- Clear risk factors exist for completed suicide (see next). The closer the patient attempting suicide approximates to these demographics, the greater the relative risk. However, the absolute risk is low and estimate of the risk in a particular case relies on assessment of the individual act and the mental state.

Assessment

The initial management of the patient following overdose or other deliberate self-harm will be completed by specialist toxicologists or general medical/surgical specialists. Early psychiatric assessment may be required for various reasons, including advice regarding psychiatric disposition and safety in the medical setting, behavioral disturbance, drug/alcohol withdrawal, or delirium. Assessment of the suicide attempt itself should be deferred until conscious level is full. Begin with general questions, then get more specific as the therapeutic relationship is more established. Special consideration should be taken as to the sensitive nature of the interview (the experience may be difficult for the patient and family/ friends to discuss).

Psychiatric exam

Obtain a routine psychiatric exam as described in chapter 2. Be certain to obtain a complete psychiatric history, including past treatment, suicide attempts/near attempts, and family history of attempts/completion. In general, avoid terms such as "parasuicide" or "suicide gestures," which are older terms sometimes used to minimize the seriousness of the attempt.

Recent history

What were the details leading up to the suicide event? Start back as early as necessary to obtain the whole picture (e.g., precipitating factors, planning, motivation and ultimate decision to go through with attempt). Focus on **lethality** (their view of whether or not the act would end in death) and **intent** (e.g., wish to die, reasons for attempting, tactics to avoid detection, plans to reattempt, preparing/telling others). Details follow:

Features of act

- **Method**: Most attempts are by overdose with self-cutting making up most of the remainder. Use of method likely to be fatal (e.g., guns, jumping, hanging) is often indicative of clear intent to die.
- **Patient's belief in the lethality of the method**: Did the patient believe that that method (e.g., combination of tablets) was likely to be fatal? Serious suicidal intent can be associated with medically trivial attempts (especially in children)—and vice versa.
- **Length of planning**: Was the act impulsive, or planned in advance (for how long)?
- **Triggers**: Was there a clear precipitant (e.g., family discord, legal problems, bereavement)? Were they intoxicated at the time? Was there any direct "gain" (e.g., patient in legal custody now receiving special treatment)?
- **Final acts**: Was there a suicide note? Did they make any other "acts of closure" (e.g., setting affairs in order, arranging for the care of children)? These acts may indicate a higher intent level.
- **Precautions to avoid discovery**: Where did the act take place? Would they have anticipated being found? Did they signal or tell their intentions to another? Was anyone else actually present at the time? Did they take precautions to avoid discovery?
- **Previous similar acts**: Is this act a repeat of a previous non-fatal act? Are there any different or similar features?
- **Actions after act**: What did they do after the act? How did they end up coming to hospital?

Current mental state

- **Attitude now to survival**: How do they feel about the situation now? Are they relieved or disappointed to be alive? What are their plans after they leave the hospital? Do they have ongoing wish to die? How do they feel about the future and what plans (if any) do they have?
- **Affective symptoms**: Current mood symptoms. Recent symptoms of low mood, anhedonia, and hopelessness? Biological depressive features.
- **Substance use problems**: Evidence for current drug or alcohol use, abuse or dependence (obtain full history).
- **Co-morbid mental illnesses**: Enquire directly about other symptoms of psychiatric illness (including current adequacy of treatment).
- **Risk to others**: Is there any evidence of intent to harm anyone else? Did the attempt put anyone else at risk (e.g., children left unattended, driver in opposing car)?

Personal and past medical/psychiatric history

With children/adolescents, always include parents/family in assessment.

- **Recent life events**: Describe recent loss or change of events (e.g., bereavements, job loss, relationship changes; in children/adolescents, a disruption in family stability, school, friendships).
- **Current life situation**: State of current significant relationships (in children/adolescents, include parents and peers). Type and security of job. Presence of legal/criminal problems. Presence of academic problems.
- **Previous or current psychiatric diagnoses and treatment**: Clarify with hospital records and obtain a collateral history (consent is needed to do this).
- **Physical health problems** Clarify with records or PCP if required.

Risk factors for completed suicide

Socio-demographic factors

- Male sex.
- Older adolescent/young adult & elderly.
- "Disconnected": Single, divorced, or widowed; living alone, poor social support, abuse, neglect; unemployed or low socioeconomic class.
- Family history of suicide attempt.
- Recent bereavement.
- Access to lethal methods (e.g., firearms).

Personal/mental health factors

- Previous attempt.
- Any mental disorder (greatest risk in mood disorders, psychosis, PTSD, personality disorders, eating disorders). 90% of those who complete suicide have a psychiatric disorder.
- Dependence on alcohol or drugs.
- Recent inpatient psychiatric treatment (especially in two weeks following discharge).

Protective factors

- Sense of connectedness: To family, school, religion.
- Sense of purpose: In school, in family, with positive peers.
- Availability of support, supervision.

Management after an attempt

Safety first Once informed of the consultation for a postsuicide assessment, verify that the primary team is monitoring the safety of the patient. If the patient is still feeling suicidal or is displaying unsafe behaviors, a trained assistant may be required to sit with the patient to monitor for impulsive or aggressive acts, or actions leading to another suicide attempt. If these concerns are still present after psychiatric assessment, the assistant may be continued 24 hours a day until disposition to an inpatient unit.

Gather details Start with general questions, then focus on specific details. Learn the step-by-step details, including the thoughts that lead up to the attempt, what happened that the person began the attempt/ continued the attempt/efforts to abort the attempt, as well as specific details of the attempt itself, and the moments after the attempt leading to the hospitalization.

Reasons for act Only a minority of patients presenting after an attempt have evidence of clear intent to die. Assessment will reveal a mixture of the following types of case:

- Those whose intent was unequivocally to die but were prevented by discovery, chance, or overestimation of the lethality of the method.
- Those who were ambivalent whether they lived or died, "letting the chips fall as they may."
- Those whose act was impulsive and "in the heat of the moment" in response to an immediate stressor.
- Those whose actions were designed to communicate distress—the classical "cry for help."
- Those attempting to escape from intolerable symptoms or an intolerable situation.
- Those whose intent is later unclear even to themselves.
- Those whose actions were manipulative in nature and designed to provoke changed behavior from others (this should not be assumed by a consultation-liaison psychiatrist, but is a possibility in rare cases).

Differential diagnoses

There may initially be **diagnostic confusion** with the following groups: (1) deliberate overdoses of drugs taken for intoxicating effect; (2) deliberate self-harm (e.g., wrist cutting), which is a repetitive, ritualistic action whose intent is to relieve tension, not to kill or seriously injure; (3) accidental overdoses of prescribed or OTC medication. The first and second may merit psychiatric evaluation in their own right and the third should be examined carefully for evidence of post hoc rationalization of an attempt.

Assessment aims

By the end of assessment you should aim to answer the following questions:

- **Is there ongoing suicidal intent?** Evidenced by: continuing stated wish to die; ambivalence about survival; sense of hopelessness toward future; clear intent to die at time of act.
- **Is there evidence of psychiatric illness** (diagnosed by psychiatric exam)? Be alert to co-morbid substance use and to the combination of an acute stressor on the background of a chronic condition.
- **Are there nonmental health issues that can be addressed?** Many patients will reveal stressors such as: family or relationship difficulties; emotional problems (particularly relating to previous abuse; school or employment problems; debt; legal problems; problems related to immigration). They can be directed to appropriate local services as part of their disposition.

Management

Disposition Often it is the job of the consultation-liaison psychiatrist to arrange the disposition of care for patients after suicide attempt. Appropriate follow-up depends on the severity (e.g., inpatient or intensive outpatient), as well as type of disorder (e.g., referral to clinician/inpatient unit for treatment of psychiatric illness; referral to drug and alcohol services for alcohol abuse; referral to more specialized mental health treatment programs such as an eating disorders unit).

- **Ongoing suicidal intent or need for acute management**: In many cases this will be managed by admission to a psychiatric inpatient unit, on an involuntary commitment if necessary.
- **Psychiatric illness**: Evaluate, educate, and consider treatment options for primary and co-morbid psychiatric illnesses.
- **Patients already known to mental health services**: Focus on close liaison with their usual treatment team to create a joint management plan.
- **Patients with a new diagnoses**: Focus should be on integrating with an appropriate service for follow-up, rather than necessarily starting new treatments. Short-term community outreach from liaison psychiatry can "bridge" the patient to the general services. Try to ensure follow-up is as soon as possible, even if nonurgent, as otherwise non-attendance is very high and risk for re-attempt during this time may also be high.
- **Considering inpatient admission**: If the patient is not safe (e.g., still feels suicidal), then inpatient psychiatric treatment is clearly necessary. However, for both new and established psychiatric illnesses, admission will sometimes be indicated after an attempt *even where there is no ongoing suicidal intent*. There are many reasons for this, including seriousness of attempt or acute condition, or to allow for a period of inpatient assessment, evaluation, and treatment of current psychiatric illness. However, patients are often best served by the least restrictive environment (e.g., intensive or routine outpatient). All details must be considered before deferring to outpatient care (details of the suicide attempt, family and other support, solidly established and effective outpatient care, likelihood of compliance with plan).

In all cases, discuss and agree on a management plan with patient and the treatment team. In most cases, discuss the results with their PCP (obtain consent prior to discussing the case with other providers). Provide emergency crisis information giving details of emergency psychiatric service and telephone contact for emergency counseling/support services. *Ensure that weapons are removed from the home and any other locations where the patient may have access.*

Goals for all cases Established safety plan, weapon removal, treatment adherence, close supervision, increased hopefulness, and continued and frequent contact.

Encourage outpatient care when appropriate A small minority of patients attend emergency services repeatedly with deliberate self-harm without suicidal intent. A management plan for such patients should be agreed on by the treatment team on a case-by-case basis. The aim is to provide appropriate support and treatment while avoiding maladaptive behaviors (e.g., using the hospital system as a primary mean of treatment without utilizing treatment from less restrictive environments).

Summary of risk factors for suicide attempts[2]

Proximal risk factors Those that are happening now as risk factors (AID ILL).
- Agitation—Anxiety, agitation, EPS/akathesia, insomnia (some factor of agitation).
- Ideation—Active ideation with a plan.
- Depression/Decline—Depression and decline (health, illness), hopelessness.
- Instability—Acute substance use, affective lability, mixed state or rapid cycling, brain injury.
- Loss—Of relationship, work, health, or function.
- Lethal agent—Availability of a gun.

Distal risk factors In the background, happens over time, can't say about risk right now (SAD DADS).
- Suicidal history—Personal or in family.
- Aggression and impulsivity.
- Difficult course—Poor treatment response, co-morbid, severe disorder.
- Difficult patient—Nonadherent.
- Abuse and trauma history.
- Disconnection from support, work, relationships (chronically isolated, not acute).
- Substance or alcohol abuse.

Recommended further reading

1 Kessler, R.C., Borges, G., Walters, E. (1999). Prevalence of and risk factors for lifetime suicide attempts in the national co-morbidity survey. *Arch Gen Psychiatry* **56**, 617–626.

2 Brent, D., Poling, K., Goldstein, T. *Therefore Choose Life: A Clinical Approach to the Care of the Depressed and Suicidal Adolescent*. New York: Guildford Press, in press.

3 Kessler. R.C. *et al.* (2005). Trends in suicide ideation, plans, gestures, and attempts in the United States, 1990–1992 to 2001–2003. *JAMA* **293**: 2487–2495.

4 Joe, S. *et al.* (2006). Prevalence of and risk factors for lifetime suicide attempts among blacks in the United States. *JAMA* **296**: 2112–2123.

Assessment prior to solid organ or bone marrow transplantation

For patients with a disease of a solid organ (heart, lung, kidney, liver, bowel, pancreas) or a leukemia, a transplantation offers the prospect of significant improvement in length and quality of life. Unfortunately, the supply of donor organs is less than the number of potential recipients. Because of this, patients requiring a variety of transplantations will suffer declining health while awaiting transplantation and 10–20% of listed patients will die while awaiting transplant. This places a responsibility on the assessing team to consider carefully each potential candidate for listing for transplantation in order to ensure the best use of the donor organs.

Psychiatric assessment of patients prior to listing for transplantation may be anticipatory and routine, or may be requested in the following situations:

• Fulminant organ failure following intentional ingestion (e.g., acetaminophen orparacetamol in livers).
• Liver disease secondary to alcoholic liver disease (ALD).
• Patients/families with history of mental illness.
• Patients with previous or current drug misuse.
• Patients/families with history of nonadherence.
• Patients/families with significant psychosocial disruption.
• Living related donor.

The involvement of the psychiatrist in the assessment prior to listing for transplantation should in no sense be a moral judgment about the patient's or family's suitability. The issues are whether there are psychiatric (biopsychosocial) factors that would jeopardize the survival of the donor organ. The psychiatric opinion may have the most profound implications for the patient or family and so assessment should be as thorough as time allows. In addition to taking psychiatric, psychosocial and developmental history and MSE, family members, PCP (if available), and hospital case records should be consulted.

Fulminant organ failure following ingestion

The issue is whether there is ongoing intent to die or refuse transplant (which would normally preclude transplantation) or whether there is a history of repeated overdoses in the past; significant psychiatric disorder; or ongoing drug or alcohol misuse (which would be relative contraindications).

Liver disease secondary to alcoholic liver disease (ALD)

Suitably selected patients transplanted for ALD have similar outcomes in terms of survival and quality of life to patients transplanted for other indications. Units will have individual policies regarding these patients which should be consulted if available. The issue is whether the patient, who has already damaged one liver, will damage a second. There is a wider issue of maintaining the public confidence in the appropriate use of donated organs.

For liver disease secondary to ALD, consider:
- How long have they been abstinent (is there independent verification of this)?
- Do they accept alcohol as the cause of liver failure?
- Do they undertake to remain abstinent post-transplant?
- Do they have a history of dependence or harmful use?
- What is their history of involvement in alcohol treatment services and in the past, how have they responded to relapse?
- When were they told that their drinking was causing liver damage, and what was their response?

Given the above findings and your routine psychiatric assessment, the transplant team will seek your opinion as to:
- The patient' psychiatric diagnosis.
- Risk of relapse.
- Risk of re-establishing harmful/dependant drinking.
- The potential for successful intervention should this occur.

History of mental illness/drug misuse

Generally speaking, a diagnosis of mental disorder (other than progressive dementia) does not preclude transplant. The important issues are whether the mental disorder will affect compliance or longer-term mortality in its own right. Close liaison with the patient's normal psychiatrist is clearly crucial here. Ongoing substance dependence is generally a contraindication to transplantation and should be addressed before listing.

History of nonadherence to treatment/psychosocial disruption

Nonadherence with treatment may be the reason for a patient's need for transplant, or places the patient at risk for future morbidity or mortality and the loss of a donated organ if not recognized early in assessment. Past medical records and discussions with past treatment teams will provide information regarding this area of risk for a given patient or family. In addition, pretransplant evaluation by multiple team members, including behavioral health, should identify psychosocial factors that place a patient or family at risk for nonadherence, and provide the team an opportunity to be proactive to increase the likelihood of future adherence and transplant success.

Living-related donors

This type of transplant uses organs or tissues from a matched and usually biologically related donor. Examples include bone marrow, kidney or sections of liver or lung. In this case, the donor may be an additional focus of evaluation, with the goal of determining informed consent and the absence of coercion.

Medically unexplained symptoms

A substantial proportion of patients presenting to primary care offices and medical hospitals have symptoms which do not fit any known medical diagnosis. When the symptoms are vague, transient, and do not affect the person's functioning, often no treatment is necessary. However, these symptoms can be severe and disabling, resulting in numerous medical hospitalizations and substantial morbidity. Consultation-liaison psychiatrists help is most often requested when the symptoms do not conform to any known medical disorder, when the pattern of symptoms or behavior make it unlikely to be medically driven (e.g., bilateral tonic-clonic "seizures" in a conscious individual), or when the intensity of pain or other symptoms appears grossly out of proportion to physical findings, particularly in pain syndromes. The CL psychiatrist role in these cases is to assess for psychiatric disorders and guide both the medical team and patient toward treatment options in a nonjudgmental and constructive fashion. This section will focus on the diagnosis and management of symptoms that are relatively discrete in presentation and not consciously produced.

Common presentations and referrals

Patients can present to any specialty with unexplained symptoms, but the most common sources of psychiatric referrals in medical hospitals include:
- Cardiology referrals for atypical chest pain.
- GI Medicine consultations for diarrhea, constipation, and/or abdominal pain of unknown etiology.
- Gynecology referrals for chronic pelvic pain.
- Medicine/Pulmonary referrals for unexplained shortness of breath, including inability to wean from a ventilator.
- Neurology referrals for tension headaches, pseudoseizures, and unexplained weakness or loss of sensation.

Assessment

The initial assessment includes a thorough review of medical records and a discussion with the primary team about the chronology of the patient's symptoms, tests performed, and the reasons they believe the symptoms are "psychosomatic" in origin. In addition to a comprehensive evaluation of psychiatric symptoms, the consultative interview should also focus on the patient's understanding of their illness and any connection they have observed between emotions, events in their lives, and the intensity of their symptoms. This discussion should be conducted in an exploratory fashion, without suggesting that the symptoms are "all in their head".

Explaining the CL psychiatric exam to the medical patient

Patients are usually willing to discuss the psychological distress associated with being ill. However, they may feel angry and insulted by the notion that they are "faking" their illness. As such, it is prudent for the primary team to explain the consult and its purpose prior to the CL psychiatric exam visit. Thoughtfully word your initial contact with patients to avoid alienating them. Collateral information from friends, family, and their primary care physician will help establish whether the patient is obtaining primary or secondary gain from being ill, as well as the chronology of the patient's symptoms and associated stressors.

Management principles of medically unexplained symptoms

The primary approach to treating patients with medically unexplained symptoms involves:

- Avoid confrontation: Remember that these disorders are likely unconscious (i.e., the patients are not actively aware they are somehow creating/exacerbating the symptoms—it is below their level of conscious awareness). Most attempts to force the patient to recognize that they are producing symptoms will result in loss of their trust and alliance.
- Work with the medical team to avoid counter-transference and limit polypharmacy. Patients with unexplained illnesses are often difficult, time-consuming, and frustrating to the medical staff. Educate staff about the unconscious nature of these illnesses and the important role they can play in recovery. Recognize that multiple ineffective medications may have been added early in the course of their illness and may now be withdrawn.
- Treat underlying psychiatric disorders: In addition to treating conditions that meet DSM-IV-TR criteria, look to treat the atypical anxiety and depression described in the following sections, and consider empiric use of antidepressants if symptoms persist. Alternative treatments such as physiotherapy, increased activity/exercise, massage therapy, acupuncture, and hypnosis should be considered.
- Arrange regular noncontingent medical follow-up: As the patient's unexplained medical symptoms may persist due to secondary gain from medical attention, arrange frequent medical appointments (about every six weeks), which are not contingent on the patient's experience of symptoms.
- Encourage psychiatric follow-up: This allows the patient to explore the underlying psychiatric issues that may be expressed with somatic symptoms, and it transfers some of the dependency needs of the patient from the medical system to their therapist or psychiatrist.

Differential diagnosis of medically unexplained symptoms

The differential diagnosis for relatively acute, isolated, medically unexplained symptoms includes:

- Uncommon medical syndromes which have not yet been diagnosed.
- Symptoms directly related to psychiatric disorders such as depression, panic attacks, and psychosis.
- Conversion disorder.
- Pain disorders.
- Somatization disorder.
- Factitious disorder.
- Factitious dosorder by proxy.
- Malingering.

As stated earlier, it is important not to fall into the dichotomy of assigning medical versus psychiatric causes to somatic symptoms, as these syndromes often involve a component of learned behavior. Patients are likely to have had pain, seizures, or other symptoms of a medical illness prior to, or concurrent with, their current presentation. Medical practice has shifted to encourage psychiatric involvement in these cases prior to exhausting all medical testing. This minimizes the perception that psychiatric consultation is a reaction to the team "giving up," and creates a more collaborative environment.

Probably the most frequent causes of medically unexplained symptoms are atypical presentations of depression and anxiety. Depression, particularly in the elderly, can present with a predominance of medical symptoms, particularly pain, GI complaints, weakness, loss of appetite and insomnia. Similarly, many unexplained cases of chest pain and shortness of breath can be attributed to anxiety such as atypical panic attacks. The primary difference between these anxiety symptoms and panic disorder is that many of these cases have a less discrete onset and offset, have limited symptoms, and/or may have clear environmental triggers (e.g., whenever a ventilator patient starts a weaning trial they become more short of breath).

Psychotic disorders can present with somatic symptoms as part of the schizophrenia spectrum, although the psychiatric diagnosis of these individuals has often been established at an earlier point. The greater difficulty for patients presenting with psychotic symptoms lies in identifying delusional disorders of the somatic type, which frequently presents with few symptoms other than physical complaints.

Conversion disorders are in some ways prototypical of this group of illnesses, and have been well described for decades. The primary feature of conversion disorder is the unconscious production of neurological symptoms affecting motor or sensory systems. This may include classical "hysterical paralysis," sensory loss (often in nonphysiological patterns), or the development of atypical seizures (either by pattern or lack of concurrent EEG findings). The course of conversion disorders is quite variable, often with abrupt onset, variable duration, and high probability of recurrence.

Individuals with pain disorders may have pain that is solely attributed to their medical conditions, but frequently develop pain related to both medical and psychological factors.

Finally, a patient with medically unexplained symptoms may have a life-long history of medical concerns as part of somatization disorder, or may be consciously producing symptoms in order to achieve primary or secondary gains (as part of a factitious disorder or malingering). Given the differences in treatment for these patients, these syndromes are covered elsewhere in this chapter 📖 *p. 967* and *972*.

Somatization disorder

Somatization disorder is a disorder of multiple medically unexplained symptoms, affecting multiple organ systems, presenting before the age of 40. It is usually chronic in adults. In children, it usually involves one or a few organ systems, often for shorter periods of time (undifferentiated somatoform disorder or somatoform disorder nos). In all ages, it is associated with significant psychological distress, functional impairment, and repeated presentations to medical services. Full blown somatization disorder or "Briquet's syndrome" probably represents the severe end of a continuum of abnormal illness behavior.

Clinical features

Patients will have long, complex medical histories ("fat/large-file" patients), although at interview may minimize all but the most recent symptomatology. Symptoms may occur in any system and are to some extent suggestible. The most frequent symptoms are non-specific and atypical. There may be discrepancy between the subjective and objective findings (e.g., reports of intractable pain in a patient observed by nursing staff to be joking with relatives). Symptoms are usually concentrated in one system at a time but may move to another system after exhausting diagnostic possibilities in the previous. Life of the patient revolves around the illness as does family life.

Diagnosis is usually only suspected after negative findings begin to emerge as normal medical practice is to take complaints at face value. There is excessive use of medical service and alternative therapies. Chronic cases will have had large numbers of diagnostic procedures and surgical or medical treatments. There is a high risk of iatrogenic harm and iatrogenic substance dependence. Hostility and frustration can be felt on both sides of the doctor-patient relationship. There may be "doctor-shopping" and "splitting" of the attitudes of staff caring for them. Psychological approaches to treatment are hampered by ongoing investigations of ever rarer diagnostic possibilities and by the attribution of symptoms to fictitious but "named" medical entities.

Two-thirds of patients will meet criteria for another psychiatric disorder, most commonly major depressive or anxiety disorders. There is also association with personality disorder and substance abuse. They characteristically deny emotional symptoms or attribute them directly to physical handicaps—"the only reason I'm depressed is this constant pain."

Etiology

Observable clinical association with childhood illnesses in the patient or the family, and a history of parental anxiety toward illness. Increased frequency of somatization disorder in first degree relatives. Possible neuropsychiatric basis to the disorder with faulty assessment of normal somatic sensory input. Association with childhood physical and sexual abuse.

Epidemiology

Lifetime prevalence of ~0.2%. Markedly higher rate in particular populations. Female:male ratio 5:1. Age of onset varies from childhood to early 30s.

Differential diagnosis

Undiagnosed physical illness, particularly those with variable, multisystem presentations (e.g., SLE, AIDS, porphyria, tuberculosis, multiple sclerosis). Onset of multiple symptoms for the first time in patients over 40 should be presumed to be due to unexposed physical disease. Psychiatric disorder: major affective and psychotic illnesses may initially present with predominately somatic complaints. Diagnosis is by examination of other psychopathology. However, many of somatization disorder patients exhibit psychiatric and medical co-morbidity.

Other somatoform disorders: Distinguish from hypochondriasis (presence of firm belief in particular disorder), pain disorder (pain rather than other symptoms is prominent), conversion disorder (functional neurological loss without multisystem complaints), factitious disorder (intentional production or feigning of physical symptoms to assume sick role) and malingering (intentional production of false or grossly exaggerated physical symptoms with external incentives). In practice the main distinction is between the full and severe somatization disorder and somatization as a symptom of other disorders.

Assessment

(See earlier in this chapter 📖 p. 962.) Establish reasons for referral, experience of illness, attitudes to symptoms, personal and psychiatric history, family perspective.

Initial management

(See earlier in this chapter 📖 p. 962.) Make, document, and communicate the diagnosis. Acknowledge symptom severity and experience of distress as real but emphasize negative investigations and lack of structural abnormality. Reassure patient of continuing care. Attempt to reframe symptoms as emotional. Assess for and treat psychiatric co-morbidity as appropriate. Reduce and stop unnecessary drugs. Consider case conference involving PCP and treating physicians. Educate parents/family.

Ongoing management

- Regular review and management by single, named doctor preferably the PCP.
- Reviews should be at planned and agreed upon frequency, avoiding emergency consultations.
- Symptoms should be examined and explored with a view to their emotional "meaning."
- Avoid tests "to rule out disease"; investigate objective signs only.
- All secondary referrals made through one individual.
- Disseminate management plan.
- These patients can exhaust a doctor's resources—plan to share the burden over time.

Some evidence for the effectiveness of patient education in symptom re-attribution, brief contact psychotherapy, group therapy, or cognitive behavior therapy (CBT) if the patient can be engaged in this.

Prognosis

Poor in the full disorder; tendency is for chronic morbidity with periods of relative remission. Treatment of psychiatric co-morbidity and reduction of iatrogenic harm will reduce overall morbidity. Key for recovery in children and adolescents is rehabilitation and return to usual activities as soon as possible.

Conversion disorder

The loss or disturbance of normal motor or sensory function which initially appears to have a neurological or other physical cause but is attributed to a psychological cause. This disorder was initially explained by psychodynamic mechanisms—repression of unacceptable conscious impulses and their "conversion" to physical symptoms, sometimes with symbolic meaning. In ICD and DSM, the presumed psychodynamic mechanisms are not part of the diagnosis. The initiation or worsening of the symptom or deficit is preceded by conflicts or stressors. Symptoms are not produced intentionally and the presence of "secondary gain" is not part of the diagnosis. Per DSM-IV-TR, symptoms cannot be fully explained by a medical condition or the direct effects of a substance or as a culturally sanctioned behavior or experience. Conversion disorders are classified with the somatoform disorders in DSM-IV-TR.

Clinical features

Vary depending on the area affected but the following are commonly seen:

Paralysis

One or more limbs or one side of the face or body may be affected. Flaccid paralysis is common initially but severe, established cases may develop contractures. Often active movement of the limb is impossible during examination but synergistic movement is observed (e.g., Hoover's test: the patient is unable to raise the affected limb from the couch but is able to raise the unaffected limb against resistance with demonstrable pressing down of the heel on the "affected" side).

Loss of speech (aphonia)

There may be complete loss of speech, or loss of all but whispered speech. There is no defect in comprehension and writing is unimpaired (and becomes the main method of communication). Laryngeal examination is normal and the patient's vocal cords can be fully opposed while coughing.

Sensory loss

The area of loss will cover the patient's beliefs about anatomical structure rather than reality (e.g., "glove" distribution, marked "midline splitting").

Pseudoseizures

Nonepileptic seizures are found most commonly in those with genuine epilepsy. Pseudoseizures generally occur only in the presence of an audience. No injury is sustained on falling to the ground, tongue biting and incontinence are rare. The "seizure" consists of generalized shaking, rather than regular clonic contractions, and there is no postictal confusion or prolactin rise. This is the most common presentation of conversion disorder in children and adolescents.

Etiology

Not known, but hypotheses include:

- Psychological—an expression of an underlying or unconscious conflict.
- Biological —precipitated by excessive cortical arousal.
- Family systems—modeling behavior; presence of enmeshment, overprotection, rigidity and a lack of conflict resolution.
- Learning theory—learning the benefits of the "sick role." At high risk may be an abused child who cannot disclose.
- Sociocultural—more accepted way to ask for help.

Diagnosis

The diagnosis will usually be suspected when physical or neurological findings do not conform to known anatomical pathways and physiological mechanisms. It is established by (1) excluding underlying disease, or demonstrating minor disorder insufficient to account for the symptoms; (2) finding of "positive signs" (e.g., demonstration of function thought to be absent or capturing a pseudoseizure on a video EEG); (3) a convincing psychological explanation for the deficit.

Additionally helpful though nonspecific is a prior history of conversion symptoms or recurrent somatic complaints or disorder, family or individual stress and psychopathology (recent stress, grief, sexual abuse) or the presence of a symptom model.

Differential diagnosis

Includes:

- Multiple medical diagnoses (e.g., migraines, temporal lobe epilepsy, CNS tumors, MS, myopathies, SLE). Dual diagnosis present in up to one-third of conversion disorders.
- Anxiety, depression. Diagnosis not made if symptom is better accounted for by another diagnosis.
- Somatoform disorders.
- Dissociative disorders.
- Malingering and factitious disorder.

Treatment

Education and formulation presented in a conference with the primary treatment team. Be supportive and nonjudgmental, using positive statements ("we have good news for you") rather than negative ("we couldn't find anything; it's all in your head"). No controlled treatment studies. CBT, IPT, supportive psychotherapy, family therapy, biofeedback all potentially helpful. Treat psychiatric co-morbidity.

Prognosis

For acute conversion symptoms, especially those with a clear precipitant, the prognosis is good, with expectation of complete resolution of symptoms (70–90% resolution at follow-up). In children and adolescents, conversion disorder usually occurs suddenly and temporarily. Outcomes are poorer for longer-lasting and well-established symptoms in the presence of chronic stressors.

Factitious disorder (Munchausen's syndrome)

In factitious disorder, patients intentionally falsify their symptoms and past history and fabricate signs of physical or mental disorder with the primary aim of assuming the sick role and obtaining medical attention and treatment. The diagnostic features are the intentional and conscious production of signs, falsification, or exaggeration of the history and the lack of gain beyond medical attention and treatment.

Three distinct subgroups are seen.

- Wandering: Mostly males who move from hospital to hospital, job to job, place to place, producing dramatic and fantastic stories. There may be aggression or antisocial PD and co-morbid alcohol or drug problems.
- Nonwandering: Mostly females; more stable lifestyles and less dramatic presentations. Often in paramedical professions; overlap with chronic somatization disorder. Association with borderline PD.
- By proxy: Mostly female. Mothers, caregivers, or paramedical and nursing staff who simulate or prolong illness in their dependants—here the clinical focus must be on the prevention of further harm to the dependant. Most victims are infants or young children. In children, this is a form of child abuse, and must be treated as such.

Additional qualifiers attached to diagnosis include predominantly physical features, predominantly psychological features or both.

The behaviors can mimic any physical or psychiatric illness. Behaviors include: self-induced infections, simulated illnesses, interference with existing lesions, self-medication, altering records, reporting false physical or psychiatric symptomatology. Early diagnosis reduces iatrogenic morbidity and is facilitated by: awareness of the possibility; a neutral interviewing style using open rather than closed questions; alertness to inconsistencies and abnormalities in presentation; use of other available information sources; and careful medical record keeping. Videotaping in the hospital has been used successfully to establish a diagnosis with certainty, especially in factitious disorder by proxy.

Differential diagnosis

Any genuine medical or psychiatric disorder. Somatization disorder (no conscious production of symptoms and no fabrication of history), malingering (secondary gain for the patient e.g., compensation, avoiding army service, avoiding detention), substance misuse (also gain, e.g., the prescription of the abused drug), hypochondriasis, psychotic and depressive illness (associated features of the primary mental illness).

Etiology

Unknown. There may be a background of childhood sexual abuse or childhood emotional neglect, a disrupted family or marriage. Probably more common in women and those with a nursing or paramedical background. Association with personality disorder, often borderline.

Management

There are no validated treatments. Patients are often reluctant to consider psychiatric assessment and may leave once their story is questioned. Management in these cases is directed toward reducing iatrogenic harm caused by inappropriate treatments and medications.

In the case of factitious disorder by proxy, when suspicions are high, child protective services should be contacted, and appropriate steps to protect the child should be taken.

- Direct challenge: Easier if there is direct evidence of feigned illness; the patient is informed that staff are aware of the intent to feign illness and the evidence is produced. This should be in a nonpunitive manner with offer of ongoing support.
- Indirect challenge: Here the aim is to allow the patient a face-saving "way out", while preventing further inappropriate investigation and intervention. One example is the "double bind", "if this doesn't work then the illness is factitious."
- Systemic change: Here the understanding is that there is no possibility of change in the individual and the focus is on changing the approach of the health care system to assessing them in order to minimize harm. These strategies can include dissemination of the patient's usual presentation and distinguishing marks to regional hospitals, "black-listing," "Munchausen's registers," etc. Because these strategies potentially break confidentiality and can decrease the risk of detecting genuine illness, they should be drawn up in a multidisciplinary fashion involving senior staff, with legal input.

Pain disorder

In pain disorder, associated with psychological factors with or without general medical condition, there is a complaint of persistent severe and distressing pain which is not explained or not adequately explained by a general medical condition. The causation of the symptom is attributed to psychological factors. This disorder is diagnosed where the disorder is not better explained by somatization disorder, another psychiatric diagnosis, or psychological factors affecting general medical condition.

All pain is a subjective sensation and its severity and quality as experienced in an individual is dependant on a complex mix of factors including the situation, the degree of arousal, the affective state, the beliefs about the source, and meaning of the pain. The experience of pain is modified by its chronicity and associations. There is a "two-way" relationship between affective state, with pain predisposing to anxiety and depressive illness, while anxiety and depressive illness tend to worsen the subjective experience of pain.

Co-morbidity

In common with the other somatoform disorders there is substantial overlap with major depression (~40% in pain clinic patients) and anxiety disorders. Substance abuse (including iatrogenic opiate dependency) and personality disorder patients are overrepresented.

Epidemiology

No population data are available. The prevalence of patients with medically unexplained pain varies by clinical setting; higher in inpatient settings, particularly surgery, and highest in pain clinic patients.

Differential diagnosis

Factitious disorder, malingering, psychological factors affecting medical condition, substance abuse, and a host of medical diagnoses in which pain may be a central feature, such as sickle cell anemia.

Assessment

History from patient and informants, length of history (may be minimized), relationship to life events, general somatization, experience of illness, family attitude to illness, periods of employment, associated morbidity, treatments, beliefs about cause, co-morbid psychiatric symptoms.

Management

(See the beginning of this chapter for more details). It is important to recognize and treat occult co-morbid depression. It is often helpful to adopt a theoretical approach: "let's see what works," and to resist pressure for "all or nothing" cure or a move to investigation by another specialty. Opiates are not generally effective in chronic pain of this type and add the risk of dependence. Psychological treatments: these are directed toward enabling the patient to manage and "live with" the pain, rather than aspiring to eliminate it completely; can include relaxation training, biofeedback, hypnosis, group work, CBT. Pain clinics: these are generally anesthetist-led with variable psychiatric provision. They offer a range of physical treatments such as: antidepressants, TENS, anticonvulsants, and local or regional nerve blocks.

Mental disorders due to general medical conditions

All psychiatric illnesses are by their nature organic—that is, they involve abnormalities of normal brain structure or function. The term "organic illness" in modern psychiatric classification, however, refers to those conditions with demonstrable effects in CNS function, either due to primary CNS pathology (e.g., temporal lobe seizures; CVA, TBI, MS) or the indirect effects of systemic illness over CNS physiology (e.g., electrolyte disturbances; inflammatory cytokines; steroid-induced psychosis; pain). Substance-misuse-related organic disorders are discussed in the substance-misuse chapter. Specific diagnostic criteria for mental disorder due to a general medical condition can be found in the DSM IV TR. The reader is encouraged to review these criteria. This section briefly discusses common traumatic, inflammatory, degenerative, infective, and metabolic conditions that may manifest as mental disorders.

Many psychiatric symptoms and disorders can have an organic etiology. For this reason, every patient who presents with psychiatric symptomatology requires a thorough history, review of systems and physical examination, including neurological examination. Laboratory investigations should follow as guided by findings in physical and neurological examination and clinical history. Mental health patients have been identified as an at-risk population and general physical health status can have significant effects over the course and presentation of primary psychiatric disorders. Acute exacerbation of otherwise stable or treatment refractory psychiatric patients should also prompt the clinician for examination of possible systemic illness.

Clinicians, particularly the psychiatric consultant, should strive for thorough biopsychosocial diagnostic and treatment formulations. Below are listed common organic causes of psychiatric syndromes (for delirium see 📖 *pp. 978–39*; dementia see 📖 *pp. 152–70*; for amnestic disorders see 📖 *pp. 448* and *174*):

Organic causes of depression

- Neurological (CVA, epilepsy, Parkinson's disease, brain tumor, dementia, MS, Huntington's disease, head injury).
- Infectious (HIV and related opportunistic infections, EBV/CMV infectious mononucleosis, Lyme).
- Endocrine and metabolic (hypothyroidism, hyperprolactenemia, Cushing's, Addison's disease, parathyroid disease, vitamin deficiencies).
- Cardiac disease (MI, cardiac bypass surgery, CHF).
- Systemic lupus erythematosus (SLE), rheumatoid arthritis, cancer.
- Medications (analgesics, antihypertensives, L-dopa, anticonvulsants, benzodiazepines [BDZs], antibiotics, steroids, OCP, cytotoxics, cimetidine).
- Drugs of abuse (alcohol, BDZs, cannabis, cocaine, opioids)/toxins.

Organic causes of mania

- Neurological (CVA, epilepsy, brain tumor, head injury, MS).
- Endocrine (hyperthyroidism, steroid producing tumors).

- Medications (steroids, antidepressants, INH, cytotoxics).
- Drugs of abuse (cannabis, cocaine, amphetamines)/toxins.

Organic causes of anxiety

- Neurological (epilepsy, dementia, head injury, CVA, brain tumor, MS, Parkinson''s disease).
- Pulmonary (COPD).
- Cardiac (arrhythmias, CHF, angina, mitral valve prolapse).
- Hyperthyroidism, hypoglycemia, metabolic acidosis/alkalosis, pheochromocytoma.
- Medications (antidepressants, antihypertensives, antiarrythmics (e.g., adenosine, flumazenil).
- Drugs of abuse (alcohol, benzodiazepines, caffeine, cannabis, cocaine, LSD, ecstasy, amphetamines).

Organic causes of psychosis

- Neurological (epilepsy, head injury, brain tumor; dementia, encephalitis e.g., HSV, HIV, neurosyphilis, brain abscess, CVA).
- Endocrine (hyper/hypothyroidism, Cushing's, hyperparathyroidism, Addison's disease).
- Metabolic (uremia, electrolyte disturbance, porphyria).
- SLE ("lupus psychosis").
- Medications (steroids, L-dopa, INH, anticholinergics, antihypertensives, anticonvulsants, stimulants).
- Drugs of abuse (cocaine, LSD, cannabis, PCP, amphetamines, opioids).
- Toxins (i.e., organophosphates, heavy metals).

Organic causes of catatonia

- Neurological (neoplasm, CVA, encephalitis, dementia, Parkinson's).
- Metabolic (hypokalemia, hypercalcemia, homocystinuria, hepatic encephalopathy).
- Medications (e.g., neuropleptics, depolarizing agents).

Organic causes of personality change

- Neurological (frontal lobe or right hemispheric lesions, Huntington's, epilepsy, encephalitis, prion disease, dementia).
- Metabolic (thyroid disease, hypoglycemia, adrenal disease).
- SLE.
- Medications (steroids, antidepressants, mood stabilizers, neuroleptics and atypical antipsychotics, stimulants).
- Drugs of abuse.

Acute confusional states (delirium)

Key features

A stereotyped response of the brain to a variety of insults, very commonly seen in hospital inpatients. It is a clinical syndrome of fluctuating global cognitive impairment associated with behavioral abnormalities. Like other acute organ failures it is more common in those with chronic impairment of that organ.

Epidemiology

Extremely common in medical and surgical inpatients (10–20%). Risk factors include: extremes of age; pre-existing dementia; sensory impairment; stroke; mental illness; metabolic abnormalities; burn victims and multiple trauma; serious physical illness; perioperative period (especially cardiac); emergency procedures and prolonged operations; polypharmacy; alcohol and benzodiazepine dependence. Carries significant morbidity and mortality and is associated with prolonged lengths of stay.

Clinical features

- Impaired level of consciousness with reduced ability to direct, sustain, and shift attention.
- Global impairment of cognition with disorientation, and impairment of recent memory and abstract thinking.
- Disturbance in sleep/wake cycle; excessive dreaming with persistence of experience during wakefulness.
- Psychomotor disturbances including agitation or hypoactivity.
- Emotional lability.
- Perceptual distortions, illusions, and hallucinations—characteristically visual.
- Speech may be rambling, incoherent, and thought disordered.
- There may be poorly developed paranoid delusions.
- Most commonly: Onset of clinical features is rapid with fluctuations in severity over minutes and hours (even back to apparent normality).

Differential diagnosis

Mood disorder; psychotic illness (new major mental disorder very much less likely than delirium in a hospitalized patient, particularly if elderly); postictal; dementia (characteristically has insidious onset with stable course and clear consciousness—clarify functional level prior to admission). Pick's disease (acute onset rapidly deteriorating dementia); acute intoxication.

Etiology

This is typically multifactorial and the most likely cause varies with the clinical setting in which the patient presents. Theorized that multiple etiologies lead to final common neuronal pathway affecting cholinergic and dopaminergic systems in the prefrontal, nondominant parietal and fusiform cortex and anterior thalami.

Common etiologies of delirium

- Intracranial: CVA (especially RMC a. territory), traumatic head injury, encephalitis, primary or metastatic tumor; raised ICP.
- Metabolic: Hypoxia, dehydration, anemia, electrolyte disturbance, hepatic encephalopathy, uremia, cardiac failure, hypothermia.
- Endocrine: pituitary, thyroid, parathyroid or adrenal diseases, hypoglycemia, diabetes mellitus, vitamin deficiencies (thiamine, B_{12}, folate, nicotinic acid).
- Infectious: UTI, chest infection, abscess, cellulites, bacteremia.
- Substance intoxication or withdrawal: Alcohol, BDZs, anticholinergics, psychotropics, lithium, antihypertensives, diuretics, anticonvulsants, digoxin, steroids, NSAIDs.
- Pain: Fecal impaction, restraints or immobility.

Course and prognosis

Delirium usually has a sudden onset, usually lasts less than one week, and resolves quickly once the medical etiology is resolved. There is often patchy amnesia for the period of delirium but patients can be aware of the experience. Associated with medical treatment challenge and high mortality (estimated to be up to 50% at 1 yr). Causes significant disruption of therapeutic milieu in hospital units.

Assessment

Delirium is a Medical Emergency—attend promptly. Review time-course of condition with nursing and medical staff and review notes including medication administration records and available laboratory data. Assess medical history and history of present illness for premorbid functional level and concomitant risk factors.

EEG

This may be useful if diagnosis is in doubt.
- Diffuse slowing of background activity common to most causes of delirium.
- Low voltage fast activity seen in alcohol and benzodiazepine withdrawal.
- Other patterns may be indicative of other process (nonconvulsive status, acute confusional migraine).

Management

- Identify and treat precipitating cause. Prevent complications and support functional needs.
- In most cases, symptomatic management with pharmacological (e.g., low dose antipsychotics) and environmental measures (e.g., stimulus modification, reassurance) should not be delayed by investigations of main etiology.
- Asses for adequacy of pain control.
- Provide education and support to staff.
- Avoid sedation unless severely agitated or necessary to minimize risk to patient or to facilitate investigation/treatment.
- Consider use of BDZs early in the course of suspected alcohol or BDZ withdrawal syndrome.
- Regular clinical review and follow-up (MMSE useful in daily monitoring cognitive improvement at follow-up).

Psychiatric issues in the chronically ill

According to the Centers for Disease Control, "Chronic diseases—such as heart disease, cancer, and diabetes—are the leading causes of death and disability in the United States. These diseases account for 7 of every 10 deaths and affect the quality of life of 90 million Americans."

Advances in medical sciences and overall improvements in nutrition, public health, and social services have increased life expectancy in the general population as well as survivability in patients with chronic "organic" disease. This has, in turn, challenged health service organizations and individual clinicians to adequately assess and intervene in the myriad of biological, psychological and social needs of the chronically ill population.

Psychiatric co-morbidity

Inpatient based studies have found no significant increased prevalence of psychiatric co-morbidities in chronically v. acutely ill patients, with the presence of life-threatening illness being the major factor affecting the prevalence of concomitant psychiatric disease. In contrast, population and family medicine practice based studies have found higher rates of depression, anxiety, and other psychiatric co-morbidities in chronically ill patients when compared to the general population. The presence of mood and other mental disorders in medically ill patients is well recognized as a significant factor leading to increased health care resource utilization and is associated with lower scores in multiple quality of life measurements.

Pediatric population

The clinician working with pediatric populations faces additional challenges in assessing and intervening in a child with chronic illness and the impact that it may have on the patient and her caretakers. Biological factors in children include, but are not limited to, increased sensitivity to medication side-effects/polypharmacy and limited information on drug metabolism of most psychotropics. Illness specific risk factors to be assessed in the process of psychosocial diagnostic and therapeutic formulation include:

Formulation of risk factors for chronic illness
- Onset: specific vulnerabilities based on developmental stage (e.g., six months–five years; early adolescence).
- Etiology: environmental exposure or inherited genes—provide specific stressors on family (i.e., rational responsibility v. guilt).
- Diagnosis: uncertainty of diagnosis or misdiagnosis negatively affects the family/medical provider relationship.
- Deformity: (including chronic pain), negatively affects development.
- Disability: of self-image, social and financial supports, and achievement of sociocognitive developmental tasks. MR population carries higher risk of abuse and neglect.
- Prognosis: negative prognosis carries greater risk to adaptive emotional development. MH provider may assist patient, families, and other medical providers in copping with realistic expectations.

Multiple or frequent hospitalizations can also increase the risk of a negative impact on a child and his family. Other dynamic factors to be considered during clinical assessment and intervention strategies include: sociocultural context of hospitalizations and significance of illness, parents/family adaptive abilities and support systems, and the child's developmental capabilities to cope with illness.

Specific illnesses

The reader is referred to published texts on child and adolescent psychiatry for a more comprehensive discussion, including specific issues in target populations such as cystic fibrosis, insulin-dependent diabetes, epilepsy/CNS disorder, and oncology. The reader is also referred to this book's section on psychiatry in the terminally ill/end of life care, and on the practice of psychiatry in a hospital setting for other useful information.

End-of-life care

Psychiatry has an important role to play in assuring excellent care of terminally ill patients. Rates of anxiety and depression are high both in terminal patients and their families. In addition to treating these symptoms, psychiatrists may be called on to help balance potential delirium resulting from pain meds and other palliative treatments. This section covers issues faced by CL psychiatrists in examining and treating dying patients, including personal, diagnostic, and therapeutic challenges.

Personal issues for the CL psychiatrist

As psychiatrists, we are privileged to share intimate moments with our patients, including helping them to cope with the powerful emotions experienced during the last phases of life. CL psychiatrists can use their interview skills to help the patient express their understanding of their illness, their preferences about whether to pursue aggressive medical treatment, and their fears and concerns about death. We can also help patients and their families to conduct "life-reviews" to help understand what the patients have valued in their life, and to help the patient determine their goals and wishes at this stage. This process not only elicits powerful emotions from patients, but from ourselves and other members of the health-care team. Many of us have a strong instinct to "fix the problem," and are uncomfortable with accepting the inevitability of death. Pay attention to your own emotions and beliefs, and don't hesitate to talk with other mental health professionals and staff who routinely work in palliative care in order to stave off feelings of failure or despair. Being with patients through this intense time will often feel rewarding, particularly if you help the patient to feel they have been heard and suffering has been kept to a minimum.

Diagnostic issues and barriers to care

Despite the high rate of psychiatric symptoms in hospitalized patients, particularly in terminal patients, psychiatrists remain underutilized as part of palliative care. This likely stems from a number of issues, including a sense that the patient's emotional symptoms are "understandable" and therefore, not treatable; the desire not to "stigmatize" an otherwise psychiatrically healthy patient; and the difficulty in distinguishing somatic symptoms of depression and anxiety from physical symptoms of advanced disease.

Diagnosis and treatment?

As discussed earlier in this chapter, one of the challenges in CL psychiatry is to determine whether to diagnose and treat depression and anxiety when some or all of the symptoms can be confounded by their medical condition. These include but are not limited to symptoms such as fatigue, sleep and appetite disturbance, and poor concentration. The primary diagnostic approaches are to use either an inclusive approach (counting symptoms even if they overlap with medical symptoms), an exclusive approach (using only symptoms that are relatively specific for depression), or a substitutive approach (adding relatively specific symptoms such as tearfulness, hopelessness, and social isolation to help determine whether the patient requires treatment). In general, we have advocated for a substitutive approach; however, even these symptoms can be difficult to assess in dying patients.

Feelings of hopelessness

Terminal patients may feel "hopeless." They may choose not to interact with certain family or friends because it is fatiguing or they don't wish to be remembered as ill or weak. Activities that previously gave the patient pleasure may be impossible or feel frivolous. We would, therefore, suggest that a symptom-based, relatively inclusive approach be utilized in terminal patients, with an emphasis on relieving suffering. Particular attention needs to be given to the issue of suicide, as a desire for death may be one of the strongest indicators of depression and unrelieved suffering. Rates of suicide are high in terminal patients. It is important, however, not to interpret all thoughts of death and dying as "suicidal." Most terminal patients have thoughts that they might be better off dead if they get to a point where they are in unremitting pain or they have no "quality of life."

Treatment strategies

Treatment goals for psychiatric disorders in terminally ill patients are relatively focused on relieving distress, with less emphasis on achieving remission. As in other psychiatric populations, choice of antidepressant medication is frequently guided by side-effect profiles and potential drug interaction.

- For example, patients with cachexia and sleep disturbance may receive mirtazapine because of its efficacy in improving those symptoms. In addition, given the relative time pressure of treating terminal patients, antidepressants may be combined with psychostimulants in patients with anergia, amotivation, or anhedonia.

Anxiety symptoms are frequently treated with antidepressants and benzodiazepines; however, narcotics and neuroleptics may play a greater role in reducing anxiety in patients with dyspnea or severe pain. In all cases, attention needs to be paid to balancing the need to reduce distress and/or pain against potential cognitive deterioration or suppression of respiratory drive that may be caused by the treatment itself.

Delirium

Delirium is also frequently seen in terminally ill patients. Whereas the primary approach for most delirious patients is to identify and treat the underlying cause, this may not be a reasonable goal in severely ill patients in whom the disease causes direct CNS effects or those in whom pain relief will require some loss of cognitive clarity. Both pharmacologic and behavioral interventions may be useful to minimize the distress caused by their confusion. Medication strategies are similar to those with other cases of delirium (see earlier section in this chapter, 📖 p. 978), with a greater emphasis on prophylactic treatment with neuroleptics/antipsychotics to decrease agitation and possibly confusion. Behavioral measures may include: decreasing stimulation such as excessive noise and lights, which may confuse patients and increase paranoia; asking family members to be present when possible to provide reassurance and comfort; decreasing the emphasis on frequent reorientation and cognitive testing; and informing patients of blood draws and other care before it occurs.

It may be human nature to avoid talking about death and dying, and we find difficulty in caring for terminal patients. It reminds us of our own mortality, and we may feel uncomfortable treating someone when there appears to be nothing to "fix". Although challenging personally, diagnostically, and therapeutically, psychiatric care of terminal patients can be extremely rewarding for the treatment team, patients, and families.

Psychotherapy

Introduction

Psychotherapy has been called the "talking cure"—a means of examining dysfunctional thoughts, feelings, and behaviors, with the aim of understanding and changing them. This examination can take place using many different techniques. The various forms of psychotherapy differ in how they conceptualize symptoms and their development, and the methods they use to treat the attendant disorders. Regardless of the modality, the relationship between patient and therapist is the key to any successful treatment. All psychotherapies also take place within a structure or frame that is agreed upon between patient and therapist. This frame includes such elements as the time, place, and frequency of meetings, payment, contact outside sessions, and the role and responsibilities of the therapist and patient. In its broadest sense—understanding symptoms and effecting their improvement by means of a therapeutic relationship—psychotherapy is at the heart of all medical and, therefore, all psychiatric treatment.

Types of psychotherapy

Supportive psychotherapy

Though informed by psychoanalytic understanding, this therapy focuses on the use of direct measures to improve symptoms, develop and increase self-esteem, and support ego functioning and adaptive defense mechanisms. This form of therapy aims to help patients better cope with symptoms and solve problems, rather than to achieve fundamental behavioral change. While supportive techniques may be used as part of many other modalities, supportive psychotherapy is preferred where patient factors such as severe crisis, poor anxiety and frustration tolerance, lack of psychological mindedness and capacity for self-observation, disorganized thoughts and behavior, limited intelligence, impaired reality testing, poor affective and impulse control, and impaired relational ability preclude more expressive therapies. Supportive psychotherapy is the most widely practiced form of individual psychotherapy.

Expressive psychotherapy

This exists on the opposite end of a continuum with supportive psychotherapy. Based on psychoanalytic principles, this form of treatment aims to effect changes in an individual's dysfunctional thinking and behavior by exploring underlying causes, the unconscious mind, childhood experience, and the quality and nature of relationships. The relationship between patient and therapist receives particularly close examination. Expressive psychotherapy is more useful in patients who are highly motivated, are able to tolerate frustration and anxiety, have good impulse control, can form meaningful relationships, and are capable of insight and abstract thought.

Cognitive/behavioral therapies

These are based on learning and cognitive theory. The focus in these therapies is the "here and now." Current thoughts and behaviors are closely examined and modified as needed to improve symptoms. Unconscious processes, childhood experience, and the specific nature of the

therapist-patient relationship receive little or no attention. Cognitive and behavioral therapies are generally more structured than other therapeutic modalities, and often take place over a brief, predetermined period of time. These therapies are useful in a wide range of disorders.
• Examples include exposure with response prevention for the treatment of obsessive-compulsive disorder.

Psychotherapeutic training

As a psychiatric trainee, you are required to gain competency in five areas of psychotherapy: supportive psychotherapy, psychodynamic psychotherapy, brief psychotherapies, cognitive behavior therapy, and combined psychopharmacology and psychotherapy. Training generally consists of formal didactic instruction, experience working with a range of patients, and regular supervision with practiced individuals. It is only through the process of conducting therapy under supervision that you will really understand psychotherapeutic techniques. These notes on general concepts and specific psychotherapies aim to familiarize you with theories, guide your referrals, and assist you in explaining the process to patients.

Recommended further reading

Dewan, M., Steenbarger, B., Greenburg, R. *The Art and Science of Brief Psychotherapies.* Arlington, VA: American Psychiatric Publishing, 2004.

Winston, A., Rosenthal, R., Pinsker, H. *Introduction to Supportive Psychotherapy.* Arlington, VA: American Psychiatric Publishing, 2004.

Gabbard, G.O. *Psychodynamic Psychiatry in Clinical Practice,* 3rd ed. Washington, DC: American Psychiatric Press, 2000.

Assessment for psychotherapy

Psychotherapeutic methods can be useful in the treatment of many psychiatric illnesses, including mild to moderate depressive illness, anxiety disorders, behavioral disorders, and personality disorders. Specific therapies also have a place in the management of learning disability, sexual problems, substance misuse, and chronic psychotic symptoms. They are generally contraindicated in the treatment of acute psychosis, severe depressive illness, dementia/delirium, and conditions where there is acute suicide risk. The assessment of a patient for psychotherapy has two major goals: establishing a therapeutic relationship, and obtaining a careful history. The history should explore the nature, duration, and severity of the presenting problem, past psychiatric history and treatment, significant interpersonal relationships, level of and changes in functioning, and basic psychological structure.

Psychological factors in assessment for psychotherapy
"Psychological-mindedness"
Refers to the capacity for insight and to understand problems in psychological terms. If lacking, a supportive (v. expressive/exploratory) emphasis is preferred.

Motivation for insight and change
Requires a degree of introspectiveness, average intelligence, and verbal fluency. Where these are not present, supportive strategies may be more helpful.

Adequate "ego strength"
Important when choosing exploratory psychotherapies. Includes the ability to sustain feelings and fantasies without impulsively acting upon them, being overwhelmed by anxiety, or losing the capacity to continue the dialogue. The individual with good ego strength is better able to maintain a therapeutic alliance, and reality testing is not compromised by psychosis or severe depression.

Ability to form and sustain relationships
Where there is inability to enter into trusting relationships (e.g., in paranoid personality disorder) or where there is inability to maintain relationship boundaries (e.g., in borderline personality disorder), this may preclude exploratory methods.

Ability to tolerate change and a degree of frustration
As with any potentially powerful treatment, psychotherapy (especially more exploratory methods) has the potential to exacerbate symptoms, particularly as maladaptive coping mechanisms are examined and changed.

Selection of psychotherapeutic method
Local availability
In practice, one determinant of therapy choice is often the availability of skilled therapists in a particular modality.

Practitioner experience
Where the treating psychiatrist also provides the psychotherapy, his or her area of expertise may determine choice of psychotherapeutic method.

Illness factors
While the exact suitability of the various therapeutic modalities to specific illnesses has yet to be clearly established, research shows that some therapies are beneficial for particular disorders (e.g., behavior therapy for specific phobias, cognitive behavior therapy for depression).

Patient choice
Patients may express a preference for a particular therapeutic model because of previous positive experience or having read or been told about the approach. A method that makes sense to the patient given their understanding of their symptoms is preferred.

Introduction to dynamic therapies

Dynamic therapies, including psychoanalysis (📖 *p. 1006*) and psycho-dynamic psychotherapy (📖 *p. 1008*) are derived from the psychoanalytic principles and practice of Sigmund Freud and his followers. Any therapy involving the gradual exploration with the patient of conflicts not previously accessible to the conscious mind can be considered a dynamic psychotherapy.

Rationale

The theoretical basis for dynamic therapies is that "neurotic conflicts," unconscious conflicts resulting in anxiety, can lead to psychopathology. The individual's previous experiences and relationships that are relevant to these conflicts and the powerful associated emotions will emerge during therapy. Awareness of these unconscious conflicts, as well as associated desires and symbolic meanings, can bring understanding of the emotional state of a patient, as well as relief from symptoms.

How illness is viewed

Both mental illness and normal psychological development are understood using psychoanalytic theories. While a typical descriptive assessment of a patient by a psychiatrist may categorize patients into similar groups using diagnostic criteria, a dynamic assessment of a patient uses psychoanalytic theory to explore the unique layout of the individual patient's conscious and unconscious mind.

Psychoanalytic theories have been repeatedly refined, revised, and challenged over the last century. However, the basic principles and techniques of dynamic psychotherapies remain similar. Indeed, while psychotherapists were historically separated by the core theories in which they believed, many contemporary dynamic psychotherapists find themselves choosing which theory to apply based on the clinical situation and needs of their patients. A brief overview of these theories is provided in the basic psychoanalytic theory section (📖 *pp. 992–94*).

Efficacy and limitations of dynamic therapies

There is some clinical research suggestive of benefits in expressed symptoms and decreased need for medication, as well as long-term and enduring improvements associated with length and completeness of treatment. The volume, validity, and reliability of the evidence, however, is limited. Some clinicians criticize all dynamic therapies because they have arisen primarily from theory and clinical observations instead of evidence-based medicine. This may not reflect on the inefficiency of psychodynamic therapies as much as it reflects the inherent difficulties in designing the research studies. There is a lack of standardization in diagnosis, method, control groups, and improvement measures, reflecting the diversity of many factors in the psychotherapeutic trials, including techniques, background of practitioners, and illnesses treated. Nonetheless, the future may bring more evidence-based medicine to support dynamic therapies, both alone and in combination with psychotropic medications. Studies may also show more support for the theories behind psychodynamic therapies. There is already experimental psychological research to support the concept that mental activity can be unconscious, such as the studies of the emotional effect of subliminal messages on research subjects.

While dynamic therapies do not have the biological side-effects of psychiatric medications, they are not free of safety risk These therapies aid in increasing the insight of the patient, which may involve the removal of defense mechanisms that play a protective role (p. 995), and, therefore, must be done with caution.

- For example, an abuse victim may undergo painful emotions when recalling trauma in therapy.

The risks and benefits of such phenomena are a subject of study and controversy, although most dynamic therapists would agree that patient readiness determines when to explore painful experiences in therapy.

Dynamic therapies are not indicated for all patients (see p. 1006). Freud himself explained that psychoanalysis was not an appropriate plan of cure for patients with psychoses. Even if insight can be improved, this may not improve outcome. In young patients with schizophrenia, for example, improved insight, in the form of awareness of illness, may actually be correlated with an increased rate of suicide.

The intensive frequency of dynamic therapy provides another limitation.

- For example, this creates an increased demand on time for patients, challenges for compliance, and increased cost (with more accessibility to wealthy populations).

While most insurance plans have some coverage, typically intensive therapy involves patient payment of some sort. Defenders of dynamic therapies will claim that the emphasis on insight, psychosocial issues, and the patient-therapist relationship makes these therapies more satisfying to the patient and worth the cost.

Basic psychoanalytic theory (1)

One principle common to all dynamic therapies is that overt symptoms may be the external expression of unconscious conflict. Symptoms continue, despite the suffering they cause to the individual because of the benefit of excluding unacceptable ideas from the conscious mind. Freud called this benefit to the individual "primary gain." More contemporary explanations have expanded this principle by describing other unconscious processes that can be expressed with symptoms, including absent or weakened sense of self and internal representations of relationships (📖 p. 1002).

Introduction to Freudian theory

Freud explained that traumatic experiences, particularly those in early life, give rise to psychological conflict. The greater part of mental activity is unconscious, and the conscious mind is protected from the experience of this conflict by inherent defenses, designed to decrease "unpleasure" and to diminish anxiety. These defenses are developmentally appropriate, but their continuation into adult life results in either psychological symptoms or in a diminished ability for personal growth and fulfillment. Conflict can be examined with regard to the anxiety itself, the defense, or the underlying wish or memory.

Freud first demonstrated the usefulness of exploring unconscious conflict in the treatment of patients with "hysteria" a historical diagnosis that was only given to women, characterized by paralysis, convulsions, somnambulism, hallucinations, as well as loss of speech, sensations, or memory. The symptoms could not be explained by underlying organic disease. (This presentation was very similar to the modern-day diagnosis of conversion disorder—📖 see p. 970). Freud conceived of "hysterical" symptoms as arising as an indirect result of a previous traumatic event in the patient's life. The memory of this trauma was painful and gave rise to unacceptable contradictions in the patient's beliefs about themselves. Although the memory of the experience was not recalled directly, the powerful associated emotional response, called "nervous excitation," was expressed as hysterical symptoms, sometimes with symbolic connection to the initial traumatic event.

The details of the traumatic events could often be accessed by the therapist during hypnosis. The hysterical symptoms could be treated by forcing the memory of the experience into consciousness, resulting in "abreaction," an emotional release or catharsis.

A brief history of Sigmund Freud

Freud made a huge contribution to our understanding of the mind, but many of his ideas are now so much a part of our general world view that it is easy to overlook their originality during this time.

Freud was born in 1856 in Moravia (now part of the Czech republic, but then part of the Austro-Hungarian Empire). He moved to Vienna when he was a child and lived there until his last year, leaving for England in 1938. On entering medical training he was influenced by "scientific empiricism"—the belief that through careful observation the un-understandable could be understood. He began laboratory work on the physiology of the nervous system under Brücke, later entering clinical medical practice after his marriage in 1882. He chose neurology as his specialty and studied in Paris. There he was exposed to the ideas of Charcot, who interested Freud in the study of "hysterical" patients under hypnosis.

Returning to Vienna, Freud began collaboration with Josef Breuer on the study of "hysteria." The subsequent development of psychoanalysis was prompted by the case of "Anna O.," treated by Breuer between 1880 and 1882. This patient, a 21-year-old woman, presented with a range of hysterical symptoms including paralysis, visual loss, cough, and abrupt personality change. These symptoms had developed while her father was terminally ill. Breuer observed that her symptoms resolved during hypnotic trances. Breuer also noted that not only did the symptoms recur after the sessions ended but that after he terminated the treatment relationship she suffered a full-blown relapse. Breuer wrote up the case after discussing it with Freud. Later they published *Studies in Hysteria*.

Experience during his clinical practice in the 1890s led Freud to develop the ideas of repression of unacceptable memories and their expression as hysterical symptoms. Freud later realized that in the majority of cases the memories were unacceptable because they evoked sexualized fantasy toward parental figures. Freud described these ideas in "The Interpretation of Dreams," published in 1900. It described the basis of his psychoanalytic technique including analysis of the content of dreams, descriptions of defense mechanisms, and his topographical model of the mind (📖 *p. 1004*).

Although Freud's early insights tended to stem directly from clinical experience, his later ideas were more theoretical and related to developing a complete understanding of the normal and abnormal development of mind, such as his drive theory (📖 *p. 994*)

In 1905 he published *Three Essays on the Theory of Sexuality*, describing his theories regarding childhood development (📖 *p. 1000*). *The Ego and the Id*, published in 1923, saw the expansion of the topographical model with the structural model of the mind (📖 *p. 994*). He described the production of anxiety symptoms by unconscious conflict in *Inhibitions, Symptoms and Anxiety* in 1926.

Freud's repeated revision of his own theories was mirrored by repeated disagreements and splits in the psychotherapeutic movement and the formation of the separate psychotherapeutic school of object relations therapists (📖 *p. 1002*). Freud died from cancer in England in 1939 after fleeing Vienna following the rise to power of the Nazis. His daughter Anna continued to refine and publicize her father's work.

Basic psychoanalytic theory (2)

Freudian theories of symptom development

Topographical model of the mind

In this early model the mind consists of the unconscious, the preconscious, and the conscious. Only those ideas and memories in the conscious mind are within awareness. The preconscious contains those ideas and memories capable of becoming conscious. The preconscious performs a censorship function by examining these ideas and memories and sending those that are unacceptable back to the unconscious ("repression"). The unconscious mind acts according to the "pleasure principle"—the avoidance of pain and the seeking of gratification. This is modified by the "reality principle" of the conscious mind, that gratification often must be postponed in order to obtain other forms of pleasure. Freud's psychoanalytic techniques would attempt to interpret unconscious content based on access to preconscious content, such as free associations, the expression of dreams, transference, and "parapraxes" (slip of the tongue; see 🕮 *p. 1007*).

Structural model of the mind

This served to explain aspects of the unconscious left out from the earlier topographic model. The mind was compartmentalized into the Id, the Ego, and the Superego. The Id, entirely unconscious, pursues its own desires in the interest of discharging tension and is heedless of external reality or moral constraints. A new born baby's mind is conceived as all Id. The Ego is mostly conscious, emerges during infancy and is the personality that moderates the desires of the Id and the Superego. The Superego (the "conscience"), is the conscious and unconscious internalization of the morals and strictures of society, which provides judgments on what behaviors are acceptable and which are "bad." When the Ego is unable to successfully moderate between the Id and Superego, it may defend the individual's sense of self by repressing the impulse to the unconscious, where its presence may produce disturbance.

Drive theory

Freud postulated the existence of basic drives, which included the "libido" the sexual drive (🕮 *p. 1000*) and the "eros" and "thanatos" (the drives toward life and death). He described the "pleasure principle," the drive to avoid pain and experience pleasure as well as its modification through the "reality principle."

Transference reactions

Freud noted that some patients developed powerful feelings toward him and called this phenomenon "transference."

Transference

The unconscious development, in the patient, of feelings and patterns of behavior toward the therapist, which partly recapitulate earlier life relationships.

Counter-transference
Describes the equivalent reaction in the therapist toward the patient. The examination of transference and counter-transference is a central part of dynamic psychotherapies and guides diagnostic formulation and the exploration of the patient's neurosis (see 📖 *p. 1006*).

Introduction to defense mechanisms

Freud's concept of "repression" was considered a "defense mechanism" because it protected the ego from painful emotions that come from conflict between the conscious mind and unconscious desires. Subsequently, a number of other defense mechanisms were described by his daughter Anna and others who followed. Defense mechanisms were viewed as developing to prevent conflict between the conscious mind and the unconscious desires. In theory, defense mechanisms are a normal process, and they can become more mature as the mind does. Therefore, all healthy individuals are expected to exhibit defense mechanisms throughout their life. Mental illness and personality disorders are often characterized by the perseverance of more primitive defense mechanisms. Therefore, the following list of defense mechanisms is divided into immature defenses, commonly seen in early childhood and mental illness, neurotic defenses, commonly seen in older children or adults experiencing stress or anxiety, and mature defenses, commonly seen in highly functioning adults.

Basic psychoanalytic theory (3)—defense mechanisms

(See Introduction to defense mechanisms, 📖 p. 995)

Primitive defense mechanisms

Denial
Remaining unaware of difficult events or truths to accept by unconsciously disregarding information.

Projection
Attributing one's own internal unacceptable ideas and impulses to an external target, such as another individual, and reacting accordingly.

Projective identification
Behaving toward another individual in a manner that causes them to take on one's own internal unacceptable ideas and impulses. Not to be confused with projection: During projection an individual with a certain emotion might *perceive* someone else as feeling the same way, but in projective identification, the individual might cause someone else to feel that same emotion.

Idealization
Perceiving others as ideal or superhuman in order to avoid conflicting feelings about them.

Splitting
Separating polarized and contradicting perceptions of self or others in order to disregard awareness of both simultaneously. (A patient believing that a doctor is "the best doctor they have ever had" at one point, and "the worst doctor they have ever had" at another).

Dissociation
Parting from usual sense or perceptions of reality, often in order to avoid being conscious of helplessness in the context of a painful experience. May be perceived as an "out-of-body experience."

Acting out
Externally exhibiting impulsive behaviors that reveal unconscious desires (A child's temper tantrum).

Regression
Responding to emotional stresses by reverting to a level of functioning of a previous maturational point.

Neurotic defense mechanisms

Repression
Preventing unacceptable aspects of internal reality from coming to conscious attention. (In adult life, no longer being consciously aware of past episodes of childhood sexual abuse). The associated emotional reaction may remain in the conscious mind but divorced from its accompanying idea or experience.

Introjection

Attributing another's unacceptable ideas and impulses to oneself through internalization, and reacting accordingly. Note that Freud's theory on depression suggests that it is caused by introjection of the aspects of others that make the depressed patient feel anger, leading to "anger turned inward."

Identification

Taking on the characteristics, feelings, and/or behaviors of someone else as one's own. (A young girl may dress in her mother's clothes during normal development). Differs from introjection in a similar manner to the way projective identification differs from projection. Whereas in introjection, one may perceive themselves as being like someone else, in identification, one may actually feel the way someone else does, and become more like the other person.

Intellectualization

Focusing on abstract concepts, logic, and other forms of intellectual reasoning to avoid facing painful emotions. (A victim of a traumatic abuse experience may discuss the statistics of abuse instead of talking about the particular experience).

Isolation of affect

Separating an experience from the painful emotions associated with it. (A victim describing a traumatic abuse experience without displaying any of the affect the experience has evoked).

Rationalization

Justifying feelings or behaviors with a plausible and more acceptable explanation, rather than examining the unacceptable explanation known to the unconscious mind. (A mourner stating that the deceased person is "In a better place now" in order to ease feelings of guilt associated with the death).

Sexualization

Attaching sexual feelings to an experience to avoid painful feelings associated with the experience.

Reaction formation

Externally expressing attitudes and behaviors that are the opposite of the unacceptable internal impulses. (Being extra kind and polite to a person to avoid expressing anger toward that person).

Undoing

Performing an action that has the effect of unconsciously "cancelling out" an unacceptable internal impulse or previous experience. The action symbolizes the opposite outcome of the impulse or experience. (A victim previously assaulted on a rainy day excessively using a hairdrier).

Displacement
Transferring the emotional response to a particular person (or experience) to someone else (or experience) that in some way resembles the original but may not be associated with as much conflict or risk. (A boy feeling anger toward a man who reminds him of his father, rather than feeling anger toward his father).

Mature defense mechanisms

Suppression
Making a conscious decision not to attend to painful feelings or thoughts.

Humor
Finding funny or ironic aspects of an unpleasant experience in order to explore the experience without the painful emotions typically attached to it.

Altruism
Attending to the needs of others above one's own needs.

Anticipation
Intentionally neglecting one's immediate needs in order to prepare for future needs or experiences.

Compensation
Developing abilities in one area in response to a deficit in another.

Sublimation
Expressing unacceptable internal impulses in socially acceptable ways. (Swinging a baseball bat in a batting cage as an outlet for feelings of aggression).

Basic psychoanalytic theory (4)

Freud's theory of psychosexual development

Freud believed that the unconscious psychological conflicts which produced morbidity most often arose in the first six years of life. He theorized that everyone is born with an instinctive sex drive called the libido, a primary source of tension if unsatisfied. He developed a theory that attempted to explain the development of the libido during infancy and childhood. He visualized four phases, characterized by particular satisfactions and conflicts. Along the way, infants progressed from a state of primary narcissism, in which they find gratification in their own body processes, to "object love," in which they can more clearly separate themselves from other "objects" or people. Inability to resolve conflicts at a particular stage could lead to arrested sexual development, or fixation. If an adult "regresses," or returns to an earlier fixated state, it could result in neurotic symptoms.

Phase; age (approx.)	Source of pleasure	Conflicts
Oral phase; Birth–18 mos.	Suckling and investigation of objects by placing them in the mouth.	Love for breast of nursing mother v. "aggressive" urge to bite or spit.
Anal phase; 18–30 mos.	Anal sensations and the ability to withhold and to appropriately produce feces.	Need to control sphincter enough to avoid shame of making a mess (related to pleasing authority and keeping orderly), but not so much that there is fecal retention.
Phallic phase; 30–48 mos.	Manipulation of the penis.	Boys: Exhibitionism v. rivalry with father. Girls: "Penis envy" leading to feelings of inferiority. (Note: This theory has been rejected or modified by many modern dynamic theorists.)
Oedipal phase; 48 mos.–6 years	Fantasies of opposite sex parent.	Boys: Love for mother v. fear of castration by father, leading to "castration anxiety." Boys unconscious desires were characterized by "oedipal complex," taken from the story "Oedipus Rex" by the ancient Greek playwright, Sophocles (430 BC) in which the main character unknowingly kills his father and marries his mother.

(Contd.)

Phase; age (approx.)	Source of pleasure	Conflicts
		Girls: Desire for a baby leads to attachment to father as someone who potentially can give her one. Called the "Electra Complex."
Latency phase; 6 years until puberty	Period of relative quiescence of sexual thoughts	The anxieties from the previous phase are repressed.
Genital phase; Period of mature adult sexuality		Improper resolution of previous phases may be manifest in symbolic ways.

Later developments in ego psychology

Freud's theories of unconscious conflict (📖 p. 992) were eventually referred to as "ego psychology." Several of those who studied with Freud made contributions themselves.

Anna Freud (1895–1982)

Although Freud recognized the importance of unconscious defenses in response to anxiety, the first systematic account of these mechanisms was written by Freud's daughter Anna in *The Ego and the Mechanisms of Defense* in 1936. She also helped to develop the study of child psychoanalysis.

Carl Jung (1865–1961)

Expanded Freud's drive theory to include drives other than sexual. Believed the unconscious mind included the "collective unconscious," in which humankind's shared mythological and symbolic past is represented in the unconscious mind of an individual. Described the representational symbols incorporated into the collective unconscious as "archetypes." Described personality types as "introverted" and "extroverted."

Erik Erikson (1902–1994)

Expanded Freud's developmental theory by explaining that there were not only sexual conflicts at each phase but also a conflict related to how individuals adapts to their social environment, leading to a "psychosocial crisis."

Freud's phase	Psychosocial conflict
Oral phase	Trust v. mistrust
Anal phase	Autonomy v. shame and doubt
Oedipal phase	Initiative v. guilt
Latent phase	Industry v. inferiority

Alfred Adler(1870–1937)

Theorized that all people are born with an "inferiority complex," an unconscious sense of inadequacy. Tied this to Freud's Oedipal complex theory by claiming that the Oedipal drives of children remain unsatisfied, which adds to their inferiority complex.

Basic psychoanalytic theory (5)

Object relations theory

Relationships between individuals often form the context in which unconscious drives are formed. Object relations theorists have suggested that an internal representation of one experience in a relationship can become part of the unconscious mind. During the experience, the mind internalizes:

- A representation of the other person in the relationship as if it were a prototypical person, called an "object." (The term "object" here refers to the person as he or she is internally represented.).
- The emotions evoked by the experience.
- The role of the self in the experience.

These three components join together to form an "object relationship."

- For example, infants may internalize the relationship with their mother in a moment when she is perceived as caring and providing nurture as a "positive" object relationship.

However, when his/her mother is needed and not available, the relationship may be internalized as a "negative" object relationship. The theorists claim that seeking objects is the primary objective of unconscious drives, rather than reducing tension, as suggested previously by Freud.

Melanie Klein (1882–1960)

A founder of the object relations movement, demonstrated that a child's unconscious conflicts can be understood by observing the child at play. While her resulting developmental theories are not widely accepted by contemporary psychologists, play therapy is still commonly practiced. She emphasized primitive defense mechanisms such as projection, introjection, and splitting (📖 p. 996).

Donald W. Winnicott (1897–1971)

Another object relations theorist, studied the infant's growth of a sense of self. He described the "transitional object," which was an item such as a pacifier or blanket that aided with the infant's transition to independence by replacing the object of the mother in the positive mother-infant object relationship. He described the "good-enough mother" to refer to the minimum environment needed for healthy psychological development.

Margaret Mahler (1897–1985)

Went beyond the developmental theories of Freud and Erikson (📖 pp. 1000–11) by using object relations theory along with empirical research of developing children. Like Winnicott, she explored how children make their transition from dependence to independence, a process she called "separation-individuation," with four separate phases:

- Differentiation, 6–10 months. Infants gradually become aware of their mother as a separate object from themselves.
- Practicing, 10–16 months. Infants spend limited time away from their mothers exploring their surroundings.
- Rapprochement, 16–24 months. The child goes through a new level of awareness of separation between themselves and their mother that intensifies feelings of vulnerability when left alone.

- Consolidation of individuality, 2–3 years and beyond. The child develops a sense of individuality and "object constancy," meaning that objects continue to exist when not in the view of the child.

Self psychology theory

While object relations theory emphasizes how relationships can be internalized, self psychology theory, led by Heinz Kohut (1913–1981), expands on object relations by identifying "mirroring" and "idealizing" as key object relationships needed in infancy and childhood for a complete sense of self. Mirroring occurs when a mother (or parental object) shows her approval of a child in the way she reacts to the child's age-appropriate performances. Idealizing occurs when the child perceives the parental object as all-knowing and able to do anything. The role of the parent becomes internalized into the child's personality as a "selfobject."

Kohut's theory opposes Freud's theory that narcissism is outgrown (see 📖 p. 1000) and instead maintains that narcissistic processes themselves mature as a process of normal development. The therapist may find, however, in examining transference and counter-transference of pathologically narcissistic patients, that they are still using immature defense mechanisms to obtain missing self-objects. Kohut believed that if there is a deficiency in mirroring and idealizing self-objects, it can lead to an incomplete sense of self. This can result in narcissistic personality disorder (📖 p. 548), in which immature defense mechanisms, such as projective identification (📖 p. 996), are maintained into adulthood. To give a clinical example, a patient may act in an entitled and grandiose manner because they feel worthless inside and wish to be fully nurtured by only the most "ideal" of therapists to compensate. In turn, by feeling pressured to act caring toward an ungrateful patient, the therapist may feel some of the patient's low self-worth, thus completing the process of projective identification.

Basic psychoanalytic theory (6)

Other contributions to psychoanalytic theory

Harry Stack Sullivan (1892–1949)

Used data from observation of the therapeutic process itself to clarify and expand the role of the therapist, who he referred to as a "participant observer." Whereas Freud himself had discovered difficulties in using his typical psychoanalytic techniques with psychotic patients, Sullivan proposed therapeutic methods for even the most psychotic patients.

Carl Rogers (1902–1987)

Worked on therapeutic technique like Sullivan. He conceived "client-centered therapy." He felt that the therapeutic attributes of genuineness, unconditional positive regard, and accurate empathy could help patients achieve what he called "self-actualization," a complete sense of self, which was beneficial to their recovery.

John Bowlby (1907–1990)

Worked on "attachment theory," which has been based on empirical research such as measuring infants' behaviors when separated from and then reunited with their mothers. Attachment theory stresses the importance of the feelings of closeness and security an infant develops with the caregiver as well as the role the caregiver plays in helping the infant to form these feelings.

Psychoanalysis

Indications and contraindications

(See general indication for psychotherapy, 📖 pp. 986–89, and Efficacy and limitations of dynamic therapies 📖 p. 990). Psychoanalysis is commonly elected by the patient rather than prescribed. It is rarely reserved only for specific mental illnesses. In fact, those with relatively sound mental health may find it improves the quality of their lives over time. Psychoanalysis is commonly used in patients where there are anxious or emotional symptoms, such as mild to moderate depressive symptoms, somatic symptoms, and dissociative symptoms. Psychoanalysis may be a good choice for patients who are looking for change, motivated to explore past experiences, and are emotionally stable and willing to re-experience some pain in doing so.

Psychoanalysis is relatively contraindicated for drug or alcohol dependence, suicidality, or harmful/violent behaviors, psychotic illness, severe depressive features, limited cognitive ability or concrete thinking, poor insight, or poor judgment.

Techniques

Psychoanalysis is an intense therapy that usually involves one to five 50-minute sessions per week. Therapy may last for years. Psychoanalysis typically features more traditional techniques to attempt to interpret unconscious content, including free associations, transference, the expression of dreams, "parapraxes" and symbolism of neurotic symptoms. The therapist will then choose appropriate moments to reveal these interpretations to the patient.

Free association

The patient agrees to reveal everything that comes to mind, no matter how embarrassing or socially unacceptable (i.e., "speaking without self-censorship"). Traditionally the patient is speaking in a reclining position with minimal eye contact with the therapist. The therapist assumes a position of neutrality, in which emotional support and directive advice is withheld. Areas where free association "breaks down" and areas of resistance to pursue associative thought may represent conflicts that are important to explore.

Exploration of transference/counter-transference

(See Transference reactions, 📖 p. 994) The intense and frequent nature of psychoanalysis often results in a patient forming powerful feelings toward a therapist. Important repressed aspects of past relationships and defense mechanisms used by the patient in current relationships find expression in the transference relationship. Through a process called "abstinence," psychoanalysts, through monitoring their own counter-transference, attempt to avoid fulfilling the patient's unconscious expectations that they will act like the people from their past.

Examination of dreams

Dreams are traditionally viewed as being formed by a mix of daytime memories, nocturnal stimuli, and representations of unconscious desires, which are then theoretically distorted by the ego to protect us from conscious knowledge of the content. The actual, or "latent" dream is eventually reconstructed from the "manifest" dream, the portions of the dream that patients remember in therapy, by a process of symbolization and elaboration which can expose the hidden unconscious desires.

Examination of parapraxes
A parapraxis is a slip of the tongue, which today is often referred to as a "Freudian slip". Occasionally it reveals unconscious desires, particularly in affect-laden situations.

Examination of symbolism
Individual patient neurotic symptoms may have symbolic meaning in the context of the patient's history, which can be usefully explored. Symbolism may also be analyzed in child psychotherapy when observing play and drawings.

Interpretation
Expression of the therapist's understanding of the meaning of what is occurring in therapy. Interpretations commonly include descriptions of defense mechanisms or explanations for current anxiety in the context of underlying desires.

Phases of treatment
Early sessions
The psychoanalyst will typically explain methods of therapy, establish ground rules, and produce a psychodynamic formulation of the case. The therapist will assess patient suitability and motivation while exploring potential risk factors.

Middle sessions
As the patient progresses in psychoanalysis, the therapist, who will typically work with a supervisor, identifies unconscious defense mechanisms, key conflicts, personality structure, and defects in personal development.

Later sessions
The therapist may use more interpretive techniques, which may increase anxiety. Regression and resistance, transference and counter-transference may also emerge.

Training
Involves education in psychoanalytic history, theory, and practice, extensive supervised case work, and personal psychoanalysis for the therapists themselves. Many major U.S. cities have a local psychoanalytic institute that may offer formal psychoanalytic training to those with doctoral or masters degrees in mental health and two years of clinical experience. Training usually consists of a five-year postgraduate curriculum specifically in psychoanalysis. For physicians, this training would typically be completed after completion of a psychiatric residency program. Most institutes also offer supervision and classes for therapists who are interested in dynamic psychotherapy, but have not chosen the five-year psychoanalytic program.

Psychodynamic psychotherapy

Psychodynamic psychotherapy is an intervention where the concepts of symptom development are based on those of psychoanalysis (p. 994), but the methods of therapy are adjusted for a reduced frequency of sessions and decreased number of total sessions. Supporters of this type of therapy claim that insights and opportunity for change and growth available from long-term psychoanalysis can be achieved in a shorter time frame, and that introducing directive elements and focus on particular topics does not necessarily reduce overall treatment effectiveness.

Indications and contraindications

See general indication for psychotherapy (pp. 986–90) and efficacy and limitations of dynamic therapy (p. 990). Indications and contraindications are similar to those of psychoanalysis (p. 1006), with particular emphasis on the ability and motivation to form a collaborative relationship with a therapist.

Techniques

Psychodynamic psychotherapy is modified from psychoanalysis in that it involves "active therapy," where the therapist attempts to guide free association on more focused topics, such as the goals, specific anxieties, and defenses of the patient. It can vary in length depending on both the therapist and the needs of the patient. It may be significantly more brief than psychoanalysis, often lasting only 20–25 sessions with the termination date decided at outset ("brief psychodynamic psychotherapy"). The frequency may only be 1–2 sessions a week. The therapist usually helps the patient to identify and explore a currently active problem. The methods employed are similar to those of psychoanalysis (p. 1006), but with therapist-patient eye contact and more verbal interaction from the therapist. Both transference and counter-transference give the therapist valuable information about the nature of past relationships (see p. 1006). The therapist will help the patient to explore symptom precipitants and associated early trauma and avoidance. The therapist may guide therapy by use of interpretation at an earlier point than in psychoanalysis.

In the case of patients with more severe mental illness, such as psychosis, or in acute crisis or decompensation, these techniques are sometimes further modified to be less focused on improving insight, and instead, the emphasis is more supportive, particularly focusing on encouraging the expression of emotions.

This therapy is sometimes combined with psychopharmacology.

Phases of treatment

Initial assessment

Diagnosis, including consideration of appropriateness of this method of therapy in this patient. Consideration of appropriate use of medication in cases of combined psychotherapy-psychopharmacology.

Early sessions

Identification of main problems, goals, and issues. Limited comments from therapist. Usually there is positive transference due to expectation of "magical" change. Identification of main defenses, coping styles, and ability to accept and work with interpretations.

Middle sessions
Exploring present emotions and emotions evoked by past experiences. Exploration of transference, counter-transference, and resistance with supervisor.

Closing sessions
Exploring anticipation of termination. Arrangements for aftercare.

Training
Often involves similar routine to training for pschoanalysis, including psycho-education in psychoanalytic history, theory, and practice; supervised case work; and personal psychoanalysis. Local psychoanalytic institutes may offer courses varying in length and time commitment.

Later developments

Jung: Expanded drive theory to include drives other than sexual. Ideas of "collective unconscious" and personality archetypes. Ideas of extro-version and introversion.

Klein: Theories of childhood development including primitive defense mechanisms such as "splitting." Methods of play therapy.

Winnicott: Object relations theory—gratification through relationships as well as through satisfaction of desires. Described transitional objects and the idea of the "Good enough mother."

Erikson: Described alternative model of psychosocial development based on the crises at each developmental stage.

Rogers: Client-centered therapy. Importance of therapeutic attributes of genuineness, unconditional positive regard, and accurate empathy.

Berne: Transactional analysis. Examination of "games" and "scripts," which characterize relationships.

Group therapy

Group psychotherapy is a form of treatment in which selected individuals are purposefully brought together under the guidance of a trained therapist with the goal of reducing distress, increasing coping, and improving relationships. Group methods were first developed in the early 20th century following observations of beneficial group effects with TB patients. Group psychotherapy allows group members to interact with one another and with the therapist, to identify difficulties in those interactions, and to change dysfunctional patterns. Like individual psychotherapy, the term group psychotherapy encompasses a range of modalities, settings, and techniques.

Groups may be homogeneous or heterogeneous (e.g., in terms of diagnosis, age, gender), and may vary as to the frequency and duration of meetings, whether the therapist is actively involved or more supervisory, whether the membership is closed or open after the group starts, whether they are time-limited or ongoing. The basic tasks of the therapist include making decisions about the aforementioned factors, formulating goals, preparing patients for the therapy, and building and maintaining a therapeutic environment that promotes group interaction.

Group therapy generally requires that members are able to carry out the task of interacting in a group, have problem areas that are compatible with the goals of the group, and are motivated for change. While most patients may benefit from some form of group therapy, exclusion criteria include inability to comply with the group norms for acceptable behavior, inability to tolerate the group setting (e.g., extreme paranoia), severe incompatibility with one or more group members, tendency to assume the deviant role.[1] As already noted, there are multiple forms of group therapy in practice today, with different theoretical orientations, methods, and goals. Some major categories are outlined below.

Types of groups

- *Supportive groups* Focus on promoting and strengthening adaptive defenses, giving advice, providing encouragement. Goals include re-establishing and/or maintaining function, improving coping. May be useful in psychotic disorders, anxiety disorders.
- *Problem-focused groups* Can include alcohol or drug dependence, paraphilias, anger management. Focus is on mutual support and group examination of strategies for change. Peers may be experts at identifying resistance and rationalization for avoiding change in other group members.
- *Psychodynamic groups* Techniques include close examination of transference, counter-transference, resistance, and unconscious conflict. May be a more individual focused therapy in a group setting, or therapy of the group as a whole. Goal is lasting change through modification of personality factors.
- *Cognitive-behavioral groups* Useful where the goal is modification of dysfunctional behaviors, such as in anxiety and eating disorders.

1 Hales, R.E., Yudofsky, S.C. *The American Psychiatric Publishing Textbook of Clinical Psychiatry* 4th ed. Arlington, Virginia: American Psychiatric Publishing, 2003.

Focus is on specific symptoms rather than on nature of interpersonal interactions. Therapist takes an active and central role.

- *Activity groups* Generally helpful for patients with intellectual impairment, severe and persistent mental illness. Examples include art, music, computing, etc. Can foster social skills and adaptive behaviors. Helpful for psychosocial and vocational rehabilitation.
- *Self-help groups* Strictly speaking, not a form of group therapy, though may have beneficial therapeutic effects. Groups tend to be organized around a specific problem, have strong peer support and group cohesion, and be led from within the group. Examples include Alcoholics Anonymous, Narcotics Anonymous, Overeaters Anonymous.

Techniques

- Free-ranging discussion.
- Psycho-education.
- Group specific process: mirroring (duplication of experience), amplification (increase in emotional resonance by sharing), catharsis (supported ventilation of emotion).
- Analysis of group dynamics.
- Clarification/interpretation/confrontation with individuals.
- Group therapeutic factors described by Yalom[2] are : installation of hope, universality, imparting information, altruism, corrective recapitulation of the primary family group, development of socializing techniques, imitation of adaptive behavior, interpersonal learning, group cohesion, catharsis, existential factors.

Phases of therapy

Early sessions

Set-up and engagement, formulation of rules and establishment of goals, focus on leader.

Middle sessions

Adaptation, potential for conflict, examination of authority, establishment of intimacy and group cohesion

Closing sessions

Negotiation of termination, review of goals, reflection on experience of group.

2 Yalom, I. *The Theory and Practice of Group Psychotherapy*. New York: Basic Books, 1995.

Basic learning theory

Behavioral psychology is a method for understanding the development of knowledge and behaviors in organisms. In an individual organism these are shaped by environmental influences and can change as a result of experience. Learning theory concerns the testing of methods to produce behavioral adaption through changing environmental influences. The two basic learning processes are classical (Pavlovian) conditioning—learning what goes with what, and operant (Skinnerian) conditioning—learning to obtain reward and avoid punishment.

Classical conditioning

Focus on the responses that are automatic and involuntary, responses that are not deliberate and do not require effort. In the initial experiment, Pavlov presented a dog with food, which produced the response of salivation. Here the food is the unconditioned stimulus (US) and the salivation is the unconditioned response (UR). A neutral stimulus such as a bell ringing is not associated with any unconditioned response. However if a bell is rung immediately before the food is presented, after a number of repetitions the dog will salivate in response to the bell alone. Now the bell is a conditioned stimulus (CS) producing a conditioned response (CR), the salivation.

Stimulus generalization

Automatic process in which the subject generalizes from a conditioned stimulus (CS) to other neutral stimuli. The subject then demonstrates the same conditioned response (CR) to these similar stimuli.

Higher order conditioning

Deliberate process in which conditioned trails cause the subject to demonstrate the (CR) to new stimuli by pairing them with the (CS).

Classical extinction

Results from repeatedly presenting the (CS) without the (US). When the tone (CS) is repeatedly presented without the meat powder (US) the dog eventually stops salivating to the tone (i.e., the conditioned response is extinguished).

Spontaneous recovery

During extinction trials, following a rest period, stimulus, the conditioned response (CR) to the conditioned stimulus (CS) often briefly reappears. This reappearance is known as spontaneous recovery.

Habituation

The subject becomes accustomed to and less responsive to the (US) after repeated exposure.
- For example, a person moves next to an airport and becomes accustomed to the noise of airplanes taking off and landing (US) that after a few weeks, she no longer startles (UR) and wakens when the planes come and go.

Techniques based on classical conditioning concepts

Systematic desensitization (📖 p. 1015)

Presentation of situations more and more similar to the CS are paired with relaxation techniques, in order to eventually break the association between the CS and the CR.

Flooding (📖 p. 1015)

Presentation of the full CS without the possibility of withdrawal from the situation. The initial unpleasant experience of the CR gradually diminishes.

Operant conditioning

The experimental techniques and rules of operant conditioning were developed by Thorndike and refined by Skinner. The basic principles of operant conditioning are that if a response to a stimulus produces positive consequences for the individual it will tend to be repeated; however, if it is followed by negative consequences, it will tend not to be repeated. In the original experiments rats were placed in a box containing a lever which, when pressed delivered a pellet of food. Eventually the rat would press the lever and be rewarded. The rat would then press the lever with increasing frequency. (Note: operant conditioning does not rely on insight on the part of the rat.)

Positive reinforcement

In an attempt to increase the likelihood of a behavior occurring in the future, an operant response is followed by the presentation of an appealing stimulus. Example: If you stroke a cat's fur in a manner that is pleasing to the cat, it will purr. The cat's purring may act as a positive reinforcer, causing you to stroke the cat's fur in the same manner in the future.

Negative reinforcement

In an attempt to increase the likelihood of a behavior occurring in the future, an operant response is followed by the removal of an aversive stimulus. Example: When a child says "please" and "thank you" to his parents, the child may not have to engage in his least favorite chore of taking out the garbage. Therefore, not having to take out the garbage will act as the negative reinforcer and increase the likelihood of the child saying "please" and "thank you" in the future.

Positive punishment

In an attempt to decrease the likelihood of a behavior occurring in the future, an operant response is followed by the presentation of an aversive stimulus. Example: If you stroke a cat's fur in a manner that the cat finds unpleasant, the cat may attempt to bite you. Therefore, the presentation of the cat's bite will act as a positive punishment and decrease the likelihood that you will stroke the cat in that same manner in the future.

Negative punishment

In an attempt to decrease the likelihood of a behavior occurring in the future, an operant response is followed by the removal of an appeasing stimulus. Example: When a child talks back to his/her parents, the child may lose the privilege of watching his or her favorite television program.

Therefore, the loss of television privileges will act as a negative punishment and decrease the likelihood of the child talking back in the future.

Operant extinction

Results from ceasing to reinforce behavior that has previously been reinforced. Withholding reinforcement will usually result in increased behaviors (response burst). Over time unreinforced behavior will be extinguished.

Stimulus dscrimination

Occurs when a subject begins to emit the target behavior in the presence of stimuli similar to but not exactly the same discriminative stimulus. For example, a child who gets attention by whining in the presence of his grandfather may also whine in the presence of other elderly males, expecting reinforcement.

Response generalization

Refers to performing a behavior similar but not identical to the one that has been previously reinforced. Example: a cat does a trick and is reinforced with a toy. Later the cat does a different trick (similar, but not identical) hoping to be reinforced.

Prompting

This is cuing a person to perform a specified behavior. For example, to teach a child good manners, a parent may prompt the child with the instruction, "Say please." Over time, the parent gradually reduces the prompt to, "What do you say?" and eventually to just a look. This gradual reduction in prompting is known as fading.

Shaping

This is used to increase the number of behaviors in a person's behavior repertoire, the behaviors that a particular person, at a particular time, is capable of performing. For example, an autistic child is taught to say her name by being prompted, "Say Kristina." She is initially reinforced for simply making any utterance, then for making the "k" sound, until at last she is able to say her full name.

Chaining

This is usually used in combination with shaping to link together a series of functionally related responses, which are associated with a stimulus condition. Each behavior in the sequence is mildly reinforced and serves as a cue to perform the next behavior in the chain. The major reinforcement occurs at the end of the chain. An example is going to a football game, which involves several steps, including finding a game of interest, driving to the game, finding a parking spot, buying tickets, and finally watching the football game (major reinforcement). Every step must be reinforced or else the chain will stop.

Techniques based on operant conditioning concepts

- Behavior modification (📖 *p. 1015*).
- Aversion therapy (📖 *p. 1015*).

Behavior therapy

Techniques based on learning theory are utilized in order to extinguish maladaptive behaviors and substitute adaptive ones.

Systematic desensitization

Holds as a central tenant the principle of reciprocal inhibition (i.e., anxiety and relaxation cannot coexist). Systematic graded exposure to the source of anxiety is coupled with the use of relaxation techniques (the "desensitization" component). Effective for simple phobias, but less so for other phobic/anxiety disorders (e.g., agoraphobia). Process in a typical case is as follows:

- Patient identifies the specific fear (e.g., cats).
- Patient and therapist develop hierarchy of situations provoking increasing levels of anxiety (e.g., stroking a cat on one's knee > touching a cat > having a cat in the room > looking at pictures of cats > thinking about cats).
- Patient is instructed in relaxation technique.
- Patient experiences the lowest item on the hierarchy while practicing the relaxation technique and remains exposed to the item until the anxiety has diminished.
- The process is repeated until the item no longer produces anxiety.
- The next item in the hierarchy is tackled in similar fashion.

Flooding/implosive therapy

High levels of anxiety cannot be maintained for long periods, and a process of "exhaustion" occurs. By exposing the patient to the phobic object and preventing the usual escape or avoidance, there is extinction of the usual (maladaptive) anxiety response. This may be done in vivo (flooding) or in imagination (implosion).

Behavior modification

Based on operant conditioning. Behavior may be shaped toward the desired final modification through the rewarding of small, achievable intermediate steps. This can be utilized in behavioral disturbance in children and patients with learning disability. Other forms of behavioral modification include the more explicit use of secondary reinforcement, such as "token economy," in which socially desirable/acceptable behaviors are rewarded with tokens that can be exchanged for other material items or privileges, or "star charts" where children's good behavior is rewarded when a certain level is achieved.

Aversion therapy and covert sensitization

The use of negative reinforcement (the unpleasant consequence of a particular behavior) to inhibit the usual maladaptive behavioral response (extinction). True "aversion" therapy (e.g., previously used to treat sexual deviancy) is not used today, however, covert techniques (e.g., the use of Antabuse in alcohol dependency) can be (at least partially) effective.

Cognitive behavior therapy

The theory, basic structure and method of Cognitive behavior therapy (CBT) was developed by Aaron Beck and outlined in a series of papers published in the 1960s.[1] CBT development was prompted by the observation that patients referred for psychotherapy often held ingrained, negatively skewed views of themselves, their future, and their environment. Treatment is based on the idea that disorder is caused not by life events, but by the view the patient takes of life events. It is a short-term, collaborative therapy, focused on current problems, whose goals are symptom relief and development of new skills.

Rationale

Behaviors and emotions are determined by the person's cognitions. Some pathological emotions are a result of "cognitive errors." Although underlying emotions are not amenable to examination and behavioral change, the cognitions are. If the person can be helped to understand the connection between cognitive errors and distressing emotion, he/she can try methods of change. CBT aims to, "change the way you feel by changing the way you think."

How illness is viewed

In some personality types and in mental illness there are errors in the perception of risk, logical errors, and errors in the processing of information (i.e., cognitive distortions). These distortions relate to self, world, and future (Beck''s cognitive triad). The model is: events ~ faulty cognitive appraisal ~ emotional response ~ maladaptive behavior ~ (behaviors/emotions) = pathology. Cognitive errors thus lead to dysphoria and maladaptive behavior. These errors originate in childhood learning, internalized family/cultural attitude, and early traumatic experiences. The cognitive model is a guide for therapy, not a comprehensive model of illness causation, and it does not exclude neurochemical or other factors as important in symptom development nor does it preclude the use of pharmacological treatments.

General elements of CBT

- Collaborative empiricism.
- Problem-oriented focus.
- Short-term for uncomplicated disorders.
- Structured methods.
- Psycho-education.
- Homework.

Techniques

The therapist is very active in CBT. The patient and the therapist are viewed as working together in a spirit of scientific inquiry to explore the problem and possible solutions—"collaborative empiricism," The therapist role is to assist the patient in: monitoring cognitions, identifying cognitive errors, and understanding maladaptive schema. The patient and therapist work together to explore strategies to challenge and change these negative cognitions and examine the resultant symptomatic effects.

CBT makes use of behavioral, cognitive, and experimental techniques to treat patients.

Behavioral techniques used in CBT
- Breathing training.
- Activity and pleasant event scheduling.
- Graded task assignments.
- Exposure and response prevention.
- Relaxation training.
- Coping cards.
- Rehearsal.

Cognitive techniques used in CBT
- Socratic questioning.
- Examining the evidence.
- Examining advantages and disadvantages.
- Imagery.
- Role play.
- Rehearsal.
- Generating rational alternatives.
- Identifying cognitive errors.
- Thought change records.
- Guided discovery.

Phases of treatment

A short-term treatment, with the initial assessment being followed by 6–20, one-hour-long sessions. Clinical attention is primarily focused on events in the "here and now." Each session generally proceeds as follows: deal with emergencies; jointly set agenda; review homework task; feedback; focus on specific items guided by current problems; suggestion of cognitive or behavioral techniques to challenge automatic thoughts/core schema; give homework.

Indications and contraindications

CBT is considered an active treatment requiring patient understanding and collaboration. Patients should, therefore, be motivated and be able to link thought and emotions. In addition to the general contraindications to psychotherapy (📖 *pp. 986–9*), CBT is contraindicated in LD and dementia. Indicated in:
- Mild to moderate depressive illness.
- Eating disorders (anorexia nervosa, bulimia nervosa, and binge eating disorder).
- Anxiety disorders.
- Bipolar disorder (reduce risk of relapse).
- Substance abuse disorders.
- Schizophrenia and other chronic psychotic disorders as an adjunct to pharmacotherapy.
- Chronic medical conditions such as fibromyalgia, chronic fatigue, pain.

Efficacy

There is good evidence for effectiveness in depressive illness, eating disorders and anxiety disorders. CBT is at least as effective as pharmacotherapy[2] in mild to moderate depression and may be more effective in long-term follow-up (e.g., at preventing relapse).

Cognitive errors

CBT identifies two levels of cognitive errors: automatic thoughts and core schemas. Automatic thoughts can be perpetuated by never being challenged consciously or by novel experience. Schemas are a person's "rules" for behaving, based on fundamental beliefs and shaped by previous (and current) experiences.

Automatic thoughts

- Selective abstraction.
- Arbitrary inference.
- All or nothing thinking.
- Magnification/minimization.
- Personalisation.
- Catastrophic thinking.
- Overgeneralization.

Fundamental beliefs (in schema)

Basic rules for making sense of environmental information (e.g., "a person must do everything right to be successful," "a good person always retains emotional control").

Recommended further reading

1 Wright, J.H. (2006). Cognitive behavior therapy: Basic principles and recent advances. *Focus* **4**(2), 173–178.

2 Dobson, K.S. (1989). A meta-analysis of the efficacy of cognitive therapy for depression. *J Consult Clin Psychol* **57**, 414–419.

Interpersonal psychotherapy

Interpersonal psychotherapy (IPT) is a time-limited, manual-based treatment developed based on concepts from the interpersonal school (Harry Stack Sullivan) by Klerman and Weissman in the 1970s for the treatment of depression. The idea for its development followed the observation that the psychosocial problems noted in their depressed clinic patients were not being addressed adequately by pharmacotherapy alone. Their goal was to develop a practical, short-term psychotherapy which could be used in conjunction with medication and which could be taught to a variety of health care professionals such as nurses and social workers as well as psychologists and psychiatrists.

Rationale

IPT focuses on the way in which depression is expressed in the current interpersonal sphere of the patient, i.e., in the "here and now," not on past traumas, early-life events, or distorted cognitions (such as in psychodynamic psychotherapy or CBT). IPT makes no attempt to differentiate whether the cause of depression is biological or psychosocial, in fact, psycho-education about both is key and, the concomitant use of antidepressant medication is encouraged when indicated. The social sphere of the depressed patient is recognized to be:

- The place where the depression is expressed and where it impacts others.
- A potential contributor to the onset of the depression.
- A place to begin to ask how the patient might act differently that could lead to improved mood regardless of the cause of the depression.

How illness is viewed

Depressive symptoms consistent with DSM-IV descriptors, regardless of their etiology, are viewed as modifiable through the application of IPT techniques. Depressive symptoms are tallied each week and improvement is linked to changes in attitude or behavior the patient is making toward better coping in one of four broad areas: role transition (such as graduating from school, marriage, job change, childbearing or retirement), role disputes (in current relationships with spouses, lovers, other family members, or in the workplace), unresolved grief (due to the death of another human being) or interpersonal deficits (longstanding difficulties sustaining mutually satisfying relationships). Reducing depressive symptoms Is the goal. No attempt is made to alter personality traits in this short-term approach.

Techniques

After a thorough psychiatric assessment, patients must agree to a contract to meet weekly for 12–16 one-hour individual sessions. This is an important component that brings conscious and unconscious pressure to continuing working before "time runs out." A focus in one of the four areas outlined above is mutually agreed upon and specific techniques for each focus are utilized as outlined in the manual. The focus is steadfastly maintained with the goal of making concerted progress, and this may require the therapist to preclude taking up other issues that occur during the therapy. Depressive symptom reduction is reviewed weekly and linked to changes in attitude or behavior. The role of IPT therapists is defined as an active advocate and a facilitator to encourage the patients to see their problems from different perspectives, to make attempts at changes and to return to discuss their successes or failures at subsequent weekly sessions. Transference interpretations are avoided in order to keep the patient focused on how to negotiate better with people in their current life outside of therapy. This, together with the short-term nature of the treatment and the required sustainment of a focus tends to fully occupy the patient's attention and allows for the planned termination to be completed without the transference issues making withdrawal from the therapist more complicated.

Phases of treatment

- Phase I (sessions 1–2): perform a thorough psychiatric interview and assess the need for psychiatric medication to be used concomitantly if indicated; contract for 12–16 sessions, allow patients to adopt the "sick role" because functioning when depressed cannot be expected to be as usual; systematically elicit a complete interpersonal inventory of all important persons in patient's life; and finally, establish a focus for the treatment as described earlier.
- Phase II (sessions 3–12) commence work on the focus per the specific techniques outlined in the IPT manual such as facilitation of the grieving process, mourning the loss of the old role and learning to embrace the challenges of the new role in the role transition focus, or determining whether a role conflict is in the impasse, renegotiation or dissolution phase with specific techniques for dealing with each. Review progress in depressive symptom reduction weekly. Review overall progress at the "halfway point," which encourages sustained effort before "time runs out."
- Phase III: (final 3–4 sessions) anticipate termination as scheduled from the outset in the contract with encouragement to continue to apply what has been learned and experimented with by the patient in their real-life interpersonal sphere. The IPT therapist points out that progress toward better coping (leading to reduced depressive symptoms) has been "earned" by the patient who did the work of changing. The IPT therapist reminds the patients that the therapist's own role was merely to facilitate what the patient now knows they can do for themselves.

Indications

Nonpsychotic depressive disorders. Adaptations of IPT have been applied to various subgroups such as adolescents, geriatric patients, primary care clinic patients, and patients with HIV, bulimia, panic disorder, bipolar disorder, dysthymic disorder, bereavement, postpartum depression, social phobia and insomnia. Modifications of IPT for groups, couples therapy, maintenance therapy, and via telephone have been developed.

IPT is not indicated for treating substance abuse or personality disorders.

Efficacy

Several randomized controlled trials (RCTs) in adults, adolescents, elders, and primary care patients have demonstrated efficacy for IPT either alone or in combination with antidepressant medication.

Dialectical behavior therapy

- Dialectical behavior therapy (DBT), developed by Marsha Linehan and her colleagues, was originally designed for the severe and chronic, multidiagnosed, difficult-to-treat patient with both Axis I and Axis II disorders, especially borderline personality disorder (BPD).
- DBT is a complex treatment that combines cognitive-behavioral interventions with Eastern contemplative practice and shares common elements with psychodynamic, client-centered, Gestalt, paradoxical and strategic approaches.
- DBT is the first empirically supported psychosocial treatment for chronically parasuicidal adult women diagnosed with borderline personality disorder. At this point, seven randomized controlled trials have supported the efficacy of DBT, including studies in other patient populations (e.g., substance abusers) for whom DBT has been adapted.
- Dialectical philosophy provides the theoretical foundation for many of DBTs treatment strategies:
  - Reality is seen not as one absolute truth, but as a system that must take into account many apparently contradictory realities, and that is continually evolving.
  - The multiple tensions and contradictions that emerge during the treatment of patients with BPD, many of whom are chronically suicidal, are referred to as "dialectics," or "dialectical dilemmas."
- DBT's "Assumptions About Borderline Patients" provide an example of the dialectical approach to reality. One of the important assumptions outlined by Linehan is that, "patients are doing the best that they can"; however, another basic assumption is that, "patients need to do better, try harder, and be more motivated to change." Although seemingly contradictory, both assumptions are seen as reflecting important truths, and a successful (and "dialectical") approach must accept the validity of both statements, and must eventually include both to yield an effective clinical approach. DBT focuses on finding the middle path or synthesis to theses dilemmas or as is sometimes described, "the middle path."

How illness is viewed

A combination of early and chronic exposure to an, "invalidating environment" and currently poorly understood biological factors leaves some individuals with abnormal emotional reactions to life events and interpersonal crises. They also lack the effective skills to cope with their own emotional responses (less "emotional regulation") and a habitual pattern of maladaptive behaviors (e.g., self-harm).

An invalidating environment is understood as one which:
- Indiscriminately rejects communication of private experiences and self-generated behaviors.
- Punishes emotional displays and intermittently reinforces emotional escalation.
- Oversimplifies ease of problem solving and meeting goals.

Techniques

Hierarchical view of treatment targets

- Target I: Reduction in life- threatening behaviors. This category includes any self-injurious behavior (SIB) or suicidal attempt with or without the intent to die.
- Target II: Reduction in therapy-interfering behaviors. This category includes any behavior from the patient and/or therapist that interferes with treatment, such as being late for a session, not completing homework, not calling for phone coaching etc.
- Target III: Reduction in quality-of-life interfering behaviors. This category includes interpersonal conflicts, financial difficulties, Axis I pathology, and anything not targeted on the two previous categories.

Cognitive and behavioral methods

Person of and relationship with, the therapist seen as the main "reinforcer" of adaptive behavior and in-therapy analysis of maladaptive behavior seen as aversive.

DBT involves a variety of approaches: individual therapy group skills training (emotional understanding, tolerance of distress, Eastern meditation techniques), availability of the therapist for telephone contact between appointments.

Key techniques include

- Validation (recognizing distress and behaviors as legitimate and understandable but ultimately harmful).
- Problem solving (agreeing with patient that there is a more appropriate approach, given all the evidence).

Phases of treatment

Assessment orientation and commitment to therapy

Commitment to therapy for specific period. Aim at reduction of SIB and suicidal behaviors. Specific attention to those behaviors, which inhibit successful therapy. Attendance at other therapies as directed.

- Stage 1: Focuses on suicide and SIB prevention with recording of episodes, exploration of internal and external antecedents. Weekly DBT skills group introduces basic skills (e.g., "mindfulness training," focusing on the "here and now," and learning to tolerate aversive states). SIB may be viewed as understandable in the context of the patient's current situation but the therapist always argues on the side of life and ways of making it more tolerable.
- Stage 2: Focuses on emotional processing of previous traumatic experiences. Underlying historical causes of dysfunction. Memories of abuse. Flashbacks. Exposure and distress tolerance techniques.
- Stage 3: Aims to develop self-esteem and establish future goals. Self-esteem and adaptive behaviors are individual agreed goals.

Motivational interviewing

Motivational interviewing (MI), which evolved from Dr William Miller's experience with the treatment of problem drinkers, later elaborated, by Dr Rollnick and Dr Miller, is defined as a patient-centered approach that has been gathering increased interest not just in the field of addiction but also in the field of general psychiatry and behavioral medicine. MI is described by Miller and Rollnick as "a particular way to help people recognize and do something about their present and potential problems." MI is a blend of principles drawn from motivational psychology, Rogerian therapy, and the stages of change model of recovery, built upon the assumption that motivation is a behavior and a state of readiness for change rather than a personality trait, which has long been the traditional view. While MI is patient centered in that it focuses on what the patients wants, thinks, and feels, and it is the patient that does most of the talking there is a "meeting between experts." MI differs from other patient-centered approaches in that it is directive. This means that there is a clear goal of exploring and resolving the patient's ambivalence about the behavior change. Interviewing in MI means "looking together."

Rationale and theoretical basis

The conceptualization of motivation as a state that is open to change is in major contrast to traditional approaches that view motivation as an attribute to personality, and denial and resistance as something to be dealt with through confrontation and high demand. In fact, to a significant extent, motivation for change is transactional, reflected in and affected by interpersonal interaction. Adopting an aggressive and confrontational approach is likely to produce defensive responses from patients such as arguing and interrupting, which may then be interpreted by the therapist as denial or resistance, thus creating a "self-fulfilling prophecy." Motivation and instigation to change often emerge in the context of an empathic interpersonal communication. The transtheoretical model of change provides a framework for understanding the change process and MI provides a means of facilitating this change process. MI aims to alter how the patient sees, feels, and means to respond to the problematic behavior. Ambivalence is at the center of this. Ambivalence is conceptualized as a principal obstacle and MI focuses on helping the patient to make decisions about and commit to change. Once the patient has made this commitment, change often proceeds swiftly without further interventions.

Principles and techniques

Rollnick and Miller distinguish between the "spirit" of MI and the specific MI techniques. Within the spirit of MI, readiness to change is seen as a result of the interpersonal interaction and change comes from within rather than being imposed. Therefore, it is the patient's task to articulate and resolve his or her own ambivalence and the therapist's role is to facilitate the understanding of ambivalence and eventually its resolution. The four principles of MI are the following:

- Express empathy: An empathic style is fundamental to MI. The attitude must be one of acceptance and belief that ambivalence is normal.
- Develop discrepancy: The therapist highlights discrepancy between the patient's present situation and where he/she would want to be.
- Roll with resistance: The therapist never hits the resistance head on but merely shifts approach.
- Support self-efficacy: The therapist supports the patient's belief in his or her ability to make a change. In this way, the patient is seen as a valuable resource in finding solutions to problems.

Typically, the MI therapist uses a variety of techniques to help increase intrinsic motivation for change, and these techniques are divided into two categories: microskills and strategies.

Microskills function to initiate and facilitate the engagement process. They include: open-ended questioning, reflective listening, using affirmations, and summarizing the patient's statements in a balanced way. The use of microskills is essential for the creation of a collaborative relationship.

The strategies involve increasingly directive techniques for building intrinsic motivation for change. The therapist may construct decisional balance matrices to elicit the patient's perceptions of the costs and benefits of status quo or change. The strategies help the patient move from a position of establishing his or her motivation for change to strengthening his or her commitment to attempt the change.

Phases of treatment

MI is typically offered in one to four sessions. MI in its various forms including adaptations has been applied both as a stand-alone intervention and as a preparation for treatment in a range of settings. This includes health setting such as the general hospital ward, emergency department, and general medical practice. Phase 1 is about building motivation for change and its goal is to resolve ambivalence and to build motivation for change. Phase 2 involves strengthening commitment to change and developing a plan to accomplish it.

Applications of MI

- Substance use disorders.
- Co-occurring disorders.
- Medication and treatment adherence.
- Criminal justice populations.
- Behavioral medicine.
- HIV risk behavior.
- Eating disorders and obesity.
- Health promotion.

Efficacy

Many studies reporting on the outcome of MI particularly in the area of alcohol abuse have made attempts to ensure that therapists adhere to the intervention protocol by evaluating the therapist's behavior as well as the patient's outcome. The greatest support for the efficacy of MI comes from the treatment of problem drinkers and from smoking cessation studies.

Phases of MI

Phase 1: Building motivation for change
- Importance of change.
- Microskills.
- Eliciting change talk.
- Enhancing confidence.
- Ambivalence diminishes but does not usually disappear.

Phase 2: Strengthening commitment to change
- Recognizing readiness for change.
- Negotiating a change plan.
- Transition into action-focused counseling.

Recommended further reading

Miller, W.R. and Rollnick, S. *Motivational Interviewing: Preparing People for Change*, 2nd ed.. New York: The Guilford Press, 2000.

Family therapy

Family therapy (FT) is a form of psychotherapy that evolved over the last 50 years and was "created" by several different psychotherapists. For that reason, several "schools" of FT exist today, each of which differs regarding how the initial sessions are run and how much control is expected from the family therapist. All forms of FT share the belief that the family environment is closely linked to the existence and expression of psychopathology within families. Another central assumption of FT is that healthy families are able to tolerate changes over the years and adapt because they communicate clearly and honestly. FT's main goal is to bring families closer to this state of healthy self-regulation. FT can use techniques and concepts derived from other forms of psychotherapy (psychodynamic, cognitive, behavioral, etc.). It is frequently combined with parent management training (📖 p. 1029).

Indications

FT can be used as the main treatment for several psychiatric diagnoses (oppositional defiant disorder, parent child relational disorder, adjustment disorders in children and adolescents) or combined with other forms of treatment (for attention-deficit hyperactivity disorder [ADHD] and anxiety disorders, combined with medication when necessary).

Techniques

• Reframing. The family therapist rewords what family member says, stressing a point (usually the positive aspect) of the family member's relationship.
• Help the family to see the rules that govern family relationships—explicit rules are harder to follow.
• The family therapist may suggest a family member to behave differently or perhaps even to continue a certain behavior (this can have a paradoxical effect and lead to behavioral changes).
• Techniques derived from group therapy: psychodrama etc.
• Prescribed homework at the end of the sessions: family members are instructed to either observe a specific way they communicate or behave and/or to experiment with a new way of interacting.

Duration

Extremely varied. Treatment can be as short as 1 or 2 sessions or take 12–24 weekly sessions or more. It is usually shorter than forms of long-term psychotherapy like psychodynamic psychotherapy.

Parent management training

Parent management training (PMT) has, until very recently, been described as a group of treatment procedures in which parents are trained to modify their child's behavior. More recent definitions of PMT encompass its broader power in improving the communication within families. PMT is not simply about generically changing a child's behavior, which is achieved mostly by improving the quality of communication within the family. More importantly PMT helps foster meaningful mutual understanding within the families, and helps create an environment that fosters healthier psychological development for children.

The treatment is conducted primarily with the parents (both parents when possible, but it can be conducted only with one parent or caregiver). PMT can be offered as its own therapeutic intervention, as one component of family therapy, or can be combined with pharmacological treatments (as in the case of children with ADHD). Significantly, the therapist works only with the parents, and therefore all the changes in a child's behaviors are mediated by the changes in the ways that parents/caregivers communicate with their children. Typically PMT is offered in 8–25 weekly sessions. It can be offered in very different settings—from school meetings to pediatricians offices, or can even be integrated into psychiatric practice. The main goal of PMT is to help parents promote prosocial behaviors and decrease deviant behavior for their children. To accomplish that, the parents are trained to identify and conceptualize their children's problem behaviors in new ways. Hands-on practices/rehearsals are typically part of the training.

Parents are taught to use positive reinforcement contingently, frequently and immediately when children demonstrate "good" behaviors. Mild punishment can also be used, but harsh or severe punishments are usually discouraged.

PMT is the main component of the treatment of children with oppositional behavior disorder. It is helpful in the treatment of ADHD. It has been recognized more recently to also be very helpful in the treatment of children with anxiety disorders. Its preventive potential has also been demonstrated, as PMT decrease the chance of children evolving with delinquent and antisocial behaviors when their parents receive the intervention.

Cross-cultural psychiatry

Introduction

Currently, multitudes of people live in the United States, bringing more diversity with each day. Hispanics and African Americans each account for about 12% of those who reside in the United States. Asians comprise 3.3% and 2.3% are Native Indian, Alaska Native, Pacific Islanders, and those of two or more races (U.S. Census Bureau). It is projected that by 2050, roughly 50% of the American population will be non-Hispanic White while Hispanics will amount to about 24.4%, African Americans comprising 14.6%, Asians 8.0%, and Native American, Alaska Native, Pacific Islanders, and those of two or more races amounting to 5.3% (U.S. Census Bureau). America is quickly becoming more diverse.

Not only does ethnic and racial diversity exist but so does diversity in gender, sexual preference, geographic location, age, occupation, marital status, socioeconomic status, education, migration history, and religious and spiritual affiliation. While this country has thrived on the variety of peoples that inhabit it, mental health care providers have a particularly challenging role of providing care that is culturally competent. The issue of culturally competent care is so important that in 2001, the Office of the Surgeon General released in a supplement to the Report on Mental Health entitled, "Mental Health: Culture, Race, and Ethnicity" discussing the growing crisis of inadequate mental health services for the country's ethnic minorities.[1] When compared to Whites, minorities have less access to and availability of mental health services. They are less likely to receive services and when they do receive services, those services are likely of poorer quality. Minorities are also underrepresented in mental health research.

In order better to understand cultural psychiatry, it is important to understand some basic definitions. Culturally bound syndromes are defined in a separate section at the end of this chapter.

Culture

Culture is defined as a set of meanings, behavioral norms, and values used by members of a particular society as they construct their unique view of the world. These values or reference points include areas such as social relationships, language, nonverbal expression of thoughts and emotions, religious beliefs, moral thought, technology, and financial philosophy. Culture is not a static notion but one that changes as it is taught by one generation to the next.[2]

Race

Used to refer to a group of people who supposedly share similar physiologic, biologic, and genetic underpinnings[2] (e.g., African, Caucasian).

---

1 http://www.surgeongeneral.gov/library/mentalhealth/cre/execsummary-2.html
2 Group for the Advancement of Psychiatry: *Cultural Assessment in Clinical Psychiatry*. Washington, DC: American Psychiatric Publishing, 2002.

Ethnicity

Subjective sense of belonging to a group of people with a common origin and with shared social and cultural beliefs and practices.[2] These people share a common history and origin. It may imply nationality, geographic location, and religious beliefs (e.g., Vietnamese American, Russian Jewish, and Ethiopian).[3]

Cultural psychiatry

The discipline that deals with the description, definition, assessment, and management of all psychiatric conditions with respected to the influence of cultural factors in a bio-psycho-social context while using concepts and instruments from social and biological sciences to advance a full understanding of psychopathology and its treatment.[2]

In order to better evaluate the effect that culture has on a patient and their illness. Caregivers need to have more than a rudimentary understanding of the patient's culture; it is vital to recognize the role patients feel they play within their cultures and the role of culture in their lives. The Cultural Formulation is a tool, found in the DSM-IV-TR. It identifies five major areas that are crucial in evaluating the cultural influences on mental health. More details about the Cultural Formulation are provided later in this chapter.

It is also imperative is to know and understand cultural bound syndromes. unlike DSM diagnoses that can be found worldwide, such syndromes are usually specific to different localities or ethnic groups. Such culturally bound syndromes may or may not correspond to diagnostic categories in the DSM-IV-TR. It is important to know such syndromes in order for clinicians to make a culturally appropriate diagnosis. The DSM lists several of these syndromes, many of which can be found in the glossary at the end of this chapter.

3 Ton, H. and Lim, R.F. "The Assessment of Culturally Diverse Individuals." *Clinical Manual of Cultural Psychiatry*. Washington, DC: APPI, 2006.

Incorporating cultural competency into the psychiatric assessment

- Do not assume anything about the patients' cultural identities.[1]
- Use an interpreter—clinicians should use a non-family interpreter if the language is not the clinician's native language. This includes sign language.

Many nuances of speech and culture within speech (e.g., slang words) can be missed, and such nuances are important to understanding the complete patient, especially in psychiatry. As such, all efforts must be undertaken to find an appropriate interpreter. The following web sites can be useful in obtaining an interpreter:

- languagefon.com
- certifiedlanguages.com
- 1-800-translate.com
- languageline.com

In urgent situations, however, a family member could be utilized for interpretation as a last resort. Please be aware that patients may not be able to discuss their issues openly because the problems may be too traumatic or embarrassing to discuss with any translator present or there may be fear of repercussions if the interpreter is a known or unknown perpetrator of domestic violence.

Consider the culture

- Elicit/encourage patients to describe what part of identity is important to them while explaining your own perspectives of illness.
- Assess symptoms that patients are comfortable expressing to create initial rapport. For examples, in many cultures, patients may be more comfortable expressing somatic complaints than psychiatric complaints.
- In order to better understand the cultural context of the patient's illness, one can ask, "How would your friends, family, community, or those who know you best (and/or are most like you) explain what is happening?"
- Always inquire about the patient's previous and current level of functioning.

---

1 Caraballo, A., Hamid, H., Lee, J.R., McQuery, J., Rho, Y., Kramer, E.J., Lim, R.F., & Lu, F. "A Resident's Guide to the Cultural Formulation": *Clinical Manual of Cultural Psychiatry*. Washington, DC: APPI, 2006.

Cultural formulation of psychiatric disorders[1]

Cultural identity
- Ethnic or cultural reference group (including sexual orientation, socioeconomic status, religion, relationship status, age).
- Degree of involvement in culture of origin.
- Degree of involvement in host culture.
- Aspects of identity that are important to them.
- Migration history (if applicable)—reasons for migration, losses, trauma, and previous role within family and society.
- Language abilities, use and preferences.

Cultural explanation of the individual's illness
- Predominant idioms of distress.
- Meaning of perceived severity of symptoms in relation to social norms.
- Perceived causes or explanatory models to explain illness—how would family/friend/community/those who know you best and/or are most like you explain what is occurring.
- Current preferences for and past experiences of professional care.

Cultural factors related to psychosocial, environmental and functionality factors
- Social stressors.
- Social supports—role of religion and kin networks, identify who is a major support for the patient.
- Levels of functioning and disability—viewed by patient, family and community (previous and current).
- Environment level of acceptance, respect felt in this country by patient and family, special/sacred places, if a community that he/she can identify with has been found (and if it is important for the patient to find one).

Cultural elements of the relationship between the individual and the clinician
- Examined culture, social status, differences, languages.
- Maintain ongoing assessment.
- Beware of transference and counter-transference issues.
- Consider the patient's motivation for seeking treatment.
- Consider need for cultural consultation.

Overall cultural assessment for diagnosis and care
- Assess cultural considerations and its influence on comprehensive diagnosis and care.

---

1 Cultural Formulation compiled from the following sources: *DSM IV-TR*, *Clinical Manual of Cultural Psychiatry*, and Group for the Advancement of Psychiatry: *Cultural Assessment in Clinical Psychiatry*.

Cultural context and the presentation of psychiatric disorders

Schizophrenia

Some apparently psychotic experiences may be normal when viewed within a cultural context. This applies to delusions (e.g., belief in magic, spirits, or demons) and hallucinations (e.g., seeing "auras," or divine entities, hearing God's voice). Other evidence of apparent psychosis, such as disorganized speech, may actually reflect local variations in language syntax, or the fact that the person is not completely fluent in the language used by the interviewer. Differences in nonverbal communication (e.g., eye contact, facial expression, body language) may also be misinterpreted (what is expected in one culture may be rude in another culture). Historically there has been a tendency in the United States and United Kingdom to diagnose schizophrenia more readily in certain cultural groups (e.g., Afro-Caribbeans). It has been argued by some that this does not reflect differences in the incidence of schizophrenia, but rather a lack of understanding of cultural differences. Some symptoms of schizophrenia (e.g., catatonia) are more common in non-Western countries, and even among Western countries the diagnosis of brief psychoses varies (e.g., for boufée deliriante- see 📖 p. 1040).

Mania

Often used colloquially to mean "changes in normal behavior," rather than its DSM definition. It may be difficult to distinguish periods of frenzied activity (e.g., in amok—see 📖 p. 1040) from increased activity, energy, and reduced need for sleep in a manic episode.

Depression

Cultural expressions of depressive symptoms vary across populations. In some cultures there is greater emphasis on somatic terms e.g., "nerves" or "headaches" (Mediterranean cultures); "problems of the heart" (Middle East); "imbalance," "weakness," or "tiredness" (China and Asia). This often makes the use of Western diagnostic classifications difficult, as symptoms may cross diagnostic boundaries (e.g., mood, anxiety, somatoform disorders). Equally difficult may be the interpretation of culturally normal explanations for symptom causation—which may appear delusional (e.g., spirit possession), or associated somatic symptoms that need to be distinguished from actual hallucinations.

Anxiety and stress-related disorders

Agoraphobia

Social sanctions against members of certain populations (e.g., women) appearing in public may be confused with agoraphobic symptoms.

Panic attacks

In some cultures these may be interpreted as evidence of magic or witchcraft (particularly when they come "out of the blue").

OCD

Religious and cultural beliefs influence the content of obsessions and nature of compulsions. It may be difficult to assess the significance of ritualistic behaviors unless the clinician has knowledge of cultural customs.

PTSD

Immigrants may have emigrated to escape military conflict or particularly harsh regimes. They may have experienced significant traumatic events, but may be unwilling (or unable) to discuss them because of language problems or fears of being sent back.

Somatization disorder

Common types of somatic symptoms vary across cultures (and genders within cultures). These reflect the principal concerns of the population (or individual) e.g., worms/insects in the scalp/under the skin—seen in South-East Asia and Africa; concern about semen loss—seen in India (see Dhat) and China (see Shenkui).

Conversion and dissociative disorders

More common in rural populations and "less educated" societies, and may be culturally normal. Certain religious rituals involve alteration in consciousness (including trance states), beliefs in spirit possession, and varieties of socially sanctioned behaviors that could be viewed as conversion or dissociative disorders (e.g., falling out, spell, zar). "Running" subtypes of culture-bound syndromes have symptoms that would meet criteria for dissociative fugue.

Anorexia nervosa

Cultural influences that promote thinness as the ideal of body shape are more prevalent in Western societies with an abundance of food. Immigrants from other cultural backgrounds may assimilate this ideal, or may present with primary symptoms other than disturbed body image and fear of weight gain (e.g., stomach pains, lack of enjoyment of food).

Alcohol and substance misuse

Cultural factors heavily influence the availability, patterns of use, attitudes about, and even the physiological or behavioral effects of alcohol and other substances.

Alcohol

Social, family, and religious attitudes toward the use of alcohol may all influence patterns of use and the likelihood of developing alcohol-related problems. Although it is difficult to separate cause from effect, low levels of education, unemployment, and low social status are all associated with increased misuse of alcohol. In some populations (e.g., Japanese and Chinese) up to 50% may have a deficiency of aldehyde dehydrogenase (complete absence in 10%), with low rates of alcohol problems in these populations because the physiological effects of consuming alcohol may be extremely unpleasant (e.g., flushing and palpitations due to accumulation of acetylaldehyde). How individuals behave when intoxicated may also be culturally determined, e.g., aggressive and antisocial behavior (typified by "soccer hooligans") not seen in cultures where alcohol is more of a "social lubricant," despite levels of alcohol consumption being similar.

Other substances

Use of hallucinogens and other drugs may be culturally acceptable when used as part of religious rituals (e.g., peyote in the Native American Church, cannabis in Rastafarianism). Equally, secular movements, typified by the hippie movements of the 1960s and 1970s, or more recently the dance or rave culture, provide a context in which psychedelic experiences (e.g., induced by LSD or MDMA) may be experienced without any adverse social sanctions.

Culture-bound syndromes

Culture-bound or culture-specific syndromes cover an extensive range of disorders occurring in particular localities or ethnic groups. The behavioral manifestations or subjective experiences particular to these disorders may or may not correspond to diagnostic categories in DSM-IV-TR or ICD-10. They are usually considered to be illnesses and generally have local names. They also include culturally accepted idioms or explanatory mechanisms of illness that differ from Western idioms and outside of their cultural setting may be mistaken for psychiatric symptoms. Awareness of culture-bound syndromes is important to allow psychiatrists and physicians to make culturally appropriate diagnoses.

Amafufunyane

See ufufunyane below.

Amok

[Malaysia, Laos, Philippines, Polynesia (cafard or cathard), Papua New Guinea, and Puerto Rico (mal de pelea), United States (going postal), and among the Navajo (iich'aa)].

Amok is the Malayan word meaning "to engage furiously in battle" and is typically prevalent only in males. It is often precipitated by a perceived slight or insult, which is followed by a sudden outburst of wild rage causing the person to run madly about with a weapon and attack or kill people and animals before being overpowered and sometimes committing suicide. Often preceded by a period of preoccupation, brooding, and mild depression. Afterwards, the person feels exhausted and amnesic. He/she eventually returns to the premorbid state. An attack can last for a few hours, and it may be attributed to magical possession by demons and evil spirits. Some instances of amok may occur during a brief psychotic episode or constitute the onset or an exacerbation of a chronic psychotic process.

Bilis and cólera

(also referred to as muina—Latino Groups).

Underlying cause of these syndromes is thought to be strongly experienced anger or rage (bilis and cólera literally translate as "bile"). Anger is viewed among many Latino groups as a particularly powerful emotion that can have direct effects on the body and can exacerbate existing symptoms. The major effects of anger are the disturbance of core body balances (which are understood as a balance between hot and cold valences in the body and between the material and spiritual aspects of the body). Syndromes can include acute nervous tension, headache, trembling, screaming, stomach disturbances, and, in more severe cases, loss of consciousness. Chronic fatigue may result from acute episode.

Bouffée deliriante

(West Africa and Haiti).

This French term refers to a sudden outburst of agitated and aggressive behavior, marked confusion, and psychomotor excitement. It may sometimes be accompanied by visual and auditory hallucinations or paranoid ideation. These episodes may resemble an episode of brief psychotic disorder.

Curanderismo

(Mexican Americans and other Spanish-speaking people).

Folk medicine in which the healers (curanderos [male] or curannderas [female] use a combination of herbal infusions, dramatic healing rituals, and prayers to treat a variety of physical and psychological symptoms including embrujo (witchcraft), empacho (intestinal distress), mal ojo (evil eye), mal puesto (hexing), mollera caída, (sunken fontanel, see 📖 *p. 1040*) and susto (soul loss, see 📖 *p. 1044*).

Dhat

(India, also jiryan), Sri Lanka (sukra prameha), and China (shen-k'uei).

A folk diagnostic term used to refer to severe anxiety and hypochondriacal concerns associated with the discharge of semen, whitish discoloration of the urine, and feeling of weakness and exhaustion. Traditional remedies consist of herbal tonics to restore semen/humoral balance.

Falling out/blacking out

(Southern United States and Caribbean groups).

Episodes are preceded by feelings of dizziness or "swimming" in the head and characterized by an individual's eyes being open but the person claims an inability to see. The person usually hears and understands what is occurring around him/her but feel powerless to move. This may correspond to a diagnosis of conversion disorder or a dissociative disorder.

Ghost sickness

(Native Americans).

A preoccupation with death and the deceased (sometimes associated with witchcraft) frequently observed among members of many Native American tribes. Various symptoms can be attributed to ghost sickness, including bad dreams, weakness, feelings of danger, loss of appetite, fainting, dizziness, fear, anxiety, hallucinations, loss of consciousness, confusion, feeling of futility, and a sense of suffocation. May be triggered by a death and afflicted individuals feel that the ghost of a dead person is torturing them.

Hwa-byung

(also known as wool-hwa-byung; in Korea as "anger syndrome").

Attributed to the suppression of anger. Symptoms include insomnia, fatigue, panic, fear of impending death, dysphoric affect, indigestion, anorexia, dyspnea, palpitations, generalized aches and pains, and a feeling of a mass in the epigastrium. The belief is related to ideas of bodily imbalances caused by anger.

Koro

[possible Malaysian origin, Chinese (shuk yang, shook yong, & suo yang), Assam (jinjinia bemar), and Thailand (rok-joo)].

Refers to an episode of sudden and intense anxiety such that the penis (or, in females, the vulva and nipples) will recede into the body and possibly cause death. Usually occurs in young, single males. Prodromal depersonalization usually occurs and elaborate measure may be taken to prevent the genitals from retracting (e.g., grasping of genitals, splints or other devices, herbal remedies, or fellatio). Precipitants may include coitus, cold exposure, fears concerning sexual virility, tales of people dying from the illness, and eating spoiled food. Koro at times occurs in localized epidemic forms in East Asian areas. This diagnosis is included in the Chinese Classification of Mental Disorders, Second Edition.

Lata, latah

[Malay, Siberian groups (amurakh, irkunii, ikota, olan, myriachit, and menketi), Thailand (bah tschi & baah-ji), Ainu, Sakhlin, Japan (imu), and Philippines (mali-mali & silok).]

In Malaysia, it presents more frequently in middle-aged women. The syndrome includes hypersensitivity to fright, often with echopraxia, echolalia, command obedience, and dissociative or trancelike behavior. It is caused by a sudden stimulus that suspends all normal activity. It may be a symptom of disease (e.g., acute psychosis, conversion/dissociative state) or be an isolated behavioral abnormality.

Locura

(Latinos in United States & South America).

Used to refer to a severe form of chronic psychosis. The syndrome is attributed to an inherited vulnerability, to the effect of multiple life difficulties, or to a combination of both factors. Symptoms exhibited by person with locura include incoherence, agitation, auditory and visual hallucinations, inability to follow rules of social interactions, unpredictability and possible violence.

Mollera caída, "fallen fontanel syndrome"

(Latino populations in the Americas).

Seen in infants less than one year old. Signs of the illness were listlessness, fever, diarrhea, and sunken eyes and were actually thought to be secondary to the depressed fontanel. In fact the depressed fontanel usually resulted from infection or malnutrition. The illness was cured by curanderismo with herbs, teas, and pastes.

Nerfiza, nerves, nervios

(Latino populations in United States, Latin America, Egypt, Northern Europe) (Similar to nevra in Greece).

Chronic somatic, emotional, and behavioral symptoms (e.g., headache, sleep problems, reduced appetite, nausea, fatigue, dizziness, paraesthesia, anxiety, concentration difficulties, and emotional lability/distress). More common in women, associated with anger, emotional distress, low self-esteem. Usually treated with traditional herbal teas, "nerve pills," rest, isolation, and increased family support.

Piblokto, pibloktoq

(Polar Eskimo women) "Arctic hysteria."

An acute dissociative state (lasting about 30 min.) following the actual (or symbolic) loss of someone or something important to the individual. Usually mild irritability or withdrawal precedes impulsive or dangerous acts (e.g., screaming, tearing off of clothes, breaking furniture, shouting obscenities, eating feces, or rushing out into the snow). May be followed by convulsions and coma (lasting up to 12 hours) with associated amnesia. Although some researchers have suggested it may be due to hypocalcaemia and tetany, it is most probably an anxiety state.

Qi-gong psychotic reaction

(China) "Exercise of vital energy."

An acute episode characterized by dissociative, paranoid, or other symptoms after participation in the health-enhancing practice of qi-gong.

Rootwork

(Haiti and Sub-Saharan Africa) associated syndromes: voodoo death (Haiti), mal puesto or brujeira (Latin America), and hex.

A variety of complaints attributed to hexing, witchcraft, sorcery, voodoo, or the evil influence of another person. Symptoms include anxiety, GI complaints, and fear of being poisoned or killed. Can result in death.

Sangue dormido, "sleeping blood"

(Cape Verde Islanders).

Somatic symptoms including pain, numbness, tremor, paralysis, convulsions, blindness, and increased risk of heart attack, infection, and miscarriage.

Shenjing shuairuo

(China) or neurasthenia.

Symptoms include: fatigue, irritability, poor concentration/memory, sleep disturbance, and other somatic symptoms (dizziness, headaches, pain, GI upset, sexual dysfunction, and other signs of autonomic dysfunction). Most cases would meet criteria for depressive or anxiety disorders.

Shen-k'uei (Taiwan), shenkui (China)

Similar to dhat and jiryan (India), and sukra prameha (Sri Lanka.).

Anxiety and panic with somatic complaints, especially sexual dysfunction (premature ejaculation and impotence). Symptoms are attributed to excessive semen loss from sexual activity or "white turbid urine," which reduces "vital energy." It is viewed as a life-threatening condition and described in areas with a Chinese ethnic population.

Shin-byung

(Korea).

Possession (dissociative) state attributed to ancestral spirits with associated anxiety/fear and somatic complaints (generalized weakness, dizziness, insomnia, loss of appetite, and GI problems).

Shinkeishitsu

(Japan).

A syndrome that is manifested by obsessions, perfectionism, ambivalence, social withdrawal, fatigue, and hypochondriasis.

Spell

(Southern United States).

A trance state in which individuals "communicate" with deceased relatives or with spirits, often accompanied by brief periods of personality change. In context, "spells" are culturally normal.

Susto, espanto, "magic fright"

(Peru) (See curanderismo who treat this condition).

Also seen in Latinos of the United States, Mexico, and other Central/South America. Related syndromes: lanti (Philippines), malgri (Aborigines of Australia), mogo laya (New Guinea), narahati (Iran), and saladera (in regions around the Amazon). Fright or fear of loss of soul. An acute anxiety state, seen in children and adolescents but also adults, usually following an acute stressor or violent (often supernatural) fright. Symptoms can occur days to years after an event. Symptoms: by anxiety, agitation, lack of motivation or interest, sleep disturbance, changes in appetite, other somatic symptoms, and a belief that the soul has been, or will be, stolen from the body.

Tabanka

(Trinidad).

Depression associated with a high rate of suicide that is seen in men abandoned by their wives.

Taijin kyofusho

(Japan).

Intense fear and guilt that one's appearance or behaviors displease, embarrass, or are offensive to others. Prominent in younger people and similar to the Western concept of social phobia.

Ufufuyane (singular), Amafufunyane (plural), saka

(Kenya, Southern Africa; Bantu, Zulu; and affiliated groups) May be related to aluro (Nigeria), phii pob (Thailand), and zar (Egypt, Ethiopia, Sudan).

Anxiety state attributed to the effects of magical potions (given to them by rejected lovers) or spirit possession, with characteristic sobbing, repeated neologisms, paralysis, trance-like states, or loss of consciousness. Seen in young, unmarried women, who may also experience nightmares with sexual themes, and rarely episodes of temporary blindness.

Zar

(East and North Africa, the Middle East e.g., Ethiopia, Somalia, Sudan, Egypt, and Iran), Somalian women (Sar).

Dissociative symptoms including shouting, laughing, head banging, singing, weeping, and other demonstrative behaviors. The person believes they are possessed by a spirit, and may develop a long-term relationship with the spirit. Other symptoms may include apathy, withdrawal, refusal to eat, and refusal to carry out tasks of daily living. Such behavior may be regarded as culturally normal.

Recommended further reading

American Psychiatric Association (APA). *Diagnostic and Statistical Manual of Mental Disorders*, 4th ed., Text Revision. Washington, DC: APA, 2000.
Group for the Advancement of Psychiatry: *Cultural Assessment in Clinical Psychiatry*. Washington, DC: American Psychiatry Publishing, 2002.

Therapeutic issues

Medication adherence

Is adherence important?

- It has been estimated that only one-third of patients prescribed medication actually adhere to the treatment plan (this applies to all medical problems, not just psychiatric problems) and that around 80% of psychiatric admissions relate to medication nonadherence. Adherence is a particular problem when the illness runs a chronic course and requires the patient to be on medication for life (e.g., diabetes, ischemic heart disease [IHD], pulmonary disease, schizophrenia).
- Patients with schizophrenia who comply with a sufficient dosage of antipsychotic medication have only about one-fifth the risk of relapse compared to patients who do not take their medication.
- There is good evidence that prophylactic lithium treatment of bipolar disorder reduces the likelihood of (particularly manic) relapse, as well as the risk of suicide.
- Continuation of antidepressant treatment for at least six months after symptom resolution significantly reduces the risk of further depressive episodes in unipolar depression.

Reasons for nonadherence

It is important to realize that the patient may have understandable reasons for being reluctant to take prescribed medication. Uncovering these reasons may help in negotiation and developing strategies to improve the situation.

- Continued symptoms of the underlying disorder (e.g., delusions, amotivation, impaired insight, disorganization) or co-morbid disorders (e.g., substance use).
- Negative feelings about being on medication.
- Stigma associated with taking medication.
- Side-effects.
- Forgetting (i.e., due to cognitive impairment, disorganized thought process).
- Lack of understanding of medication administration instructions.
- Inability to read.
- Belief that medication is not working
- Improvement in condition resulting in belief that medication is no longer needed.
- Failure to obtain or renew prescription.
- Continued symptoms of the underlying disorder (e.g., delusions, lack of motivation, impaired insight, disorganization) or co-morbid disorders (e.g., substance misuse, personality disorder).

Strategies to improve adherence
Education
- Promote insight and understanding about the illness and the benefits of treatment.
- Provide information about the medication, how to take it, possible side-effects, the length of time needed to see benefits, and the potential problems of suddenly stopping.
- Discuss the reasons for prophylactic or continued treatment, especially when patient is feeling better (i.e., to reduce risk of relapse and improve long term outcome).
- Encourage open discussion with patient of pros and cons of suggested treatment plan.
- Encourage frank discussion about potentially embarrassing issues that may lead to nonadherence (i.e., sexual side-effects).
- Regularly ask about and document side-effects.
- Promote insight and understanding about the illness and the benefits of treatment.

Sensible prescribing
- Simplify drug regimen—use a single dose when available.
- Minimize side-effects by using medication with lowest potential for side-effects and using lowest therapeutic dose.
- If side-effects are problematic, consider a change to an alternative preparation or prescribe additional agents to counter significant problems.
- Rational medication choice based on individual acceptability of side-effects.
- Provide clear communication of any changes in regimen both to patient and primary care team.
- Consider use of depot medication, especially when patient has a history of nonadherence.
- Regularly review the need for continued medication.

Practical measures
- Provide written information to patient, especially when regimen is complex or when change of dose or medication is planned.
- Help patients establish a daily routine for taking medication.
- Use a pillbox.
- Consider contacting the patient's pharmacy for assistance with packaging of medication (i.e., large print instructions, individual dosing packs).
- Supervised administration (i.e., by a relative, at the clinic).
- Active monitoring (i.e., pill count, blood levels).

Weight gain with psychiatric medication

General points

Weight gain is a significant cause of nonadherence with psychiatric medication, and patients often complain about increases in weight, even when clinicians may regard it as "clinically insignificant." Effects on general health, self-esteem, and social embarrassment should not be overlooked.

Antipsychotics

Proposed mechanisms

Sedation (reduced activity), thirst (anticholinergic side-effects), reduced metabolism, fluid retention, endocrine effects (increased prolactin, altered cortisol, altered insulin secretion, peripheral insulin resistance), central antipsychotic-induced leptin resistance (changes in "set-point" weight), and altered neurotransmitters (5-HT$_{2A-C}$ blockade, histamine H1 affinity, D$_2$ blockade, central a1 stimulation, CCK changes) have all been proposed.

Increased risk

Female, young age, low baseline bodyweight, previous pattern of overeating, narcissistic traits, family or personal history of obesity.

Effects of specific agents (see opposite).

Management[1]

- Personal/family history of obesity.
- Warn patient of possibility.
- Baseline weight, height (BMI) and waist circumference; repeat monthly until three months and then quarterly.
- Baseline BP, fasting plasma glucose and lipid profile; repeat at 12 weeks and then yearly.
- Encourage "healthy diet" (involve dietician if necessary), regular physical exercise, avoid high-calorie fluids.
- Use lowest therapeutic dose, introduce medication increases slowly, choose agents with lower weight-gain propensity (see opposite).
- Consider adjunctive prescribing (e.g., clozapine plus Abilify®, to allow lowering of clozapine dose). Metformin, topiramate, orlistat, silbutramine, rimonabant.

Antidepressants

Proposed mechanisms

Reduced metabolism, carbohydrate craving (note; may be a symptom of depression itself), central serotonin and norepinephrine mechanisms in regulating food intake (appetite/satiety).

Effects of specific agents (see opposite).

---

1 Consensus Statement. Consensus development conference on Antipsychotic Drugs and Obesity and Diabetes (2004). *Diabetes Care* **27**(2), 596–600.

Management
- General advice about diet and exercise.
- Use lowest therapeutic dose.
- Consider switching to alternative antidepressant.
- Adjunctive prescribing (e.g., naltrexone, ranitidine at night (may reduce "midnight snacks").

Lithium[2]
Proposed mechanisms
Increased intake of high calorie drinks, hypothyroidism, increased insulin secretion, direct central appetite stimulation, water retention, hormonal changes (higher frequency of weight gain in females).

Management
Counseling and advice about diet and exercise, use of low-calorie drinks, avoidance of salty foods (or adding salt to foods).

Other mood stabilizers
Carbamazepine
Weight gain due to increased appetite.

Valproate
Substantial weight gain, which may be due to central leptin resistance; insulin resistance, hormonal mechanisms.

Topiramate
Slight weight loss.

Weight gain over 10 weeks with antipsychotics

Antipsychotic	Average weight gain (kg)
Pimozide	−2.7
Placebo	−1.0
Trifluoperazine	0.3
Ziprasidone	0.3
Haloperidol	0.5
Polypharmacy	0.5
Loxapine	0.7
Nondrug controls	0.8
Fluphenazine	1.1
Risperidone	1.7
Quetiapine	2.5
Thioridazine	2.8
Thiothixene	2.9
Sertindole	2.9
Chlorpromazine	4.2
Olanzapine	4.2
Clozapine	5.7

Allison and Casey (2001). *J Clin Psychiatry* **62**(suppl 7), 22–31.

2 Baptista, T. (1995). Lithium and body weight gain. *Pharmacopsychiatry* **28**, 35–44.

Weight changes with antidepressants

SSRIs Fluoxetine, sertraline, fluvoxamine, citalopram, escitalopram: no short-term weight change; slight weight gain long-term; paroxetine, moderate weight gain.

TCAs marked weight gain (amitriptyline > imipramine > clomipramine); desipramine, moderate weight gain.

MAOIs/RIMAs Rarely weight gain (selegiline); slight weight gain (moclobemide).

Others mirtazapine, trazodone; marked weight gain; duloxetine, slight weight gain; venlafaxine: no change; buproprion, weight loss.

Hyperprolactinemia with antipsychotics

Description

Secretion of prolactin (PRL) by the pituitary is under inhibitory control via dopamine from the hypothalamus. Blockade of dopamine D_2 receptors by antipsychotics can raise prolactin levels, leading to symptoms of hyperprolactinemia in both men (erectile dysfunction, loss of libido, and hypogonadism) and women (amenorrhea, galactorrhea, gynecomastia, infertility, loss of libido, acne and hirsutism); possible decrease in bone mineral density in both groups.

Differential diagnosis

Physiological pregnancy, stress; *pharmacological* antidepressants, antihypertensives (verapamil), cimetidine, ranitidine, oral contraceptives; Diseases of the pituitary (e.g., prolactin secreting pituitary adenomas) or hypothalamus, severe primary hypothyroidism, liver cirrhosis, end-stage renal disease, stress, high-dose estrogens, chronic cocaine use, opiates.

Investigations

- Check for signs of chest wall irritation (which can promote galactorrhea and raise prolactin) and signs of a sellar mass (including checking visual fields).
- Serum levels of TSH (exclude hypothyroidism), creatinine (exclude renal failure), and PRL (may be raised due to stress, after eating, or postictally).
  Note: patients may be symptomatic even when PRL in the normal range (i.e., it is the relative increase in PRL that matters, not just the absolute increase).
- Consider CT/MRI and/or a referral to endocrinology.

Management

- Exclude other possible etiologies.
- Consider a change of medication to a prolactin-sparing antipsychotic (e.g., clozapine, olanzapine, aripiprazole) or reduction in dose if the patient's mental state is stable (monitor closely).
- If problems persist or medication changes are precluded (or not tolerated), consider referral to endocrinology for consideration of other treatments: hormone replacement, bromocriptine, cabergolide etc.
- Premenopausal women should be advised about resumption of normal menstrual cycle (and return of fertility) when changing antipsychotics, and the use of contraception should be discussed.

Note: asymptomatic hyperprolactinemia does not necessarily warrant (in itself) changes to medication.

Sexual dysfunction and psychiatric medication

The degree of sexual dysfunction experienced by patients taking psychiatric medication may be a major source of distress and a significant reason for nonadherence. Clinicians are notoriously poor at inquiring about these problems, despite reports that patients regard sexual side-effects as the most troublesome of all medication-related problems.

Antidepressants

Rates of sexual dysfunction seen in clinical practice (commonly altered desire, delayed ejaculation and orgasmic dysfunction; in males erectile dysfunction) may be higher than those reported in product information. Clomipramine, SSRIs (paroxetine, sertraline, citalopram, fluoxetine), and venlafaxine appear to be most likely to cause sexual dysfunction of some form (30–60%). Other TCAs show intermediate risk of dysfunction (10–30%). Bupropion and moclobemide appear much less likely to cause problems (≤10%). Mirtazapine appears possibly to have the lowest rates of sexual side-effects.[1] Problems of reduced libido appear to be associated with SSRIs, whereas TCAs tend to cause (more troublesome) difficulties with sexual performance.

Management[2]

- "Watchful waiting"—to see if symptoms subside.
- Dose decrease to find effective dose without side-effects.
- Addition of another agent to counteract the sexual side-effects (combination with e.g., mirtazapine, buspirone, bupropion; or "as required" e.g., sildenafil, tadalafil, yohimbine).
- Switch to another agent known to have fewer adverse sexual effects (e.g., mirtazapine, bupropion).

Antipsychotics

The prevalence of sexual dysfunction associated with antipsychotics medication ranges from 40–70%, with reports of problems in all groups of antipsychotic medication (while antipsychotics often restore sexual functioning, they may impair sexual performance; in males, erectile, ejaculatory; in males and females, orgasmic dysfunction).[3]

- Dysfunction may be related to sedation; dopamine blockade, autonomic side-effects, hyperprolactinemia, serotonergic effects of novel agents.
- The dose of medication, use of anticholinergics, and co-morbid depression and SSRI use are significant associations.
- Thioridazine can cause "dry" or "retrograde" ejaculation (semen may be present in the urine).
- Clozapine and quetiapine seem to have the lowest risk of sexual side-effects.

1 Gregorian, R.S., Golden, K.A., Bahce, A., *et al.* (2002). Antidepressant-induced sexual dysfunction. *Annals of Pharmacotherapy* **36**, 1577–1589.

2 Taylor, M.J., Rudkin, L., Hawton, K. (2005). Strategies for managing antidepressant-induced sexual dysfunction: Systematic review of randomized controlled trials. *J Affective Disorders* **88**, 241–254.

3 Wirshing, D.A., Pierre, J.M., Marder, S.R., *et al.* (2002). Sexual side effects of novel antipsychotic medications. *Schizophrenia Research* **56**, 25–30.

Management
- Dose reduction where possible.
- Reduction or discontinuation of drugs with anticholinergic effects.
- Consider switching to alternative agent (e.g., quetiapine, clozapine, aripiprazole).

Mood stabilizers

Lithium therapy may impair desire and arousal, but does not appear to have a major impact on patient self-satisfaction or subjective sense of pleasure during sexual activity.[4] Although the occurrence of sexual dysfunction is estimated as 10–30%, it is usually mild, not a source of distress, and does not lead to noncompliance.

Carbamazepine and phenytoin both increase prolactin and decrease dehydroepiandrosterone and other adrenal androgen levels, making sexual dysfunction likely.

Valproate inhibits steroid hormone metabolism, predisposes to phenotypic signs of hyperandrogenism-hirsutism, and is associated with sexual dysfunction as well.

4 Aizenberg, D., Sigler, M., Zemishlany, Z., Weizman, A. (1996). Lithium and male sexual function in affective patients. *Clinical Neuropharmacology* **19**, 515–519.

Priapism

Priapism[1] is defined as a sustained, painful erection that cannot be relieved by sexual intercourse or masturbation, and that is frequently unrelated to sexual desire. Stasis of blood for more than several hours leads to increased blood viscosity, deoxygenation, and, ultimately, irreversible fibrosis of tissue. Thus, priapism is a urologic emergency requiring immediate intervention.[2] (Clitoral priapism, although rare, has also been reported.[3])

Trazodone

About 30% of reported cases of priapism are drug-induced, with 80% of those cases involving trazodone. Trazodone-induced priapism is rare, occurring in less than 0.1% of patients taking the drug. It typically is seen within the first month of therapy, occurs in all age groups, and may occur even with low daily doses of 50–100mg.

Other drugs

Antidepressants (phenelzine, SSRIs, buproprion, buspirone), Antipsychotics (haloperidol, clozapine, zuclopenthixol), prazosin, nifedipine, phenytoin, sildenafil, recreational drugs (cocaine, marijuana, ETOH), and intracavernosal injection of vasoactive drugs.

Management

Because trazodone-induced priapism is understood to be due to alpha$_1$-adrenergic blockade, pharmacologic treatment is preferred since it carries no risk of permanent sequelae.

- Patients must be aware of the possibility of priapism when taking trazodone, and treatment must be given quickly to minimize the risk of permanent impotence.
- Priapism is a urologic emergency: Treatment within four hours of occurrence carries best prognosis, otherwise upward of 50% of patients will retain some form of erectile dysfunction.
- Nonsurgical treatment: Evacuation of old blood from the corpora cavernosa, irrigation with α_1-adrenergic agonist. Preferred agent: phenylephrine (the most selective and potent alpha$_1$-adrenergic vasoconstrictor); onset of action less than 1 minute and duration of 7–20 minutes; several intermittent injections of 0.1mg/ml solution may be necessary (continuously monitor BP and HR).
- Surgery: creation of shunt between corpus cavernosum and glans, corpus spongiosum, deep dorsal, or saphenous vein.

---

1 "Priapus," the son of Zeus and Aphrodite, was a god with an enormous penis who symbolized the Earth's fertility.
2 Cherian, J., Rao, A.R., Thwaini, A., Kapasi, F., Shergill, I.S., Samman, R. (2006). Medical and surgical management of priapism. *Postgrad Med J* **82**, 89–94.
3 Patel, A.G., Mukherji, K., Lee, A. (1996). Priapism associated with psychotropic drugs. *British Journal of Hospital Medicine* **55**, 315–319.

Patient counseling

Although rare, priapism is a serious medical emergency that requires immediate intervention. Since most patients would not attribute the prolonged erection to trazodone, patient counseling about its possibility is necessary for all men beginning therapy with the drug. They should be advised to report prolonged or painful erections to their doctor immediately.

Antipsychotic-induced parkinsonism

Description

A frequent adverse effect found in full form in at least 20% of patients treated with antipsychotic medication. Generally occurs within four weeks of treatment and is a major cause of noncompliance. Examination (📖 p. 242) is generally sufficient to detect the onset of symptoms and should be carried out frequently in the first three months of treatment. Monitoring may help establish the minimally effective dose of antipsychotic needed by individual patients, reducing discomfort and improving compliance.

Symptoms/signs

Characterized by resting tremor, rigidity, and bradykinesia; the presentation is similar to that of idiopathic Parkinson's disease (PD; 📖 p. 198), although bradykinesia may be less prominent and symptoms are usually bilateral, but may be asymmetrical.

Pathophysiology

D_2 receptor blockade in the nigrostriatal pathway.

Differential diagnosis

Many drugs have been associated with parkinsonism (see opposite) and some may increase the likelihood of problems (e.g., prednisolone). Other differentials include: idiopathic PD, dementia (e.g., DLB), negative symptoms of schizophrenia, psychomotor retardation (e.g., in depression).

Treatment

Several strategies may be used, including:
- Dose reduction.
- Switching to another antipsychotic agent e.g., olanzapine, quetiapine, clozapine.
- Use of anticholinergic agents (e.g., biperiden, benztropine) or amantadine.

Anticholinergic agents are often used in younger patients. However, older patients may not be able to tolerate the side-effects of blurred vision, dry mouth, constipation, urinary retention, and particularly cognitive impairment. This has led to the use of amantadine, which is better tolerated, or more frequent use of the newer antipsychotics, especially when patients already have early signs of PD.
- When treatment is by depot, there is some evidence that flupenthixol and where available pipothiazine palmitate, or zuclopenthixol decanoate may be better tolerated. Risperidone depot is also available, but also bears a risk of inducing parkinsonian symptoms.

Follow-up

- If anticholinergics have been used, the need for continued treatment ought to be kept under review.
- Their slow withdrawal should be attempted after the acute phase of treatment, or following any lowering of antipsychotic dose, as drug-induced parkinsonism tends to resolve over time and additional medication may no longer be needed.

Drugs reported to cause parkinsonism

- Antidepressants (e.g., SSRIs, MAOIs, TCAs).
- Lithium.
- Anticonvulsants (e.g., carbamazepine, valproate).
- Analgesics (e.g., NSAIDs, opiates).
- Drugs of abuse (e.g., cocaine, PCP).
- Cardiovascular drugs (e.g., amiodarone, diazoxide, diltiazem, methyldopa, nifedipine, tocainide).
- GI drugs (e.g., cimetidine, domperidone, metoclopramide, prochlorperazine).
- Anti-infection drugs (e.g., acyclovir, cephaloridine, chloroquine).
- Respiratory drugs (e.g., antihistamines, salbutamol, terbutaline).
- Hormones (e.g., medroxyprogesterone).
- Cytotoxics (e.g., cyclosporin, interferons).
- Others (e.g., cyclizine, ondansetron, levodopa, tetrabenazine).

Akathisia

Description

Akathisia (Greek, literally "unable to sit") usually occurs in the context of antipsychotic treatment, although SSRIs have also been implicated. It may manifest in acute, chronic, withdrawal-related, or tardive (late-onset) forms. It is an unpleasant, distressing side-effect of medication and may be confused with agitation or worsening of psychiatric symptoms. When it is severe, patients may act aggressively, leading to inappropriate increases in antipsychotic medication. Careful assessment, including detailed history and review of medication, is essential.

Symptoms/signs

Although there is no universally accepted definition of akathisia, the disorder characteristically manifests with:

- A subjective component—a feeling of inner restlessness or tension (with the drive to engage in motor activity, especially lower limbs and trunk); attentional dysfunction, anxiety, discomfort; also, depression, paranoia, impulsivity.[1]
- An objective component—movements: such as pacing constantly; inability to stand, sit, or lie still; rocking; crossing/uncrossing legs.

Pathophysiology

Not yet fully understood. Theories include: dopaminergic/noradrenergic interactions (e.g., inhibition of presynaptic D_2 heteroreceptors on NA nerve terminals, with net increase in NA release), imbalance of dopaminergic/cholinergic transmission (causing compensatory increased norepinephrine [NA] or serotonin [5HT] release), and low serum iron/ferritin.

Epidemiology

Prevalence ranges reported in patients with schizophrenia on older antipsychotic medication are quoted as 41% (mild symptoms), 21% (moderate-severe symptoms), up to 24% (for chronic symptoms (inpatient population)). For newer antipsychotic agents, the reported incidence is up to 6%.

Risk factors

Use of high-dose and/or high-potency antipsychotics, chronic use of antipsychotics, rapid increase/sudden withdrawal of antipsychotics, use of depot intramuscular preparations, history of organic brain disease (e.g., dementia, alcoholism, HIV), history of previous akathisia, concomitant use of predisposing drugs (e.g., SSRIs, calcium-channel antagonists).

Differential diagnosis

Anxiety/agitation (primary or secondary to other psychiatric disorders), other withdrawal/discontinuation syndromes, acute confusional states, encephalitis/meningitis, parkinsonism/dystonia/dyskinesia, serotonin syndrome (early symptoms), toxicity due to other drugs (e.g., recreational drugs—amphetamine, MDMA, cocaine; antidepressants; antihistamines;

---

1 Kim, J-H., Lee, B.C., Park, H-J., Ahn, Y.M., Kang, U.G., Kim, Y.S. (2002). Subjective emotional experience and cognitive impairment in drug-induced akathisia. *Comprehensive Psychiatry* **43**(6), 456–462.

sympathomimetics; salicylate), restless legs syndrome, iron deficiency anemia, endocrine disorders (e.g., thyrotoxicosis, hypo/hyperglycemia, phaeochromocytoma).

Investigations

General blood screen (CBC w/diff, LFTs, 'lytes, glucose, TSH).

Management

- Review history/medication to identify possible causative agent(s).
- Reduce dose or slow increase of potential causative agent.
- If antipsychotic related, consider use of less EPS-prone drug (e.g., olanzapine, quetiapine).
- If symptoms persist, consider specific treatment: first line—propranolol, initially 30mg/d (usual range 30–120mg/d); or pindolol, betaxolol, metoprolol.
- If patient has history of hypotension, diabetes, or associated parkinsonism (or propranolol ineffective) consider use of anticholinergic agents (e.g., benztropine, biperiden).
- If ineffective, consider adding or changing to a benzodiazepine (e.g., clonazepam, diazepam, lorazepam).
- For unresponsive, predominantly anxious/agitated patient (without hypotension) consider clonidine 0.2–0.8mg/d (may be sedative).
- Other possible agents include amantadine, buspirone (may also worsen symptoms), tryptophan, levetriracetam, or even iron supplements.

Course/prognosis

Most cases will respond to treatment and usually the response will be seen after a few days. Chronic or tardive cases may be more difficult to treat, and it should be borne in mind that therapeutic benefit (e.g., of propranolol) can take up to three months.

Follow-up

- Once the akathisia has settled, any specific treatment ought to be kept under review.
- Slow withdrawal of any additional agent should be attempted after a few weeks (in the case of benzodiazepines) or after several months (for other agents).
- If akathisia recurs, long-term therapy may be necessary. However, little data exists for agents other than propranolol (although original optimism for long-term benefit has not been borne out) or anticholinergics.
- The need for continued use of high-dose, high-potency antipsychotics should also be reviewed in the light of any change in the clinical presentation of the primary psychiatric disorder.

Drugs reported to cause akathisia

Antipsychotics (usually high-potency): chlorpromazine (less likely), clozapine (rare), haloperidol, olanzapine prochlorperazine, promazine, risperidone (withdrawal), aripiprazole, thioridazine (less likely), trifluoperazine, trimeprazine, trifluoperazine, zuclopenthixol.

Antidepressants: citalopram, fluoxetine, sertraline, fluvoxamine, imipramine (and other TCAs), mianserin, paroxetine, venlafaxine (withdrawal).

Anxiolytics: alprazolam, buspirone, lorazepam.

Others: diltiazem, verapamil, alpha-interferon, levodopa, lithium, melatonin (withdrawal), metoclopramide, ondansetron.

Tardive dyskinesia

Description

Late onset (months, years, mean = 7 years) involuntary, repetitive, pur-poseless movements, occurring with long-term antipsychotic treatment (although also has been reported in untreated patients with schizophrenia). Also associated with bupropion, buspirone, clomipramine, doxepin, diphenhydramine, fluoxetine, fluvoxamine, lithium, metoclopramide, and phenytoin.

Symptoms/signs

Perioral movements are the most common (e.g., tongue, lips, jaw), hence the alternative terms: oral-lingual, orofacial, oro-bucco-facial, or buccal-lingual-masticatory dyskinesia. Other movements may include: axial—trunk twisting, torticollis, retrocollis, shoulder shrugging, pelvic thrusting; limbs—rapid movements of the fingers or legs, hand clenching (and sometimes slower, choreiform movements). Symptoms can be suppressed consciously or through voluntary actions, worsen with distraction, are exacerbated by stress and antiparkinsonian agents, and disappear during sleep.

Pathophysiology

Not yet fully understood. Theories include: dopaminergic/cholinergic imbalance, up-regulation/supersensitivity of postsynaptic DA receptors in the basal ganglia following chronic blockade, GABA hypofunction leading to enhanced DA transmission, neurodegeneration through free-radical and excitatory mechanisms, genetic vulnerability.

Epidemiology

Prevalence is about 24% of chronically treated patients but may be as high as 70% in the "high risk" population.

Risk factors

Old age, female (1.7:1), history of acute EPS, chronic use of antipsychotics (particularly in high dose), change/cessation of chronic treatment (especially intermittent treatment), concomitant anticholinergic treatment elderly, history of organic brain disease (e.g., dementia, learning disability, epilepsy), previous head injury, alcoholism, co-morbid mood disorder, negative symptoms of schizophrenia, diabetes mellitus, concomitant use of predisposing drugs (e.g., antidepressants, stimulants).

Differential diagnosis

Tic disorders, Parkinson's disease, hereditary choreas (Huntington's/ Sydenham's chorea, Wilson's disease), basal ganglia or cerebellar strokes, other drugs (e.g., levodopa, amphetamines, cocaine, lithium, tricyclic antidepressants), psychogenic.

Management

- Review history/medication to identify possible causative agent(s).
- Reduce dose of potential causative agent, to achieve minimum effective dose that adequately controls psychotic symptoms.

- Anticholinergic agents will exacerbate the problem and should also be slowly reduced and stopped if possible.
- If residual symptoms can be tolerated, it is best to "wait and see," before considering addition of any specific treatment, because TD tends to improve with time.
- If residual symptoms are severe, interfere significantly with functional abilities, or may be life threatening, then temporarily raising the dose of antipsychotic may give immediate relief, while addition of a specific treatment may be commenced (dose of antipsychotic should then be reduced again).
- First line: switch to less EPS-prone "atypical or newer antipsychotic" (e.g., olanzapine, quetiapine).
- Other possible strategies:
  - Dopamine agonists (e.g., low-dose bromocriptine 0.75–7.5mg/d, L-dopa, amantadine).
  - Biogenic amine (DA) depleting agent: Reserpine 0.25mg/d to start, titrated to 0.75–4mg/d.
  - Benzodiazepines (e.g., clonazepam).
  - Adrenergic agents (e.g., propranolol, clonidine).
  - Calcium-channel blockers (e.g., nifedipine (high doses), verapamil, diltiazem).
  - Anticonvulsants (e.g., valproate, gabapentin).
  - Antioxidants (e.g., vitamin E [efficacy disputed]).
  - Other (e.g., baclofen, buspirone (high dose), levetiracetam, pyridoxine, donepezil).
  - Injections of botulinum-toxin.
- If the symptoms are severe and nonresponsive to other strategies, then consider clozapine (reportedly effective in up to 43% of refractory cases), ECT has also been (anecdotally) shown to be effective.

Course/prognosis

- Symptoms may not progress, 25% show a fluctuating course, 10% improve. After 5–10 years, about 50% show improvement of 50% or more, even without treatment.
- Most cases will respond to treatment although a balance may need to be struck between reduction in dyskinesia v. control of psychotic symptoms.

Follow-up

- Residual symptoms should be closely monitored.
- The need for continued antipsychotic treatment should also be regularly reviewed.
- Ensure that occurrence of TD and treatment strategy clearly recorded in case notes.

Acute dystonic reaction

Description

Acute reaction following exposure to antipsychotic medication with sustained, often painful muscular spasms, producing twisted abnormal postures, often within days of therapy initiation.

Etiology

Unknown. Related to dopamine-receptor blockade, although the delay between blockade and onset of symptomatology suggests involvement of additional mechanisms, such as secondary dopamine-receptor hyper-sensitivity.

Incidence

Two to three percent of patients exposed to all antipsychotics (up to 50% with high-potency drugs in "high-risk" individuals).

Risk factors

Previous/family history of dystonia, younger age group,[1] males > females (most likely due to use of higher doses of antipsychotics in men), liver failure, clinically severe schizophrenia (esp. with marked negative symptoms), use of high-potency antipsychotics (up to 10%; for other agents see opposite).

Onset

50% of cases occur within 48 hrs, rising to 90% within 5 days.

Symptoms/signs

Frequency of occurrence of dystonias: neck (30%), tongue (17%), jaw (15%), oculogyric crisis (neck arched and eye rolled back: 6%), opisthotonus (body arching: 3.5%). Usually more generalized in younger patients (may be confused with seizures, especially in children) and more localized (head and neck) in older patients.

Course

May fluctuate over hours, but most last minutes to hours without treatment.

Differential diagnosis

May be mistaken for bizarre behavior motivated by psychotic symptoms or even histrionic personality traits.

Management

- Discontinue suspected agent.
- Emergency treatment with IM/IV anticholinergic agents (e.g., biperiden 2mg po initially, then twice daily, benztropine 1–2mg IV, then 1–2mg orally twice daily).

---

1 Note: In contrast with most medication side-effects, acute dystonias are more common in the young than the elderly. This may be related to asymptomatic loss of dopaminergic neurons in later life.

- Continue use of anticholinergic for 1–2 days, unless antipsychotic clinically needed—then concomitant anticholinergic should be continued, but tapered off after 2–3 weeks (long-term treatment may predispose to TD).
- Adverse reactions of anticholinergics, such as memory impairment, blurred vision, and dry mouth, may occur.
- Alternative treatment includes use of amantadine (fewer SEs than other agents).
- Routine prophylaxis should be considered for patients with a history of previous drug-induced dystonic reaction.

Agents reported to cause dystonias

Antipsychotics

Clozapine (rare/abrupt withdrawal), flupentixol decanoate, haloperidol (decanoate), olanzapine (rare), risperidone (rare), aripiprazole, thioridazine, fluphenazine; most other "typical" or older antipsychotics.

Other psychotropics

TCAs, benztropine (rare), bupropion, buspirone, carbamazepine, cocaine (+ withdrawal), disulfiram (rare), fluoxetine, midazolam, paroxetine, phenelzine, sertraline.

Other (mostly rare/isolated cases)

Amiodarone, diphenhydramine, domperidone, ergotamine, indomethacin, metoclopramide, nifedipine, penicillamine, prochlorperazine, promethazine, propranolol, sumatriptan.

Neuroleptic malignant syndrome

Description

A rare, life-threatening, idiosyncratic reaction to antipsychotic (and other i.e., antidepressant) medication (see opposite), characterized by: fever, muscular rigidity and akinesia, altered mental status, and autonomic dysfunction. Rhabdomyolysis and renal failure may ensue.[1]

Note: psychiatric emergency; if diagnosed in a psychiatric setting, transfer patient to acute medical services where intensive monitoring and treatment are available.

Pathophysiology

Theories: to DA activity in the CNS—i.e., striatum (rigidity), hypothalamus (thermoregulation)—by blockade of D_2-receptors or DA availability; impaired Ca^{2+} mobilization in muscle cells leads to rigidity (like malignant hyperthermia[2]); sympathetic nervous system activation or dysfunction.

Epidemiology

Incidence 0.07–0.2% (pooled data); M:F = 2:1.

Mortality

5–20%: death usually due to respiratory failure, cardiovascular collapse, myoglobinuric renal failure, arrhythmias, or DIC.

Morbidity

Rhabdomyolysis, aspiration pneumonia, renal failure, seizures, arrhythmias, DIC, respiratory failure, worsening of primary psychiatric disorder (due to withdrawal of antipsychotics).

Symptoms/signs

Hyperthermia (>38C), muscular rigidity, confusion/ agitation/altered level of consciousness, tachycardia, tachypnoea, hyper/ hypotension, diaphoresis/ sialorrhea, tremor, incontinence/retention/obstruction, CK/urinary myoglobin, leukocytosis, metabolic acidosis.

Risk factors

Ambient temperature; dehydration; patient agitation or catatonia; rapid antipsychotic initiation/dose escalation; withdrawal of antiparkinsonian medication; use of high-potency agents/depot IM preparations; history of organic brain disease (e.g., dementia, alcoholism), affective disorder, previous NMS; predisposing drugs (e.g., lithium, anticholinergic agents); elderly more susceptible, especially to higher doses.

---

1 Kipps, C.M., Fung, V.S.C., Grattan-Smith, P., de Moore, G.M., Morris, J.G.L. (2004). Movement disorders emergencies. *Movement Disorders* **20**(3), 322–334.

2 A rare disorder associated with exposure to inhaled anaesthetics and succinylcholine. Genetic linkage found on chromosome 19. Possibly due to a muscle membrane defect, leading to increase in intracellular Ca and intense muscle contractions. Temperature rises rapidly (up to 1 C/5 mins).

Differential diagnosis

(Lethal) catatonia (see next); sepsis; malignant hyperthermia; encephalitis/meningitis; heat exhaustion; parkinsonism/acute dystonia; serotonergic syndrome; toxicity due to other drugs (e.g., amphetamine, MDMA, cocaine, phencyclidine, antidepressants, antihistamines, sympathomimetics, salicylates); DTs; rhabdomyolysis; haemorrhagic stroke; tetanus; pheochromocytoma; strychnine, CO poisoning.

Investigations

CBC w/diff, blood cultures, LFTs, renal functions including 'lytes, protein; calcium and phosphate levels, serum CPK, urine myoglobin, ABGs, coagulation studies, serum/urine toxicology, CXR (if aspiration suspected), ECG; consider head CT (intracranial cause), LP (to exclude meningitis).

Management

• Stop any agents thought to be causative (especially antipsychotics); in mild cases this may be all that is required.
• Benzodiazepines for acute behavioral disturbance (📖 p. 1100) (Note: use of restraint and I/M injection may complicate the interpretation of serum CK).
• Supportive measures: monitor patient in acute medical setting, oxygen, correct volume depletion/hypotension with IV fluids, reduce the temperature (e.g., cooling blankets, antipyretics, cooled IV fluids, ice packs, evaporative cooling, ice-water enema).
• Rhabdomyolysis—vigorous hydration and alkalinization of the urine using IV sodium bicarbonate to prevent renal failure.
• Pharmacotherapy to reduce rigidity—dantrolene (IV 0.8–2.5mg/kg qds; po 50–100mg bd); Second line: bromocriptine (po 2.5–10mg tds, increase to max. 60mg/day); amantadine (po 100–200mg bd); Third line: lorazepam (up to 5mg), nifedipine; also consider ECT (Note: risk of fatal arrhythmias).

Course

May last 7–10 days after stopping oral antipsychotics and up to 21 days after depot antipsychotics (e.g., fluphenazine).

Prognosis

In the absence of rhabdomyolysis, renal failure, or aspiration pneumonia, and with good supportive care, prognosis is good.

Follow-up

Monitor closely for residual symptoms. One-third or more patients relapse with reintroduction of antipsychotic therapy. Thus, once symptoms have settled allow 2+wks (if possible) before restarting medication (use low-dose, low-potency, or newer "atypical" agents, avoid lithium). Consider prophylaxis (bromocriptine). Inform patient about risk of recurrence if given antipsychotic medication. Ensure this is recorded prominently in their medical notes.

Drugs reported to cause symptoms characteristic of NMS

Antipsychotics: chlorpromazine, clozapine (rarely), flupenthixol, fluphenazine, haloperidol, loxapine, olanzapine, promazine, quetiapine (rarely), risperidone, thioridazine.

Antiparkinsonian agents: amantadine (+withdrawal), anticholinergics (withdrawal), levodopa (+withdrawal).

Antidepressants: amoxapine, clomipramine, desipramine, phenelzine, trimipramine, venlafaxine.

Other: carbamazepine (+withdrawal), ganciclovir, ferrous sulphate, lithium, methylphenidate, metoclopramide, oral contraceptives.

Differentiating NMS from catatonia

Feature	NMS	Catatonia
Patient taking antipsychotics	Usually	Not usually
Catatonic symptoms:		
Echo phenomena	Rare	Yes
Ambitendency	Rare	Yes
Posturing	Rare	Yes
Hyperthermia	Usually before stupor	Usually before/during severe agitation
Muscle rigidity	Yes	Yes
Raised WCC	Yes	No
Raised CK	Yes	Yes

Serotonin syndrome

Key features

Serotonin syndrome (SS) is a rare but potentially fatal syndrome occurring in the context of initiation or dose increase of a serotonergic agent, characterized by altered mental state, agitation, tremor, shivering, diarrhea, hyperreflexia, myoclonus, ataxia, and hyperthermia. Although SSRIs are commonly linked to SS, many other drugs (e.g., amphetamines, MAOIs, TCAs, lithium) have the potential of causing hyperserotonergic symptoms. SS can occur as a result of overdose, drug combinations (including over-the-counter medications), and rarely with therapeutic doses.

Pathophysiology

A variety of mechanisms can potentially increase the quantity or activity of serotonin: ↑production of serotonin due to ↑availability of precursors (L-tryptophan containing substances); ↓metabolism of serotonin (MAOIs, selegiline); ↑release of stored serotonin (amphetamine, cocaine, fenfluramine, MDMA, meperidine); reuptake inhibition (SSRIs, TCAs, SNRIs, NaSSAs, MDMA, dextromethorphan, meperidine, St. John's wort); direct stimulation of serotonin receptors (buspirone, LSD); unknown mechanisms (lithium).

Epidemiology

Incidence around 1% for SSRIs (moderate/major symptoms; mild symptoms may be common, but tend to go unreported); mortality <1 in 1000 cases.

Symptoms/signs (see opposite)

Psychiatric/neurological: confusion, agitation, coma. Neuromuscular myoclonus, rigidity, tremors (including shivering), hyperreflexia (usually lower rather than upper limbs), ataxia. Autonomic Hyperthermia (may be due to prolonged seizure activity, rigidity, or muscular hyperactivity), GI upset (nausea, diarrhea), mydriasis, tachycardia, hyper/hypotension.

Differential diagnosis

NMS, malignant hyperthermia, infections (encephalitis/meningitis/sepsis), metabolic disturbances, substance abuse (cocaine)/withdrawal/overdose (LSD, PCP).

Investigations

CBC, 'lytes, LFTs, glucose, pH, chemistry panel (including calcium, magnesium, phosphate, anion gap), CK, drug toxicology screen, CXR (if evidence of respiratory distress/possible aspiration), ECG monitoring (arrhythmia/conduction problems—prolonged QRS or QTc interval).

Treatment

If severe, requires immediate transfer to emergency department for inpatient supportive treatment and active management including airway, breathing and circulation (ABCs); intravenous fluids; and hemodynamic monitoring.

If overdose, consider gastric lavage and/or activated charcoal.

IV access to allow volume correction (dehydration: insensible fluid loss due to hyperthermia) and reduce risk of rhabdomyolysis.

Rhabdomyolysis should be dealt with quickly, with emphasis on maintaining a high urine output combined with alkalinization using sodium bicarbonate (target urine pH of 6). If necessary, reduce the temperature (e.g., cooling blankets, antipyretics, cooled IV fluids, ice packs, evaporative cooling, ice-water enema).

Pharmacotherapy

Agitation, seizures, and muscular rigidity/ myoclonus best managed using a benzodiazepine (e.g., lorazepam IV (slow) 1–2mg every 30 mins; clonazepam). Serotonin receptor antagonists may be considered in selected cases (e.g., cyproheptadine po 4–8mg every 2–4 hrs (max 0.5mg/kg/d), chlorpromazine (risk of reduced seizure threshold), mirtazepine, methysergide, propranolol (mild 5HT antagonist)). Antihypertensives are usually unnecessary unless the hypertension is persistent and clinically significant (e.g., nitroglycerin IV 2mg/kg/min).

Course and prognosis

Onset is usually acute, However, recurrent mild symptoms may occur for weeks before the appearance of severe symptoms. Most cases resolve without sequelae within 24–36 hours with adequate supportive measures. Following an SSRI overdose, a patient who remains asymptomatic for several hours is unlikely to need further medical management.

Sternbach's diagnostic criteria[1]

- Other potential causes excluded (e.g., infection, metabolic, substance abuse, withdrawal).
- No concurrent antipsychotic dose changes prior to symptom onset.
- At least three of the following:
  - Agitation/restlessness.
  - Diaphoresis.
  - Diarrhoea.
  - Fever.
  - Muscle rigidity (usually lower extremities predominating).
  - Hyperreflexia.
  - Ataxia.
  - Mental state changes (confusion, hypomania).
  - Myoclonus.
  - Shivering.
  - Tremor.

Distinguishing SS from NMS

Although the clinical presentation of these two syndromes is very similar (i.e., autonomic dysfunction, alteration of mental status, rigidity, and hyperthermia), differentiation is very important as specific management may differ (e.g., use of chlorpromazine in SS, which may worsen NMS).

	NMS	**SS**
Associated Rx	Antipsychotics (Idiosyncratic/normal dose)	Serotonergic agents (OD/drug combination)
Onset	Slow (days to weeks)	Rapid
Progression	Slow (24–72 hrs)	Rapid
Muscle rigidity	Severe ("lead pipe")	Less severe
Activity	Bradykinesia	Hyperkinesia

Recommended further reading

1 Sternbach, H. (1991). The serotonin syndrome. *AJP* **148**, 705–13.

SSRI[1] withdrawal (discontinuation) syndrome[2]

The incidence and prevalence of this syndrome are currently unknown. Rates of occurrence vary from 12 to 85%, depending both on the SSRI used and the underlying condition being treated. The few available discontinuation studies indicate minor forms of the syndrome may be common and severe forms unusual. There may be less risk with certain drugs (e.g., fluoxetine, perhaps due to longer half-life) and possibly greater risk with paroxetine (perhaps due to cholinergic rebound), although symptoms of discontinuation have been reported with all the SSRIs.

Clinical features

Neurologic symptoms

Most common: dizziness, vertigo, lightheadedness, and gait instability.

Somatic complaints

Nausea/emesis, fatigue and headache; insomnia. Less frequently reported: shock-like sensations, paresthesia, visual disturbances, diarrhea, flulike symptoms (myalgias and chills).

Nonspecific symptoms

Agitation, impaired concentration, vivid dreams, depersonalization, irritability, and suicidal thoughts have also been reported.

Course and duration

Usually develop after one month of SSRI treatment, within two to five days after SSRI discontinuation or dose reduction depending on the half-life of the SSRI being used. If untreated, duration is variable (one to several weeks) and ranges from mild-moderate intensity in most patients, to extremely distressing in a small number.

Etiology

The biological mechanisms underlying this syndrome are not well understood, although an acute decrease in synaptic serotonin in the face of down-regulated or desensitized serotonin receptors has been postulated.

Risk factors

Appears to be idiosyncratic with no specific associations with age, sex, diagnosis, or dose of SSRI (both low and high doses have been reported).

---

1 The "special case" for differentiating an "SSRI discontinuation syndrome" is debatable, since withdrawal syndromes have been described with most antidepressants including TCAs and SNRIs (venlafaxine)—all with similar symptoms to those described for SSRIs. In general, gradual tapering of antidepressants is recommended and abrupt stopping should be avoided (see 📖 p.307).

2 Zajecka, J., Tracy, K.A., Mitchell, S. (1997). Discontinuation symptoms after treatment with serotonin reuptake inhibitors: a literature review. *Journal of Clinical Psychiatry* **58**, 291–297 (& suppl. 7).

Differential diagnosis

The syndrome may be easily confused with recurrence of symptoms after inadequate duration of SSRI treatment, particularly in the anxiety disorders. Other possibilities (e.g., infection, metabolic, withdrawal from drugs of abuse/alcohol) should be excluded. If the syndrome occurs when cross-tapering from one SSRI to another antidepressant, be aware of the possibility of serotonin syndrome (see 📖 *p. 1070*).

Management

- Gradually tapering SSRIs may help reduce the risk of developing the syndrome. However, guidelines on the optimum rates of dose reduction are at best empirical (see 📖 *p. 307*) and a cautious approach is advised (slowly over a number of weeks).
- If severe, re-introduction of the SSRI rapidly resolves the symptoms. However, the syndrome may recur in up to 75% of patients when the same SSRI is later discontinued.
- Awareness of some of the more unusual symptoms, such as dizziness and shock-like sensations, and education of patients prior to stopping or tapering an SSRI, should prevent unnecessary and expensive medical investigations.
- When symptoms are mild-moderate and short-lived they can generally be tolerated by the patient, allowing for successful discontinuation of the SSRI.
- Additionally, some clinicians have seen success in recommending dietary supplementation of choline, lecithin, and B complex in patients discontinuing SSRIs.

Hyponatremia and antidepressants

Key features

Low serum sodium is a rare, idiosyncratic side-effect of antidepressants, which may have serious consequences if undiagnosed.

Etiology

Incompletely understood, but probably due to the syndrome of inappropriate antidiuretic hormone (SIADH).

Risk factors

Previous SIADH/history of hyponatremia; advanced age (>80yrs); co-morbidity: diabetes mellitus, hypertension, impaired renal function, COPD; other medication (e.g., diuretics).

Clinical features

Depend on the severity, duration, and rate of change in serum sodium. May be asymptomatic, or display symptoms and signs (e.g., lethargy, confusion, nausea, weight loss, muscle cramps/weakness, hypertension, cardiac failure, edema, seizures).

Investigations

(Serum Na^+<125mmol/l), 24-hr urine collection (urinary Na^+>20mmol/l and osmolality>100mosml/kg). Alternatively there may be low plasma osmolality (<260mmol/kg) without hypovolemia, edema, or diuretics.

Differential diagnosis

Malignancy e.g., lung small-cell; pancreas; prostate; lymphoma. CNS disorders e.g., meningoencephalitis; abscess; stroke; subarachnoid/subdural hemorrhage; head injury; Guillain-Barré; vasculitis. Respiratory disorders e.g., TB; pneumonia; abscess; aspergillosis. Metabolic disease e.g., porphyria; trauma. Drugs e.g., opiates; chlorpropramide; cytotoxic agents.

Management

- Prevention: Baseline 'lytes prior to commencing antidepressant, with monitoring for those at high risk (initially monthly, or after any dose change, once treatment dose established, every 3 to 6 months).
- Treatment:
  - Withdraw suspected agent immediately.
  - If serum Na^+ is <125mmol/l, refer to specialist medical care (to eliminate other possible causes, and to treat more intensively—e.g., with fluid restriction and occasionally with demeclocycline). There is a risk of developing central pontine myelinolysis with rapid correction of levels of 120mmol/l or lower.
  - If serum Na^+>125mmol/l, continue to monitor "lytes daily until >135mmol/l.
  - consider alternative antidepressant (usually from a different class at a low dose, gradual increasing with close monitoring) or, if treatment urgent, ECT may be an option.

Paradoxical reactions to benzodiazepines[1]

Key features

Paradoxical or "disinhibitory" reactions to BDZs occur in a minority of patients (less than 1% of general population) and are characterized by acute excitement and altered mental state sometimes featuring:

- Increased anxiety.
- Vivid dreams.
- Hyperactivity.
- Sexual disinhibition.
- Hostility and rage ("aggressive dyscontrol").

Recognition is important as behavioral disturbance may be exacerbated by inappropriate use of higher doses of BDZs. Of note, similar types of reaction are described for most CNS depressants (e.g., alcohol, barbiturates).

Etiology

Incompletely understood; theories include: "release behavior" due to loss of frontal lobe inhibition through GABA$_A$ mechanism; BDZ related reduction in 5HT neurotransmission; BDZ related reduction in ACh neurotransmission: potential idiosyncratic transient inverse agonist effect of shorter half-life BDZs in susceptible individuals.

Risk factors

Children, learning disability, history of brain injury, dementia, borderline PD, antisocial PD, history of aggression/poor impulse control, family/personal history of paradoxical reaction, use of high-dose/high-potency relatively short half-life BDZs (e.g., alprazolam, clonazepam, flunitrazepam, triazolam), IV/intranasal administration.

Management

- Nurse in safe environment, with constant supervision.
- Use sedative antipsychotic or sedative antihistamine to treat acute behavioral disturbance if necessary.
- If the disinhibition is transient and associated with the use of a relatively short acting (i.e., lorazepam, clonazepam), BDZ, the administration of a longer half life BDZ (i.e., diazepam), may reduce the disinhibition.
- In extreme cases consider use of IV flumazenil (may require repeated doses).
- Clearly record occurrence of paradoxical reaction so that future episodes of acute behavioral disturbance are managed appropriately.

Recommended further reading

1 Paton, C. (2002). Benzodiazepines and disinhibition: a review. *Psychiatric Bulletin* **26**, 460–462.

Prescribing for patients with cardiovascular disease

General points

The importance of psychiatric treatment in patients with cardiovascular disease is undeniable. Depression is now included among the risk factors for MI. In considering a suitable psychotropic drug, the main issues revolve around the propensity of that drug to interact with other medications the patient may be taking, to affect blood pressure, or lead to cardiac conduction problems (see opposite). Due to the unpredictability of drug interactions, polypharmacy is best avoided.

Specific contraindications

Thioridazine is most cardiotoxic, BDZs in pulmonary insufficiency, disulfiram and lithium in heart failure or sick sinus syndrome, most psychotropics interact with warfarin.

Myocardial infarction

Antidepressants
Primary use of SSRIs is preferred given their studied safety and efficacy. May start at any point post-MI if clinical circumstances support it.

Antipsychotics
High doses should be avoided; phenothiazines are generally more hypotensive than butyrophenones; clozapine should be used with caution in the 1st year post MI; of the newer antipsychotics, olanzapine may offer best risk-benefit balance but also carries the highest association with the metabolic syndrome.

Heart failure

Where possible, hypotensive agents (β-blockers, clozapine, risperidone, TCAs) and drugs causing fluid retention (carbamazepine, lithium) should be avoided. Ziprasidone and quetiapine may be used with low starting doses and careful titration.

Angina/IHD

Avoid hypotensive agents and those known to cause tachycardia (phenothiazines, clozapine, risperidone).

Hypertension

Avoid agents that may raise blood pressure (low-dose TCAs, phenothiazines, clozapine, high-dose venlafaxine, bupropion).

Arrhythmias

Antidepressants
SSRIs should be first choice (but not fluvoxamine or citalopram). Bupropion may also be an option.

Antipsychotics

High doses should be avoided; risperidone may be least likely to cause conduction problems. Avoid ziprasidone, clozapine, quetiapine, and phenothiazines (especially thioridazine).

Psychostimulants

Psychostimulants (e.g., methylphenidate) may prove acutely toxic in many of these circumstances. Caution should be applied in particular when there has been a recent negative event (uncontrolled HTN/CHF/tachycardia, or recent MI). Absolute contraindications are motor tics/Tourette's, glaucoma, and recent MAOI use. Dextroamphetamine should be avoided.

Mood stabilizers

Lithium and carbamazepine are best to avoid. Other anticonvulsants (valproate, lamotrigine, gabapentin) are all considered "heart-safe."

The QT^c question

Awareness of QT prolongation, as measured by the corrected QT interval (QT^c), has been heightened because of the potential (but relatively rare) risk of fatal arrhythmias (e.g., torsade de pointes), highlighted recently by the withdrawal of thioridazine as a first-line antipsychotic (and now contraindicated in patients with a history of, or at risk of, arrhythmias) and the restricted use of droperidol.

QT^c is derived by dividing the QT interval by the square root of the cycle length i.e.:

$$QT^c = \frac{QT}{\sqrt{(R-R)}}$$

Normal QT^c: is 380–420ms; if prolonged to 450ms—some concern; if >500–520ms—"at risk."

Causes of prolonged QT interval: acute myocardial ischemia, myocarditis, bradycardia (e.g., AV block), head injury, hypothermia, electrolyte imbalance (K$^+$, Ca^{2+}, Mg^{2+}), congenital, sotalol, quinidine, antihistamines, macrolides (e.g., erythromycin), amiodarone, antipsychotics (especially phenothiazines, ziprasidone, quetiapine in OD), antidepressants (esp. TCAs).

General advice: good practice dictates use of routine ECG prior to commencement of antipsychotic medication (especially ziprasidone, pimozide, zotepine, thioridazine, and other phenothiazines), and regular monitoring, particularly with use of high doses (📕 *p. 239*).

Prescribing for patients with liver disease

General points
- Almost all psychotropic drugs are metabolized by the liver.
- Exceptions to this rule include lithium, gabapentin and paliperidone, which have minimal (or no) liver metabolism.
- Most drugs are highly protein bound (with the exception of citalopram) and plasma levels may be increased in liver disease.
- In liver disease, when using drugs with high first-pass clearance (e.g., imipramine, amitriptyline, desipramine, doxepin, haloperidol), initial doses should be low.
- When possible, phenothiazines (e.g., chlorpromazine) and hydrazine MAOIs (may be hepatotoxic) should be avoided.
- If in doubt, closely monitor LFTs, particularly during dose changes, but remember that LFTs can lead to inaccurate interpretation in the setting of severe liver disease.

Antidepressants (always start with lowest possible dose)
- TCAs: Best evidence for use of imipramine.
- SSRIs: No clear preference among agents; avoid nefazodone.
- MAOIs: When clinically necessary, use 30–50% usual dose.
- Others: Venlafaxine (use 50% usual dose), mirtazepine (cautious use).

Antipsychotics
- Best evidence for haloperidol (considered "drug of choice").
- Few problems reported for flupenthixol/zuclopenthixol.
- Clozapine dose should be kept low (some evidence of hepatotoxicity).
- For the newer agents recommendations suggest:
  - Olanzapine (up to 7.5mg) may be safe (but does induce transaminases).
  - Risperidone doses should be kept low (start 0.5mg bid, max 4mg/d).
  - Quetiapine is extensively metabolized (hence start low—25mg).
  - Aripiprazole and ziprasidone have no recommended adjustments.

Mood stabilizers
- Lithium is the "drug of choice," with gabapentin as second choice.
- Valproate is contraindicated in severe liver disease, but may be used with caution in mild to moderate impairment.
- Similarly, caution should be exercised with carbamazepine.
- Lamotrigine is contraindicated in severe disease.
- Topiramate has decreased urinary excretion in patients with liver disease so use caution.

Anxiolytics
- Use LOT medications (lorazepam, oxazepam, temazepam) as they are conjugated by glucuronidation (spared in liver disease).
- Clonazepam should be used as a long-acting agent.

Prescribing for patients with renal impairment

General points

- Renal impairment generally leads to accumulation of drugs (or active metabolites) that are predominantly cleared by the kidney. This will lead to higher serum levels, and increased risk of dose-related side-effects (e.g., postural hypotension, sedation, EPSEs).
- Hence, all psychotropics should be started at a low (or divided) dose, increased slowly, and carefully monitored (for efficacy and tolerability).
- When patients are receiving dialysis, seek specific advice from manufacturer—dosages should usually be reduced by at least 50% and dosing separated in time from dialysis itself.

Classification of chronic renal failure (CRF)

CRF may be classified as mild (GFR 30–50ml/min), moderate (GFR 10–29ml/min), severe (GFR <10ml/min), or end-stage (GFR <5ml/min).

Antidepressants

- In severe renal failure, avoid fluoxetine, paroxetine, and venlafaxine (unless the patient is on dialysis).
- Otherwise cautious use, beginning low and gradually increasing the dose is advised.
- No specific therapeutic dose adjustments are necessary for MAOIs (except for isocarboxazid), meclobamide, mianserin, tryptophan, trazodone, or TCAs.

Antipsychotics

- Lower doses are recommended to avoid dose-related side-effects (particularly with the phenothiazines and paliperidone, which may be best avoided).
- Clozapine is contraindicated in severe renal impairment.
- Greater care is necessary with risperidone, and ziprasidone (may be best to avoid).
- Loxapine appears to have few specific problems.
- Some authorities recommend haloperidol, but accumulation is possible, so careful monitoring is still necessary.

Mood stabilizers

- Lithium is relatively contraindicated in renal failure. However, its use may often be necessary, and dose reduction (e.g., to 50–75% for mild-moderate and 25–50% for severe renal failure) with close monitoring of plasma levels is recommended. In dialysis, 600mg × 3/wk (after dialysis) has been shown to maintain therapeutic plasma levels.
- No specific problems are reported for valproate or carbamazepine, although in severe renal failure, serum levels should be monitored.
- Gabapentin requires specific dose adjustments and manufacturer's recommendations should be sought.

- Lamotrigine should be used cautiously, particularly in severe renal impairment.
- Topiramate requires dose reduction to 50% in moderate-severe renal failure.

Anxiolytics/hypnotics

- BDZs (with the exception of chlordiazepoxide) tend to accumulate, with increasing CNS side-effects (particularly sedation)—hence use low doses.
- Buspirone is contraindicated in moderate-severe renal failure.
- β-blockers should be started at low dose as they may complicate renal failure by reducing renal blood flow.
- Zolpidem and zaleplon require no dosage adjustment. However, the half-life of zolpidem may be doubled in renal failure.

Others

- Anticholinergics, disulfiram—cautious use.
- Acamprosate—contraindicated if serum creatinine >120µmol/l.
- Anticholinesterases—no reported problems.

Estimating glomerular filtration rate (GFR)

Creatinine clearance is a measure of GFR, the volume of fluid filtered by the glomeruli per minute (ml/min). Normal value is approx. 125ml/min. Urine is collected over a 24-hr period for urinary creatinine (mmol/l), along with a blood sample for serum creatinine (µmol/l).

Urine creatinine concentration = u mmol/l
Plasma creatinine concentration = p µmol/l
24-hr urine volume = vmls

$$\text{Creatinine clearance (ml/min)} = (u \times 0.7) \times \left(\frac{v}{p}\right)$$

NB: Always check the units are correct for each variable in the equation.
   For an estimate of creatinine clearance* based only on the serum creatinine, the following formula can be used:

$$\text{Creatinine clearance (ml/min)} = \frac{(140 - \text{age in year}) \times (\text{wt in kg})}{72 \text{ serum creatinine in mg/dl}}$$

NB: To convert µmol/l to mg/dl, divide µmol/l by 88.4.

* For women, the above estimate should be multiplied by 0.85. This estimate assumes stable renal function, absence of obesity and/or edema.

Prescribing for patients with epilepsy

General points

In considering a suitable psychotropic there are two related considerations:
- The propensity of that drug to interact with other medications the patient may be taking (justifying serum monitoring where possible),
- The risk of lowering seizure threshold and exacerbating the condition.

As these effects appear dose related, the daily dose of any drug should be kept as low as possible. Greater caution is necessary when:
- Other psychotropics are also being given,
- Patients may be withdrawing from CNS depressants (e.g., BDZs, barbiturates, or alcohol).

Antidepressants

- All TCAs appear to lower seizure threshold, although there appears to be greater risk with amitriptyline and clomipramine.
- Tetracyclics (maprotiline and amoxapine) also appear proconvulsant, as does bupropion.
- The other antidepressants appear less likely to cause problems, and a usual first choice is often an SSRI (care should be exercised as they can slow the metabolism of anti-epileptic drugs).

Antipsychotics

- Greatest risk of seizures is associated with the use of phenothiazines (especially chlorpromazine), loxapine, olanzapine, and particularly clozapine.
- The risk of seizures with clozapine rises from 1% (at doses <300mg/d), to 2.7% (300–600mg/d), to 4.4% (>600mg/d). EEG changes are seen in up to 75% of people taking clozapine, with 40% showing paroxysmal discharges.[1] Because of this risk, it is quite common to cover high doses of clozapine with concomitant use of valproate. Hence, greater caution is needed when clozapine is used in individuals with epilepsy.
- Lowest risk is associated with haloperidol, pimozide, quetiapine, ziprasidone, aripiprazole and risperidone.

Mood stabilizers

- Lithium does cause seizures in overdose. However, therapeutic doses appear safe.
- If in doubt, anticonvulsants provide useful alternatives and may serve to treat both mood and epilepsy symptoms.

Anxiolytics/hypnotics

- Generally these drugs are anticonvulsant.
- Exceptions include buspirone, zolpidem, and β-blockers, although there is no evidence that they are epileptogenic.

---

1 Pacia, S.V. and Devinsky, O. (1994). Clozapine-related seizures: experience with 5,629 patients. *Neurology* **44**, 2247–2249.

Others
- Anticholinergics, acamprosate—no reported problems.
- Disulfiram—caution recommended.
- Anticholinesterases—care is needed with donepezil and rivastigmine. However, galantamine appears safe.

Plasma level monitoring

There are a limited number of drugs with well-established plasma levels that equate with efficacy. Plasma monitoring is a regular procedure only for lithium therapy. However, there may be a number of other reasons for requesting plasma levels (bear in mind that assays for specific drugs may not be locally available and may need special arrangements). Many psychiatric drugs have marked variations in metabolism, or large numbers of active metabolites, making plasma levels difficult to interpret.

Reasons for monitoring

- Established therapeutic plasma levels (see below).
- Monitoring of any changes in plasma level that might affect efficacy (e.g., due to drug interactions, intercurrent illness, pregnancy, or altered pharmacokinetics over time).
- Clinical evidence of toxicity (e.g., lithium, anticonvulsants).
- When there is doubt about patient compliance (e.g., lack of effect despite adequate or even high-dose treatment).
- For cases in which the patient may be unable to report adverse effects (e.g., children, severe LD, dementia).
- After overdose, to confirm it is safe to restart medication.

Reference ranges for selected drugs

Lithium (see 📖 p. 376)	0.8–1.2mmol/L (0.6–0.8mmol/L—as an augmentative agent)
Valproate (see 📖 p. 382)	50–125mg/L
Carbamazepine (see 📖 p. 384)	4–12mg/L (>7mg/L may be more efficacious in BAD)
Clozapine (see 📖 p. 244)	350–500mcg/L (0.35–0.5mg/L)
Nortriptyline	50–150mcg/L

Psychiatric emergencies and difficult situations

Dealing with psychiatric emergencies

Psychiatric emergencies arise in a variety of settings, from those as clinically exposing to the psychiatrist as a 1:1 office setting, to heavily staffed environments like an emergency room (ER). One's response will necessarily vary depending on both the nature of the problem and the available staff and resources. In the 1:1 setting, one has to primarily establish personal safety, only then initiating an intervention with the patient. In an ER setting, however, the role of the psychiatrist will shift to leading the intervention itself and directing the behavior of nursing and clinical staff, as well as of safety or security staff that might be available. Be familiar with procedures in place for the management of both behavioral and medical emergencies in your hospital, clinic, office, or other site of practice, as well as with methods of accessing emergency medical services.

Basic principles

Safety of patient, staff, and others

A central idea in managing psychiatric emergencies is that safety is continuously assessed. This includes not only the immediate safety of the patient, but yours and any involved (or even proximate) third parties. Suspicion of medical etiologies of psychiatric emergencies as well as acute medical problems, such as overdose, which need immediate attention, should be assessed.

Due to the vital importance of safety, be familiar with the best means to access emergency psychiatric and/or medical assessment and stabilization. Assess the need for assistance by security or police and the most efficient means of accessing such help.

Assessment: balancing quality of care with efficiency

Any emergent psychiatric assessment should combine efficiency and quality, balancing each as fits the particular case. Quality of care should be maximized in accordance with the particular setting under which one is working. The quality of care of other patients in a busy emergency room setting, however, must also be taken into consideration and attention in time and effort be paid to each case in a reasonable fashion. An obvious inpatient admission of a well-known patient, for example, may require far less "face time" than an unknown patient whose crisis needs to be stabilized sufficiently to be referred to an ambulatory level of care.

Never rush to judgments

Assess each case carefully and gather information from additional sources when possible. Slow down the pace of evaluations as is necessary; commonly, collateral information not obtained from the "first round" of interviewing can be absolutely critical to decision making.

While disposition planning can and should start as early in the evaluation process as possible, it is a dynamic process as more information is gathered. As such, postpone deciding final plans and disposition until the end of the assessment.

Explain to the patient the general process of evaluation, as orientation can be helpful in comforting and stabilizing the patient. Do this throughout the assessment process, also taking responsibility for making sure that patients and those accompanying them are never left for long periods of time wondering, "What is going on?"

Standard model of basic assessment

Each case being assessed should involve the following components:

Triage

A patient presents with a chief complaint or question. Typically front-line staff such as triage nurses, secretaries, registration personnel, depending on the setting, may have first contact with a patient. You, as the psychiatrist, may also have first contact with a patient. In some settings, additional clinical information (risk screening, medications, medical problems, vital signs, allergies, substance abuse history, etc.) is gathered at this stage as well.

Communication

Any triage information gathered by front-line staff should be communicated to the representative of the team in charge of the case (e.g., the ER attending or the consulting psychiatrist), in a time-efficient manner, focusing on the presenting problem and any acute factors.

Prioritizing

Depending upon information obtained at triage, some cases or situations may need addressing before others as more urgent action may be required (e.g., suicidal ideation, withdrawal from substances, acute medical problems, etc.).

Consultation

Should problems requiring more immediate consultation arise, such as an acute medical condition, address this as urgently as necessary via appropriate consultation, and have access numbers at your disposal. Consult senior colleagues or administrators if necessary. Should an imminent safety situation arise, urgent consultation with safety/security staff and nursing may become needed in order to coordinate the crisis intervention.

Intervention

Always be mindful of whether and when interventions such as medications or restraint/seclusion are necessary and implement as appropriate. (see next section).

Patient interview

The evaluation phase generally begins with the patient interview when possible. Interviewing staff and gathering collateral information is necessary, but the thoroughness of interview must be balanced with the triage level of the current case, expediency, and addressing the needs of others for whose care you are responsible.

Collateral information-gathering

After patient interview, decide which sources of collateral information are necessary in order to complete the assessment. This may include record review, live interviews, or telephone interviews.

Case formulation

This is the heart of any assessment, and if working with a team, have a conference with other team members to arrive at a consensus formulation and plan. In case of disagreement, the team member who is ultimately responsible for the case, often the psychiatrist, is expected to have final decision-making authority. If necessary, obtain consultation from a senior colleague or administrator.

Treatment planning

This would routinely involve disposition and treatment recommendations. Discuss with patient (and their family, if warranted) and attempt to arrive at a consensus. If another clinician has done the principal interviewing, your discussion with the patient at this point should also be used to confirm the findings that are determining the level of care recommended.

Disagreements

In case of patient's or others' disagreement with recommendations, discuss in an empathic manner. Guiding principals should be safety issues and standards of care. Attitude throughout assessment process should be empathic. If consensus cannot be reached, make final recommendations and, if necessary, refer involved parties to appropriate departments for grievance resolution. When rapid intervention is required in response to a patient (who has been established as dangerous or grossly dysfunctional) demanding to leave, it can be effective to replace reflexive limit-setting (or even threats!) with matter-of-fact yet empathic statements underscoring your desire to help them, as well as how they and their loved ones deserve that we not dismiss their dangerousness or problems now. In all cases, familiarize yourself with institutional and legal standards for handling mental health care in emergency situations.

What to do if called to a crisis situation—negotiation principles

Initial actions
- Speak with staff who summoned you.
- Obtain as much information as possible, until clear decisions can be made.
- Clarify your role and what is expected of you.

Attitudes
- Attempt to put the patient at ease by orienting them to who you are and why you were asked to intervene.
- A consistently calm demeanor can be reassuring to both patient and others.

Communication

Verbal communication

Listen empathically and actively to the patient, and respond with empathic statements, reassuring statements, and clarifying questions. Some patients need to vent, even loudly. Not rushing to set limits with them immediately can sometimes allow them to calm down by themselves. Try instead: "I can see that you're upset . . . .How can I help you?"

Nonverbal communication

Use comforting nonverbal communication with the patient such as head nodding, eye contact, or smiling as means of communicating a supportive, nonthreatening presence to the patient. Pay attention to cues from the patient that may suggest potential aggressive behaviors such as fist clenching, rocking, leaning, and teeth gritting.

Assessment and intervention for aggressive behavior

Aggression

Includes verbal aggression such as screaming, growling, and threatening, as well as physical aggression such as violence toward self and others and property destruction.

Triaging acute and emergent situations

In the most extreme circumstances such as a person standing on a roof or threatening others with a firearm, the situation should be considered an urgent police or security matter and the appropriate authorities contacted, depending upon the setting and situation. You are never to be expected to risk your own life or well-being in order to deal with emergent situations such as these.

Less urgent but emergency situations

Should immediate police or 911 intervention as above not be necessary, then adopt the general framework outlined in the previous section which can be used for assessing and addressing aggressive behavior.

Rapid understanding of etiology

Throughout the emergency situation, the assessor must continually attempt to gain an understanding of the etiology of the behavior. The differential may be wide and intervention may be necessary before any clarification is possible.

Immediate interventions

Depending on the circumstances, the following immediate interventions may prove necessary: manual or mechanical restraint; locked or open seclusion; either injectable (IM or IV) or oral medication; environmental changes such as giving space to pace or "cool down" or isolating from destabilizing stimuli; or verbal calming techniques such as orienting, explaining, or reassuring lines of questioning. Use physical space to separate any "warring" parties. The least restrictive, patient-accepted methods are always preferred. Patients may be willing to accept the method proposed, especially if it is part of a predetermined safety plan. Nonetheless, dangerous situations may arise where more restrictive means (e.g., seclusion, restraint) are required for the safety of the patient, the staff, and other individuals present in the area.

Restraint

Be familiar with institutional policies regarding threshold for such an intervention. When possible, attempt the least restrictive means (e.g., offering oral medication/other intervention first. During the use of restraints, one person on the team should act as leader and continuously communicate with the patient what is happening and why.

Seclusion

Again, typically offers of medication are to be made prior to this intervention. Be familiar with policies regarding the use of seclusion; there are typically institutional/legal regulations regarding the implementation, documentation, and monitoring prior to, during, and after the use of seclusion or restraints.

Medication interventions for aggressive behavior

These are covered in the subsequent section on, "severe behavioral disturbance, 🕮 *pp. 1100–12*" The basic principles are as follows:
- Offer oral medication first. Inform the patient about the risks/benefits/side-effects of the medication offered, and why it may help the current situation.
- IM medication should only be used when the harm to self or others is imminent or in process (check with your local rules). IV medication is typically not recommended.
- Use the least amount of medication necessary to help the patient to control their behavior.
- Don't confuse the tranquillizing (calming), effects of medication with the sedative (hypnotic or sleep inducing) effects.

Aftercare

- Respiration, pulse and blood pressure should be monitored frequently (e.g., within an hour of the drug's administration and regularly thereafter). Monitor for acute dystonia.

- All patients placed in seclusion or restraint should be monitored on a one-to-one basis for the duration of the intervention and, in general, released as soon as clinically possible.
- Most aggressive patients can "contract" to maintain safe behavior fairly soon after a seclusion or restraint has occurred, with the possible exception of intoxicated, personality-disordered, acutely psychotic, manic, delirious, brain-injured and/or the more severely mentally retarded. Remember that fatalities and serious injuries have resulted in the context of emergency restraint (this includes patients and staff).
- All patients who undergo seclusion or restraint should be assessed for urgent medication intervention as outlined above.

Managing suicide attempts in hospital

Attempted overdose

In psychiatric wards, the most likely means of attempted self-poisoning involves building up a stock of prescribed medication or bringing tablets to be taken at a later date (e.g., while out on pass). Often patients will volunteer to trusted staff that they have taken an overdose, or staff will notice the patient appears overtly drowsy and when challenged the patient admits to overdose.

- Try to ascertain the type and quantity of medication taken (look for empty bottles, medication strips, etc.).
- Establish the likely time-frame.
- If patient is unconscious, significantly drowsy, or at medical risk, arrange immediate transfer to emergency medical services (Call a "code" if appropriate).
  - Inform medical team of patient's diagnosis, current mental state, current status (informal/formal) any other regular medications.
  - A comprehensive drug panel is often ordered. Contact your local Poison Control Center for more details on management for the drug(s) in question (e.g., 1-800-222-1222).
- If patient is asymptomatic, but significant overdose is suspected, arrange immediate transfer to emergency services.
  - Do not try to induce vomiting.
  - If available, consider giving activated charcoal (single dose of 50g with water) to reduce absorption (esp. if NSAIDs/acetaminophen).
- If patient is asymptomatic, and significant overdose unlikely:
  - Monitor closely (general observations, level of consciousness, evidence of nausea/vomiting, other possible signs of poisoning).
  - If acetaminophen or salicylate (aspirin) suspected: perform routine bloods (CBC, 'lytes, LFTs, HCO$_3$, INR) and request specific blood levels (4 hr postingestion for acetaminophen),
  - If other psychiatric medications may have been taken, consider urgent blood levels (e.g., lithium, anticonvulsants see 📖 p. 1086),
  - Be aware that baseline LFTs may be abnormal in patients on antipsychotic or antidepressant medication.
- If in doubt, get advice, or arrange for medical assessment.

Self-injurious behavior

Most episodes of self-injurious behavior involve superficial self-inflicted injury (e.g., scratching, cutting, burning, scalding etc.) to the body or limbs. There may also be other forms including intentional blunt trauma or exposure to harmful substances. To avoid secondary reinforcement of behavior, these may be easily treated on the ward instead of using medical consultation services.

- Any significant injuries (e.g., stabbing, deep lacerations) should be referred to emergency medical services, with the patient returning to the psychiatric ward as soon as medically fit.

- Medical advice should also be sought if:
  - You do not feel sufficiently competent to suture minor lacerations.
  - Lacerations are to the face/other vulnerable areas (e.g., genitals) or where you cannot confirm absence of damage to deeper structures (e.g., nerves, blood vessels, tendons).
  - The patient has swallowed/inserted sharp objects into their body (e.g., vagina, anus).
  - The patient has ingested potentially harmful chemicals.

Attempted hanging

Most victims of attempted hangings in hospitals do not use a strong enough noose or sufficient drop height to cause death through spinal cord injury ("judicial hanging"). Cerebral hypoxia through asphyxiation is the probable cause of death and should be the primary concern in treatment of this patient population.

On being summoned to the scene

- Support the patient's weight (if possible enlist help).
- Loosen/cut off ligature.
- Lower patient to flat surface, ensuring external stabilization of the neck and begin usual basic resuscitation (Call a code, ABCs, IV access, etc.).
- Emergency airway management is a priority:
  - Where available, administer 100% O_2.
  - If competent and indicated: use nasal or oral endotracheal intubation.
- Assess conscious level, full neurological examination, and degree of injury to soft tissues of the neck.
- Arrange transfer to emergency medical services as soon as possible.

Points to note

- Aggressive resuscitation and treatment of postanoxic brain injury is indicated even in patients without evident neurological signs.
- Cervical spine fractures should be considered if there is a possibility of a several foot drop or evidence of focal neurological deficit.
- Injury to the anterior soft tissues of the neck may cause respiratory obstruction. Close attention to the development of pulmonary complications is required.

Attempted asphyxiation

- Remove source (ligature, plastic bag, etc.).
- Give 100% O_2.
- If prolonged period of anoxia or impaired conscious level, arrange immediate transfer to emergency medical services.

After the event

Patient

- Once the patient is fit for interview, formally assess mental state and conduct assessment of further suicide risk (📖 p. 954).
- Establish level of observation necessary to ensure patient's safety, clearly communicate your decision to staff, and make a record in the patient's notes. (Note: hospitals policy may vary, but levels of observation will range from timed checks (e.g., every 15mins) to having a member of staff within arm's length of the patient 24hrs/day based upon the clinical facts of each individual case.

Staff

- Carefully document the event per your facility's policy. It may be necessary to arrange a specific, "critical incident review" (at a later date) or an "M&M" (morbidity and mortality) conference where all staff involved participate in a confidential debriefing session. This is not to establish blame, but rather to review policy and to consider what measures (if any) might be taken to prevent similar events occurring in the future.

Severe behavioral disturbance

This covers a vast range of presentations, but will usually represent a qualitative acute change in a person's normal behavior, that manifests primarily behavior problems e.g., shouting, screaming, increased activity (often disruptive/intrusive), aggressive outbursts, threatening violence (to others or self).

In extreme circumstances (e.g., person threatening to commit suicide by jumping from a height (out of a window, off a roof), where the person has an offensive weapon, or a hostage situation), this is a police matter and your responsibility does not extend to risking your own or other people's lives in trying to deal with the situation.

Common causes

- Acute confusional states/delirium (🕮 p. 978).
- Drug/alcohol intoxication.
- Acute symptoms of psychiatric disorder, mania (🕮 p. 347) schizophrenia/ other psychotic disorders (🕮 p. 210).
- "Challenging behavior" in brain-injured or MR patients (🕮 p. 932).
- Behavior unrelated to primary psychiatric disorder—this may reflect personality disorder, abnormal personality traits, or situational stressors (e.g., frustration).

General approach

- Sources of information will vary depending on the setting (e.g., inpatient psychiatric hospital, in outpatient settings, emergency assessment of new patient). Try to establish the context in which the behavior has arisen.
- Follow the general principles outlined in the first section of this chapter (🕮 p. 1088).
- Look for evidence of possible psychiatric disorder.
- Look for evidence of possible physical disorder.
- Try to establish any possible triggers for the behavior-environmental/ interpersonal stressors, use of drugs/alcohol, etc.

Management

This will depend on assessment made:
- If organic medical cause suspected:
  - Follow management of delirium (🕮 p. 979).
  - Consider use of sedative medication (see opposite) to allow proper examination if absolutely necessary, facilitate transfer to medical care (if indicated), or to allow active (urgent) medical management.
- If psychiatric cause suspected:
  - Consider pharmacological management of acute behavioral disturbance (see opposite).
  - Consider need for involuntary commitment.
  - Review current management plan, including observation level.
- If no medical or psychiatric cause suspected, and behavior is dangerous or seriously compromising patient care, inform security or the police to have person removed from the premises (and possibly charged if a criminal offense has been committed e.g., assault, damage to property).

Pharmacological approach to severe behavioral disturbance[1]

Consider the following medications for calming the acutely aggressive or self-injurious patient: Monitor very closely for side-effects (e.g., NMS, EPS). Use tablets when possible—save liquids or disintegrating tabs for those who can't swallow well, or are suspected of "cheeking" (hiding medication in their mouth to avoid taking it or to sell/trade later). Most meds are "off label" for this purpose. Special populations have unique prescribing considerations.

Oral

Always offer the patient the option of taking oral medication first (before IM) unless the risk is too high and there is immediate risk to self or others.

Medication options include

- Haloperidol (Haldol®): Liquid 2.5mg–10mg po (2.5mg dose initially, 5mg if very severe), repeated at a minimum of 30–60 minute intervals to a maximum of 20mg in 24 hours)
- Risperidone (Risperdal®): M-tab orally dissolving tablets 0.5–1mg po (if severe with a history of tolerance to this drug, a 2mg dose may be used initially), repeated at a minimum of 30–60-minute intervals to a maximum of 6mg in 24 hours). Monitor for EPS. Avoid atypical antipsychotics in dementia-related psychosis.
- Olanzapine (Zyprexa®): Zydis® orally disintegrating tablets 2.5mg–10mg po (5mg dose initially, repeated at a minimum of 30–60 minute intervals to a maximum of 20mg in 24 hours). Avoid atypical antipsychotics in dementia-related psychosis.

Any of these with or without

- Lorazepam 1–2mg po (see warning below), (1mg dose initially, repeated at a minimum of 30–60 minute intervals to a maximum of 4mg in 24 hours)

Intramuscular (IM) Injection

If the patient refuses medication or is too unwell to have a further discussion but needs calming, you may need to give medication by injection.

Medication options include:

- Haloperidol 5–10mg IM with benztropine 1–2mg IM; repeat in 1–2 hours as necessary; be observant for signs of acute dystonic reactions. Maximum 20mg Haloperidol in 24 hours. Haloperidol, in small doses, is the treatment of choice if patient intoxicated, but not having symptoms of withdrawal.
- Lorazepam 1–2mg IM either alone or in combination with above haloperidol and benztropine. Have flumazenil (Romazicon®) available should excess sedation or respiratory suppression occur (although beware of potential for seizure and autonomic hyperactivity in alcohol or tranquilizer-dependent patients). Also beware of giving benzodiazepines if alcohol intoxication or delirium suspected due to

synergistic sedation and possible respiratory suppression (conversely, one must also watch for signs of alcohol or benzodiazepine withdrawal in even intoxicated patients, since heavy tolerance could lead to significant withdrawal risk at levels just below what it takes to intoxicate a given patient).

- Olanzapine 5–10mg IM; repeat in 1–2 hours as necessary. Olanzapine IM may not be given with lorapzepam. Benztropine is not required

Other possibilities

- Ziprasidone 10–20mg IM; Usefulness limited as should not be given without a prior EKG. Do not use if the patient has an increased corrected QT interval.
- Chlorpromazine 25–50mg IM; be mindful of postural hypotension and sterile abscesses. Only use if nothing else is available.

Recommended further reading

1 Battaglia, J. (2005), Pharmacological management of acute agitation. *Drugs* **65**(9), 1207–1222.

The catatonic patient

Catatonia is a syndrome consisting of several motor and behavioral symptoms that could be a part of several psychiatric and medical disorders. It has been consistently described since the beginning of the 19th century but some clinicians feel that recently catatonia is less commonly seen in clinical practice, or even that the syndrome no longer exists[1]. Others believe that catatonia is still fairly prevalent, especially in hospitalized patients, but is not being recognized and, subsequently is under treated[2].

In general, this clinical presentation is a cause for concern, particularly when a previously alert and oriented patient becomes mute and immobile. The bizarre motor presentations (e.g., posturing) may also raise concerns about a serious acute medical or neurological problem (hence these patients may be encountered in a consultation and liaison setting), and it is important that signs of catatonia are recognized. Equally, the "excited" forms may be associated with sudden death ("lethal" or "malignant" catatonia), which may be preventable with timely interventions.

Clinical presentation

Characteristic signs
- Mutism.
- Stupor.
- Posturing (catalepsy).
- Waxy flexibility.
- Negativism.
- Mannerisms.
- Automatic obedience.
- Echophenomena (echopraxia, echolalia).
- Stereotypy.

Typical forms
- Retarded (stuporous).
- Excited (delirious mania).

Common causes

Psychiatric conditions
Mood disorder
More commonly associated with mania (accounts for up to 50% of cases) than depression. Often referred to as manic (or depressive) stupor (or excitement).
Schizophrenia
10–15% of cases ("Catatonic schizophrenia," 📖 *p. 211*).

Medication and drug-related: (antipsychotics, dopaminergic drug withdrawal; benzodiazepine withdrawal, opiate intoxication).

Neurological conditions
- Postencephalitic states.
- Parkinsonism.
- Seizure disorder (e.g., nonconvulsive status epilepticus).
- Bilateral globus pallidus disease.

- Lesions of the thalamus or parietal lobes.
- Frontal lobe disease.
- General paresis.
- Space-occupying lesions.

General medical conditions
- Delirium of any etiology.
- Metabolic disturbances.
- Endocrine disorders.
- Viral infections (including HIV).
- Typhoid fever.
- Heat stroke.
- Autoimmune disorders.

Differential diagnosis
- Elective or selective mutism (📖 p. 739) is usually associated with pre-existing personality disorder, clear stressor, no other catatonic features, and is unresponsive to lorazepam.
- Stroke: Mutism associated with focal neurological signs and other stroke risk factors. "Locked-in syndrome" (lesions of ventral pons and cerebellum) is characterized by mutism and total immobility (except for vertical eye movements and blinking). The patient will often try to communicate.
- Stiff-person syndrome: Progressive rigidity with painful spasms brought on by touch, noise, or emotional stimuli (may respond to benzodiazepines or baclofen, the latter can induce catatonia).
- Malignant hyperthermia: Occurs following exposure to anaesthetics and muscle relaxants in genetically predisposed individuals (📖 p. 332).
- Akinetic parkinsonism: Usually, in patients with a history of parkinsonian symptoms and dementia and depression—may display mutism, immobility, and posturing. May respond to anticholinergics, not benzodiazepines.

Other recognized catatonia (and catatonia-like) subtypes
- Malignant (febrile, pernicious) catatonia: acute onset of excitement, delirium, fever, autonomic instability, and catalepsy. May be fatal if untreated.
- Neuroleptic malignant syndrome (NMS)—📖 pp. 238, 1066.
- Serotonin syndrome (SS)—📖 p. 1070.

Management
Assessment
- Full history (often from third-party sources), including recent drug exposure, recent stressors, known medical/psychiatric conditions.
- Physical examination (including full neurological status).
- Laboratory studies—CBC, UA, LFTs, Chem 7, TFTs, cortisol, prolactin, consider CT/MRI and EEG.

Treatment

- Symptomatic treatment of catatonia will allow you to assess any underlying disorder more fully (i.e., you will actually be able to talk to the patient).
- Best evidence for use of benzodiazepines (e.g., lorazepam 0.5mg–1mg PO/IM/IV—if effective, given regularly thereafter), barbiturates (e.g., amobarbital 50–100mg), and ECT.
- Alone or in combination these effectively relieve catatonic symptoms regardless of severity or etiology in 70—80% of cases.[3, 4]
- Address any underlying medical, neurological or psychiatric disorder.

Recommended further reading

1 Mahendra, B. (1981). Editorial: Where have all the catatonics gone? *Psychol Med* **11**, 669–671.
2 Fink, M., Tayler, M.A. (2003). *Catatonia: A Clinician's Guide to Diagnosis and Treatment.* Cambridge: Cambridge University Press, 📖 pp. 10–11.
3 Bush, G., Fink, M., Petrides, G., et al. (1996). Catatonia II: treatment with lorazepam and electroconvulsive therapy. *Acta Psychiatr Scand* **93**, 137–143.
4 Ungvari, G.S., Kau, L.S., Wai-Kwong, T., Shing, N.F. (2001). The pharmacological treatment of catatonia: an overview. *Eur Arch Psychiatry Clin Neurosci* **251** (suppl 1), 31–34.

Medication or drug-related problems requiring immediate action

There are a number of presentations related to both prescribed and recreational drugs that may present acutely and require urgent attention. These include:

Prescribed medication
- Acute dystonic reaction (📖 p. 1062).
- Neuroleptic malignant syndrome (📖 p. 1066).
- Serotonin syndrome (📖 p. 1070).
- Lithium toxicity (📖 p. 380).
- Clozapine-related agranulocytosis (📖 p. 248).
- Paradoxical reactions to benzodiazepines (📖 p. 1077).

Recreation drugs
- Acute opiate withdrawal (📖 pp. 651–3).
- Acute benzodiazepine withdrawal (📖 pp. 645–9).
- Acute alcohol withdrawal (📖 pp. 633–37).

The challenging patient—general principles

In the context of psychiatric (and other medical) settings, certain patients present with behaviors that are usually viewed as maladaptive and include:

- Inappropriate or unreasonable demands.
- More of your time than any other patient receives.
- Wanting to deal with a specific doctor.
- Only willing to accept one particular course of action (e.g., admission to hospital, a specific medication or other form of treatment).
- Behavioral consequences of failing to have these demands met.
- Claims of additional symptoms they failed to mention previously.
- Vague or explicit threats of self-harm or harm to others, filing formal complaints, litigation, or violence.
- Passive resistance (refusal to leave until satisfied with outcome of consultation).
- Verbal or physical abuse of staff or damage to property.
- Actual formal complaints relating to treatment (received or refused), or false accusations of misconduct against medical staff.

Key points

- Patients DO have the right to expect appropriate assessment, care, and relief of distress.
- Doctors DO have the right to refuse a course of action they judge to be inappropriate.
- Action should always be a response to clinical need (based on a thorough assessment, diagnosis, and best evidence for management), NOT threats or other manipulative behaviors.
- It is entirely possible that a patient who demonstrates challenging behavior *does* have a genuine problem (it might be that they really need help, but that their way of seeking help is inappropriate).
- Some of the most challenging patients tend to present at "awkward" times (e.g., the end of the working day, early hours of the morning, weekends, holidays, shift change)—this may be intentional.
- Admitting a patient to hospital for further assessment when they make vague threats to self or others, their story is inconsistent or they are unable to contract reliably for safety is not necessarily a failure—some patients are very good at engineering this outcome. It may, though, reinforce inappropriate coping behaviors for the patient in the future.
- If you have any doubts about what course of action to take, consult a senior colleague and discuss the case with them.

Management principles

New case: make a full assessment to establish

- Psychiatric diagnosis and level of risk (to self and others).
- Whether other agencies need to be involved (e.g., specific services: drug and alcohol problems; social work: housing/benefits/social supports; counselling: for specific issue—debt/employment/bereavement/alleged abuse).

- Ask the patient what they think is the main problem.
- Ask the patient what they were hoping you could do for them, e.g:
  - Advice about what course of action to take.
  - Wanting their problem to be "taken seriously."
  - Wanting to be admitted to hospital (see below).
  - Wanting a specific treatment.
- Discuss with them your opinion of the best course of action, and establish whether they are willing to accept any alternatives offered (e.g., other services, outpatient treatment).

The "frequent flyer"/chronic case

- Do not take short cuts—always fully assess current mental state and make a risk assessment, no matter who frequently this patient has presented and been evaluated by you or your colleagues in the recent past.
- Whenever available, always check previous notes, treatment plans plan, or "alerts" agreed upon by outpatient treatment teams about how to deal with the particular patient when in crisis.
- Establish the reason for presenting, "Why now?" (i.e., what has changed in their current situation).
- Ask yourself, "Is the clinical presentation significantly different so as to warrant a change to the previously agreed treatment plan?"
- If not, go with what has been laid out in the treatment plan.
- Use extra caution and judgment when asked for a "private" consultation with a patient of the opposite sex; to make "special" arrangements; and rarely, if ever, give out personal information or allow patients to contact you directly.

Pitfalls (and how to avoid them)

- Try not to take your own frustrations (e.g., being busy, feeling "dumped on" by other colleagues, lack of sleep, lack of information, vague histories) into an interview with a patient—your job is to make an objective assessment of the person's mental state and to treat each case you see on its own merits.
- Try not to allow any preconceptions or the opinions of other colleagues influence your assessment of the current problems the patient presents with (people and situations change with time, and what may have been true in the past may no longer be the case).
- Watch out for the patient who appeals to your vanity by saying things like: "You're much better than that other doctor I saw … I can really talk to you … I feel you really understand …" They probably initially said the same things to "that other doctor" too!
- Do not be drawn into being openly critical of other colleagues; remember you are only hearing one side of the story. Maintain a healthy regard for the professionalism of those you work with—respect their opinions (even if you might not agree with them).
- If you encounter a particularly challenging patient, enlist the support of a colleague and conduct the assessment jointly.

The challenging patient—specific situations

Patient demanding medication

There are two common scenarios where there is an urgent need for medications (most others can wait for the patient's regular provider):

- The patient who is acutely unwell and requires admission to hospital anyway (e.g., with acute confusion, acute psychotic symptoms, severe depression, high risk of suicide).
- The patient who is known and has genuinely run out of their usual medication (for whom a small supply may be dispensed to tide them over until they can obtain a refill on their prescription).

Patient demanding immediate admission

- Clarify what the patient hopes to achieve by admission, and decide whether this could be reasonably achieved, or if other services would better meet these requests.
- If the patient is demanding admission due to a chemical dependence, emphasize the need for clear motivation to remain abstinent, and offer referral to specialty programs (see Chapter 15).
- Always ask about any recent legal trouble since it is not uncommon for the hospital to be sought as a "sanctuary" from an impending court hearing (but also remember this can be a significant stressor for patients with current psychiatric problems).

Demanding relatives/other advocates

- Assess the patient on their own initially, but allow those attending with the patient to have their say (this may clarify the "why now" question, particularly if it involves the breakdown of usual social supports).
- Ask the patient for their written consent to discuss the outcome of your consultation with family and treatment providers to avoid misunderstandings and improve compliance with the proposed treatment plan.
- If a patient is dissatisfied with the outcome of your consultation, they may try a number of ways to change your mind; they may even explicitly say: "What do I have to do to convince you that ..." before resorting to other behaviors.
- This type of response only serves to confirm any suspicions of attempted manipulation and should be documented as such in your note, verbatim if possible.
- Stick to your original management plan, and if the patient becomes passively, verbally or physically aggressive, clearly inform them of the standards for admission to your facility.
- Equally, any specific threats of violence toward individuals present during the interview or elsewhere should be dealt with seriously and the hospital security and the police (and the individual concerned) should be informed. However, since this is a breach in patient's confidentiality, you should thoroughly and carefully document the situation and the rationale for the chosen course of action.

Suspected factitious disorder

- Try to obtain corroboration of the patient's story (or confirmation of your suspicions) from third-party sources (e.g., PCP, relatives, previous notes by other providers and other utilized treatment facilities).
- If your suspicions are confirmed, directly provide this information back to the patient and your supervisor. Clearly inform them of what course of action you plan to take (e.g., recording this in their notes, informing other agencies, etc.).
- Do not feel "defeated" if you decide to admit them to hospital. Record your suspicions in your note and inform the inpatient psychiatric team that the reason for admission is to assess how clinically significant the reported symptoms are (it will soon become clear in an inpatient unit environment and it may take time to obtain 3rd party sources). Carefully evaluate, as individuals with factitious disorder may have actual medical or psychiatric illnesses.

Patient threatening suicide by telephone

- Try to elicit useful information before continuing the conversation (name, where they are calling from, what they plan to do, risk to anyone else).
- Keep the person talking.
- If you judge the patient to be at high risk of suicide, encourage them to come to hospital—if they refuse or are unable to do so, you must petition the appropriate authorities for their involuntary transportation to and evaluation at an emergency room, in accordance with the legal procedures in place for your particular state, county, municipality, etc.
- If the patient refuses to give you any information, inform the police who may have other means to determine the source of the call and respond.
- Always document phone calls in the same way you would any other patient contact (see below).

Documentation and communication

- Clearly document your assessment, any discussion with senior colleagues, the outcome, and any treatment plan that has been agreed upon.
- Record the agreement/disagreement of the patient and any other persons attending with them.
- If appropriate, provide the patient with written instructions (e.g., appointment details, directions, other contact numbers) to ensure clear communication.
- Ensure that you have informed any other interested parties (e.g., case managers, social workers, therapists, psychiatrists, and other providers who are either already involved with the patient or have referred them to you for an assessment).
- If the assessment occurs after business hours, make arrangements for information to be passed on to the relevant parties in the morning of the following business day (ideally try to do this yourself).

- If you have suggested outpatient follow-up for a new patient, make sure you have a means of contacting the patient, to allow the relevant service to make arrangements to see them as planned.
- If you think it is likely the patient will present again to other services, inform them of your contact with the patient and the outcome of your assessment.

Looking after your own mental health

Let's face it—your job can be difficult. As a mental health provider, you are exposed to countless daily stressors, challenging patient encounters, and demanding professional obligations. It is virtually impossible to provide good patient care, let alone enjoy the reasons that drew you to this career in the first place, when you yourself are suffering.

Symptoms to be aware of
- Difficulty sleeping.
- Change in appetite.
- Feeling impatient or irritable.
- Difficulty concentrating or making decisions.
- Increased use of alcohol or tobacco.
- Finding less enjoyment in pleasurable activities.
- Being unable to relax or "switch off."
- Feeling fatigued or having difficulty getting out of bed.
- Feeling chronically overwhelmed or overemotional.
- Feeling dispassionate or hostile toward patients.
- Feeling tense (may manifest as recurrent headache, muscle tension, GI upset, heart racing, or other somatic symptoms).

Developing good habits
- Learn to relax: according to the American Academy of Family Physicians, up to two-thirds of all office visits to family doctors are for stress related symptoms. Release stress by learning methods of progressive relaxation, or simply setting aside time to unwind.
- Practice good sleep hygiene: live life less frantically by going to bed at a regular hour and getting up 15–20 minutes earlier to prevent the feeling of "always being in a rush."
- Take regular breaks: even when work is busy, try to give yourself a 5–10 minute break every few hours. This includes healthy meal breaks (away from work).
- Escape the pager: in the day and age of being always obtainable, it is a good idea to be "unobtainable" once or twice a week, to give yourself time to be alone and reflect.
- Exercise: there is no doubt that regular physical activity can help reduce levels of stress. It can also help keep you fit, prevent heart disease, control weight, improve sleep, and improve mood.
- Avoid substance use: tobacco and other recreational drugs are best avoided. Caffeine and alcohol should be used only in moderation.
- Develop nonwork related interests: finding a pursuit that has no deadlines, no pressures, and which can be picked up or left easily can allow you to forget about your usual stresses (e.g., exercise, reading, meditation, yoga, painting, etc.)
- Respect times of stress: allow time to cope with major life events (e.g., major events for a family member or friend, divorce or marital discord, natural disaster, or other loss), even when you perceive them as positive (promotion at work, birth of a child, move to a new home).

- Reach out to significant others: whether confiding in a friend, playing with your children, or scheduling a date night with your partner, be sure to take time to foster relationships that are important to you.

Organizing your own medical care

- Establish yourself with a Primary Care Physician!
- Allow yourself to benefit from the same standards of care (including specialist referral, if this is deemed necessary) you would expect for your patients.
- If you are having difficulties related to stress, anxiety, depression, or use of substances, consult your PCP sooner rather than later.
- Be willing to take advice. In particular, do not rely on your own judgment of your ability to continue working.
- If your PCP suggests speaking to a psychiatrist or therapist, and you feel uncomfortable with being seen locally, ask for an out-of-area consultation.
- Utilize other sources of help and advice—both informal (peers, friends, family, self-help books) and formal (see below). Remember you are certainly not the first doctor to feel the strain of this profession!

Sources of support and advice

- The National Suicide Prevention Lifeline is a federally funded, 24-hour, toll-free service available to anyone in a serious mental health crisis. Your call is free and confidential at 1-800-273-TALK (8255). Also available for the hearing-impaired at 1-800-799-4889.
- The Substance Abuse and Mental Health Services Administration (SAMHSA), an agency of the U.S. Department of Health and Human Services has a Toll-Free Referral Helpline at 1-800-662-HELP (4357) to link individuals with community-based mental health and/or substance abuse treatment services. Resources are also available online at www.mentalhealth.samhsa.gov

The mental health of doctors

"Quis custodiet ipsos custodes?"
("Who will watch the watchmen?" or "Who cares for the caregivers?)"
In general, doctors enjoy relatively good health, with a lower prevalence of smoking, cardiovascular disease, cancer, and a longer life expectancy than the general population. With respect to mental health, however, physicians sometimes fall short in caring for their own mental well-being.

- It is estimated that approximately 10–15% of all physicians will face personal obstacles that ultimately affect their ability to practice medicine at some point in their careers.
- Resident physicians are at greater risk than the general population for developing stress-related or mental health problems. In a 2002 survey of internal medicine trainees, 40% of female residents and 32% of male residents reported 4–5 symptoms of depression. Overwhelming and untreated depression, anxiety, and drug and alcohol misuse may be significant contributory factors to decreased work productivity, sleep deprivation, inability to maintain attention, decreased empathy, poor decision making capacity, and occupational dysfunction.
- Furthermore, untreated depression and substance abuse are two of the strongest predictors for physician suicide. And sadly, physicians have been shown to have a substantially lower risk of mortality compared to the general population for all causes of death except suicide. Specialties over-represented include anesthesia, medicine, emergency medicine, and psychiatry.

Why are doctors more likely to have mental health problems?

Individual factors
- Personality—many of the qualities that make us "good doctors" also increase our risk for psychiatric problems: (e.g., perfectionism, ambitiousness, self-sacrifice, low tolerance of uncertainty, difficulty expressing emotions, excessive devotion to work to the exclusion of leisure activities).
- Coping styles—e.g., intellectualization, minimization, rationalization, self-criticism, denial, acting out (e.g., drugs & alcohol), desire to appear competent to others.

Occupational factors
- Long work hours and sleep deprivation.
- Exposure to potentially traumatic events (e.g., patient deaths, ethical dilemmas, etc.).
- Lack of support from senior colleagues.
- Competing needs of patients and family.
- Increasing expectations with diminishing resources.
- Professional and geographic isolation.
- Symptom concealment due to fears of loss of medical license or exposure to stigmatization.

What to do if you suspect a colleague has a problem

As a physician, you have taken an oath. It is your ethical and moral obligation to protect patients against harm and act in the best interest of your colleagues. Not to intervene in a timely manner could both put patients at risk and potentially deny a potentially life-saving treatment for your fellow colleague. A staged approach generally works best:

- In most cases, the first step is to confirm your suspicions by speaking directly to the colleague in question. Such a discussion enables you to provide compassionate support, gather information, assess whether he or she recognizes the problem, and, if appropriate, urge him or her to seek help.
- If the colleague is a superior or someone you would feel uncomfortable approaching directly, however, it is advisable to speak to an impartial senior colleague (i.e., residency training director for physicians in training) in order to seek further advice as how to proceed.
- In the case of a colleague who continues to practice despite reasonable offers of assistance and referral, it may be necessary to report the impaired physician to a hospital peer review body, state physician health program, and/or the state licensing or disciplinary board. The Federation of State Physician Health Programs has a central office at the AMA headquarters in Chicago. State-specific information and resources may be obtained online at http://www.fsphp.org by calling 312-464-4574.

"The Sick Physician"

In a landmark policy paper prepared by the AMA Council on Mental Health, "The Sick Physician: Impairment by Psychiatric Disorders, Including Alcoholism and Drug Dependence," the AMA acknowledged physician impairment. In 1974, model legislation was developed that offered a therapeutic alternative to discipline, recognizing alcoholism and other drug addictions as illnesses. The AMA held a Physician Health Conference in April 1975 and a second in 1977 where it officially recognized the psychiatrically disturbed physician. A flurry of articles published in the late 1970s increased education and awareness about physician addiction. By 1980, less than a decade after the AMA's policy paper, "all but three of the 54 U.S. medical societies of all states and jurisdictions had authorized or implemented impaired physician programs." Today, all states have responded and developed programs that provide many different levels of service to physicians in need.

Excerpt from the Federation of State Physician Health Programs web site: http://www.fsphp.org

Integrative medicine and psychiatry

Integrative medicine in psychiatry

Introduction

What is "integrative medicine" and how does it apply to psychiatry? The theoretical foundation for integrative medicine dates back thousands of years. Its foundation is integration of the mind, body, and spirit. This is combined with an "openness to us[e] alternative or complementary therapies that have a record of safety and efficacy but are outside of the conventional biomedical model."[1]

Generally speaking, integrative medicine works at the interface of "alternative" and "conventional" medicine. Integrative medicine is becoming increasingly popular with patients, researchers, and some training institutions. As such, the current status of integrative medicine in psychiatry is reviewed in this chapter.

What is considered integrative medicine is constantly changing as we learn more about the safety and efficacy of different treatment modalities. For example, cognitive behavior therapy, one of the most utilized therapies in psychiatry today, was once considered a controversial alternative to conventional treatment.

Integrative medicine seeks to engage the patient and encourage personal responsibility for care by using less invasive, more self-reflective techniques.

Integrative medicine is frequently referred to by other names, such as complementary and alternative medicine (CAM). For the purpose of this chapter, integrative medicine and CAM will be used interchangeably.

Use of integrative medicine/CAM with mainstream medicine

While physicians may vary in their acceptance of integrative medicine in their practice, the increasing demand for these services cannot be ignored. Studies report about 40% of all U.S. citizens have tried some kind of CAM therapy, and of those who used CAM, about 40% have tried two or more kinds. The most popular CAM is currently herbal medicine[2]. "Factors associated with highest rates of CAM use were ages 40–64, female gender, non-black/non-Hispanic race, and annual income of $65,000 or higher."[3] Regarding psychiatric care, about 10% of psychiatric patients utilize CAM, and having psychological distress or a mental illness is reported with increased likelihood of CAM utilization.[3]

Patients may seek integrative medicine therapy for any psychiatric illness or symptoms, and may view the treatment as adjunctive or in place of traditional psychiatric care. Research in integrative medicine has increased in response to this undeniable interest.

- For example, in 1998, the federal government established a division within the National institute's of health (NIH) called The National Center for Complementary and Alternative Medicine (NCCAM). The mission of NCCAM was to fund and advance scientific research on CAM. In 2006, congress appropriated over 122 million dollars in funding for NCCAM. There are also multiple other associations known to fund research in integrative medicine/CAM.

Barriers to integrative medicine treatment

There are several barriers to obtaining and utilizing integrative medicine treatments. For example:

Practitioners

The training, credentialing, and monitoring of integrative medicine practitioners varies widely from none to strict federal standards. Such standards may be known to the practitioners, but are rarely evident to the patient. As such, patients may not receive comparable treatment, or may not know where to go to find qualified integrative medicine/CAM providers.

Cost

Another factor is cost. Some integrative medicine treatments are covered by insurance companies, but most are not. The costs involved with a course of integrative medicine treatment can contrast from pennies to hundreds of dollars per treatment. This limits certain integrative medicine treatments to those with the independent financial means to cover the costs.

Medical clinics and integrative medicine

There are also several limitations for clinicians interested in becoming proficient in an integrative medicine modality. Training may involve considerable travel and expense. The equipment required may be an additional cost burden. Reimbursement may be limited, and the patient base may not be able to afford the full cost of the treatment. Liability and malpractice related to referral, treatment, and delay of conventional medicine must also be considered.

Approach to the patient requesting or inquiring about integrative medicine/CAM treatment modalities

Patients and family may come to practitioners asking for alternatives to conventional treatment. Their reasons for asking about integrative medicine are usually varied. Be open and inquire about their interest. They may seek something that seems "natural" or "safe." Review their motivation for integrative medicine treatment (sometimes, seeking integrative medicine/CAM may be a method of denying the reality or severity of an illness). As with any treatment plan, help patients/ families make the choice that is right for them by explaining the risks, benefits, and alternatives.

The "ABC Approach" for advising patients who inquire about alternative therapies[1] is one method to facilitate discussion of integrative medicine/CAM in treatment:

Ask, don't tell

Be open. Ask what they want to treat, what they have tried, and what they are currently interested in.

Be willing to listen to learn

Be respectful, open and receptive. Know the limits of your knowledge, and be willing to learn information about the treatment requested by your patient.

Communicate, collaborate

Know the skilled practitioners and specialists in your area. Communicate with them and your patient throughout the therapeutic treatment.

Diagnose

Utilize the standard of care for diagnosis, and share this information with the integrative medicine practitioner.

Explain and explore options and preferences

Balance the patient's wishes with the obligation to disclose by thoroughly explaining the risks, benefits, and alternatives for treatment options. Be certain the patient has all of the information on the conventional treatment as well as the integrative medicine treatment before they make a decision (e.g., possible interactions, risks of withholding approved treatment choices, limitations of the unapproved treatments). Refer to a supervisor or specialist as needed.

Recommended further reading

1 Sierpina, V.S. Integrative Health Care, Complementary and Alternative Therapies for the Whole Person. New York: FA Davis Company, 2001.
2 Simon, G.E., Cherkin, D.C., Sherman, K.J. Eisenberg, D.M., Deyo, R.A., Davis, R.B. Mental health visits to complementary and alternative medicine providers. *General Hospital Psychiatry.* **26**(3), 171–177, 2004.
3 Tindle, H.A., Davis, R.B., Phillips, R.S., Eisenberg, D.M. Trends in use of complementary and alternative medicine by US adults: 1997–2002. *Alternative Therapies in Health & Medicine.* **11**(1), 42–49, 2005.

Biochemical approaches (1)

What some call health, if purchased by perpetual anxiety about diet, isn't much better than tedious disease. —George Denison Prentice

Since 1994 herbs along with dietary supplements, botanicals, and vitamins have been classified legally as dietary supplements. As such, there is no FDA approval needed unless a claim to disease treatment is made. Subsequently, there exist a wide variety of supplements in regards to quality, origin and standardization. There are also limited safety and efficacy studies, although many of these substances have been used by indigenous cultures for hundreds or thousands of years. There has been widely increased use of herbal/supplements in the United States, mostly for the number of chronic illnesses that are increasing as the population ages. One of the biggest reasons that herbal-nutritional therapies are sought out is that there is a perceived low risk-benefit ratio. However, one must take into account that risks are inherent in ingestion of any substance, and there are potential additive or subtractive effects on both the therapeutic or toxic effects of drugs or herbs. Another major consideration is the risk inherent if treatment results in the withholding of a proven therapy (e.g. antipsychotic medications in schizophrenia).

The following is a basic summary of popular biochemical integrative medicine approaches that may come up in psychiatric practice. They are not FDA approved for any treatment, but are listed by potential efficacy. Review the current standards and research prior to consulting on the use and risks of these supplements.

Good evidence for efficacy

Omega-3 fatty acids

A large percent of the human brain is composed of lipids that must be obtained through the diet (essential). These can either be in the form of omega-3 or omega-6 polyunsaturated fatty acids. Important, nutritionally essential omega-3 fatty acids are alpha-linolenic acid (ALA), eicosapentaenoic acid (EPA) and docosahexaenoic acid (DHA).

Omega-3 fatty acids have been shown to have metabolites that are less inflammatory and thrombogenic than those of omega-6. Found predominantly in algae and plankton, as well as the fish that eat them (mackerel, sardines, salmon, tuna). Also found in some grains, seeds (flaxseed), Omega-6 fatty acids are found predominantly in grains, grain fed animals, and vegetable oils. It is believed that the western diet, with approximate 15:1 ratio of omega-6 to omega-3, is at great odds with the 1:1 ratio in the diet of our ancestors at the time of human evolution. As such, some view omega-3 intake as supplementation to correct a nutritional deficit. At the neuronal level, they act to facilitate neurotransmission.

A 2006 APA subcommittee found omega-3 fatty acids, namely EPA and DHA, have an overall protective effect in mood disorders. Meta-analyses show statistically significant effects in bipolar disorder and depression. A recent double-blind placebo-controlled trial showed efficacy in pediatric depression. No consistent effects were noted in schizophrenia. Associated with mild GI side-effects, may prolong bleeding time (increased bleeding risk with warfarin, aspirin). Caution is warranted in consuming large amounts of larger, slow-growing fish due to risk of mercury toxicity, especially in the pediatric/child-bearing population. Available as supplements of EPA or DHA, most commercial brands containing a 2:1 ratio of EPA:DHA. Some research has demonstrated better psychoactive effects with EPA. Recommended dose 1–2g/day.

St. John's wort

Hypericum perforatum. An herb, the main active ingredient of which is most likely hyperforin (also contains hypericin). Considered a first-line antidepressant in many European countries (and recently becoming popular in the United States).

Has been found in several meta-analyses to be as efficacious as TCAs in the treatment of mild to moderate depression, though there are conflicting reports. Also used in anxiety, chronic fatigue, AIDS. Thought to exert effects through serotonin reuptake inhibition, in-vitro studies have shown weak MAO-inhibition, norepinephrine and dopamine reuptake inhibition, as well as antiretroviral activity.

Is metabolized through CYP p450 as well as P-glycoproteins. Induces CYP enzymes including 3A4 thereby decreasing plasma levels of benzodiazepines, barbiturates, valproate, amitryptiline, warfarin, digoxin, and protease inhibitors. Can also interact with antiepileptics, antivirals and antibiotics. Increased bleeding risk with oral contraceptives. Risk of serotonin syndrome when used concomitantly with antidepressants, also carries risk of inducing mania in patients with bipolar depression. Usual dose 300mg tid standardized to 3% hypericin, taken with food to prevent GI upset.

L-tryptophan

An essential amino acid precursor of serotonin, as well as melatonin. Also similar is 5-hydroxytryptophan, an intermediary between L-tryptophan and serotonin. Is indicated for specialist use as an adjunct for treatment-resistant depression (lasting more than two years). Some evidence of efficacy for sleep. Common adverse effects include drowsiness, headache, nausea, and dizziness. In addition, there exists the rare possibility of eosinophilia-myalgia syndrome, possibly due to tryptophan interference with histamine metabolism. Therefore, monitoring of blood counts is necessary. Sometimes used with a peripheral decarboxylase inhibitor (PDI) such as carbidopa, to avoid peripheral conversion of 5-HTP into serotonin. Usual dose L-tryptophan 1g tid, increased to maximum 6g/d.

Kava kava

The root extract of a pepper plant, Piper Methysticum from Polynesia. Active ingredients are Kava Lactones. Tea, extract or leaves are used as a sedative/hypnotic, anxiolytic, and a sleep aid. Potentiates GABA transmission, and thus can have an additive effect with benzodiazepines, increased liver toxicity with ethanol. Usual side-effects of mild GI distress, with risk of possible uterine atony in pregnancy. Several instances of hepatotoxicity reported related to Kava ingestion, including several fatalities. The hepatic adverse event rate had been found to compare favorably to those of the benzodiazepines,[1] however additional fatalities have since occurred and safety is uncertain. It has since been banned for sale in the EU, and is no longer recommended for use by the FDA pending further investigation. Usual dose 50–70mg purified kavalactones.

Saw palmetto

The extract of berries of American Dwarf Palm. Has been found to be efficacious for use in benign prostatic hyperplasia and has antiandrogenic effects. Side-effects of sexual dysfunction, fatigue. One case report of acute pancreatitis and hepatitis. Shown to cause increased INR with warfarin.

Recommended further reading

1 Hanson, E., *et al.* (2007). Use of Complementary and Alternative Medicine among Children Diagnosed with Autism Spectrum Disorder. *J Autism Dev Disord,* **37**(4): 628–637.
2 Fugh-Berman, A. (2000). Herb–drug Interactions. *The Lancet,* **355**: 134–138.

Biochemical approaches (2)

Some evidence for efficacy

Gluten-free casein-free (GFCF) diet

It has been theorized that peptides derived from casein (milk products) and gluten (wheat products) enter the bloodstream as a result of abnormal intestinal permeability secondary to inflammation in the gut and are associated with abnormal activity of opioids in the brain. Investigated primarily in autistim spectrum disorders, where increased levels of CSF opioids and urinary peptides have been found. As a result as many as 15% of autistic children have been placed on this type of diet, and a recent survey showed 38% of autistic children at a developmental medicine clinic to be on some type of dietary restriction.[1] Several uncontrolled trials have shown efficacy, however a 2003 Cochrane review found only one study that met inclusion criteria. This study failed to show significant change in cognitive skills, linguistic ability or motor ability, but did show a reduction in autistic traits.[2] A 2006 double blind placebo controlled study failed to show any significant effects.[3]

Ginko biloba

Extract taken from the leaves of the Ginko tree, active ingredients are flavenoid glycosides, terpene lactones. Some studies have shown moderate effects sizes in the treatment of dementia and intermittent claudication, with mixed results in studies on memory and tinnitus. It acts as an antioxidant and membrane stabilizer and been shown to inhibit platelet activating factor. Interactions with warfarin, aspirin, acetaminophen. The major concern is that it has been shown to increase risk of GI bleed. Can cause GI upset, headache, rash.

Black cohosh

Extract taken from roots of Cimicifuga Racemosa herb. May be of benefit in the treatment of menopausal symptoms, larger studies pending. Side-effects of nausea, vomiting, headaches, overall very tolerable. There have been reports of hepatotoxicity, but to date, no direct association has been made. Mechanism unknown, investigations into estrogenic activity negative to date.

Echinacea

Echinacea angustifolia, E. purpurea E. Pallida. Obtained from the root of the plant, with many potential active ingredients. Most commonly treatment is prevention of upper respiratory tract infections. Cochrane review in upper respiratory infection was inconclusive. Relatively safe with reports of allergic reactions.

Yohimbine

An alkaloid derived from the bark of the Yohimbe tree Pausinystalia yohimbe, available as a prescription medicine as well as available over the counter via bark extract. It acts as a presynaptic alpha-2 antagonist, is known to raise blood pressure, and is sometimes used to treat erectile dysfunction. Known to cause hypertension when used with TCAs.

No strong evidence at this time

Ginseng

Asian/Chinese variety, Panax Ginseng. Active ingredients are Ginsenosides, with a wide array of claims made. Believed to act as CNS stimulant as well as immune modulant. No proven efficacy. There have been several case reports of ginseng inducing mania in patients on MAO-I. Caution is also warranted for taking with an SSRI or TCA. Decreases plasma warfarin and INR. Caution with other species: Korean ginseng may increase blood pressure; Russian or Siberian ginseng may raise digoxin concentrations.

Garlic

Allium sativum. Has been considered antimicrobial and immune enhancing, some also claim cardiovascular benefit. Can decrease CYP2E1 activity. No significant psychotropic interactions. Shown to decrease plasma levels of saquinovir, and increases INR when used with warfarin.

Ginger

Zingiber officinale. Commonly used as a digestive aid, antinauseant and anti-inflammatory. It is contraindicated in patients with bleeding disorders.

On the horizon

Valerian

Valeriana officinalis. Used as sedative and known to Galen (~150AD). GABAergic activity, with some sedative efficacy shown. Recent inconclusive review. Cases of hepatotoxicity with long-term use.

Passion flower

Passiflora incarnate. Partial benzodiazepine agonist. One study found equal efficacy to oxazepam (a benzodiazepine),[4] more studies needed.

SAM-E

S-Adenosylmethionine. With folate, facilitates methylation of many neurotransmitters. Two RCTs have shown effectiveness in depression comparable to imipramine. May induce mania in bipolar depression.

Selenium

An antioxidant known to assist conversion of t4 to t3. Low levels have been associated with depressed mood, with possible dose-dependent mood improvement with supplementation. No clinical trials at this time.

Glyconutrients

Supplementation of diet with specific mono- and polysaccharides. Thought to enhance immune, endocrine and overall bodily function. The body uses sugars attached to proteins or lipids for cell signaling and trafficking. Although there are over 200 naturally occurring monosaccharides, the body primarily uses less than a dozen (e.g. glucose, mannose, galactose, xylose, N-acetylglucosamine) and many of these, unlike glucose, are not found in the modern western diet to any great extent.

Vitamin E

An antioxidant, thought to possibly be useful in tardive dyskinesia (TD), based on the thought that TD is a result of oxidative damage from neuroleptics. A systematic review of 10 randomized controlled trials (RCTs) failed to show improvement in TD with vitamin E, but did show efficacy in protection from further degeneration.[5] Also question of efficacy in Alzheimers with an inconclusive Cochrane review. A 2005 Cochrane meta-analysis of high dose (>400 i.u./day) vitamin E showed an increase in all-cause mortality.

Recommended further reading

1 Clouatre, D.L. (April 2004). Kava kava: examining new reports of toxicity. *Toxicology Letters*, **150**, 85–96.
2 Knivsberg, A-M., et al. (2002). A randomized, controlled study of dietary intervention in autistic syndromes. *Nutritional Neuroscience* **5**(4): 251–261.
3 Elder, J.H. et al. (2006). The gluten-free, casein-free diet in autism: Results of a preliminary double blind clinical trial. *Journal of Autism and Developmental Disorders* **36**(3).
4 Akhondzadeh, S., Naghavi, H. R., Vazirian, M., et al. (2001). Passionflower in the treatment of generalized anxiety: a pilot double-blind RCTwith oxazepam. *J Clin. Pharm and Therapeutics*, **26**, 363–367.
5 Soares, K.V.S., McGrath, J.J. (2003). Vitamin E for neuroleptic-induced tardive dyskinesia. *Cochrane Library Cochrane Library*, issue 6. Oxford: Update Software.

Mind-body therapies

Eye Movement Desensitization and Reprocessing (EMDR)

EMDR is an "information-processing" therapy that integrates elements of other psychotherapies including psychodynamic, cognitive-behavioral, exposure, and body-based into a standardized set of procedures and clinical protocols. While originally designed to alleviate the distress associated with traumatic memories, EMDR has been advanced as a treatment for a variety of anxiety disorders and more. In this intervention, a patient focuses on a disturbing image and associated emotions and cognitions, while the therapist initiates saccadic eye movements by having the patient track a visual focal point (usually an index finger) in horizontal movements, or otherwise invokes alternate stimulation of the right and left brain hemispheres through visual, auditory, or kinesthetic cues. Positive results have been obtained repeatedly, although mechanism has not been elucidated so it is unclear if hemispheric stimulation is key to its efficacy. A recent study found sustained reduction in PTSD symptoms (75% in adults, 33% in children) at six months post-EMDR treatment.[1] These results were not seen with fluoxetine treatment alone.

EMDR is currently recommended in guidelines for treatment of PTSD by American Psychiatric Association,[2] U.S. Dept of Veterans Affairs & DOD,[3] as well as international treatment guidelines[4] (e.g., U.K., France, Sweden, Netherlands, Northern Ireland, and Israel).

Hypnosis[4]

Hypnosis can be defined as "the induction of a state of mind in which a person's normal critical or skeptical nature is bypassed, allowing for acceptance of suggestions." While the media view of hypnosis ranges widely, it is felt to be more of a natural state that involves changing the perception of the brain—not a purely suggestible or sleep-like trance. In the hypnotic state, patients are alert, focused, and continue to feel emotions. The technique is started by choosing a target behavior or symptom. During hypnosis, the patient is guided into a state of relaxation, with an enhanced focus, and typically includes distraction or replacement. The goal is to redirect your thoughts to a preferred, controlled outcome. It is different from meditation in that hypnosis specifically focuses on this outcome as the goal of treatment.

Hypnosis has been reported useful in a number of medical and psychiatric conditions. Practicing with guidance can be essential for efficacy of outcome. Possible adverse reactions are usually related to improper technique, and include drowsiness, anxiety, stiffness, headaches, and masking true symptoms. Because techniques and methods are so variable and influenced by therapeutic alliance, proper research is challenging.

Biofeedback

Biofeedback involves the use of an external device, typically technologic, to bring into awareness a person's physiologic activity for the purpose of addressing a physical or mental health condition. Most commonly used modalities include skin temperature, electromyography (EMG), and skin conductance. All of these systems are affected by chronic stress and stress reactivity. By increasing awareness of the physiologic activity, one can learn approaches that change that activity with concomitant change in stress response. The greatest usage has been in behavioral medicine, for general health problems such as migraines and abdominal pain. The therapeutic benefit may derive from a direct autonomic effect on these systems as well as modulation of the stress-pain cycle. There is a smaller body of literature on biofeedback for anxiety disorders and as with other mind-body approaches. Practice is essential.

Heart rate variability training

Heart rate variability (HRV), reflecting the beat-to-beat variation in the heart rate, has been found to provide a window into our autonomics. Respiratory sinus arrhythmia (RSA) is the normal variation in heart rate seen with our breathing cycle. Rhythmic breathing, utilized in yoga and meditation results in augmentation of this RSA pattern, which is largely vagally mediated. Biofeedback utilizing HRV can be used to easily teach a person to attain a relaxed and focused state. Using slow paced breathing, e.g. at six cycles per minute, a person learns to reach coherence, reflecting a smooth rhythmic pattern in the heart rate tracing. This technique can be coupled with therapy exercises to achieve greater awareness of affective states and management of emotions. While this has been studied most with cardiac and COPD patients, there is great potential for benefit with patients with anxiety and depressive disorders.

EEG biofeedback[6]

EEG Biofeedback, also known as neurofeedback, stems from the evolving field of associating psychiatric illness with functional brain abnormalities. This special kind of biofeedback uses the same principles described above, but utilizes brain waves as measured by EEG scalp leads. The patient's brain wave activity is compared in some way (for example, to a database from normative samples), and the abnormal readings are the focus of the therapy. The patient uses visual or auditory cues to learn how to normalize their abnormal EEG readings, and this may facilitate effective neuronal communication. Improvement is (in theory) the result of actual change in the brain function, which is created by facilitation of the neuronal communication. While investigations continue, currently neurofeedback has been reported to be effective for ADHD and epilepsy, possibly effective for anxiety, phobias, and PTSD, but less support for its use in depression and OCD despite several studies in this area. While the side-effects are felt to be minimal, the long term effects of neurofeedback are not known at this time.

Recommended further reading

1 Van der Kolk, B., et al. (2007). A randomized clinical trial of EMDR, fluoxetine and pill placebo in the treatment of PTSD: Treatment effects and long-term maintenance. *Journal of Clin. Psych* **68**, 37–46.

2 Ursano, R.J. et al. (2004). Practice Guideline for the Treatment of Patients with Acute Stress Disorder and Posttraumatic Stress Disorder, American Association Practice Guidelines, 57–59.

3 http://www.oqp.med.va.gov/cpg/PTSD/PTSD_Base.htm

4 http://www.emdria.org/

5 Stewart, J.H. Hyposis in contemporacy medicine. Mayo Clinic Proc. April 2005; **80**(4), 511–524.

6 Hammond, D.C. (2005). Neurofeed back with anxiety and affective disorders. *Child Adolesc psychaitric Clin N Am*, **14**: 105–123.

Biomechanical approaches

Chiropractic medicine[1]

Chiropractic techniques date back to ancient times, but modern chiropractic principles were founded by Daniel David Palmer in 1895. The focus of chiropractic is treatment of neuromusculoskeletal (NMS) pain and injury using "chiropractic adjustment." First, chiropractors diagnose the problem using examination, imaging, and sometimes lab work. Then the practitioners apply hands-on manipulation techniques to areas of hypomobility over a series of prescribed visits. Their focused technique is felt to enhance mobility to the area over time, thus providing improved function. They may also recommend rehabilitation or lifestyle changes. Chiropractic techniques have been studied and been shown effective for several NMS dysfunctions, and are often covered by insurance companies.

Doctors of chiropractic medicine are licensed in all 50 states. Training usually involves premedical education and 4 to 5 years of education/training at a chiropractic college. Possible side-effects are limited, but include soreness, aching, and general discomfort, which usually subsides after several hours. A thorough screen to rule out potential contraindications (e.g. cauda equina syndrome, herniation, carotid artery disease, certain neuropathies or malignancies) is suggested prior to treatment.

Osteopathic medicine[2]

Osteopathic medicine is an augmented field of conventional medicine founded by in 1874 by Andrew Taylor Still, M.D. The training is similar to allopathic (M.D.) schools, but places additional emphasis on the biopsychosocial "whole person" approach. In addition, doctors of osteopathic medicine (D.O.s) receive extensive training on the hands-on diagnosis and treatment of NMS disorders, including manipulation and muscle therapy techniques. This technique is referred to as Osteopathic Manipulation Therapy (OMT) and can have risks and side-effects similar to chiropractic techniques.

The foundation of osteopathic teachings is integration of the mind, body, and spirit, and the interrelationship of this with structure, function, and disease state. There is an inherent focus on disease prevention and facilitation of the body's natural ability to heal itself. While such concepts are more mainstream today, these principles have been the core foundation for D.O.s for over 130 years. Osteopathic medicine has gained increasing popularity, with a 67% increase in the number of D.O.s since 1990.

As part of this philosophy, all D.O.s are trained as primary care physicians first, usually including a traditional internship followed by residency. 65% of D.O.s practice in some area of primary care. D.O.s are fully licensed physicians whose entrance, training, and credentialing requirements are comparable to their M.D. peers. Currently, there is a movement to expand the understanding and benefit of the philosophy through research.

Craniosacral therapy[3, 4]

Craniosacral therapy (CST) is based on the principle that there is an inherent rhythmical flow of cerebrospinal fluid that can be palpated by gently placing hands on the head and sacral region. Furthermore, disruptions in the flow may result in pain and dysfunction such as headache or emotional dysfunction. The concept was founded by William G. Sutherland, D.O. and recently advanced into a treatment modality by John Upledger, D.O.[3]

CST may be practiced by a variety of practitioners, including chiropractors, osteopaths, massage therapists, and others. Training and competency of practitioners also varies widely, and competency in this treatment takes much practice and patience. Research in this area is limited with low power and variable results.[4] Before undergoing CST, full medical evaluation of the patient should be completed to rule out medical etiology of symptoms. For example, individuals with increased intracranial pressure or aneurysm should not receive CST.

Side-effects are rarely reported, but could include discomfort or change in mood. Current interests include advancing the understanding of CST and using EEG and neurofeedback to better understand CST.

Recommended further reading

1 www.amerchiro.org
2 www.osteopathic.org
3 http://www.upledger.com
4 Moran, R.W., Gibbons, P. (2001). Intraexaminer and interexaminer reliability for palpation of the cranial rhythmic impulse at the head and sacrum. *Journal of Manipulative & Physiological Therapeutics*. **24**(3), 183–190.

Bioenergetic therapies

Acupuncture

Involves the insertion of fine needles into different parts of the body to correct the imbalance of energy (chi) in the body, based on Chinese philosophy of Yin and Yang and the Five Elements, used for greater than 3000 years. Styles range from traditional/classical, auricular (ear), trigger point, single point, and electrical. Some evidence for use in the following: depression[1] (including depression in pregnancy per a randomized-controlled pilot study), anxiety with insomnia (increases nocturnal melatonin secretion and reduces insomnia and anxiety[2]), obesity (appetite suppression and lipolithic effects), substance use disorders (mixed results, adjunctive seems warranted), and smoking cessation[3] (no strong evidence supporting its use yet, but genetic polymorphism appears related to response). Demonstrated to be safe in the hands of a competent practitioner.[4] More research is warranted.

Spiritual and religious practices

Spiritual and religious practices make up an ancient and widely used intervention for alleviating illness and promoting good health. Distant healing (including spiritual healing, mental healing, faith healing, Reiki healing, psychic healing, intercessory prayer) can be defined as a conscious, dedicated act of mentation attempting to benefit another person's physical or emotional well-being at a distance. The efficacy as a treatment for various medical conditions has been studied and approximately 57% of trials showed a positive treatment effect.[5] Religious involvement is positively associated with a variety of health outcomes, with attendance at religious services most strongly related to physical health, mental health, and mortality in community-based samples. There is limited evidence (cross-sectional data only) suggesting that religious participation is associated with higher levels of immune functioning.[6] Clinical samples show faith-based coping as the most powerful predictor of recovery and survival. However, there is evidence that there are both "positive" and "negative" forms of religious coping. A study of a chronic pain population showed that forgiveness, negative religious coping, daily spiritual experiences, religious support, and self-rankings of religious/spiritual intensity significantly predicted mental health status.[7]

Therapeutic touch and healing touch

Therapeutic touch (TT) and healing touch (HT) are "biofield" or "energy-based" therapies used to promote relaxation, reduce pain and anxiety, and facilitate the body's natural restorative processes. TT is described as a contemporary interpretation of several ancient healing practices, an intentionally directed process of energy exchange during which the practitioner uses the hands as a focus for facilitating healing. The intervention is administered with the intention of enabling people to repattern their energy in the direction of health. Meta-analytic review raised many concerns regarding the quality of TT research to date.[8] Similarly, many positive results of HT have been reported, but none of the findings have been conclusive, mostly due to research and reporting problems with the studies.[9]

Homeopathy

A German physician Samuel Hahnemann developed homeopathy in the late 1800's after noting that cinchona bark used to treat malaria, when ingested, gave symptoms similar to malaria. This led to his founding homeopathy (from Greek *omeos* meaning similar, and *pathos* meaning suffering). This demonstrates homeopathy's "principle of similars." To treat a symptom, a small amount of a substance is given that produces toxic syndrome similar to that condition. The belief is that illness is a result in the disruption of one's essential energetic makeup. The remedies are created using a method of serial dilution sometimes done beyond Avogadro's number (no molecules of initial substance present). Treatment is individuated, and specific to the person's individual symptom qualities and constellation. As a result, it has proven difficult to study. Four comprehensive systematic reviews of RCTs comparing homeopathy to placebo have been done, overall suggesting a benefit over placebo, but no strong conclusions. Systematic reviews of RCTs for specific indications have shown some benefit using arnica for pain, oscillococcinum for flulike syndrome, isopathic nosodes in allergy, and galphimia in allergic rhinitis.[10]

Recommended further reading

1 Smith, C.A., Hay, P.P.J. (2006). Acupuncture for Depression. Cochrane Database of Systematic Reviews, Volume (2),

2 Spence, D.W. *et al* (2005). Acupuncture increases nocturnal melatonin secretion and reduces insomnia and anxiety: A preliminary R\report. *J of Neuropsychiatry and Clinical Neurosciences* **16**, 19–28.

3 Berman, A.H. et al. (2004). Treating drug using prison inmates with auricular acupuncture: A RCT. *J of Substance Abuse Treatment* **26**, 95–102.

4 Vincent, C. (2001) The safety of acupuncture. *BMJ* **323**,:446 7–8.

5 Astin, J.A. et al. (2000). The efficacy of "distant healing": a systematic review of randomized trials. *Annals of Internal Medicine* **132**(11), 903–910.

6 Koenig, H.G., Cohen, H.J., George, L.K., Hays, J.C., Larson, D.B., Blazer, D.G. (1997). Attendance at religious services, interleukin-6, and other biological indicators of immune function in older adults. *International Journal of Psychiatry in Medicine* **257**, 233–250.

7 Rippentrop, A.E. *et al.* (2005). The relationship between religion/spirituality and physical health, mental health, and pain in a chronic pain population. *Pain* **116**, 311–321.

8 Peters, R.M. (1999). The effectiveness of therapeutic touch: a meta-analytic review. *Nursing Science Quarterly.* **12**(1), 52-61.

9 Wardell, D.W., Weymouth, K.F. (2004). Review of studies of healing touch. *J of Nursing Scholarship*, **36**(2), 147–154.

10 Jonas, W.B., Kaptchuk, T.J., Linde, K. (2003). A critical overview of homeopathy. *Ann Intern Med.* **138**:393–399.

Lifestyle modifications

Exercise

Regular exercise has long been accepted as beneficial to physical well-being, as well as preventative for chronic medical conditions (e.g. cardiac disease, hypertension, hyperlipidemia). Until recently, however, the psychological benefits of exercise were supported principally by anecdotal report. In 1999, Blumenthal et al.[1] conducted a clinical controlled study which showed that aerobic exercise in older patients with MDD yields statistically significant reductions in depressive symptoms, comparable to treatment with SSRI. Furthermore, 50 minutes of exercise per week was associated with a 50% reduction in risk of depressive symptom recurrence after six months.[2]

Indications

Mild-moderate depression and anxiety disorders.

Dosing

The public health recommendation of 30 minutes of moderate-intensity physical activity, ≥5 days a week, has shown to be effective in mild to moderate MDD, although it appears that total energy expenditure (≥17.5-kcal/kg/week) is the key factor, as opposed to exercise frequency.[3]

Risks

According to the CDC, less than 40% of U.S. adults engage in the recommended amount of physical activity at baseline (and 25% are not active at all). It is therefore important to advise previously sedentary individuals and those at risk for chronic health problems to first consult their PCP prior to initiating an exercise regimen.

Yoga

In its most authentic form, Yoga is an ancient Indian tradition of moral discipline, spirituality, and physical practice as a means to enlightenment. Archaeological evidence from the Indus valley depicts figures in yoga poses dating back to 3000 BC. Since its origins, many different schools of yoga have evolved. The most popular version adopted by Western culture, is a secular interpretation of Hatha yoga ("Forced" yoga). This form incorporates three basic elements:

- Asanas (postures).
- Pranayama (breathing exercises).
- Dhyana (meditation).

Although yoga is used widely today for its perceived mind-body benefits, the field is still lacking large clinical controlled trials. One recent small study found individuals with mild depression had significant reduction in Beck Depression scores and a trend for higher morning cortisol levels when compared to controls.[3] Recent meta-analyses and review of the literature have strengthened the evidence supporting clinical benefits of yoga for depression, anxiety, cardiovascular disease, hypertension, asthma, diabetes, osteoarthritis, and various other maladies.[4]

Mindfulness meditation

Based in Buddhist traditions from more than 2500 years ago, mindfulness meditation is considered a form of insight meditation, or Vipassana. The central philosophy behind "mindfulness" is to consciously experience moment-to-moment thoughts, emotions, and sensations with a nonjudgmental awareness. In 1979, Jon Kabat-Zinn, Ph.D. developed a formal 8-week mindfulness-based stress reduction (MBSR) program which combines training in meditation as well as hatha yoga. Today more than 200 U.S. hospital systems offer MBSR as a form of complementary medicine aimed at reducing medical symptoms and psychological distress. Although to date there are no large-scale, clinical controlled trials on MBSR, preliminary evidence is promising. In an early study, Speca et al. showed a 65% reduction of mood disturbance and a 35% reduction in stress symptoms in cancer patients after training in MBSR.[5] In a recent meta-analysis, MBSR was found to be beneficial across a broad range of disorders, some of which include: depression, anxiety, chronic pain, fibromyalgia, binge eating, cancer, and coronary artery disease. Furthermore, there have been at least two controlled studies in nonclinical populations, which have shown MBSR helpful in mitigating stress, anxiety, and dysphoria.[6]

Recommended further reading

1 Blumenthal, J.A. et al. (1999). Effects of Exercise Training on Older Patients with Major Depression. Archives of Internal Medicine **159**, 2349–2356.

2 Babyak, M. A. et al. (2000). Exercise treatment for major depression: Maintenance of therapeutic benefit at 10 months. Psychosomatic Medicine **62**, 📖 pp. 633–638.

3 Woolery, A., Myers, H., Sternlieb, B., and Zeltzer, L. (2004). A yoga intervention for young adults with elevated symptoms of depression, Altern. Ther. Health Med. **1**(2), 60–63.

4 Pilkington, K., Kirkwood, G., Rampes, H., Richardson, J. (Dec 2005). Yoga for depression: the research evidence. Journal of Affective Disorders **89**(1–3), 13–24.

5 Speca, M., Carlson, L.E., Goodey, E., Angen, M. (Sep–Oct 2000). A randomized, wait-list controlled clinical trial: the effect of a mindfulness meditation-based stress reduction program on mood and symptoms of stress in cancer outpatients. Psychosomatic Medicine. **62**(5), 613–622.

6 Grossman, P., Niemann, L., Schmidt, S., Walach, H. (Jul 2004). Mindfulness-based stress reduction and health benefits. A meta-analysis. Journal of Psychosomatic Research. **57**(1), 35–43.

Useful publications and web sites

Books and web sites by chapter topic

There are many excellent books and websites that provide further information on psychiatric topics. These references may be helpful for clinicians, trainees, and even patients and families. The following list provides a few of these helpful resources on a variety of topics, and is organized according to the book's chapter order.

General reference

General books for psychiatry

- *Diagnostic and Statistical Manual of Mental Disorders DSM-IV-TR* 4th ed., American Psychiatric Association.
- H. Kaplan, B. Sadock, V. Sadock, *Synopsis of Psychiatry: Behavioral Sciences/Clinical Psychiatry*. Lippincott Williams & Wilkins.

Pharmacology

- Alan F. Schatxberg and Charles B. Nemeroff, *Essentials of Clinical Psychopharmacology*.
- Stephen M. Stahl (2008). *Essential Psychopharmacology: Neuroscientific Basis and Practical Applications*.

Neurology

- David Myland Kaufman (Ed.) (2006). *Clinical Neurology for Psychiatrists*, 6th ed. Philadelphia: W.B. Saunders.

Web sites

- www.psych.org—American Psychiatric Association (practice guidelines, patient and provider information).
- www.nimh.nih.gov—National Institute of Mental Health with the National Institutes of Health.
- www.NARSAD.org
- www.apa.org/topics

Families

- www.mayoclinic.org
- www.nami.org—National Alliance on Mental Illness, extensive resources for patients and their families.

Financial help for patients

- www.needymeds.com
- www.cms.hhs.com
- www.insurekidsnow.gov

Thinking about psychiatry

Books

- Floyd E. Bloom, Flint Beal, and David Kupfer (Eds.). *The Dana Guide to Brain Health: A Practical Family Reference from Medical Experts*.
- David J. Kupfer, Michael B. First, Darrel A., M.D. Regier. *A Research Agenda for DSM-V*.

Psychiatric assessment
Books
- W. B. Andrew Sims. *Symptoms in the Mind: An Introduction to Descriptive Psychopathology.*
- Richard Strub and F. William Black. *The Mental Status Examination in Neurology.*
- *Diagnostic and Statistical Manual of Mental Disorders DSM-IV-TR*, 4th ed, American psychiatric Association.

Web sites
- www.behavenet.com has a DSM-IV-TR for on-line browsing.

Signs and symptoms of psychiatric illness
Books
- J. Frank, Jr. Ayd, Charles Nemeroff, David Kupfer. *Lexicon of Psychiatry, Neurology & the Neurosciences.*

Evidence-based psychiatry
Books
- Gregory E. Gray. *Concise Guide to Evidence-Based Psychiatry.*
- Helena Chmura Kraemer, Karen Kraemer Lowe, David J. Kupfer. *To Your Health: How to Understand What Research Tells Us about Risk.*
- G. Guyatt, D. Rennie. *Users' Guide to Medical Literature: A Manual for Evidence-Based Clinical Practice.*

Web sites
- Cochrane library, Cochrane database of systematic reviews, Cochrane central register of controlled trials (accessible through Ovid, Wiley InterScience and others).
- http://medlineplus.gov—An unbiased, government sponsored resource for patients and families with links to the best and most comprehensive libraries.
- www.cebm.utoronto.ca
- www.cebm.net

Organic illness
Books
- John Mellers, Simon Fleminger, Simon Lovestone, Anthony David, Michael Kopelman (2007). *Lishman's Organic Psychiatry: A Textbook of Neuropsychiatry.* Blackwell Publishing Professional.
- C. Edward Coffey, Jeffrey L. Cummings (2000). *The American Psychiatric Press Textbook of Geriatric Neuropsychiatry.* American Psychiatric Press.

Schizophrenia and related psychoses
Books
- Silvano Arieti. *Interpretation of Schizophreni* (rev. ed.)—a classic.

Web sites
- www.narsad.org—National Alliance for Research on Schizophrenia and Depression: The Mental Health Research Association. Funds research on those and other disorders.
- www.schizophreniaforum.org—sponsored by NARSAD, supported by NIMH, NIH and Department of HHS.

Depressive disorders
Books
- Michael E. Thase and Susan S. Lang. *Beating the Blues: New Approaches to Overcoming Dysthymia and Chronic Mild Depression.*

Patients and families
- Beth Andrews. *Why Are You So Sad? A child's about parental depression.*

Web sites
- http://mentalhealth.samhsa.gov/suicideprevention/
- www.depressedteens.com
- www.miminc com

Bipolar disorders
Books
- Boris Birmaher. *New Hope for Children and Teens with Bipolar Disorder.*

Anxiety and stress-related disorders
Books
- For OCD: Lee Baer. *The Imp of the Mind: Exploring the Silent Epidemic of Obsessive Bad Thoughts.*
- G.H. Eifert and J.P. Forsyth. *Treatment Manual: Acceptance & Commitment therapy for anxiety disorders.*
- Deborah C. Beidel, Samuel M. Turner. *Childhood Anxiety Disorders: A Guide to Research and Treatment.*

Web sites
- www.adaa.org

Eating disorders
Web sites
- www.nationaleatingdisorders.org

Sleep disorders
Books
- Meir Kryger, Thomas Roth, William Dement. *Principles and Practice of Sleep Medicine,* 4th ed.

Reproductive disorders and sexuality
Books
- Sarah E. Romans, Mary V. Seeman. *Women's Mental Health: A Life Cycle Approach.*

Web sites
- www.womensmentalhealth.org
- www.auanet.org—useful guidelines from the American Urological Association.
- www.urologyhealth.org—urology for patients.
- For women: Boston Women's Health Book Collective (BWHBC)'s site:
- www.ourbodiesourselves.org

Personality disorders
Books
- J. Oldham, A. Skodol, L. Bender. *The American Psychiatric Publishing Textbook of Personality Disorders.*
- M.C. Zanarini (Ed.). *Borderline Personality Disorder.*

Patients and families
- L.J. Siever, W. Frucht. *The New View of Self.* (Depression and PD from a layman's perspective using biological findings).

Web sites
- www. borderlinepersonalitydisorder.com—National Education Alliance for Borderline Personality Disorder (an NIMH sponsored organization that holds scientific seminars around the country about BPD).
- www.tara4bpd.org—treatment and research news in BPD, an advocacy organization.

Geriatric psychiatry
Books
- M.E. Agronin, G.J. Maletta (Eds.). *Principles and Practice of Geriatric Psychiatry.* Philadelphia: Lippincott Williams and Wilkins.
- D.G. Blazer, D.C. Steffens, E.W. Busse (Eds.). The American Psychiatric Publishing Textbook of Geriatric Psychiatry.
- Nancy L. Mace, Peter V. Rabins. *The 36-Hour Day: A Family Guide to Caring for Persons with Alzheimer Disease, Related Dementing Illnesses, and Memory Loss in Later Life.*
- John Herr, John Weakland. *Counseling Elders and Their Families: Practical Techniques for Applied Gerontology.*

Patients and families
- Mark D. Miller, Charles F. III Reynolds, Barry D. Lebowitz. *Living Longer Depression Free: A Family Guide to Recognizing, Treating, and Preventing Depression in Later Life.*

Web sites
- www.aagpgpa.org
- www.aarp.org

Substance abuse disorders

Books

- Marc Galanter, MD, Herbert D Kleber, MD. *Textbook of Substance Abuse Treatment.*
- Dennis C. Daley, Antoine Douaihy. *Addiction and Mood Disorders. A Guide for Clients and Families.*
- Dennis M. Donovan, G. Alan Marlatt (Eds.). *Assessment of Addictive Disorders.*
- R. Frances, S.I. Miller, A. Mack (Eds.). *Clinical Textbook of Addictive Disorders.*
- J.H. Lowinson, P. Ruiz, R.B. Millman, J.G. Langrod (Eds.). *Substance Abuse: A comprehensive textbook.*
- G. Alan Marlatt, Dennis M Donovan (Eds.). *Relapse Prevention*
- Carlo C. DiClemente. *Addiction & Change.*
- William R. Miller, Stephen Rollnick. *Motivational Interviewing.*
- K.T. Mueser, D.L. Noordsy, R.E. Drake, L Fox. *Integrated treatment for dual disorders: A guide to effective practice.*

Pateints and families

- www.alcoholics-anonymous.org
- www.al-anon.alateen.org/

Web sites

- www.drdennisdaley.com
- www.nida.gov
- www.niaa.nih.gov

Child and adolescent psychiatry

Books

- Andrés Martin, Fred R Volkmar, Melvin Lewis. *Lewis's Child and Adolescent Psychiatry A Comprehensive Textbook.*
- A. Lieberman, S. Weider, E. Fenichel (Eds) *The DC: 0–3 Casebook: A Guide to the use of ZERO TO THREES "Diagnostic Classification of Mental Health and Developmental Disorders of Infancy and Early Childhood" in Assessment and Treatment Planning. National Center for Infants, Toddlers and Families.*
- Deborah C. Beidel, Samuel M. Turner. *Childhood Anxiety Disorders: A Guide to Research and Treatment.*
- Andres Martin, Lawrence Scahill, Dennis S. Charney, James F. Leckman. *Pediatric Psychopharmacology: Principles and Practice.*
- Fred R. Volkmar, Rhea Paul, Ami Klin, Donald J. Cohen. *Handbook of Autism and Pervasive Developmental Disorders, Assessment, Interventions, and Policy.*

For parents

- Adele Faber, Elaine Mazlish. *How to Talk So Kids Will Listen & Listen So Kids Will Talk.*
- David Pruitt (Ed.). *Your Child: Emotional, Behavioral, and Cognitive Development from Birth through Preadolescence.*

Web sites
- www. aacap.org/—American Academy of Child & Adolescent Psychiatry, search for "Facts for Families"—useful handouts on ~100 topics, and in multiple languages (free).
- www.chadd.org—ADHD.
- www.bpkids.org—bipolar disorder.
- www.nichd.nih.gov/autism/, www.teacch.com/—PDD, see 📖 *p.709* for more.

Forensic psychiatry

Books
- Paul E. Mullen, Michele Pathé, Rosemary Purcell. *Stalkers and their Victims.*
- Richard Rosner. A Hodder. *Principles and Practice of Forensic Psychiatry.*
- Gary B. Melton, John Petrila, Norman G. Poythress, Christopher Slobogin. *Psychological Evaluations for the Courts*, 3rd ed., *A Handbook for Mental Health Professionals and Lawyers.*

Intellectual and developmental disabilities

Books
- Kenneth Jones. *Smith's Recognizable Patterns of Human Malformation* 6th ed.

Web sites
- www.aaidd.org—American Association on Intellectual and Developmental Disabilities.
- www.medgen.ubc.ca/wrobinson/mosaic/index.htm—Chromosomal Mosaicism information

Consult–liaison psychiatry

Books
- Michael G. Wise, James R. Rundell *The American Psychiatric Press Textbook of Consultation-Liaison Psychiatry: Psychiatry in the Medically Ill*
- Alan Stoudemire, Barry S. Fogel, Donna Greenberg. *Psychiatric Care of the Medical Patient.*
- Thomas Grisso, Paul S. Appelbaum. *Assessing Competence to Consent to Treatment: A Guide for Physicians and Other Health Professionals.*

Psychotherapy

Books
- Glen O. Gabbard. *Psychodynamic Psychiatry in Clinical Practice.*
- Glen O. Gabbard. *Long-Term Psychodynamic Psychotherapy: A Basic Text.*
- Judith S. Beck *Cognitive Therapy: Basics and Beyond.*
- Dennis Greenberger, Christine Padesky. *Mind Over Mood: Change How You Feel by Changing the Way You Think.*
- Marsha M. Linehan. *Skills Training Manual for Treating Borderline Personality Disorder.*
- Karen J Maroda. *The Power of Countertransference: Innovations in Analytic Technique*, 2nd ed.
- John M. Gottman, Nan Silver *The Seven Principles for Making Marriage Work: A Practical Guide from the Country's Foremost Relationship Expert.*

- William R. Mille, Stephen Rollnick. *Motivational Interviewing*, 2nd ed.
- Suzanne Bender, Edward Messner. *Becoming a Therapist: What Do I Say, and Why?*

Cross-cultural psychiatry
Books
- Russell F. Lim (Ed.). *Clinical Manual of Cultural Psychiatry.*
- Group for the Advancement of Psychiatry Committee on Cultural Psychiatry. *Cultural Assessment in Clinical Psychiatry: GAP Report 145.*

Web sites
- www.omhrc.gov/clas—"Assuring Cultural Competence in Health Care: Recommendations for National Standards," Health and Human Services' Office of Minority Health.
- www.surgeongeneral.gov/library/mentalhealth/cre/

Therapeutic issues
Books
- Alan F. Schatzberg, Charles B. Nemeroff. *Essentials of Clinical Psychopharmacology.*

Difficult and urgent situations
Books
- Robert Simon, Robert Hales. *Textbook of Suicide Assessment and Management.*
- John A. Chiles, Kirk D. Strosahl. *The Suicidal Patient: Principles of Assessment, Treatment, and Case Management.*

Web sites
- www.afsp.org—American Foundation for Suicide Prevention.

Integrative psychiatry
Web sites
- http://nccam.nih.gov/

Research in psychiatry and neuroscience
Web sites
- www.nimh.nih.gov/nimhhome/index.cfm—The National Institute for Mental Health.
- www.humanbrainmapping.org—The Organization for Human Brain Mapping: Advancing Understanding of the Human Brain.
- www.sobp.org—Society of Biological Psychiatry.
- www.neuropsychologycentral.com
- www.wpic.pitt.edu/research/—Western Psychiatric Institute and Clinic research page.
- www.NARSAD.org

DSM-IV-TR/ICD-10 codes

Using DSM-IV-TR

Multiaxial System for DSM-IV-TR

Axis I	Clinical Disorders
	Other Conditions That May Be a Focus of Clinical Attention
Axis II	Personality Disorders
	Mental Retardation
Axis III	General Medical Conditions
Axis IV	Psychosocial and Environmental Problems
Axis V	Global Assessment of Functioning

Global assessment of functioning

Code	Description (use intermediate codes when appropriate, e.g., 45, 68, 72)
100 to 91	Superior functioning in a wide range of activities, life's problems never seem to get out of hand, is sought out by others because of his or her many positive qualities. No symptoms.
90 to 81	Absent or minimal symptoms (e.g., mild anxiety before an exam), good functioning in all areas, interested and involved in a wide range of activities, socially effective, generally satisfied with life, no more than everyday problems or concerns (e.g., an occasional argument with family members).
80 to 71	If symptoms are present, they are transient and expectable reactions to psychosocial stressors (e.g., difficulty concentrating after family argument); no more than slight impairment in social, occupational, or school functioning (e.g., temporarily falling behind in schoolwork).
70 to 61	Some mild symptoms (e.g., depressed mood and mild insomnia) OR some difficulty in social, occupational, or school functioning (e.g., occasional truancy, or theft within the household), but generally functioning pretty well, has some meaningful interpersonal relationships.
60 to 51	Moderate symptoms (e.g., flat affect and circumstantial speech, occasional panic attacks) OR moderate difficulty in social, occupational, or school functioning (e.g., few friends, conflicts with peers or co-workers).
40 to 31	Some impairment in reality testing or communication (e.g., speech is at times illogical, obscure, or irrelevant) OR major impairment in several areas such as work or school, family relations, judgment, thinking, or mood (e.g., depressed man avoids friends, neglects family, and is unable to work; child frequently beats up younger children, is defiant at home, and is failing at school).
30 to 21	Behavior is considerably influenced by delusions or hallucinations OR serious impairment in communication or judgment (e.g., sometimes incoherent, acts grossly inappropriately, suicidal preoccupation) OR inability to function in almost all areas (e.g., stays in bed all day; no job, home, or friends).
20 to 11	Some danger of hurting self or others (e.g., suicide attempts without clear expectation of death; frequently violent; manic excitement) OR occasionally fails to maintain minimal personal hygiene (e.g., smears feces) OR gross impairment in communication (e.g., largely incoherent or mute)
10 to 1	Persistent danger of severely hurting self or others (e.g., recurrent violence) OR persistent inability to maintain minimal personal hygiene OR serious suicidal act with clear expectation of death.
0	Inadequate information.

	DSM-IV-TR code	ICD-10 code
Disorders Usually First Diagnosed in Infancy, Childhood, or Adolescence		
MENTAL RETARDATION		
Note: these are coded on Axis II	**DSM-IV-TR**	**ICD-10**
Mild Mental Retardation	317	F70.9
Moderate Mental Retardation	318.0	F71.9
Severe Mental Retardation	318.1	F72.9
Profound Mental Retardation	318.2	F73.9
Mental Retardation, Severity Unspecified	319	F79.9
LEARNING DISORDERS		
Reading Disorder	315.00	F81.0
Mathematics Disorder	315.1	F81.2
Disorder of Written Expression	315.2	F81.8
Learning Disorder NOS	315.9	F81.9
MOTOR SKILLS DISORDER		
Developmental Coordination Disorder	315.4	F82
COMMUNICATION DISORDERS		
Expressive Language Disorder	315.31	F80.1
Mixed Receptive-Expressive Language Disorder	315.32	F80.2
Phonological Disorder	315.39	F80.0
Stuttering	307.0	F98.5
Communication Disorder NOS	307.9	F80.9
PERVASIVE DEVELOPMENTAL DISORDERS		
Autistic Disorder	299.00	F84.0
Rett's Disorder	299.80	F84.2
Childhood Disintegrative Disorder	299.10	F84.3
Asperger's Disorder	299.80	F84.5
Pervasive Developmental Disorder NOS	299.80	F84.9
ATTENTION-DEFICIT AND DISRUPTIVE BEHAVIOR DISORDERS		
Attention-Deficit/Hyperactivity Disorder	314.xx	—.—
Combined Type	.01	F90.0 Combined Type
Predominantly Inattentive Type	.00	F98.8

	DSM-IV-TR code	ICD-10 code
Predominantly Hyperactive-Impulsive Type	.01	F90.0
Attention-Deficit/Hyperactivity Disorder NOS	314.9	F90.9
Conduct Disorder	312.xx	F91.8 Specify type:
Childhood-Onset Type	.81	Childhood-Onset Type
Adolescent-Onset Type	.82	Adolescent-Onset Type
Unspecified Onset	.89	__.__
Oppositional Defiant Disorder	313.81	F91.3
Disruptive Behavior Disorder NOS	312.9	F91.9

FEEDING AND EATING DISORDERS OF INFANCY OR EARLY CHILDHOOD

Pica	307.52	F98.3
Rumination Disorder	307.53	F98.2
Feeding Disorder of Infancy or Early Childhood	307.59	F98.2

TIC DISORDERS

Tourette's Disorder	307.23	F95.2
Chronic Motor or Vocal Tic Disorder	307.22	F95.1
Transient Tic Disorder Specify if: Single Episode/Recurrent	307.21	F95.0
Tic Disorder NOS	307.20	F95.9

ELIMINATION DISORDERS

__.__ Encopresis, specify as below		__.__ Encopresis
With Constipation and Overflow Incontinence	787.6	R15 (also code K59.0 constipation)
Without Constipation and Overflow Incontinence	307.7	F98.1
Enuresis (Not Due to a General Medical Condition) Specify type: Nocturnal Only/Diurnal Only/Nocturnal and Diurnal	307.6	F98.0

	DSM-IV-TR code	ICD-10 code
OTHER DISORDERS OF INFANCY, CHILDHOOD, OR ADOLESCENCE		
Separation Anxiety Disorder Specify if: Early Onset	309.21	F93.0 Specify if: Early Onset
Selective Mutism	313.23	F94.0
Reactive Attachment Disorder of Infancy or Early Childhood Specify type: Inhibited Type/ Disinhibited Type	313.89	F94.x
		.1 Inhibited Type
		.2 Disinhibited Type
Stereotypic Movement Disorder. Specify if: With Self-Injurious Behavior	307.3	F98.4
Disorder of Infancy, Childhood, or Adolescence NOS	313.9	F98.9
Delirium, Dementia, and Amnestic and Other Cognitive Disorders		
DELIRIUM		
Delirium Due to . . . [Indicate the General Medical Condition]	293.0	F05.0 [Indicate the General Medical Condition] (code F05.1 if superimposed on Dementia)
__._ Substance Intoxication Delirium (refer to Substance-Related Disorders for substance-specific codes)		__._
__._ Substance Withdrawal Delirium (refer to Substance-Related Disorders for substance-specific codes)		__._
__._ Delirium Due to Multiple Etiologies (code each of the specific etiologies)		__._
Delirium NOS	780.09	F05.9
DEMENTIA		
294.xx* Dementia of the Alzheimer's Type, With Early Onset (also code 331.0 Alzheimer's disease on Axis III)		F00.xx Dementia of the Alzheimer's Type, With Early Onset (also code G30.0 Alzheimer's Disease, With Early Onset)

	DSM-IV-TR code	ICD-10 code
.10 Without Behavioral Disturbance		.00 Uncomplicated
.11 With Behavioral Disturbance		.01 With Delusions
		.03 With Depressed Mood
		Specify if: With Behavioral Disturbance
Dementia of the Alzheimer's Type, With Late Onset (also code 331.0 Alzheimer's disease on Axis III)	294.xx*	F00.xx Dementia of the Alzheimer's Type, With Late Onset (also code G30.1 Alzheimer's Disease, With Late Onset)
Without Behavioral Disturbance	.10	.10 Uncomplicated
With Behavioral Disturbance	.11	.11 With Delusions
		.13 With Depressed Mood
		Specify if: With Behavioral Disturbance
Vascular Dementia	290.xx	F01.xx
Uncomplicated	.40	.80
With Delirium	.41	____.-
With Delusions	.42	.81
With Depressed Mood	.43	.83
Specify if: With Behavioral Disturbance		Specify if: With Behavioral Disturbance
Code presence or absence of a behavioral disturbance in the fifth digit for Dementia Due to a General Medical Condition:		
Without Behavioral Disturbance	0	
With Behavioral Disturbance	1	
Dementia Due to HIV Disease (also code 042 HIV on Axis III)	294.1x*	F02.4 (also code B22.0 HIV disease resulting in encephalopathy)
Dementia due to Head Trauma (also code 854.60 head injury on Axis III)	294.1*	F02.8 (also code S06.9 Intracranial injury)

	DSM-IV-TR code	ICD-10 code
Dementia Due to Parkinson's Disease (also code 332.0 Parkinson's disease on Axis III)	294.1x*	F02.3 (also code G20 Parkinson's disease)
Dementia Due to Huntington's Disease (also code 333.4 Huntington's disease on Axis III)	294.1x*	F02.2 (also code G10 Huntington's disease)
Dementia Due to Pick's Disease (also code 331.1 Pick's disease on Axis III)	294.1x*	F02.0 (also code G31.0 Pick's disease)
Dementia Due to Creutzfeldt-Jakob Disease (also code 046.1 Creutzfeldt-Jakob disease on Axis III)	294.1x*	F02.1 (also code A81.0 Creutzfeldt-Jakob disease)
Dementia Due to . . . [Indicate the General Medical Condition not listed above] (also code the general medical condition on Axis III)	294.1x*	F02.8
Substance-Induced Persisting Dementia (refer to Substance-Related Disorders for substance-specific codes)	___._	___._
Dementia Due to Multiple Etiologies (code each of the specific etiologies		F02.8 (instead code F00.2 for mixed Alzheimer's and Vascular Dementia)
294.8 Dementia NOS		F03

AMNESTIC DISORDERS

	DSM-IV-TR code	ICD-10 code
Amnestic Disorder Due to . . . [Indicate the General Medical Condition] Specify if: Transient/Chronic	294.0	F04
Substance-Induced Persisting Amnestic Disorder (refer to Substance-Related Disorders for substance-specific codes)	.	___._
Amnestic Disorder NOS	294.8	R41.3

OTHER COGNITIVE DISORDERS

	DSM-IV-TR code	ICD-10 code
Cognitive Disorder NOS	294.9	F06.9

Mental Disorders Due to a General Medical Condition Not Elsewhere Classified

	DSM-IV-TR code	ICD-10 code
Catatonic Disorder Due to . . . [Indicate the General Medical Condition]	293.89	F06.1

	DSM-IV-TR code	ICD-10 code
Personality Change Due to . . . [Indicate the General Medical Condition] Specify type: Labile Type/Disinhibited Type/Aggressive Type/Apathetic Type/Paranoid Type/Other Type/Combined Type/Unspecified Type	310.1	F07.0
Mental Disorder NOS Due to . . . [Indicate the General Medical Condition]	293.9	F09

Substance-Related Disorders

	DSM-IV-TR code	ICD-10 code
	The following specifiers apply to Substance Dependence as noted:	[a] The following specifiers may be applied to Substance Dependence:
	[a] With Physiological Dependence/Without Physiological Dependence	Specify if: With Physiological Dependence/ Without Physiological Dependence
	[b] Early FullRemission/ Early Partial Remission/ Sustained Full Remission/Sustained Partial Remission	Code course of Dependence in fifth character:
	[c] In a Controlled Environment	0 = Early Full Remission/Early Partial Remission
	[d] On Agonist Therapy	0 = Sustained Full Remission/ Sustained Partial Remission
	The following specifiers apply to Substance-Induced Disorders as noted: [i] With Onset During Intoxication/[W] With Onset During Withdrawal	1 = In a Controlled Environment
		2 = On Agonist Therapy
		4 = Mild/Moderate/ Severe

ALCOHOL-RELATED DISORDERS

Alcohol Use Disorders

Alcohol Dependence[a,b,c]	303.90	F10.2x Alcohol Dependence[a]

	DSM-IV-TR code	**ICD-10 code**
Alcohol Abuse	305.00	F10.1
Alcohol-Induced Disorders		
Alcohol Intoxication	303.00	F10.00
Alcohol Intoxication Delirium	291.0	F10.03 Alcohol Intoxication Delirium
Alcohol Withdrawal Delirium	291.0	F10.4
Alcohol-Induced Persisting Dementia	291.2	F10.73
Alcohol-Induced Persisting Amnestic Disorder	291.1	F10.6
Alcohol-Induced Psychotic Disorder	291.x	F10.xx
With Delusions[I,W]	.5	.51
With Hallucinations[I,W]	.3	.52
Alcohol-Induced Mood Disorder[I,W]	291.89	F10.8
Alcohol-Induced Anxiety Disorder[I,W]	291.89	F10.8
Alcohol-Induced Sexual Dysfunction[I]	291.89	F10.8
Alcohol-Induced Sleep Disorder[I,W]	291.89	F10.8
Alcohol-Related Disorder NOS	291.9	F10.9

AMPHETAMINE (OR AMPHETAMINE-LIKE)-RELATED DISORDERS

	DSM-IV-TR code	**ICD-10 code**
Amphetamine Use Disorders		
Amphetamine Dependence[a,b,c]	304.40	F15.2x Amphetamine Dependence[a]
Amphetamine Abuse	305.70	F15.1
Amphetamine-Induced Disorders		
Amphetamine Intoxication	292.89	F15.00
Specify if: With Perceptual Disturbances		F15.04
Amphetamine Withdrawal	292.0	F15.3
Amphetamine Intoxication Delirium	292.81	F15.03
Amphetamine-Induced Psychotic Disorder	292.xx	F15.xx

	DSM-IV-TR code	ICD-10 code
With Delusions[I]	.11	.51
With Hallucinations[I]	.12	.52
Amphetamine-Induced Mood Disorder[I,W]	292.84	F15.8
Amphetamine-Induced Anxiety Disorder[I]	292.89	F15.8
Amphetamine-Induced Sexual Dysfunction[I]	292.89	F15.8
Amphetamine-Induced Sleep Disorder[I,W]	292.89	F15.8
Amphetamine-Related Disorder NOS	292.9	F15.9
CAFFEINE-RELATED DISORDERS		
Caffeine-Induced Disorders		
Caffeine Intoxication	305.90	F15.00
Caffeine-Induced Anxiety Disorder[I]	292.89	F15.8
Caffeine-Induced Sleep Disorder[I]	292.89	F15.8
Caffeine-Related Disorder NOS	292.9	F15.9
CANNABIS-RELATED DISORDERS		
Cannabis Use Disorders		
Cannabis Dependence[a,b,c]	304.30	F12.2x
Cannabis Abuse	305.20	F12.1
Cannabis-Induced Disorders		
Cannabis Intoxication	292.89	F12.00
Specify if: With Perceptual Disturbances		F12.04
Cannabis Intoxication Delirium	292.81	F12.03
Cannabis-Induced Psychotic Disorder	292.xx	F12.xx
With Delusions[I]	.11	.51
With Hallucinations[I]	.12	.52
Cannabis-Induced Anxiety Disorder[I]	292.89	F12.8
Cannabis-Related Disorder NOS	292.9	F12.9
COCAINE-RELATED DISORDERS		
Cocaine Use Disorders		
Cocaine Dependence[a,b,c]	304.20	F14.2x Cocaine Dependence[a]

	DSM-IV-TR code	ICD-10 code
Cocaine Abuse	305.60	F14.1
Cocaine-Induced Disorders		
Cocaine Intoxication	292.89	F14.00
Specify if: With Perceptual Disturbances		F14.04
Cocaine Withdrawal	292.0	F14.3
Cocaine Intoxication Delirium	292.81	F14.03
Cocaine-Induced Psychotic Disorder	292.xx	F14.xx
With Delusions[I]	.11	.51
With Hallucinations[I]	.12	.52
Cocaine-Induced Mood Disorder[I,W]	292.84	F14.8
Cocaine-Induced Anxiety Disorder[I,W]	292.89	F14.8
Cocaine-Induced Sexual Dysfunction[I]	292.89	F14.8
Cocaine-Induced Sleep Disorder[I,W]	292.89	F14.8
Cocaine-Related Disorder NOS	292.9	F14.9
HALLUCINOGEN-RELATED DISORDERS		
Hallucinogen Use Disorders		
Hallucinogen Dependence[b,c]	304.50	F16.2x Hallucinogen Dependence[a]
Hallucinogen Abuse	305.30	F16.1
Hallucinogen-Induced Disorders		
Hallucinogen Intoxication	292.89	F16.00
Hallucinogen Persisting Perception Disorder (Flashbacks)	292.89	F16.70
Hallucinogen Intoxication Delirium	292.81	F16.03
Hallucinogen-Induced Psychotic Disorder	292.xx	F16.xx
With Delusions[I]	.11	.51
With Hallucinations[I]	.12	.52
Hallucinogen-Induced Mood Disorder[I]	292.84	F16.8
Hallucinogen-Induced Anxiety Disorder[I]	292.89	F16.8
Hallucinogen-Related Disorder NOS	292.9	F16.9

	DSM-IV-TR code	ICD-10 code
INHALANT-RELATED DISORDERS		
Inhalant Use Disorders		
Inhalant Dependence[b,c]	304.60	F18.2x Inhalant Dependence[a]
Inhalant Abuse	305.90	F18.1
Inhalant-Induced Disorders		
Inhalant Intoxication	292.89	F18.00
Inhalant Intoxication Delirium	292.81	F18.03
Inhalant-Induced Persisting Dementia	292.82	F18.73
Inhalant-Induced Psychotic Disorder	292.xx	F18.xx
With Delusions[I]	.11	.51
With Hallucinations[I]	.12	.52
Inhalant-Induced Mood Disorder[I]	292.84	F18.8
Inhalant-Induced Anxiety Disorder[I]	292.89	F18.8
Inhalant-Related Disorder NOS	292.9	F18.9
NICOTINE-RELATED DISORDERS		
Nicotine Use Disorder		
Nicotine Dependence[a,b]	305.1	F17.2x
Nicotine-Induced Disorder		
Nicotine Withdrawal	292.0	F17.3
Nicotine-Related Disorder NOS	292.9	F17.9
OPIOID-RELATED DISORDERS		
Opioid Use Disorders		
Opioid Dependence[a,b,c,d]	304.00	F11.2x Opioid Dependence[a]
Opioid Abuse	305.50	F11.1 Opioid Abuse
Opioid-Induced Disorders		
Opioid Intoxication	292.89	F11.00 Opioid Intoxication
Specify if: With Perceptual Disturbances		F11.04 With Perceptual Disturbances

	DSM-IV-TR code	ICD-10 code
Opioid Withdrawal	292.0	F11.3
Opioid Intoxication Delirium	292.81	F11.03
Opioid-Induced Psychotic Disorder	292.xx	F11.xx
With Delusions[I]	.11	.51
With Hallucinations[I]	.12	.52
Opioid-Induced Mood Disorder[I]	292.84	F11.8
Opioid-Induced Sexual Dysfunction[I]	292.89	F11.8
Opioid-Induced Sleep Disorder[I,W]	292.89	F11.8
Opioid-Related Disorder NOS	292.9	F11.9

PHENCYCLIDINE (OR PHENCYCLIDINE-LIKE)-RELATED DISORDERS

Phencyclidine Use Disorders		
Phencyclidine Dependence[b,c]	304.60	F19.2x Phencyclidine Dependence[a]
Phencyclidine Abuse	305.90	F19.1 Phency-clidine Abuse
Phencyclidine-Induced Disorders		
Phencyclidine Intoxication	292.89	F19.00
Specify if: With Perceptual Disturbances		F19.04
Phencyclidine Intoxication Delirium	292.81	F19.03
Phencyclidine-Induced Psychotic Disorder	292.xx	F19.xx
With Delusions[I]	.11	.51
With Hallucinations[I]	.12	.52
Phencyclidine-Induced Mood Disorder[I]	292.84	F19.8
Phencyclidine-Induced Anxiety Disorder[I]	292.89	F19.8
Phencyclidine-Related Disorder NOS	292.9	F19.9

	DSM-IV-TR code	ICD-10 code
SEDATIVE-, HYPNOTIC-, OR ANXIOLYTIC-RELATED DISORDERS		
Sedative, Hypnotic, or Anxiolytic Use Disorders		
Sedative, Hypnotic, or Anxiolytic Dependence[a,b,c]	304.10	F13.2x Sedative, Hypnotic, or Anxiolytic Dependence[a]
Sedative, Hypnotic, or Anxiolytic Abuse	305.40	F13.1 Sedative, Hypnotic, or Anxiolytic Abuse
Sedative-, Hypnotic-, or Anxiolytic-Induced Disorders		
Sedative, Hypnotic, or Anxiolytic Intoxication	292.89	F13.00
Sedative, Hypnotic, or Anxiolytic Withdrawal Specify if: With Perceptual Disturbances	292.0	F13.3
Sedative, Hypnotic, or Anxiolytic Intoxication Delirium	292.81	F13.03
Sedative, Hypnotic, or Anxiolytic Withdrawal Delirium	292.81	F13.4
Sedative-, Hypnotic-, or Anxiolytic-Induced Persisting Dementia	292.82	F13.73
Sedative-, Hypnotic-, or Anxiolytic-Induced Persisting Amnestic Disorder	292.83	F13.6
Sedative-, Hypnotic-, or Anxiolytic-Induced Psychotic Disorder	292.xx	F13.xx
With Delusions[I,W]	.11	.51
With Hallucinations[I,W]	.12	.52
Sedative-, Hypnotic-, or Anxiolytic-Induced Mood Disorder[I,W]	292.84	F13.8
Sedative-, Hypnotic-, or Anxiolytic-Induced Anxiety Disorder[W]	292.89	F13.8
Sedative-, Hypnotic-, or Anxiolytic-Induced Sexual Dysfunction[I]	292.89	F13.8

	DSM-IV-TR code	ICD-10 code
Sedative-, Hypnotic-, or Anxiolytic-Induced Sleep Disorder[I,W]	292.89	F13.8
Sedative-, Hypnotic-, or Anxiolytic-Related Disorder NOS	292.9	F13.9
POLYSUBSTANCE-RELATED DISORDER		
Polysubstance Dependence[a,b,c,d]	304.80	F19.2x Polysubstance Dependence[a]
OTHER (OR UNKNOWN) SUBSTANCE-RELATED DISORDERS		
Other (or Unknown) Substance Use Disorders		
Other (or Unknown) Substance Dependence[a,b,c,d]	304.90	F19.2x Other (or Unknown) Substance Dependence[a]
Other (or Unknown) Substance Abuse	305.90	F19.1
Other (or Unknown) Substance-Induced Disorders		
Other (or Unknown) Substance Intoxication	292.89	F19.00
Specify if: With Perceptual Disturbances		F19.04
Other (or Unknown) Substance Withdrawal	292.0	F19.3 Specify if: With Perceptual Disturbances
		F19.03 (code F19.4 if onset during withdrawal)
Other (or Unknown) Substance-Induced Delirium	292.81	
Other (or Unknown) Substance-Induced Persisting Dementia	292.82	F19.73
Other (or Unknown) Substance-Induced Persisting Amnestic Disorder	292.83	F19.6
Other (or Unknown) Substance-Induced Psychotic Disorder	292.xx	F19.xx
With Delusions[I,W]	.11	.51
With Hallucinations[I,W]	.12	.52

	DSM-IV-TR code	**ICD-10 code**
Other (or Unknown) Substance-Induced Mood Disorder[I,W]	292.84	F19.8
Other (or Unknown) Substance-Induced Anxiety Disorder[I,W]	292.89	F19.8
Other (or Unknown) Substance-Induced Sexual Dysfunction[I]	292.89	F19.8
Other (or Unknown) Substance-Induced Sleep Disorder[I,W]	292.89	F19.8
Other (or Unknown) Substance-Related Disorder NOS	292.9	F19.9
Schizophrenia and Other Psychotic Disorders		
Schizophrenia	295.xx	F20.xx
Paranoid Type	.30	.0x
Disorganized Type	.10	.1x
Catatonic Type	.20	.2x
Undifferentiated Type	.90	.3x
Residual Type	.60	.5x Residual Type
	The following Classification of Longitudinal Course applies to all subtypes of Schizophrenia: Episodic With Interepisode Residual Symptoms (specify if: With Prominent Negative Symptoms)/Episodic With No Interepisode Residual Symptoms	Code course of Schizophrenia in fifth character: 2 = Episodic With Interepisode Residual Symptoms (specify if: With Prominent Negative Symptoms) 3 = Episodic With No Interepisode Residual Symptoms
	Continuous (specify if: With Prominent Negative Symptoms)	0 = Continuous (specify if: With Prominent Negative Symptoms)
	Specify if: Single Episode In Partial Remission (specify if: With Prominent Negative Symptoms)	4 = Single Episode In Partial Remission (specify if: With Prominent Negative Symptoms)

	DSM-IV-TR code	ICD-10 code
	Specify if: Single Episode In Full Remission	5 = Single Episode In Full Remission
	Specify if: Other or Unspecified Pattern	8 = Other or Unspecified Pattern
		9 = Less than 1 year since onset of initial active-phase symptoms
Schizophreniform Disorder Specify if: Without Good Prognostic Features /With Good Prognostic Features	295.40	F20.8 Schizophreniform Disorder
Schizoaffective Disorder	295.70	F25.x Schizoaffective Disorder
Specify type: Bipolar Type		.0 Bipolar Type
Specify type: Depressive Type		.1 Depressive Type
Delusional Disorder Specify type: Erotomanic Type/Grandiose Type/Jealous Type/Persecutory Type/Somatic Type/Mixed Type/Unspecified Type	297.1	F22.0
Brief Psychotic Disorder Specify if: With Postpartum Onset	298.8	F23.xx
Specify if: With Marked Stressor(s)		.81
Specify if: Without Marked Stressor(s)		.80
Shared Psychotic Disorder	297.3	F24
Psychotic Disorder Due to . . . [Indicate the General Medical Condition]	293.xx	F06.x
With Delusions	.81	.2
With Hallucinations	.82	.0
__.__ Substance-Induced Psychotic Disorder (refer to Substance-Related Disorders for substance-specific codes) Specify if: With Onset During Intoxication/With Onset During Withdrawal	__.__	__.__
Psychotic Disorder NOS	298.9	F29 Psychotic Disorder NOS

	DSM-IV-TR code	ICD-10 code

Mood Disorders

The following specifiers apply (for current or most recent episode) to Mood Disorders as noted:

[a] Severity/Psychotic/Remission Specifiers/[b] Chronic/[c] With Catatonic Features/ [d] With Melancholic Features/[e] With Atypical Features/[f] With Postpartum Onset

The following specifiers apply to Mood Disorders as noted:

[g] With or Without Full Interepisode Recovery/[h] With Seasonal Pattern/ [i] With Rapid Cycling

DEPRESSIVE DISORDERS		
Major Depressive Disorder	296.xx	
Single Episode[a,b,c,d,e,f]	.2x	F32.x
Recurrent[a,b,c,d,e,f,g,h]	.3x	F33.x
	Code current state of Major Depressive Disorder or Bipolar I Disorder in fifth digit:	Code current state of Major Depressive Episode in fourth character:
Mild	296.x1	F33.0
Moderate	296.x2	F33.1
Severe Without Psychotic Features	296.x3	F33.2
Severe With Psychotic Features	296.x4	F33.3
	Specify: Mood-Congruent Psychotic Features/ Mood-Incongruent Psychotic Features	Specify: Mood-Congruent Psychotic Features/ Mood-Incongruent Psychotic Features
In Partial Remission	296.x5	4
In Full Remission	296.x6	5
Unspecified	296.x0	9
Dysthymic Disorder	300.4	F34.1
	Specify if: Early Onset/Late Onset	Specify if: Early Onset/Late Onset
	Specify: With Atypical Features	Specify: With Atypical Features
Depressive Disorder NOS	311	F32.9

	DSM-IV-TR code	ICD-10 code
BIPOLAR DISORDERS		
Bipolar I Disorder	296.xx	
Single Manic Episode [a,c,f] Specify if: Mixed	.0x	F30.x
		Code current state of Manic Episode in fourth character: 1 = Mild, Moderate, or Severe Without Psychotic Features; 2 = Severe With Psychotic Features; 7 = In Partial or Full Remission
Most Recent Episode Hypomanic [g,h,i]	.40	F31.0
Most Recent Episode Manic [a,c,g,h,i]	.4x	F31.x
		Code current state of Manic Episode in fourth character: 1 = Mild, Moderate, or Severe Without Psychotic Features; 2 = Severe With Psychotic Features; 7 = In Partial or Full Remission
Most Recent Episode Mixed [a,c,f,g,h,i]	.6x	F31.6
Most Recent Episode Depressed [a,b,c,d,e,f,g,h,i]	.5x	F31.x
		Code current state of Major Depressive Episode in fourth character: 3 = Mild or Moderate; 4 = Severe Without Psychotic Features; 5 = Severe With Psychotic Features; 7 = In Partial or Full Remission
Most Recent Episode Unspecified [g,h,i]	.7	F31.9
Bipolar II Disorder [a,b,c,d,e,f,g,h,i] Specify (current or most recent episode): Hypomanic/Depressed	296.89	F31.8
Cyclothymic Disorder	301.13	F34.0
Bipolar Disorder NOS	296.80	F31.9
Mood Disorder Due to . . . [Indicate the General Medical Condition]	293.83	F06.xx

	DSM-IV-TR code	ICD-10 code
Specify type: With Depressive Features/With Major Depressive-Like Episode/With Manic Features/With Mixed Features		.32 With Depressive Features
		.32 With Major Depressive-Like Episode
		.30 With Manic Features
		.33 With Mixed Features
Substance-Induced Mood Disorder (refer to Substance-Related Disorders for substance-specific codes). Specify type: With Depressive Features/With Manic Features/With Mixed Features Specify if: With Onset During Intoxication/With Onset During Withdrawal	___.__	___.__
Mood Disorder NOS	296.90	F39
Anxiety Disorders		
Panic Disorder Without Agoraphobia	300.01	F41.0
Panic Disorder With Agoraphobia	300.21	F40.01
Agoraphobia Without History of Panic Disorder	300.22	F40.00
Specific Phobia. Specify type: Animal Type/Natural Environment Type/Blood-Injection-Injury Type/ Situational Type/Other Type	300.29	F40.2
Social Phobia. Specify if: Generalized	300.23	F40.1
Obsessive-Compulsive Disorder. Specify if: With Poor Insight	300.3	F42.8
Post-traumatic Stress Disorder. Specify if: Acute/Chronic and/or With Delayed Onset	309.81	F43.1
Acute Stress Disorder	308.3	F43.0
Generalized Anxiety Disorder	300.02	F41.1
Anxiety Disorder Due to . . . [Indicate the General Medical Condition] Specify if: With Generalized Anxiety/With Panic Attacks/With Obsessive-Compulsive Symptoms	293.84	F06.4

	DSM-IV-TR code	ICD-10 code
Substance-Induced Anxiety Disorder *(refer to Substance-Related Disorders for substance-specific codes)* Specify if: With Generalized Anxiety/With Panic Attacks/With Obsessive-Compulsive Symptoms/With Phobic Symptoms. *Specify if:* With Onset During Intoxication/With Onset During Withdrawal	__.__	__.__
Anxiety Disorder NOS	300.00	F41.9
Somatoform Disorders		
Somatization Disorder	300.81	F45.0
Undifferentiated Somatoform Disorder	300.82	F45.1
Conversion Disorder. Specify type:	300.11	F44.x
With Motor Symptom or Deficit	300.11	.4
With Seizures or Convulsions	300.11	.5
With Sensory Symptom or Deficit	300.11	.6
With Mixed Presentation	300.11	.7
Pain Disorder Specify if: Acute/Chronic	307.xx	F45.4
Associated With Psychological Factors	.80	Specify type: Associated With Psychological Factors/ Associated With Both Psychological Factors and a General Medical Condition
Associated With Both Psychological Factors and a General Medical Condition	.89	
Hypochondriasis Specify if: With Poor Insight	300.7	F45.2
Body Dysmorphic Disorder	300.7	F45.2
Somatoform Disorder NOS	300.82	F45.9

	DSM-IV-TR code	ICD-10 code
Factitious Disorders		
Factitious Disorder	300.xx	F68.1 Specify type:
With Predominantly Psychological Signs and Symptoms	.16	With Predominantly Psychological Signs and Symptoms
With Predominantly Physical Signs and Symptoms	.19	With Predominantly Physical Signs and Symptoms
With Combined Psychological and Physical Signs and Symptoms	.19	With Combined Psychological and Physical Signs and Symptoms
Factitious Disorder NOS	300.19	F68.1
Dissociative Disorders		
Dissociative Amnesia	300.12	F44.0
Dissociative Fugue	300.13	F44.1
Dissociative Identity Disorder	300.14	F44.81
Depersonalization Disorder	300.6	F48.1
Dissociative Disorder NOS	300.15	F44.9
Sexual and Gender Identity Disorders		
SEXUAL DYSFUNCTIONS		
The following specifiers apply to all primary Sexual Dysfunctions: Lifelong Type/Acquired Type/Generalized Type/Situational Type/Due to Psychological Factors/Due to Combined Factors		
Sexual Desire Disorders		
Hypoactive Sexual Desire Disorder	302.71	F52.0
Sexual Aversion Disorder	302.79	F52.10
Sexual Arousal Disorders		
Female Sexual Arousal Disorder	302.72	F52.2
Male Erectile Disorder	302.72	F52.2
Orgasmic Disorders		
Female Orgasmic Disorder	302.73	F52.3
Male Orgasmic Disorder	302.74	F52.3
Premature Ejaculation	302.75	F52.4

	DSM-IV-TR code	ICD-10 code
Sexual Pain Disorders		
Dyspareunia (Not Due to a General Medical Condition)	302.76	F52.6
Vaginismus (Not Due to a General Medical Condition)	306.51	F52.5
Sexual Dysfunction Due to a General Medical Condition		
Female Hypoactive Sexual Desire Disorder Due to . . . [Indicate the General Medical Condition]	625.8	N94.8
Male Hypoactive Sexual Desire Disorder Due to . . . [Indicate the General Medical Condition]	608.89	N50.8
Male Erectile Disorder Due to . . . [Indicate the General Medical Condition]	607.84	N48.4
Female Dyspareunia Due to . . . [Indicate the General Medical Condition]	625.0	N94.1
Male Dyspareunia Due to . . . [Indicate the General Medical Condition]	608.89	N50.8
Other Female Sexual Dysfunction Due to . . . [Indicate the General Medical Condition]	625.8	N94.8
Other Male Sexual Dysfunction Due to . . . [Indicate the General Medical Condition]	608.89	N50.8
Substance-Induced Sexual Dysfunction (refer to Substance-Related Disorders for substance-specific codes) Specify if: With Impaired Desire/With Impaired Arousal/With Impaired Orgasm/With Sexual Pain. Specify if: With Onset During Intoxication	___.__	___.__
Sexual Dysfunction NOS	302.70	F52.9
PARAPHILIAS		
Exhibitionism	302.4	F65.2
Fetishism	302.81	F65.0
Frotteurism	302.89	F65.8

	DSM-IV-TR code	ICD-10 code
Pedophilia Specify if: Sexually Attracted to Males/Sexually Attracted to Females/Sexually Attracted to Both Specify if: Limited to Incest. Specify type: Exclusive Type/Nonexclusive Type	302.2	F65.4
Sexual Masochism	302.83	F65.5
Sexual Sadism	302.84	F65.5
Transvestic Fetishism Specify if: With Gender Dysphoria	302.3	F65.1
Voyeurism	302.82	F65.3
Paraphilia NOS	302.9	F65.9
GENDER IDENTITY DISORDERS		
Gender Identity Disorder. Specify if: Sexually Attracted to Males/ Sexually Attracted to Females/ Sexually Attracted to Both/ Sexually Attracted to Neither	302.xx	F64.x
in Children	.6	.2
in Adolescents or Adults	.85	.0
Gender Identity Disorder NOS	302.6	F64.9
Sexual Disorder NOS	302.9	F52.9
Eating Disorders		
Anorexia Nervosa. Specify type: Restricting Type; Binge-Eating/ Purging Type	307.1	F50.0
Bulimia Nervosa. Specify type: Purging Type/Nonpurging Type	307.51	F50.2
Eating Disorder NOS	307.50	F50.9
Sleep Disorders		
PRIMARY SLEEP DISORDERS		
Dysomnias		
Primary Insomnia	307.42	F51.0
Primary Hypersomnia. Specify if: Recurrent	307.44	F51.1
Narcolepsy	347	G47.4
Breathing-Related Sleep Disorder	780.59	G47.3

	DSM-IV-TR code	ICD-10 code
Circadian Rhythm Sleep Disorder. Specify type: Delayed Sleep Phase Type/Jet Lag Type/Shift Work Type/Unspecified Type	307.45	F51.2
Dyssomnia NOS	307.47	F51.9
Parasomnias		
Nightmare Disorder	307.47	F51.5
Sleep Terror Disorder	307.46	F51.4
Sleepwalking Disorder	307.46	F51.3
Parasomnia NOS	307.47	F51.8
SLEEP DISORDERS RELATED TO ANOTHER MENTAL DISORDER		
Insomnia Related to . . . [Indicate the Axis I or Axis II Disorder]	307.42	F51.0
Hypersomnia Related to . . . [Indicate the Axis I or Axis II Disorder]	307.44	F51.1
OTHER SLEEP DISORDERS		
Sleep Disorder Due to . . . [Indicate the General Medical Condition]	780.xx	G47.x
Insomnia Type	.52	.0
Hypersomnia Type	.54	.1
Parasomnia Type	.59	.8
Mixed Type	.59	.8
Substance-Induced Sleep Disorder (refer to Substance-Related Disorders for substance-specific codes). Specify type: Insomnia Type/Hypersomnia Type/Parasomnia Type/Mixed Type. Specify if: With Onset During Intoxication/With Onset During Withdrawal	___._	___._
Impulse-Control Disorders Not Elsewhere Classified		
Intermittent Explosive Disorder	312.34	F63.8
Kleptomania	312.32	F63.2
Pyromania	312.33	F63.1
Pathological Gambling	312.31	F63.0
Trichotillomania	312.39	F63.3
Impulse-Control Disorder NOS	312.30	F63.9

	DSM-IV-TR code	ICD-10 code
Adjustment Disorders		
Adjustment Disorder Specify if: Acute/Chronic	309.xx	F43.xx
With Depressed Mood	.0	.20
With Anxiety	.24	.28
With Mixed Anxiety and Depressed Mood	.28	.22
With Disturbance of Conduct	.3	.24
With Mixed Disturbance of Emotions and Conduct	.4	.25
Unspecified	.9	.9
Personality Disorders		
Note: these are coded on Axis II.		
Paranoid Personality Disorder	301.0	F60.0
Schizoid Personality Disorder	301.20	F60.1
Schizotypal Personality Disorder	301.22	F21
Antisocial Personality Disorder	301.7	F60.2
Borderline Personality Disorder	301.83	F60.31
Histrionic Personality Disorder	301.50	F60.4
Narcissistic Personality Disorder	301.81	F60.8
Avoidant Personality Disorder	301.82	F60.6
Dependent Personality Disorder	301.6	F60.7
Obsessive-Compulsive Personality Disorder	301.4	F60.5
Personality Disorder NOS	301.9	F60.9
Other Conditions That May Be a Focus of Clinical Attention		
PSYCHOLOGICAL FACTORS AFFECTING MEDICAL CONDITION		
. . . [Specified Psychological Factor] Affecting . . . [Indicate the General Medical Condition]	316	F54
Choose name based on nature of factors:		
Mental Disorder Affecting Medical Condition		
Psychological Symptoms Affecting Medical Condition		

	DSM-IV-TR code	ICD-10 code
Personality Traits or Coping Style Affecting Medical Condition		
Maladaptive Health Behaviors Affecting Medical Condition		
Stress-Related Physiological Response Affecting Medical Condition		
Other or Unspecified Psychological Factors Affecting Medical Condition		
MEDICATION-INDUCED MOVEMENT DISORDERS		
Neuroleptic-Induced Parkinsonism	332.1	G21.0
Neuroleptic Malignant Syndrome	333.92	G21.0
Neuroleptic-Induced Acute Dystonia	333.7	G24.0
Neuroleptic-Induced Acute Akathisia	333.99	G21.1
Neuroleptic-Induced Tardive Dyskinesia	333.82	G24.0
Medication-Induced Postural Tremor	333.1	G25.1
Medication-Induced Movement Disorder NOS	333.90	G25.9
OTHER MEDICATION-INDUCED DISORDER		
Adverse Effects of Medication NOS	995.2	T88.7
RELATIONAL PROBLEMS		
Relational Problem Related to a Mental Disorder or General Medical Condition	V61.9	Z63.7
Parent-Child Relational Problem	V61.20	Z63.8 (code Z63.1 if focus of attention is on child)
Partner Relational Problem	V61.10	Z63.0
Sibling Relational Problem	V61.8	F93.3
Relational Problem NOS	V62.81	Z63.9
PROBLEMS RELATED TO ABUSE OR NEGLECT		
Physical Abuse of Child (code 995.54 if focus of attention is on victim)	V61.21	T74.1
Sexual Abuse of Child (code 995.53 if focus of attention is on victim)	V61.21	T74.2

	DSM-IV-TR code	ICD-10 code
Neglect of Child (code 995.52 if focus of attention is on victim)	V61.21	T74.0
Physical Abuse of Adult (code 995.81 if focus of attention is on victim)	__.__	T74.1
(if by partner)	V61.12	
(if by person other than partner)	V62.83	
Sexual Abuse of Adult (code 995.83 if focus of attention is on victim)	__.__	T74.2
(if by partner)	V61.12	
(if by person other than partner)	V62.83	

ADDITIONAL CONDITIONS THAT MAY BE A FOCUS OF CLINICAL ATTENTION

	DSM-IV-TR code	ICD-10 code
Noncompliance With Treatment	V15.81	Z91.1 Noncompliance With Treatment
Malingering	V65.2	Z76.5
Adult Antisocial Behavior	V71.01	Z72.8
Child or Adolescent Antisocial Behavior	V71.02	Z72.8
Borderline Intellectual Functioning. Note: this is coded on Axis II.	V62.89	R41.8
Age-Related Cognitive Decline	780.9	R41.8
Bereavement	V62.82	Z63.4
Academic Problem	V62.3	Z55.8
Occupational Problem	V62.2	Z56.7
Identity Problem	313.82	F93.8
Religious or Spiritual Problem	V62.89	Z71.8
Acculturation Problem	V62.4	Z60.3
Phase of Life Problem	V62.89	Z60.0

Additional Codes

	DSM-IV-TR code	ICD-10 code
Unspecified Mental Disorder (non-psychotic)	300.9	F99
No Diagnosis or Condition on Axis I	V71.09	Z03.2
Diagnosis or Condition Deferred n Axis I	799.9	R69
No Diagnosis on Axis II	V71.09	Z03.2
Diagnosis Deferred on Axis II	799.9	R46.8

Index